KirstyGi

AT ON   NO

A Handbook of
Menstrual Diseases
in Chinese Medicine

A Handbook of
Menstrual Diseases
in Chinese Medicine

by
Bob Flaws

Blue Poppy Press, Inc.
Boulder CO

Published by:

BLUE POPPY PRESS
A Division of Blue Poppy Enterprises, Inc.
5441 Western Ave., Suite 2
BOULDER, CO 80301
303-447-8372

First Edition, January, 1997
Second Printing, May, 2001

ISBN 0-936185-82-1 ✓
LC 96-80188

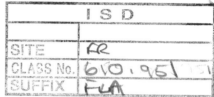

I S D	
SITE	FR
CLASS No.	610.951
SUFFIX	FLA

DISCLAIMER: The information in this book is given in good faith. However, the
author and the publishers cannot be held responsible for any error or omission. The
publishers will not accept liabilities for any injuries or damages caused to the reader
that may result from the reader's acting upon or using the content contained in this
book. The publishers make this information available to English language readers
for research and scholarly purposes only.

The publishers do not advocate nor endorse self-medication by laypersons. Chinese
medicine is a professional medicine. Laypersons interested in availing themselves of
the treatments described in this book should seek out a qualified professional
practitioner of Chinese medicine.

COMP Designation: Original work using a standard translational terminology

Printed at Thomson-Shore, Inc., Dexter, MI

10 9 8 7 6 5 4 3 2

Preface

In 1992, I published a book titled *My Sister the Moon: The Diagnosis & Treatment of Menstrual Diseases by Traditional Chinese Medicine*. When it was time to reprint that book, it was no longer the state of my art. For the last two years, I have been engaged in teaching an 18 month post-graduate course in TCM gynecology. In the process of preparing for and teaching this course, I have discovered much new and useful information in the Chinese gynecological literature and have clarified many key points in the practice of Chinese gynecology. Therefore, I have created this book to take the place of that earlier one. Because this book is substantially different from that first book and because that first book's title may have been too poetic for a clinical textbook, I have chosen to title this book simply *A Handbook of Menstrual Diseases in Chinese Medicine*.

Some of the major changes between these two books are that 1) I have added considerable new material to this edition, especially on premenstrual conditions and perimenopausal syndrome. I have also included many more formulas. 2) I have changed a significant portion of the technical terminology to more closely conform to Nigel Wiseman's in his recently released *English-Chinese Chinese-English Dictionary of Chinese Medicine*, Hunan Science & Technology Press, Changsha, 1995. 3) I have added acupuncture-moxibustion and desiccated extract protocols in appendices as well as other appendices on topics peripherally related to the TCM treatment of menstrual diseases. 4) I have changed a number of medicinal names in order to simplify their recognition and more closely correspond with those in the second, revised edition of Bensky and Gamble's *Chinese Herbal Medicine: Materia Medica*. In addition, I have corrected some mistaken medicinal identifications. And 5) I have added the English translations of the Pinyin names of formulas in order to help make their recognition easier as well. Hopefully, these additions and changes will make this book even more clinically useful for Western practitioners of Chinese gynecology.

I have been specializing in Chinese gynecology for the last 16 years. As a Chinese gynecology specialist, the bulk of my daily practice has to do with the category of diseases called *yue jing bing*. *Yue* means moon. *Jing* means channel but also refers to a river or canal. As a compound term, *yue jing* literally means moon flow. This is the most common Chinese term for menstruation which, coincidentally, also means moon or monthly flow in Latin. This category of diseases covers menstruation ahead of schedule, menstruation behind schedule, menses which are (sometimes) early, (sometimes) late, and come at no fixed schedule, scanty menstruation, profuse menstruation, menses which start and stop, menses whose amount is (sometimes) profuse, (sometimes) scanty and not fixed, painful menstruation, premenstrual or perimenstrual diseases (such as breast distention, diarrhea, fever, and body aches and which are literally referred to in Chinese as menstrual movement diseases), blocked menstruation, flooding and leaking, and perimenopausal syndrome. As Chinese medical disease categories, these complaints can be used to cover a number of Western disease categories. For instance, endometriosis as a Western disease category is covered in the Chinese medical literature by painful menstruation, menstrual movement bleeding from an orifice other than the vagina, and profuse menstruation. Therefore, if one understands the logic and methodology of the Chinese medical presentation of menstrual diseases, one can treat a number of Western disease categories not specifically included in most traditional Chinese gynecology texts.

In my experience, most menstrual diseases respond very favorably to Chinese medicine. Most menstrual complaints can be brought under control or eliminated in from three to five cycles. When this is accomplished by Chinese medicine, the cure is without the iatrogenesis which is so often a part of modern Western gynecology. Although menstrual diseases are a subcategory within the specialty of Chinese medical gynecology, most systemic diseases in women will have an adverse effect on a woman's menstruation. Therefore, by regulating the menses, one can have a broad, systemic impact on a woman's entire health. Because of the close relationship between the psyche, the endocrine system, and the immune system as described by modern Western psycho-neuro-immunology, one can treat both psychological problems and various immune disorders in women, such as chronic fatigue immune deficiency syndrome (CFIDS) and systemic lupus erythematosus (SLE), by, in large part, regulating their menses. Therefore, the regulation of menstruation should never be looked down upon as a minor endeavor.

Sun Si-miao, the famous Tang dynasty Chinese doctor, said that he would rather treat 10 men than one woman. This is because one must always take the menstrual cycle into account when diagnosing and treating women. Thus women have a whole other realm of signs and symptoms which must be taken into account. Since men do not have such monthly cycles, at first glance they may appear easier to diagnose and treat as was, it seems, Sun Si-miao's opinion. However, if one understands the mechanisms behind the menstrual cycle, I find that gynecology is an especially easy area of medicine since one gets a monthly report card on the woman's status and the progress of her therapy. The menses, rather than presenting an extra, mysterious dimension to therapy, reveal, in a very immediate and clearly read way, exactly how the woman is doing and whether therapy is going forward as expected and desired. As the early nineteenth century author of the *Yi Xue Shi Zai Yi (The Study of Medicine is Really Easy)* correctly perceived, the menses give the practitioner an eleventh question when it comes to treating women or, in other words, a whole extra category of *revelatory* signs and symptoms.

The information in this book on the Chinese medical disease causes, disease mechanisms, pattern discrimination, and treatment of menstrual diseases is taken from numerous Chinese sources described in detail in the Bibliography. I have expanded upon this material based on my own clinical experience and thought. As mentioned above, the English language translations for Chinese medical technical terms employed in this book are based on Nigel Wiseman's *English-Chinese Chinese-English Dictionary of Chinese Medicine*. In those few instances were I disagree with Wiseman's terminology, I have noted my deviation from this norm in footnotes. Mostly, I have tried to work within the terminology Wiseman has suggested. This is based on my agreement with him that our profession must develop and use a standardized professional vocabulary which accurately conveys the meaning and intent of the Chinese which is the foundation of our practice. Chinese medicine is very clear and logical *in Chinese* and much of this clarity and precision is lost in translation. Using standard translational terminology as suggested by Wiseman is one way of attempting to retain this clarity and precision. Some of the terms used may sound peculiar at first, but the reader should remember that this is a technical vocabulary and that special technical vocabularies do have to be specially learned.

The identification of materia medica is given first in Latinate pharmacological nomenclature and is based on identifications found first in Bensky and Gamble's *Chinese Herbal Medicine: Materia Medica*. When I have failed to find a medicinal in this book, secondly I have looked in Hong-yen Hsu's *Oriental Materia Medica: A Concise Guide*; third in Cloudburst Press' *A Barefoot Doctor's Manual*; fourth in Southern Materials Center's *Chinese Materia Medica*, Vol. 1-6, Taipei, and fifth in the *Zhong Yao Da Ci Dian (A Large Dictionary of Chinese Herbs)* published in the People's Republic of China. Latin identifications are then followed by the medicinals' Pinyin names in parentheses in order to make their identification less ambiguous and more definite. Regarding the Pinyin names of medicinals, I have used whatever Chinese names the Chinese authors of the texts I consulted used in their discussions of the various formulas. Therefore, there are some varying Chinese names for the same medicinal. I have retained these variations because, in many cases, they do further identify either variations of the medicinal or regional sources which can be important distinctions in the use of these medicinals. I have also translated any methods of preparing medicinals specified by my sources using Wiseman's terminology for these processing methods. For more information on the methods and uses of such prepared medicinals, readers are referred to Philippe Sionneau's *Pao Zhi: An Introduction to the Use of Processed Chinese Medicinals* also published by Blue Poppy Press.

In order to make this book more immediately usable, I have given the ingredients of each formula each time it appears under each disease category. This is so practitioners will not have to flip around from section to section looking for the ingredients in guiding formulas also discussed under other disease categories. The names of the formulas are given in Pinyin first followed by English in parentheses. Unlike many Chinese gynecology texts which only give a single or at most two guiding formulas for each pattern under each disease category, I have given a wide variety of formulas from various sources, both ancient and modern. This larger selection should give practitioners more flexibility in meeting their patients' idiosyncratic presentations. Therefore, when choosing a guiding formula, one should first insure that it is designed to treat the right pattern. This means that it treats the pattern in its entirety. In clinical practice, most patients do not present with a single textbook pattern but a pattern made up of several elements at the same time. Secondly, one should look at all the ingredients and check that these ingredients do actually treat the major signs and symptoms of the patient at hand. Even though two patients may have essentially the same pattern or patterns, they still will typically vary in terms of their signs and symptoms or at least the severity and, therefore, the clinical importance of particular signs and symptoms.

The standard of care in TCM as a specific style of Chinese medicine is individually modified prescriptions for individual patients dispensed from bulk medicinals and administered as water-based decoctions. Relying on the rote use of formulas contained in books, the use of Chinese patent medicines, or modern concentrated formulas and tinctures, one simply cannot achieve the high level of specificity and, therefore, the results of individually modified prescriptions dispensed in bulk for preparation as freshly brewed decoctions. Pills, powders, and tinctures may be easier to use, but, in my experience, they do not achieve the same clinical results as the traditional *tang* or decoction. Although they may be appropriate for the treatment of simple cases, for the consolidation of clinical results, and in some chronic conditions requiring prolonged administration, they cannot adequately replace the individually tailored prescription which is the standard of care in professional Chinese medicine.

I have specifically not included dosages for individual ingredients in the formulas given. In TCM, the study of gynecology comes only after one has studied the materia medica, formulas and prescriptions, and internal medicine. Practitioners who have already accomplished those studies should have no difficulty in deciding on an *ad hoc* basis, how much of each ingedient to use for an individual patient. Otherwise, I do not encourage the rote use of Chinese medicinal formulas by practitioners who have not undergone the appropriate preliminary training, and omitting dosages is one way of discouraging such professionally premature practice. For further information on the dosage parameters, indications, and contraindications of most of the formulas discussed herein, the reader is referred to Bensky and Barolet's *Chinese Herbal Medicine: Formulas & Strategies*.

That being said, most Western practitioners do not practice the same standard of care as in the People's Republic of China. Rather, most Western practitioners use a combination of acupuncture and moxibustion with various patent pills or desiccated, powdered extracts. Therefore, in the appendices, the reader will find acupuncture-moxibustion protocols and Chinese formulas available in powdered form. Because I practice, or at least try to practice, the same standard of care as in mainland China today, I cannot personally guarantee the effectiveness of these protocols. However, I do think that, if one is giving regular acupuncture treatments in combination with powdered Chinese medicinal extracts, those treatments may make up for the lesser potency of such powdered extracts. Nevertheless, this does not mean one should prescribe such ready-made formulas unless they have undergone professionally appropriate training in their clinical use.

As a textbook of TCM gynecology, there are only certain things this book can do. TCM clinical manuals such as this are not meant to be "the be all and end all" of information on the specialties they cover. Recent studies in educational psychology confirm that, when presenting complex new knowledge, it is important to first sketch out a schematic structure which is too simple to reflect the complex reality of the subject. Only after the student has grapsed this admittedly oversimplified outline should the teacher then go back and qualify, elaborate, and modify it in order to come closer to the real-life situation. Likewise, TCM textbooks, including this one, are only meant to be such oversimplified outlines. The material they contain is meant to be "qualified, elaborated on, and modified" by supplemental case history readings, medical essays, clinical research reports, and supervised clinical practice under the guidance of well-educated and experienced senior practitioners. However, because the Chinese case history, medical essay, and research report literature is so scanty in English, and because few Western practitioners have the opportunity to undergo prolonged clincial practice under adequate supervision, I have made this book somewhat more complex than the average Chinese gynecology text. Hopefully, it will take practitioners further than most TCM textbooks without causing confusion in beginners.

In particular in this book, I have attempted to clarify and elucidate the process of doing Chinese gynecology. Throughout this book, the abbreviation TCM for Traditional Chinese Medicine is meant as the proper name of a specific style of Chinese medicine. In fact, in Chinese, there is no such thing called Traditional Chinese Medicine. There is only Chinese medicine or *zhong yi*. This raises a certain amount of confusion in the West, since more than a single style of Chinese medicine has been taught over the last century by a variety of Asian, American, and European teachers. When I refer to TCM, I specifically mean that style of Chinese medicine currently taught at the provincial medical colleges in the People's Republic of China. TCM as a specific style of Chinese medicine is a rational methodology whose treatment is based on dual diagnosis. In each case, the practitioner is expected to make both a *bian bing* or disease discrimination and a *bian zheng* or pattern discrimination. Treatment is then given predicated upon both these two types of diagnoses. When one can formulate treatment based on such dual diagnosis, one can treat both the person as a unique individual and the disease as a discreet pathological process.

TCM as a style of Chinese medicine is a blend of rational and empirical medicines. As a rational style, the quality of its practice is dependent upon the clarity and rectitude of the practitioner's logic. The logic of Chinese medicine is based, to a very large extent, on the Chinese language. If, in this book, I have been able to make this logic more accessible and understandable to English readers, then I will account this book a success. As Albert Einstein once said:

> Theory without practice is sterile. Practice without theory is blind.

Bob Flaws
Boulder, CO
December, 1996

Table of Contents

Preface *5*

BOOK ONE: Introductory Theory

1 The Physiological Characteristics of Females 3
2 The Causes, Mechanisms & Prevention of Menstrual Disease 31
3 TCM Methodology 59
4 The Logic in the TCM Discussion of *Yue Jing Bing* 67
5 Western Disease Diagnosis & TCM Menstrual Diseases 71
6 Key Points in the TCM Diagnosis of Menstrual Disease 73
7 Key Patterns in Menstrual Diseases 97
8 Treatment Principles & Chinese Medicinals 115
9 Treatment Strategies & Expectations 137

BOOK TWO: The Diagnosis & Treatment of Menstrual Diseases

1 Menstruation Ahead of Schedule 145
2 Menstruation Behind Schedule 175
3 (Sometimes) Early, (Sometimes) Late, Menstruation at No Fixed Schedule 199
4 Profuse Menstruation 213
5 Scanty Menstruation 233
6 Flooding & Leaking 247
7 Blocked Menstruation 293
8 Painful Menstruation 337
9 Menstrual Movement Diseases 387
　Breast Distention & Pain 399
　Diarrhea and/or Vomiting 416
　Body Pain 427
　Headache 434
　Fever 447
　Vertigo & Dizziness 456
　Edema 460
　Oral *Gan* 461
　Loss of Sleep 463

Menstrual Movement Diseases (continued)

  Acne 465

  Raving & Confused Vision 469

  Dull-wittedness & Stupidity 472

  Addictive Papules (Hives or Urticaria) 473

  Flowing Drool 476

  Oral Thirst 477

  Hoarse Voice 478

  Eye Pain 481

  Lumbar Pain 482

  Suspended Vagina Pain 484

  Nosebleed 486

  Coughing Blood 492

  Bloody Stool 493

  Bloody Urine 495

10 Perimenopausal Syndrome 499

Appendix 1: Acupuncture & Moxibustion Formulas for Menstrual Diseases 537

Appendix 2: Ancient Formulas in Powdered Form for Menstrual Diseases 555

Appendix 3: Abnormalities in the Color & Consistency of the Menstrual Water . 565

Appendix 4: Li Dong-yuan's Gynecology 573

Bibliography 589

Formula Index 599

General Index 605

Book One

Introductory Theory

The Physiological Characteristics of Females

In TCM, theory comes before practice. As mentioned in the Preface, TCM as a specific style of Chinese medicine is a blend of rationale and empirical medicine. In some sense, TCM is a system or methodology for thinking about a patients' disease and then solving their clinical problem through the manipulation of the key statements of fact of Chinese medicine. In other words, it is a problem-solving methodology. It is not so much about memorizing set responses or formulas for diseases but about creating *ad hoc* treatments for unique and idiosyncratic patient presentations. In order to do this, one must first have a firm grasp of basic theory with which to think. Therefore, all Chinese TCM gynecology texts begin with a discussion of basic TCM theory as it pertains to gynecology. This basic theory usually covers the *bao gong, bao mai,* and *bao luo*, the viscera and bowels, the channels and network vessels, qi and blood, disease causes and mechanisms, and treatment principles all *vis à vis* gynecology.

Bao gong

Most Chinese gynecology books typically open with the statement that men and women are the same but that women have a uterus and, therefore, they menstruate, can conceive, and give birth to babies. All three of these activities are dependent upon women's being endowed with a uterus. In Chinese, the uterus is most commonly called the *bao gong* or wrapper palace. The *bao gong* is conceived of in TCM as an extraordinary bowel. That means that the *bao gong* is a bowel in form but a viscus in function. As a bowel, the uterus is hollow. However, as an extraordinary bowel, it stores essence similar to a viscus. On a monthly level, the uterus stores blood. After conception, the uterus stores the fetus. In addition, like a bowel, the uterus also discharges. Monthly, it discharges the blood and, at full term it discharges the fetus. A number of other classical names for the uterus underscore this dual role of both storing and discharging:

Nu zi bao	Fetal wrapper	*Bao zang*	Wrapper viscus
Zi chu	Place for fetal growth	*Chan chang*	Birth intestine
Zi gong	Fetal palace	*Zi chang*	Fetal intestine
Zi zang	Fetal viscus		

The *bao gong* is also defined as the place where essence is treasured and concealed. Therefore, in a sense, both sexes are endowed with it. In men, it is called the *jing shi*, chamber of essence, and in women it is called the *xue shi* or chamber of blood. It is also the sea of blood in women and the sea of qi/cinnabar field in men. It is the place where essence is stored in men and blood is stored in women, remembering that blood is the physical manifestation of essence in women in the same way that the ejaculate is in men. Fu Qing-zhu, the most famous premodern Chinese gynecologist, in his *Fu Qing Zhu Nu Ke (Fu Qing-zhu's Gynecology)*, emphasizes that the menstrual blood is not just blood but is, in fact, essence, when he explains:

> What's more, the menstruation is not blood but the *tian gui*. Originating in the kidneys, it is the essence of consumate yin [the kidneys], but possessed of the qi of the consumate yang [the heart]. Therefore, it is red like blood but is, in fact, not blood. This accounts for its name, the *tian gui* or heavenly water. People nowadays regard the menstrual flow as blood, but this is an incorrect assumption, [in fact,] an unshakable assumption for 1,000 years. If it were blood, why should it be named menstrual water [*jing shui*] rather than menstrual blood [*jing xue*]. This name, *jing shui,* is derived from the belief that it comes from the kidneys and is transformed by the heavenly stem *gui*. Regrettably, people accept conventional ideas without giving profound consideration to their implications and look upon [the menstruate] as blood.

Thus the wrapper palace where the essence is stored in women is the *bao gong*. (We will have more to say about the *tian gui* below.)

The uterus may be a unique or extraordinary bowel, but it is, nonetheless, connected to both the viscera and bowels, the channels and network vessels, and the qi and blood of the entire organism. The viscera and bowels are the origin of the engenderment of the qi and blood, while the channels and network vessels are the free-flowing pathways for the transportation and movement of the qi and blood. The qi and blood are the foundation of the uterus's functions of moving the menstruate, harmonizing gestation, and birthing the child. It is the qi and blood which form the menstruate and nourish the fetus. In particular, it is said that the *bao gong* is the place where the heart and kidneys connect. Although one of the definitions of an extraordinary bowel is that they do not have an interior-exterior relationship like the other bowels do with a yin viscus, nonetheless, as we will see below, the uterus does have a special relationship with the heart. In addition, the activities of the uterus are dependent upon kidney qi and the *tian gui.*

Bao mai

The *bao mai* (literally, the wrapper vessel) is a vessel which connects the uterus to the pericardium or *xin bao luo*. In this case, the pericardium is seen not as a separate viscus but merely as the network vessels wrapping the heart. In this sense, the pericardium is an extension of the heart. It is said that the *bao mai* homes to the pericardium but acts on behalf of the heart. This word homes is the same word used when speaking about one of the twelve correct or regular channels homing to a particular viscus or bowel. Therefore, it is said that the *bao mai* homes to the heart viscus but connects (literally, networks) with the *bao gong* as a bowel. This parallels the relationship between other channels and vessels which connect a yin viscus with a yang bowel.

The *bao mai's* function is to convey heart qi and blood to the uterus. It is the vessel over which heart qi sends blood down to the uterus. According to the *Nei Jing Su Wen (Inner Classic Simple Questions)*, "Failure of arrival of menstruation is due to closure of the *bao mai*." Therefore, it is said that menstruation proceeds smoothly when heart qi and heart blood flow freely to and reach the uterus unobstructed. This means that the uterus's function are normal only when and if heart function is normal.

In the Chinese literature, there is a debate about whether the *chong mai* or penetrating vessel[1] and the *bao mai* are one and the same or different. Both connect the uterus and the heart. I personally do not regard these as two separate and discreet channels. In actual fact, there are no pattern discriminations that are based on the term *bao mai*. When it comes to pattern discrimination and treatment, it is always the *chong mai* that is referred to. The *bao mai* is only a term used in theoretical and introductory discussions such as this.

Bao luo

The *bao luo* are network vessels distributed over the *bao gong* which supply and fill the *bao gong* with kidney essence. The *Nei Jing Su Wen (Inner Classic Simple Questions)* says, "The *bao luo* connect the kidneys to the uterus." It is by way of the *bao luo* that the uterus is nourished and enriched by essence. Menstruation and the ability to conceive are dependent upon both an abundance of blood sent down via the *bao mai* to the uterus and sufficient kidney essence supplied via the *bao luo*.

Taken as a whole, the *bao mai* is the pathway by which heart blood is transported down to the uterus. Whereas, the *bao luo* is the pathway by which yin essence is transported to the uterus but also from thence upward via the *chong mai/bao mai* to the heart and upper body. The uterus is the juncture between the *bao mai* and *bao luo* and, therefore, also between the heart and kidneys or the upper and lower burners. There is also a reciprocal polarity implied

---

[1]   Wiseman translates *chong mai* as thoroughfare vessel. According to the classical Chinese scholar and translator, Yang Shou-zhong, Wiseman's previous penetrating vessel is a better translation. That being said, throughout this work, I mostly use the Pinyin, *chong* or *chong mai* when referring to this vessel.

by the terms *xin bao luo* and the *bao luo gong*. In both cases there is a *bao luo*. Above there is a heart *bao luo*, while below there is a *bao luo gong*.

Disorders of the kidneys and heart may both give rise to gynecological disorders due to their connections to the uterus via the *bao mai* and *bao luo*. For instance, due to grief damaging the heart qi, qi fall may give rise to profuse menstrual bleeding. Or, during late pregnancy, due to kidney yin insufficiency, the *bao luo* may become obstructed and, therefore, kidney qi and fluids may not be able to reach the root of the tongue, thus causing late term laryngitis.

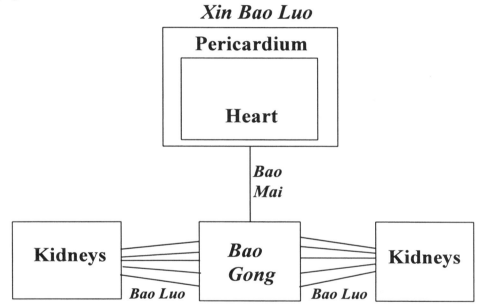

Tian gui

Tian means heaven and *gui* is the name of one of the ten heavenly stems. It is the heavenly stem which corresponds to kidney water. Thus *tian gui* means heavenly water. This term has several meanings in Chinese medicine depending upon its usage and school of thought. The onset of menstruation both at menarche and monthly is referred to as the arrival of the *tian gui* and menopause is also called the cessation of the *tian gui*. Some schools see the *tian gui* as the menstruate. Others see it as the increased vaginal discharge which precedes menstruation. However, since blood and fluids share a common source, this distinction is not important here.

If menarche is the arrival of the *tian gui*, it is important to understand why the *tian gui* arrives when it does. It says in the second chapter of the *Nei Jing Su Wen (Inner Classic Simple Questions)* that the *tian gui* arrives at two times seven or 14 years of age when the kidney qi is exuberant. To understand this statement, one must understand that blood is created out of both former (*i.e.,* prenatal) and latter heaven (*i.e.,* postnatal) sources. Prenatally, kidney essence provides a substrate for the blood. Postnatally, the blood is created out of the pure part of the impure part of water (liquids) and grains (food). The digestion or spleen-stomach function is not mature until approximately six years of age. At six years of age or so, the girl manufactures a daily surplus of qi and blood which is then stored as acquired essence during sleep at night. It is this latter heaven or acquired essence which bolsters and supports the former heaven or prenatal essence and which causes the kidney qi to become euxuberant at 14 years of age or thereabouts. At 14, the girl is manufacturing sufficient extra qi and blood and, therefore, her kidney essence and hence kidney qi is exuberant enough that, every 28 days or so, she creates such a superabundance of blood that it wells over the uterus where it is stored and is discharged as the menstruate. This is the heavenly water or *tian gui.* Yu Yao-feng, on the very first page of the *Nu Ke Ji Yao (The Collected Essentials of Gynecology),* in discussing the menstrual water, says:

> The *tian gui* is the woman's essence which follows or is dependent upon the filling of the *ren mai.* The menstrual matter is the menstrual blood which follows the filling of the *tai chong.*

It is called *tian gui* because the blood is manufactured in the heart or upper part of the body. Therefore, in terms of the cosmological metaphors of Chinese medicine, it is a liquid dependent on kidney essence which descends from heaven.

TCM theory says that three viscera participate in the creation of the blood, one from each burner—the spleen, kidneys, and heart. The spleen extracts the pure part of the food and liquids. The purest of the pure is sent up to the lungs to become the qi. The purest part of the impure is sent up to the heart to become the blood. In Chinese, the phrase, *zhuo gui xin* or the turbid gathers at the heart, refers to the heart's part in manufacturing the blood. For this to happen, the kidneys must send up some essence to act as a substrate parallel to how the kidneys send up source qi to the lungs to act as a catalyst for the creation of the qi. Therefore, the blood is finally made in the heart/upper burner from whence it is dispersed and descended in order to nourish the rest of the body. It is said that the heart turns the blood red. Red is the color of fire and the heart is the fire organ. All transformations in the body are, according to Chinese medicine, warm transformations. It is the warming and transforming function of heart qi and yang which turn the blood red.

Based on the above description of the creation of blood, the *tian gui* may fail to arrive if a) the kidney essence is prenatally insufficient, b) spleen function fails to send the pure of the impure up to the heart as a by-product of digestion, or c) the heart fails to transform this combination of digestive essence and kidney essence into blood. Similarly, menopause occurs when the decline of spleen function and kidney essence together result in the body's inability to create a monthly superabundance of blood which brims over the chalice of the uterus as menstruation. This happens at roughly seven times seven or 49 years of age because, at around 35, the *yang ming* or digestion begins to weaken and at 49 kidney essence begins to show signs of exhaustion. Because both the pre- and postnatal sources of blood production have become weak, there is no longer a superabundance of blood being produced.

This point is an extremely important one. If one merely reads the *Nei Jing Su Wen (Inner Classic Simple Questions)* and various other premodern and contemporary Chinese authors on the *tian gui*, one may get the impression that the *tian gui* is simply and solely a manifestation of kidney essence. For instance, in the Qing dynasty, Shen Yao-fang said:

> The *tian gui* is women's essence. It passes through the controlling vessel [*ren mai*] and comes. The menstruation is the channel blood. It passes through the *tai chong* and comes.

While the *Nei Jing Su Wen (Inner Classic Simple Questions)* says:

> The *tian gui* is yin essence. Now the kidneys pertain to water and the *tian gui* also pertains to water. Due to the former heaven qi accumulating to its limit and growing, the yin essence becomes the *tian gui*.

And the *Yi Xue Zheng Zhuan (Orthodox Transmission of the Study of Medicine)* states, "The menstrual water is entirely bestowed by kidney water."

However, Zhang Jing-yue (a.k.a. Zhang Jie-bin) explains:

> Menstrual water is made from the essence qi of grain and water. It harmonizes and regulates the five viscera and sprinkles the six bowels. Then it is able to enter the vessels. It continuously [flows] and comes, engendering and transforming in the spleen, homing to the heart, stored in the liver, diffused by the lungs, and discharged by the kidneys. Thus it irrigates the whole body... In women, it ascends and becomes the breast milk. It descends and gathers in the sea of blood becoming the menstrual water.

In this quote, Zhang Jing-yue clearly states that the menstrual water is not just made from kidney essence but that the viscera bowels must transform and engender blood from water and grain before the menstruate can be made. This blood circulates through the entire body, nourishing the various viscera and bowels and body tissues and functions. What is left over after these needs are met can then descend to become the menstrual water. Zheng Shou-qian, in *Nu Ke Zong Yao (Gathered Essentials of Gynecology)*, also explains the interdependence of former and latter heaven function in the creation of the menstrual water:

The *tian gui* is a general name for manifestations of men's and women's growth and development. *Tian* or heaven in regard to humans refers to former heaven [*xian tian*] whose root is the original qi [*yuan qi*]. It comes from one's father and mother and is also called heaven's true qi [*tian zhen zhi qi*]. *Ren* and *gui* are the two ancient heavenly stems associated with water. In humans, *gui* water refers to heaven's endowment of the blood vessels' yin water. This comes by way of the kidney viscus's qi transformation action and thus it is created. Therefore, the *tian gui* is made from a combination of heaven's true qi and *ren* and *gui's* water. This is then cultivated and fostered by latter heaven's cultivation and fostering of water qi materials and substances and by means of the kidneys' qi transformation activity. Thus the male essence and female blood of reproduction is produced.

All this means that, when it comes to the engenderment and transformation of the menses, one must always take into account both the former and latter heaven essences and their interrelationship.

Qi & blood, fluids & essence

Because the menstruate or *tian gui* is a superabundance of blood and because of the reciprocal relationships between the qi and blood, blood and fluids and humors, and blood and essence, it is important to be clear about these relationships. Imbalances in any of these relationships may give rise to menstrual diseases.

First of all, the qi is the commander of the blood. If the qi is weak, it will not engender and transform the blood. In other words, qi vacuity may give rise to blood vacuity and this may result in delayed, scanty, absent menstruation, or painful menstruation. If the qi is vacuous, it may also not contain the blood within its vessels. It is the qi which holds the blood within its vessels and qi vacuity often results in profuse or untimely bleeding. Further, it is the qi which moves the blood. It is said:

The qi moves the blood. If the qi moves, the blood moves. If the qi stops, the blood stops.

This means that if the qi becomes sluggish or stagnant, the blood may become static and stuck. This may also result in delayed, scanty, absent, or painful menstruation.

Concomitantly, the blood is the mother of the qi. If the blood is insufficient, the qi will lose its root and flush upward and to the exterior, coursing erratically. In this case, the qi becomes internally generated wind due to blood vacuity. If the blood becomes static and stuck, the qi may become sluggish and stagnant as well. This may cause abdominal and breast distention, premenstrual depression, and painful menstruation. Or, if blood becomes greatly vacuous, the qi and yang may desert, resulting in hemorrhaging and profuse sweating.

Since the blood and fluids share a common source, if fluids are lost or damaged due to fever, copious sweating, vomiting, or diarrhea, blood may become damaged and vacuous. This may result again in delayed, scanty, or absent menstruation. Likewise, if blood is lost or consumed, fluids may become dried and consumed. However, since qi is yang and fluids are yin, if fluids are full to repletion, this may impede the movement and transformation of qi. In terms of menstruation, this may result in phlegm obstruction and phlegm dampness causing delayed or absent menstruation, profuse menstruation, or flooding and leaking. This can also impede the qi's engenderment and transformation of the blood, thus resulting in scanty or delayed menstruation.

Since essence is manufactured from surplus qi and blood, if qi and blood become weak, essence will not be stored postnatally. Since the essence and the blood share a common source, *i.e.*, the kidneys, if essence becomes vacuous, the blood may become insufficient to support the normal arrival and volume of menstruation. Inversely, if blood is lost or its engenderment and transformation is impaired, this may result in essence not being transformed and stored. And, since blood is the manifestation of essence in women, this is especially the case in females.

Viscera & bowels

Since it is the viscera and bowels which engender and transform both the qi and blood, viscera and bowel function is also vitally important for the creation and discharge of the menstruate. There are four viscera of particular importance *vis à vis* TCM gynecology. These are the three viscera which participate in the engenderment and transformation of the blood—the spleen, kidneys, and heart—and the three viscera which control the blood—the spleen, heart, and liver. Since two of these are the same—the heart and spleen—there are four important viscera altogether in terms of the blood and menstruation.

We have discussed the creation of blood above. However, because these basic facts are so vitally important when puzzling out a pattern discrimination and creating a treatment plan, it does no harm to go over some of this material more than once. When we say that the heart, spleen, and kidneys are the three viscera which engender and transform the blood, it is important to know exactly what each viscus's role is in this process. The spleen transforms the finest essence of water and grains and upbears this to the heart. The kidneys send up essence to the heart as well. Then heart yang, which includes heart qi, transforms these two into red blood which is then sent down to the uterus via the *bao mai*.

As for the control of blood by the spleen, heart, and liver, TCM theory says that the spleen constrains the blood within its vessels. The heart moves the blood. And the liver stores the blood. In each case, it is the qi of the viscus involved which exerts its controlling function over the blood. The spleen's role in containing the blood within its vessels is well-known. The heart moves the blood downward the same way or parallel to how the lungs move the qi and fluids downward. The liver stores the blood. Because the uterus is identified with the sea of blood and the blood chamber which are also all said to store or treasure the blood, the liver is accorded an especially important role in the regulation of menstruation. In fact, since the liver stores the blood and the blood is the manifestation of the essence in women, it is said that the liver is the former heaven viscus in women in the same way that the kidneys are the former heaven viscus in men.

As mentioned above, menstruation occurs when a superabundance of blood accumulates in the uterus which then brims or wells over as the menstrual discharge. However, the flow of this blood is dependent upon the transporting function of the qi and the liver controls the coursing and discharge of the qi. Therefore, if the liver qi becomes depressed and stagnant, this can have an especially pronounced effect on the free flow of the menstruate. It may be said that the kidneys and heart nourish and enrich the uterus, but the liver controls its flow.

TCM theory has nothing particular to say about lung function *vis à vis* menstruation. The lungs do not directly participate in either the creation or the control of the blood and menstruation is primarily a blood issue in Chinese medicine. The lungs may play their part in both menstrual disease mechanisms and in the treatment of menstrual disorders, but they are usually not discussed *per se* as an important viscus in menstruation. Some few Chinese gynecology books discuss the lung qi's role in moving the blood downward, and certainly, the heart and lung qi are closely related and together form the great or chest qi. However, I believe that it is useful to distinguish between the lung qi function of downbearing and diffusing the qi and, therefore, freeing the flow of the water passageways and the heart qi's function of controlling or moving the blood.

Likewise, TCM theory does not typically discuss any of the bowels in terms of menstruation. The gallbladder, bladder, and small intestine are not accorded any direct or indirect part in the menstrual cycle. However, it is my opinion that the stomach and large intestine do merit at least some discussion. Although the stomach's participation in the creation of blood is subsumed under spleen function, upward counterflow of stomach qi may cause pre and perimenstrual nausea and vomiting and may be involved in premenstrual breast distention and pain. As we will see below, liver depression transforming heat may attack the stomach, causing depressive heat in that bowel as well. This may give rise to increased hunger and/or acne premenstrually.

The large intestine is the largest organ in the lower burner. Its free flow and function are associated with the uninhibited and smooth flow of the qi and blood of the entire contents of the lower burner. If the large intestine is not smoothly and freely flowing, this may lead to stagnation of qi within the liver and stasis of blood within the uterus. Therefore, at least therapeutically, the large intestine does deserve some mention and attention. Further, damp heat pouring downward and accumulating in the large intestine can damage the liver and kidneys. According to five phase theory, the large intestine is the mother of the kidneys. Categorized as metal, the large intestines favor dryness and are averse to dampness. Therefore, dampness can damage the large intestine which then may fail to engender the kidneys. As we have seen above, healthy, exuberant kidneys are necessary if the uterus is to function correctly and if menstruation is to occur with proper regularity.

Channels & network vessels

Just as the viscera and bowels engender and transform the qi and blood, the channels and network vessels are responsible for the circulation and disbursement of the qi and blood to the rest of the body. Of the eight extraordinary vessels, the four of particular importance in terms of menstruation are the *chong, ren, du,* and *dai*. It is said that the *chong, ren,* and *du* all arise from within the uterus, whereas the *dai* bifurcates from the *ren* and binds together all the other longitudinal channels thus regulating the flow of qi and blood between the upper and lower halves of the body. Since the *tian gui* begins in the upper body and flows down to the lower body, should the *dai mai* be either too tight or too loose, this may have an impact on the menstruation. In addition, if the *dai mai* is too loose, then this may allow fluids to percolate downward to the lower burner, there to manifest as abnormal vaginal discharge or *dai xia*. The qi transformation function of the *dai mai* is rooted in the life gate fire which expresses itself in the yang qi and warming and transforming activities of the kidneys, spleen, heart, and liver directly and indirectly in the stomach and intestines, gallbladder, bladder, and three burners.

Of these four extraordinary vessels, the two most important in terms of menstruation are the *chong* and *ren*. The *chong* or penetrating vessel is called the sea of blood and the sea of all twelve channels. The *ren* or controlling vessel is called the sea of all yin.[2] However, in terms of the relationship between the *chong* and *ren* which, at least in terms of TCM gynecology, are conceived of as a pair, the *chong* mainly contains blood and the *ren* mainly contains qi. Therefore, their relationship is based on the relationship between the qi and blood. The *chong* nourishes all the channels, remembering that the menstruate is also called *jing* or channel. It nourishes the yang above and the yin below. The *ren* controls the *bao gong*. As extraordinary vessels, the *chong* and *ren* are both dependent upon an abundance of kidney qi.

---

[2] Readers should note that Wiseman's new term for the *ren mai* is the controlling vessel. This replaces the older conception vessel.

Pathologically, the *chong* and *ren* may be *bu gu*, unsecured or not securing, *bu tiao* or unregulated/not regulating, or *sun shang* or damaged due to detriment. *Chong* and *ren bu gu* implies that the qi in the *ren* cannot constrain the blood in the *chong*. *Chong* and *ren bu tiao* means that the qi and blood are not balanced. More particularly this implies that the qi is not controlling the free flow of blood as it should. And *chong* and *ren sun shang* means that the qi and blood in these two channels have become damaged and weak, for instance through too early or too many pregnancies.

The role of the *du* or governing vessel in menstruation is a bit more abstruse. It is said that the *ren* and *du* flow ceaselessly up the back and down the front. The *ren* is the sea of yin and the *du* is the sea of yang. As we will see below, the menstrual cycle can be described as the flow of yang qi upward during the first half of the cycle and the flow of yin blood downward during the second half. Because the *ren* and *du* control this general or background circulation of yang up and yin down, the periodicity of menstruation is believed to be under the control of the *ren* and *du*. However, in TCM gynecology, little specific attention is directed at the *du mai* either diagnostically or therapeutically.

Of the twelve regular channels, the most important in TCM gynecology are the foot *tai yin* spleen, the foot *jue yin* liver, the foot *shao yin* kidney, and the foot *yang ming* stomach channels. The liver, spleen, and kidney channels all run internally through the pelvic cavity and connect with the controlling vessel and thence with the uterus. The kidney channel is believed by many to connect with the *chong mai* along its course up the ventral surface of the abdomen and the stomach channel connects with the *chong mai* at *Qi Chong* (St 30). In addition, the liver network vessels irrigates the external genitalia. In most Chinese TCM gynecology texts only the liver, spleen, and kidney channels are mentioned. However, one cannot understand premenstrual breast distention without understanding the stomach channel and its connection to the *chong*.

The following four diagrams taken from four different contemporary Chinese gynecology texts each, in their own way show how the menses are produced by the interrelated functioning of the viscera and bowels, channels and network vessels, and qi and blood.

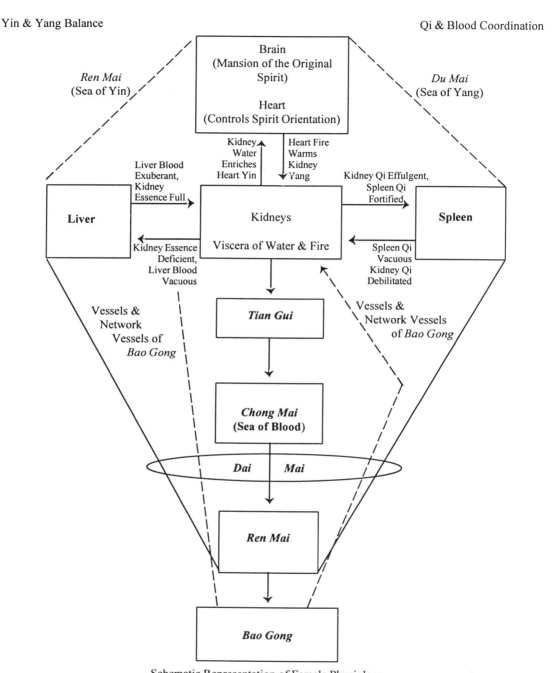

Schematic Representation of Female Physiology

(From *Fu Ke Zheng Zhi* [*Gynecological Patterns & Treatments*] by Sun Jiu-ling, Hebei People's Press, Shijiazhuang, 1983)

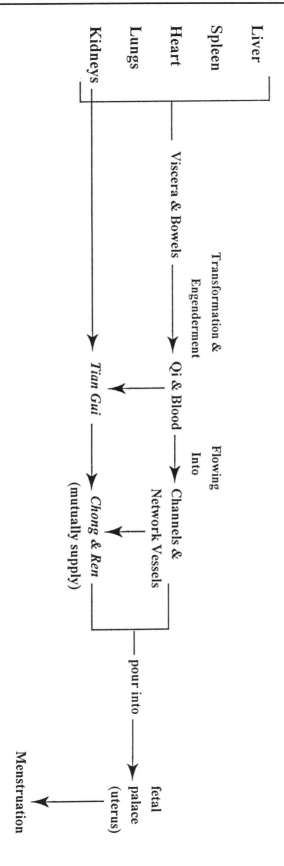

Diagram of the Mechanisms of Production of Menstruation

(From *Zhong Yi Fu Ke Xue* [*A Study of Chinese Medicine Gynecology*] by Liu Min-ru, Sichuan Science & Technology Press, Chengdu, 1992)

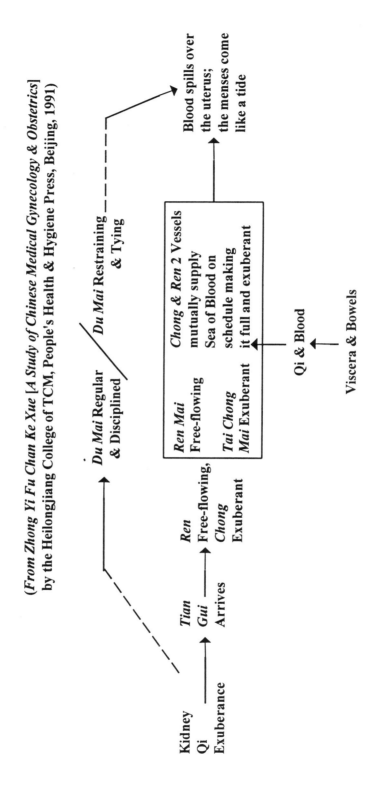

(From Zhong Yi Fu Chan Ke Xue [A Study of Chinese Medical Gynecology & Obstetrics] by the Heilongjiang College of TCM, People's Health & Hygiene Press, Beijing, 1991)

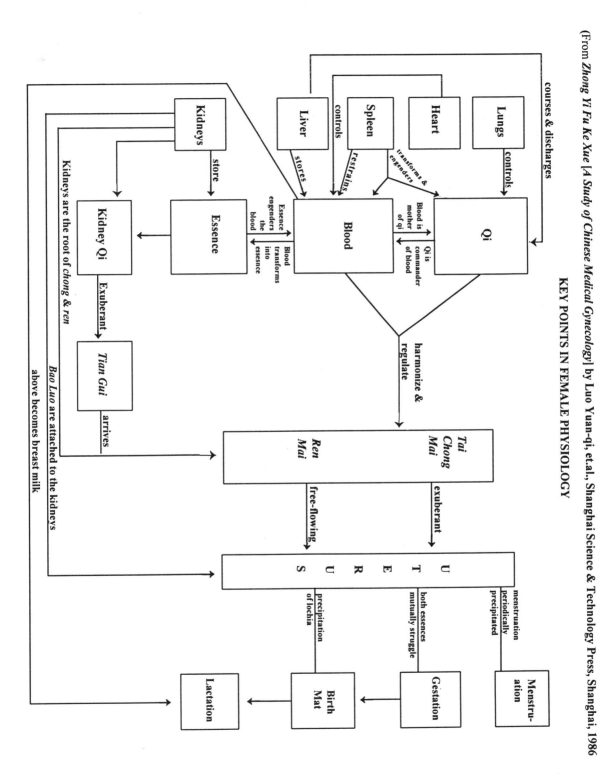

(From *Zhong Yi Fu Ke Xue [A Study of Chinese Medical Gynecology]* by Luo Yuan-qi, et.al., Shanghai Science & Technology Press, Shanghai, 1986

KEY POINTS IN FEMALE PHYSIOLOGY

The menstrual cycle

In the *Nei Jing Su Wen (Inner Classic Simple Questions)*, it says:

> At seven years of age in women, the kidney qi is exuberant and, therefore, the [second] teeth are emitted and grow. At two times seven, the *tian gui* arrives, the *ren mai* is free-flowing, the *tai chong mai* is exuberant, the menses descend periodically, and, therefore, they can have babies.

This is the *locus classicus* in the Chinese medical literature about the cause of menarche occurring at puberty and the cause of menstruation occurring periodically thereafter. To recapitulate, for menarche to occur at puberty and for the menses to descend periodically, the kidney qi must be exuberant, the controlling vessel must be freely flowing, and the penetrating vessel, *i.e.*, the sea of blood, must be exuberant. We have seen above that the exuberance of the kidneys is based on both former heaven or prenatal and latter heaven or postnatal factors. From this point of view, the monthly menstruation is due to the uterus being filled to overflowing each month. Therefore, the menses are often referred to as the

Qi, Blood, Yin & Yang
vis-a-vis Menstrual Cycle

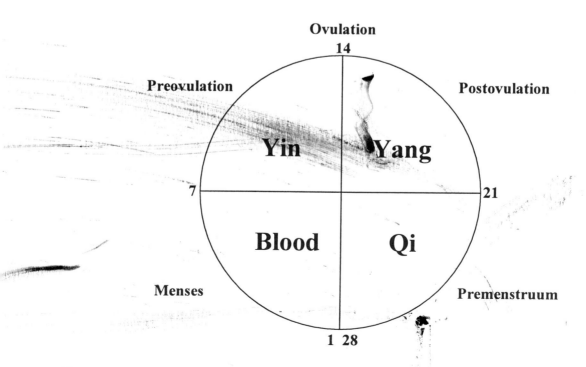

tide. This concept of tide implies the flood at high tide and the cyclicity of the tides. Li Shi-zhen said, "*Jing* means constancy." Chen Yu-cang, in *Jing Dai Zheng Zhi (Menstrual & Vaginal Discharge [Diseases] Patterns & Treatments)* glosses this by saying, "This means, like the moon, it waxes and wanes, and like the tides, it comes regularly." Chen quotes Wang Zi-heng, saying:

> Women's menstruation has a constant time. This schedule is due to the rise and fall of the whole body's yin and yang.

The rise and fall of yin and yang responsible for the menstrual cycle is made up of four approximately seven day segments. According to TCM theory, during each of these four segments, different physiological processes take place, and only if one understands these various processes can one understand why signs and symptoms appear when and as they do. Likewise, only by understanding these four segments can one apply the right therapy at the right time. These four segments of the menstrual cycle as a whole are related to the blood, yin, yang, and qi respectively.

The cycle begins on day one of the period. During the period, the blood flows down and out. The uterus that was full to overflowing becomes gradually emptied. Therefore, during the menstruation, the emphasis is on the blood and more specifically on its free flow. If the blood is not able to flow freely, even though there may be sufficient blood, there may be delayed menstruation, scanty menstruation, painful menstruation, or blocked menstruation. If the blood is freely flowing, by the end of menstruation, the sea of blood is empty.

During the second week or approximately seven days after the onset of the menses, the discharge has stopped and the blood begins to grow. The body busies itself with engendering and transforming more blood to replenish this relative yin and blood vacuity. Because blood and essence share a common source, the emphasis in this segment of the cycle is on enriching yin in order to nourish and replenish the blood.

On or around day 14, two weeks after the onset of menstruation, the blood is now again normally full. Because a basic tenet of yin-yang theory is that, when yin reaches its extreme, it transforms into yang, this exuberance of yin transforms yang. In modern TCM gynecology, this transformation of exuberant yin into yang is related to ovulation and the rise in basal body temperature that follows ovulation. Therefore, for ovulation to occur, yin must transform into yang, and thus invigorating and warming yang during this third segment of the menstrual cycle becomes extremely important.

From day 21 on to the onset of menstruation, heart qi must move the blood down to the uterus. It is the liver qi which controls the coursing and discharge of qi, including the heart qi. If the liver is depressed and, therefore, the qi stagnant, the qi may counterflow during this segment of the cycle. This then may cause any number of premenstrual signs and symptoms of counterflowing or non-freely flowing qi, such as premenstrual breast and/or lower abdominal pain and distention. In addition, if the spleen qi is vacuous and weak, it may be too weak to contain the blood accumulating in the uterus. In that case, there may be early menstruation or profuse menstruation. Therefore, during the premenstruum, the emphasis is on the rectification and fortification of the qi.

These four segments of the menstrual cycle are shown in the accompanying diagram. In addition, it should be noted that ovulation can only occur at midcycle if yin transforms into yang. On the one hand, there must be sufficient yang to catalyze this transformation, since all transformations in the human body are warm transformations. On the other, this transformation may only occur if the qi mechanism is functioning properly. The qi mechanism is the mechanism of qi transformation. This mechanism functions properly only if the qi is flowing freely. Therefore, although the main concern is the transformation of yin into yang, this transformation requires the qi to be rectified and the blood to be moving freely. If either the qi is stagnant or the blood is static, this may impede this transformative process because of their negative impact on the qi mechanism.

The main implication of this theory is that, when treating women, one should not necessarily give the same treatment no matter where their patient is in her menstrual cycle. There are more appropriate times to accomplish certain treatment principles than others. In Chinese medicine, we try to work within the cycles of change of the seasons, the weather, the moon, etc. In gynecology, we also need to take into account these four great segments of the menstrual cycle when planning and implementing treatment. For instance, blood vacuity often goes along with blood stasis, either as a cause or a result. However, quickening the blood and dispelling stasis is an attacking method of treatment. Since the blood is vacuous at the end of menstruation and, during the second segment of the cycle, the body is trying to enrich and nourish yin blood, then we know that quickening the blood and dispelling stasis may be contraindicated during this segment. Whether it is contraindicated in fact depends on what the patient is being treated for and what their actual pattern discrimination is. However, at the least, the practitioner should take relative blood and yin vacuity into account before using attacking methods either unwarrantedly, too strongly, or without simultaneously supplementing yin blood. Concrete examples of using this theory in clinical practice in order to plan or modify treatment are given below when discussing the treatment of menstrual diseases.

Basal body temperature (BBT)

In China today, the four segments of the menstrual cycle are believed to be dependent upon the kidneys. Since the kidneys are the root of yin and yang in the body and the *tian gui* is dependent upon the kidney essence, this theoretical advance makes sense. Lian Fang, in a recent article appearing in *The Journal of Chinese Medicine*, writes:

> Recent investigations on the theory of "adaptation of the human body to the natural environment" and on biorhythms have revealed that the four menstrual phases are the result of transformation of Kidney-yin and Kidney-yang. A balanced coordination between Kidney-yin and Kidney-yang is important for normal transformation of the four menstrual phases.[3]

Lian Fang then goes on to say:

> The normal changes in BBT [basal body temperature] from low to high during the four menstrual phases seem to be related with the transformation of Kidney-yin and Kidney-yang. In the post-menstrual period, there is growth of Kidney-yin and BBT is in the hypothermal phase; in the inter-menstrual period, there is transformation of Kidney-yin into Kidney-yang and BBT rapidly rises; in the pre-menstrual period, both yin and yang are exuberant and BBT persists in hyperthermal state; in the menstrual period, both yin and yang become insufficient and BBT returns to hypothermal state.[4]

The above statements imply that the basal body temperature is a function of the life gate fire. In its narrowest sense, life gate fire is none other than kidney yang, kidney fire, or true yang. However, as explained above, life gate fire directly and indirectly affects the functioning of a number of other viscera and bowels in the body which may be said to participate in the larger concept of life gate fire. This coordination of TCM theory with the modern Western medical staging of the menstrual cycle can have significant effect on TCM diagnosis and treatment. By using the BBT or basal body temperature as an indicator of which phase the woman is actually in, in comparison to where she should theoretically be based on the day of the month, one can even more efficiently and effectively balance and regulate the cycle.

According to modern Western medicine, if a normally ovulating and menstruating woman takes her basal body temperature at the same time each morning before she gets out of bed or engages in any activity, her temperature when plotted on a graph will display a biphasic

---

[3] Lian Fang, "TCM Treatment of Luteal Phase Defect", *Journal of Chinese Medicine*, UK, # 38, January 1992, p. 21

[4] Ibid., p. 21

curve made up of a hypothermal or low temperature phase and a hyperthermal or high temperature phase. The transition from low to high occurs at ovulation and is an indicator of ovulation. The rise in temperature is due to the effects of progesterone secreted from the corpus luteum after ovulation on the body's metabolism. Therefore, the hyperthermal phase is also called the luteal phase. The temperature drops 12-24 hours before the onset of menstruation due to the discontinuance of the corpus luteum's secretion of progesterone. Because the serum progesterone drops, the endometrium necroses and sheds, and thus menstruation occurs. Therefore, the hypothermal phase goes from just before the onset of menstruation to the occurrence of ovulation, while the hyperthermal phase goes from ovulation to just before the onset of menstruation, and hence, changes in basal body temperature signal either the occurrence of ovulation or the immanence of the menstruation.

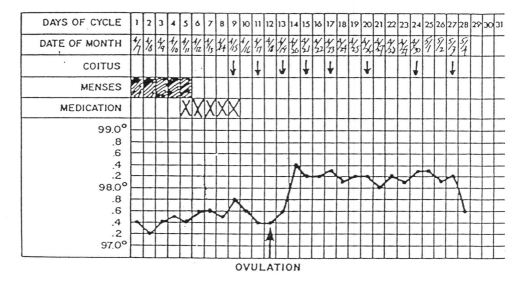

This is a typical normal biphasic basal body temperature chart. Before ovulation, temperature will be in the 97.2° to 97.4° F. range; with ovulation it will rise at least 0.5° F. The best time for intercourse is one or two days before temperature starts to rise.

The famous contemporary Chinese gynecologist, Xia Gui-cheng from Nanjing, says that a normal, biphasic bbt curve, and therefore a normal menstrual cycle, indicates that the kidney essence is sufficient, yin and yang are in harmony, and the qi and blood are uninhibited. If the bbt curve is abnormal, this then can give an indication as to the disease mechanism causing menstrual irregularities. The following indications for bbt abnormalities are based on Dr. Xia's, Cheng Jing's, and my own clinical observations.

If there is a monophasic, flat line bbt, this indicates anovulation. If the bbt is flat line and relatively low, this is due to kidney yang insufficiency. If it is flat line and relatively high, this is due to kidney yin vacuity with vacuity heat. In either case, there should be corroborating signs and symptoms, tongue and pulse.

If there is a prolonged hypothermal phase, meaning that the BBT stays low for more than 14 days, this indicates either a kidney yin vacuity or a spleen-kidney yang vacuity. If it is due to a kidney yin vacuity, this means that the enrichment and nourishment of the yin blood is slower than normal. In this case, it takes more than 14 days for the yin to become exuberant and transform into yang. However, because spleen and kidney yang are necessary to promote warm transformation, if there is a spleen-kidney yang vacuity, this may also lead to a prolonged hypothermal phase. In that case, one should look either for yin vacuity or yang vacuity signs and symptoms.

If there is an abnormally short hypothermal phase, meaning that ovulation occurs earlier than day 14 and thus also earlier than normal menstruation, this is due to the presence of evil heat. The reason why this is due to evil heat will become clear below under our discussion of menstruation ahead of schedule. In my experience, this heat may be either vacuity heat or depressive heat and one should confirm which by the accompanying signs and symptoms, tongue and pulse.

If there is an abnormally long transition phase from hypo- to hyperthermal phases lasting more than 72 hours, this may be due to kidney yang vacuity and/or liver depression qi stagnation. In the first case, there is insufficient yang qi to promote this warm transformation in an efficient manner. In the second case, liver depression qi stagnation affects the liver's coursing and discharge which, in turn, inhibits the qi mechanism. Because the qi mechanism is not functioning properly, qi transformation cannot take place freely and uninhibitedly.

If the BBT goes up normally but then sags back down, only to go up again before it finally drops just prior to the onset of menstruation, this is called a horse-shaped BBT curve. It is called this because it looks like the swayed back of an old horse. It indicates a yang qi insufficiency. There was enough yang qi, meaning spleen qi and kidney yang, to transform yin into yang and raise the BBT, but then there was not enough yang qi to keep the temperature elevated. However, after falling down, the yang qi again collects itself and again raises the BBT before it falls for good just before the onset of the menstruation.

If the BBT curve during the hyperthermal phase goes up and down irregularly like the teeth of a saw, this is called a saw-toothed curve and it means that there is a yang vacuity with loss of harmony of the heart, lungs, liver, spleen, and stomach. What this means is that there is a spleen-kidney yang vacuity with liver depression which has transformed into heat. This depressive heat in the liver has then caused the mutual engenderment of depressive heat in the heart, lungs, and stomach. When this heat is predominant, the BBT goes up, and when spleen-kidney vacuity is predominant, the BBT goes down. This is actually a common BBT curve in Western clinical practice.

If the BBT transition from hyper- to hypothermal is prolonged, meaning that it takes more than 72 hours to occur, this means that there is a spleen-kidney yang vacuity. In actuality, this is a type of shortened luteal or hyperthermal phase. What this actually means in clinical practice is that the BBT begins to decline several days before normal. It does not plunge downward as it should but slides downward over several days. Nevertheless, it should be read as essentially a shortened hyperthermal phase.

In terms of a shortened hyperthermal phase, this means that the BBT goes down too soon after ovulation. When normal, the BBT should stay high for 13 days, thus resulting in a 28 day menstrual cycle. When the BBT goes down before this, the basic indication is that the patient is suffering from a spleen-kidney yang vacuity. This should be corroborated from the accompanying signs and symptoms, tongue and pulse. Dr. Cheng says that a shortened luteal phase may also be due to either replete or vacuity heat. However, in my experience, this is only so if there is depressive heat concomitant with a spleen and possibly kidney vacuity or if there is a spleen qi and kidney yin vacuity with vacuity heat. If the luteal or hyperthermal phase only lasts 6-7 days, giving a 20-21 day cycle, this is considered extremely short. If it lasts 8-9 days, giving a 22-23 day cycle, this is considered a short hyperthermal phase. And if it lasts 10-11, giving a 24-25 day cycle, this is considered a slightly short hyperthermal phase.

Cheng Jing says that replete heat and vacuity heat may both be seen in women with a luteal phase defect and shortened hypothermal phase. In the case of replete heat, this is actually depressive heat. When depressive heat occurs in a luteal phase defect, there is, in my experience also always a spleen qi and possibly a kidney yang vacuity. It is the spleen-kidney yang vacuity which then leads to a premature decline in BBT. As for vacuity heat, it is hard to posit a logical TCM reason why this should actually result in a premature lowering of the BBT. In thinking about this, all I can say is that, in my experience, I have seen women with a shortened luteal phase with liver depression and spleen vacuity accompanied by kidney yin and yang vacuity. In those cases, there certainly were signs and symptoms of vacuity heat above, but there were also signs and symptoms of qi and yang vacuity below, and it is my opinion that that is why the BBT declines prematurely, not specifically due to the vacuity heat.

If there is blood stasis, this either causes a slow transition from hypothermal to hyperthermal or a saw-toothed hyperthermal phase. This is because static blood which is a yin accumulation impedes the free flow of qi which is yang. Because the qi must flow freely for the qi mechanism to function correctly, static blood impeding the free flow of qi may inhibit qi transformation. Likewise, static blood may cause or exacerbate liver depression qi stagnation[5] which then transforms into depressive heat.

Cold congelation is primarily associated with a prolonged follicular or hypothermal phase. This is because cold congelation is usually in the West due to kidney yang vacuity. If kidney yang is vacuous and insufficient, it cannot catalyze the transformation of yin to yang in a timely manner. If there is phlegm obstruction, there may be either a monophasic, anovulatory bbt or a shortened luteal phase. This is because phlegm is nothing other than congealed dampness and dampness is moved and transformed by yang qi. In the first case, there is insufficient yang qi to promote the transformation of yin to yang. In the second, there is insufficient yang qi to maintain the bbt high enough for long enough.

In terms of treatment, if a woman ovulates early, *i.e.*, has a shortened hypothermal phase, she will usually also have an early menstruation. If that shortened hypothermal phase is due to yin vacuity engendering vacuity heat, then it is imperative to supplement the kidneys and enrich yin during the postmenstruum or proliferative stage. This is the time when the body is trying to nourish the blood and enrich yin. If one does not supplement the kidneys and enrich yin during this phase of the menstrual cycle, then one will not stop the menses from coming early. Once ovulation has occured prematurely, then the menses will come 14 days later. This shows not only how this information regarding the menstrual cycle and the bbt can be incorporated in tcm gynecology but also how important it can be for successful treatment planning.

Why women menstruate and men do not

Although we have seen above that the main difference between men and women according to Chinese medicine is that women have a uterus and men do not and, therefore, women menstruate, conceive, and bear children, nevertheless, Tang Rong-chuan, the late Qing dynasty author of the *Xue Zheng Lun (Treatise on Bleeding Disorders)*, included in that book a discussion about why women menstruate and men do not. As the reader will see, Tang's discussion is not based on the presence of the uterus but on differences between men and women in the amount and direction of flow of the qi and blood. Although this discussion is a bit convoluted when translated into English, it is an interesting exercise in Chinese medical logic.

It is said that men are primarily qi and women are primarily blood. Because it is said that men's blood is rich while women's blood is frail, it is also said that the differences in the blood

---

[5] I regard the term *gan yu qi zhi* as a single compound term. In this case, it is liver depression which causes qi stagnation. Thus liver depression modifies qi stagnation, specifying its cause and type.

of men and women [are known by all but] that the similarities are not [widely] understood. As for the dissimilarities, women have menses and men do not. Moreover, this is the sum of the differences between men and women.

Now if the blood is the same, why do women have menses and men do not? Women are primarily blood. Blood is a species of yin and it moves downward in its circulation. It is qi that moves and circulates it [*i.e.*, the blood]. Women, being primarily blood, are always reliant upon the qi to move the blood, [since it is] qi that transforms water...

Qi and blood interact below the umbilicus within the uterus. This is called the cinnabar field in men, and the blood chamber in women. It is under the control of the liver and kidneys and is the sum combination of qi and blood. Qi is engendered from water and transforms water. Since men are primarily qi, blood enters the cinnabar field and is transformed into water by the water [itself] and is internally transformed by the blood. Since the water is unpurified, it is extremely thick and condensed, and it is this that we refer to as kidney essence.

Now a woman's qi is capable of returning and transforming water as well. However, since women are primarily blood, the qi within the blood chamber and everything is transformed into blood by the blood [itself]. So that what is changed is the blood [itself], and it is this we refer to as the menstrual flow. Nevertheless, since the qi transforms water humors within the blood, the menstrual period is [also] referred to as menstrual water. Moreover, both before and after the menstrual flow, the watery [discharge] will always have a pale color. This [is reflective of] a woman's blood division which invariably avails itself of the water of the qi division to lead the movement and circulation.

Having understood this, one understands the subtleties of the qi and water categories in men, and that, within them, there is no lack of blood or fire. Moreover, in understanding the female menstrual cycle, [one understands] the categories of blood and fire and that, within them, there is no lack of qi and water. When the essence is thin in males, this is due to a vacuity of blood, while menstrual disorders in females are due to qi stagnation.

It may be asked, [since] it has been stated that men are primarily qi, while women are primarily blood and within them [*i.e.*, these two aspects] there are changes, then how is it that the menses flow in women and not in men? The answer is this: The menstrual blood is the surplus of the blood. Now the new blood is generated from the removal of the old. According to the natural laws of all things between heaven and earth, the moon waxes and wanes and the sea has its high and low tides. [So too] is the case of a woman's blood. [In accordance with the] removal of the old and generation of the new, once the blood is full it will overflow. This is the way in which the abundance is lost monthly in women and thus menstruation is periodic. It is this which drains the blood's surplus. Blood is primarily yin and circulates downward. Therefore it drains downward, and this is the menstrual blood.

Now, in considering males, although there is no menstrual cycle to examine, the surplus is certainly drained off. Men are primarily qi, and qi itself, being primarily yang, circulates upward. Therefore, the surplus of blood is not drained downward but follows the qi in its upward circulation along the *chong* and *ren* vessels. In the upper [part of the body], these encircle the lips and cheeks. It is the beard and mustache which drains the surplus of the blood. Since women have a menstrual cycle, [the blood] in the upper part of their body does not precipitate the growth of facial hair. Since men grow facial hair, [the blood] in the lower part of the body does not initiate menstruation. Because the primary aspects of ascension and descension are varied, this is the only difference [between men and women]. This interpretation can be found in the *Nei Jing (Inner Classic)* and is not of my own invention.

In this discussion, Tang says that the menses are the discharge of surplus blood circulating downward in the woman's body. He also says that this discharge does dispel old or static blood. Further, if this old or static blood is not discharged, it will impede the engenderment of fresh blood. As Tang Rong-chuan says further down in the same chapter:

It is also said that the blood within the uterus is exchanged monthly. The old is removed and the new is engendered. The old blood is static blood. If this old blood is not removed, it will obstruct the transformative mechanism... If there is blood stasis impeding circulation, the new blood is cut off and cannot be engendered and regulated.

If we observe in the menstrual flow a removal of the old blood and an engenderment of the new, we may understand this [process. For instance,] in the study of the treatment of open sores, one must also first transform necrotic tissue before one may engender new flesh. If the necrotic tissue is not transformed, then the new blood will be cut off in this case as well and cannot be engendered or regulated. Moreover, this is also true in the case of fistulas. The open necrotic flesh should be removed and then the suppuration will stop [of its own accord]. In the treatment of blood loss, if one does not rid stasis and then seek to fortify the blood, how is this any different from attempting to treat sores by seeking to engender new flesh rather than transforming necrosis? [In both cases, treatment will be unsuccessful]. While failing to dispel stasis is one matter and the engenderment of new [blood] is a seperate matter, [yet,] in the dispelling of blood stasis, the engenderment of new blood is already achieved, and, in the engenderment of new blood, blood stasis will be dispelled on its own. In the beginning [of therapy], these are not seperate [conditions].

The downward circulation during menstruation is the removal of stasis. This is when the new blood is already germinated within the sea of blood and conception [becomes possible as well]. Even if there is no menstruation for a long period of time, one must still engender new blood afterward. If one understands this, then one understands that the treatment principle of dispelling stasis is [*i.e.*, implies] the engenderment of the new, and the principle of engendering the new also implies the dispelling of stasis.

This line of thinking introduces two seemingly contradictory conceptions of the menses. On the one hand, as we have seen above, the menses are the expression of a woman's essence, Fu Qing-zhu arguing that the menses, in fact, are not blood (although perhaps what he meant was that the menses are not *merely* blood). On the other, the menses are the discharge of old or static blood. Chen Yu-cang reiterates this point by saying, "If there is no conception, the uterus removes the old blood so that fresh blood can replace the menstruate." For Western practitioners, this sort of contradiction in Chinese medical theory can be upsetting. However, there is really no contradiction in these theories. The menstruate starts out as essence blood. If conception does not take place, then it becomes static blood if it were not otherwise discharged. In fact, there is a parallel between the proliferation of healthy endometrial tissue which then necroses and is shed if conception does not take place with the filling of the uterus with essence blood which later becomes old blood, malign, or dead blood (all synonyms in the Chinese literature for static blood) needing to be dispelled.

To recapitulate the above several theories regarding menstruation, the uterus is the organ responsible for menstruation. Qi and blood are the functional and material bases of menstruation. The viscera and bowels are the source of qi and blood engenderment and transformation. And the channels and network vessels are the avenues over which the qi and blood circulate. Thus, in order to understand the menstruation, both its healthy physiology and its pathophysiology, one must understand the characteristics of the uterus, qi and blood, viscera and bowels, and channels and network vessels in relation to the 28 day cycle of yin and yang transformation which is, in turn, characteristic of females.

Normal menstruation

As discussed above, Chinese medicine believes that normal menstruation begins around 14 years of age and ceases at around 49 or 50. However, due to the high level of nutrition available in the West, it is not uncommon for Western adolescent females to begin menstruating at 10-11 years of age. Likewise, because of good nutrition and a less physically exhausting lifestyle, Western women often do not stop menstruating until after 50. During the first year or two after the onset of menstruation, the menses may not arrive regularly or may even cease for several months. This is because the girl's ability to create a monthly superabundance of blood has not yet become fully stable. In the same way, the menstruation may not just suddenly cease at menopause but may be erratic due to fluctuations in the woman's ability to produce surplus blood.

It is also possible for some women to menstruate only once every two, three, or four months or even only once per year. If the menses come one time every two months, this is called bimonthly (literally, merged) menstruation. If it comes one time every three months, this is called stored or seasonal menstruation. And if it comes only once per year, this is called shunned menstruation. As long as the menses come at regular periods over a prolonged period of time since soon after menarche and is not regularly accompanied by any signs or symptoms of pathology, this may be considered normal for that woman and does not necessarily require treatment. Only if the menses become delayed after having been regular for a long period of time should the woman be treated for menstruation behind schedule or blocked menstruation (*i.e.*, amenorrhea). Further, it is possible for some women who have never menstruated to become pregnant. This is referred to as occult or invisible menstruation. It is also possible for a pregnant woman to continue having normal menses after conception without any danger or damage to the fetus. This is called stimulated menstruation, flourishing fetus, or dirty fetus.

The normal menstrual cycle is about 28 days in length. This is the same as the lunar cycle and this is why menstruation is called *yue jing* or moon flow. However, in individual women, it may also be normal for the menses to come anywhere between 26-35 days or even more as mentioned above. The menstrual discharge itself typically lasts from three to five days and in some women up to seven days. The normal range in volumes of blood discharged runs from 50-100ml with the amount typically less in virgins and more in sexually active women. Based on these normative values, modern TCM practitioners symbolize normal menstruation thus:

$$15 \; \frac{3 - 5}{28 - 30}$$

Fifteen means that menstruation should begin by 15 years of age. Three to five means it should last three to five days. And 28–30 means it should come every 28 to 30 days. In addition, the blood should begin red and may become somewhat dark by the end of the menses. It should also be free from clots, from specific odor, and should be neither watery nor sticky or mucousy.

Some women may consciously experience ovulation. In particular they may experience either an increase in vaginal secretions or pain. An increase in vaginal secretions is considered normal. Since the blood reaches its fullest volume at midcycle and since blood and body fluids share a common source, it is not inappropriate to have more vaginal discharge at this time. This is considered normal or physiologic *dai xia* or vaginal discharge. Some Chinese doctors do recommend, however, that one should include dampness-eliminating medicinals in ovulatory phase formulas in order to prevent accumulating dampness from impeding the qi mechanism. Ovarian or uterine pain at ovulation is not considered normal. In Western medicine, it is referred to as *mittleschmerz*. In Chinese medicine, it is said:

Tong zhi bu tong,	If there is free flow, there is no pain;
Bu tong zhi tong	If there is pain, there is no free flow.

Pain, therefore, in Chinese medicine is *always* an indication that something is amiss. *Mittleschmerz* is categorized in Chinese medicine as a species of lower abdominal pain and treated accordingly. This is why many Chinese gynecologists include medicinals in ovulatory phase formulas to quicken the blood and free the flow of the network vessels. Likewise, in Chinese medicine, midcycle or ovulatory bleeding is seen as a type of pathological bleeding and should be treated. We will discuss the mechanisms of midcycle bleeding under the heading of flooding and leaking in Book Two.

Many women also experience some premenstrual signs and symptoms. These may include slight soreness in the lumbar area, lower abdominal distention, weakness of the limbs, dizziness, headache, breast pain and distention, changes in bowel movements, cravings, emotional lability, and fatigue. When slight, these signs and symptoms disappear spontaneously upon the onset of menstruation and are not necessarily considered pathological. However, any of these signs and symptoms may be considered pathological in TCM if they become more severe, and all of them can be treated and eliminated in the majority of women. Really healthy women should have little or no prodromal signs of the approach of their menses other than a little lower abdominal distention and heaviness of the body corresponding to the fullness of blood and fluids accumulating in the abdomen.

2

The Causes, Mechanisms & Prevention of Menstrual Disease

The Causes of Menstrual Disease

According to TCM and as in the rest of Chinese medicine as a whole, the causes of menstrual diseases are categorized as internal, external, and neither internal nor external causes of disease.

External causes

TCM posits six external causes of disease or *wai yin*. These are wind, cold, heat, summerheat, dampness, and dryness. Of these, cold, dampness, and heat are three of the most likely to cause menstrual disease. Cold and dampness, either singly or in combination, can cause obstruction to the free flow of qi and blood and thus lead to congelation and stagnation in the uterus. Heat may cause either wasting of the blood after a *wen bing* or warm disease or may cause the blood to move frenetically outside its pathways. Heat and dampness may also combine and cause obstruction of and mutually entangle with the qi and blood in the lower burner. Summerheat and dryness are less often involved in menstrual pathologies.

The tendency of any of these six external evils to cause menstrual disease is, in part, dependent upon the climate in which the patient lives. For instance, I live and practice in a high plains desert in Colorado. Therefore, I most commonly see external heat as a disease causing or complicating factor in my female patients' menstrual pathologies and less often see externally invading cold and dampness. Because of this, practitioners must adjust their sights according to their patients' local environment.

Usually, when one thinks of the external causes of disease, such as wind cold, wind heat, damp cold, and damp heat *vis à vis* gynecology, one thinks of specific acute pathologies, such as flu symptoms before the onset of menstruation. However, external environmental factors do have a more subtle effect on menstruation and menstrual pathology. In clinical practice, one cannot fail to notice that women's menstrual complaints tend to run in trends. For instance, for the last two weeks, more than a half dozen of my patients have complained of extreme nipple tenderness and sensitivity. At other times, I have noticed many women's menses coming early, at other times late, and at other times, many of my patients have complained of breakthrough bleeding and spotting. I believe these trends have to do with changes in the ruling and guest qi of heaven and earth.

In Chinese medicine, the progression and transformation of these energies are described in the theories on *wu yun liu qi* or the five transports and six qi. These, in turn, are based on the ten heavenly stems and twelve earthly branches. The fact that the background or macrocosmic energies of heaven and earth have a pronounced effect on the menstruation is substantiated by the following lines from the *Nei Jing Su Wen (Inner Classic Simple Questions)*:

> If heaven and earth are warm and harmonious, this leads to the *jin shui* or menstruation being peaceful and calm. If heaven is cold and earth is chilly, this leads to the menstruation being congealed and (accompanied by) tears (due to pain). If heaven and earth are hot, this leads to the menstruation boiling and overflowing. And, if violent winds rise up, the menses may come in unexpected waves.

In these lines, the words used for menstruation are *jing shui* or, more literally, menstrual water. The effects of the macrocosmic environment are thus analogous to the effects of heat, cold, and wind on water.

Internal causes

The internal causes of disease or *nei yin* are defined in TCM as the seven affects or emotions. These are anger, fear, fright, thought, grief, melancholy, and joy. Each of these seven affects results in a particular effect on the flow of qi. For instance, anger is associated with an upward movement of qi, while fear results in a downward movement of qi. Therefore, when any of these seven affects are excessive or enduring, they may result in the erratic flow of qi. Since the qi moves the blood, such counterflow of the qi will, over time, have a negative impact on the flow of blood. Upwardly counterflowing qi may result in perimenstrual bleeding from the upper orifices. While qi stagnation may lead to blood stasis and, therefore, delayed, scanty, painful, or blocked menstruation. In addition, it is said that the seven passions all transform into fire when excess. Therefore, excessive emotional stress can cause internal and blood heat resulting in either wasting of the blood and yin fluids or boiling of the blood causing it to run frenetically outside its pathways. In the first case, there may be delayed, scanty, or blocked menstruation; in the second, early or profuse menstruation, flooding and leaking, or other types of perimenstrual pathological bleedings, such as hemafecia, hematuria, hemoptysis, or epistaxis.

In particular, anger and frustration may cause upward counterflow of qi or may transform into fire. This, in turn, may cause premenstrual headache, premenstrual breast distention and pain, and premenstrual epistaxis and hemoptysis. Disturbance of fire in the lower burner may damage the *chong* and *ren* and cause early menstruation, profuse menstruation, and flooding and leaking.

Fear and grief both tend to cause a sinking and weakening of yang qi which may result in the *chong* and *ren* becoming insecure or unable to astringe and secure the menses. This may then manifest as profuse menstruation, and flooding and leaking. Specifically in Chinese it is said that sadness causes the qi to scatter and fear causes it to descend. This scattering of qi is due to heat in the lungs caused by sadness.

Thought and worry both inhibit the dispersal of qi and tend to lead to stagnation of the qi and blood. It is said in Chinese that overthinking and worry cause the qi to knot or bind. This inhibits the function of the *chong* and *ren* and obstructs the free and uninhibited discharge of the menstruate. This may result in either delayed menstruation, scanty menstruation, blocked menstruation, painful menstruation, or the formation of nodulations.

Joy keeps the qi in harmony and the emotions at peace. Therefore, joy is not seen as a disease cause but rather as a disease remedy. Joy insures that the constructive and defensive are freely flowing and uninhibited.

In TCM, the two viscera which are believed to be the most affected by emotional excess and mental stress are the heart, the residence of the spirit and the liver, the residence of the ethereal soul. Because the heart sends the *tian gui* down to the uterus and because the liver directly controls the storage of the blood within the uterus and the free and uninhibited flow of the menstruate, it is easy to see why emotional excess and mental stress can cause or participate in the development of menstrual disease. It is also, therefore, understandable why so much of TCM's treatment of menstrual diseases is directed at the liver. As Liu He-jian of the Yuan dynasty said, "In gynecological diseases, once the *tian gui* has arrived [*i.e.*, after menarche], one should mainly treat the foot *jue yin* liver channel."

Neither internal nor external causes

The *bu nei bu wai yin* category of neither internal nor external causes of disease includes, in terms of menstrual disease, trauma, iatrogenesis, diet and lifestyle imbalances, bedroom (*i.e.*, sexual) taxation, and *chong* or parasites. Any or all of these may contribute to or cause menstrual diseases.

1. Trauma

Trauma can include blows to the pelvis, surgery and cutting or piercing wounds to the lower abdomen, and artificially induced abortions which are a species of traumatic attack on the uterus. In the West, lower abdominal surgery and abortions are often contributing causes to the development of static blood in the uterus. Surgery which causes scarring and cutting of the channels and vessels in the pelvis may result in the formation of static blood. Likewise, Chinese gynecology texts say that after an abortion, whether natural or artificial, one typically needs to address and eliminate static blood in the uterus.[6] This implies that abortions can cause static blood and this is certainly supported by my clinical experience in gathering histories from my female patients. It is not uncommon to find the development of the signs and symptoms of stagnation either occurring or worsening after abortion.

2. Iatrogenesis

In terms of iatrogenesis, oral birth control pills (OCs) typically cause both stasis and wasting of the blood. Some Chinese gynecologists go so far as to say they damage the kidneys. Further, when pelvic inflammations and infections are treated solely by antibiotics, they often leave the accompanying blood stasis untreated which then may cause a chronic, recurrent situation which further courses of antibiotics fail to address. In addition, antibiotics may cause or aggravate a yeast proliferation and thus gives rise to a "parasite" condition which may cause or complicate a number of menstrual diseases. And, intrauterine devices (IUDs) used for contraception also often cause blood stasis and heat toxins. Iatrogenesis may also include self-medication with herbs which are taken based on a disease discrimination diagnosis alone. I regularly see women who have taken one herb or another based on a friend's or folk herbalist's recommendation which has been categorically wrong for them according to TCM pattern discrimination and has worsened instead of ameliorated their condition.

3. Diet

In Chinese gynecology texts, the main emphasis in terms of faulty diet is on food stagnation due to overeating and lack of diffusion of water and grains affecting the flow of qi and blood

---

[6] Song Guang-ji & Yu Xiao-zhen, *Zhong Yi Fu Ke Shou Ce (A Handbook of Traditional Chinese Gynecology)*, 42nd, revised edition, trans. by Zhang Ting-liang & Bob Flaws, Blue Poppy Press, Boulder, CO, 1995, p. 153

due to accumulation and depression. However, this is not the most common situation one sees in the West. Diet is a major contributing factor in many Western women's menstrual pathology. Overeating damp, chilled, uncooked, fatty, and sweet foods all damage the spleen and lead to spleen vacuity. If the spleen becomes vacuous, it will lose control over either or both of its two main functions. Either it will not engender and transform the qi and blood out of the finest essence of water and grains or it will lose control over the movement and transformation of fluids. Therefore, spleen vacuity may lead to both qi and blood vacuity and the accumulation of dampness. Enduring dampness may then eventually congeal into phlegm.

Also, some women who eat a vegetarian diet may develop blood vacuity due to insufficient *wei* or heavy, nourishing "flavor" in their diet. All foods are made up of a combination of qi and *wei*. This is basically a yin-yang dichotomy. Foods with more qi tend to be aromatic, light, and relatively dry. Such foods affect the qi and stimulate function. Foods with more *wei* are heavier, denser, more nutritious, and moister. They nourish yin, blood, and bodily form. Meat, including fish and foul, eggs, and dairy products all contain a lot of *wei*. Because blood is yin in comparison to qi and because women must replace the blood they lose each month during menstruation, many women living in temperate climates and engaging in work (including thinking and reading which both consume much blood) need to eat a certain amount of animal products in order to adequately nourish their blood.

In addition, drinking coffee can cause or aggravate PMS and related conditions by transforming the essence into qi and then out-thrusting that qi upward and outward through the pores of the skin. On the one hand, this may lead to blood vacuity and kidney weakness. Blood vacuity may then manifest as scanty or delayed menstruation, while kidney vacuity may manifest as perimenstrual low back pain, cold feet, diminished sexual desire, and infertility. On the other, it may lead to or aggravate counterflow of qi. Such counterflow of qi may then lead to all sorts of PMS signs and symptoms, such as premenstrual breast pain and distention and/or headaches.

4. Work & rest

As a neither internal nor external cause, the category of work and rest covers two lifestyle imbalances causing menstrual disease. On the one hand, insufficient physical exercise may lead to inhibited flow of the qi and blood, accumulation of phlegm and dampness, and weak spleen and stomach/intestinal function. If the qi and blood do not flow freely and easily, this may lead to PMS in turn due to stagnation and counterflow. It may also lead to delayed, scanty, blocked, and painful menstruation. As we will see below, phlegm and dampness as yin depressions impede and hinder the free flow of qi and blood and lead to or worsen their stasis and stagnation. A certain amount of exercise is necessary to also keep the qi mechanism functioning properly. If the qi mechanism does not function properly, this may also result in spleen vacuity and later to qi and blood vacuity. The qi may then be too weak to move or contain the blood. While the blood may be too vacuous and insufficient to nourish the vessels and fill the uterus.

Conversely, all movement, sensation, mental/emotional, and physiological function consume qi, blood, and yin substance through their transformation into yang activity. There-fore, insufficient rest and relaxation may cause effulgence of yang and flaring of vacuity fire in combination with yin vacuity. We have seen above what happens when the qi and blood are too weak to perform their functions *vis à vis* the uterus. If there is yin vacuity, since the blood and essence share a common source, this may lead to delayed, scanty, or blocked menstruation. If yin vacuity gives rise to vacuity heat, this heat may force the blood to move frenetically outside its pathways, causing early, and/or profuse menstruation, flooding and leaking, or other pathological sorts of bleeding associated with the menstrual cycle.

5. Sexual taxation

Sexual taxation means too much sex or unbridled sexual desire. However, as a disease cause, stifled sexual desire may also lead to changes in a woman's physiology. Too much sex can consume the essence and damage the blood. Unbridled desire can cause excessive stimulation of the life gate fire, while stifled desire may cause depressive heat. Failure to orgasm likewise tends to create depressive heat. Desire is a glowing of yang and orgasm is the crescendo and release of yang. Without this release, yang desire can fulminate and smolder. In addition, sex during menstruation can cause counterflow of the qi and blood. During menstruation, the flow of qi and blood is normally down. During sexual intercourse, this flow is reversed. This causes a collision within the pelvis and may result in the formation of blood stasis. In my experience as a clinician, growth in sexual desire just before or during menstruation is due to liver depression transforming into depressive heat. Because the larger notion of the life gate fire includes the yang of the liver, liver depression-depressive heat may cause mutual flaring of life gate fire since these two are mutually engendering.

6. Parasites

Chong or parasites are not generally discussed as a cause of menstrual disease in Chinese TCM gynecology texts. However, *Candida albicans* or yeast are a species of *chong* in Chinese medicine. Usually one only encounters discussions of yeast as parasites in the Chinese TCM gynecology literature in terms of vaginal yeast infections. However, prolifer-ation of yeast may cause or aggravate an endocrine imbalance thus contributing to menstrual disorder. Often there is yeast involvement in cases of PMS, painful menstruation, perimenopausal, and other menstrual complaints whose diagnosis is complicated by spleen vacuity, dampness, and heat. When there is such a combination of spleen vacuity and damp heat, sometimes it is possible to achieve remarkable clinical results with formulas from the parasite-dispelling category. Therefore, I think that it is useful to include parasites as potential menstrual disease-causing factors.

Personally, I have found diagnosis of candidiasis as a species of *chong* to be of some importance in treating Western women. Candidiasis is aggravated by antibiotic use, hormone therapy, including OCs and estrogen replacement therapy (ERT), prednisone, and other corticosteroids, eating sugars and sweets, eating yeasted or fermented foods, such as bread, vinegar, and alcohol, and stress causing depression of the immune system. Because of the pervasive influence of these etiological factors in the West, it is no wonder that candidiasis is such a problem among Western patients when it is hardly even discussed in the Chinese literature. However, when one identifies candidiasis as a factor in a woman's overall diagnosis, that does not mean that one does not still have to do an individualized pattern discrimination. Rather, it helps define and refine that pattern discrimination, may help direct one to the proper formula or medicinals, and most defintely helps one indentify the types of foods the patient should minimize or avoid.

Sexual abuse

Sexual abuse, rape, and incest are a real problem in the West. I know of no Chinese gynecology text which discusses these as possible etiological factors in menstrual disease. However, in my experience, a portion of my female patients with various menstrual pathologies report a history of sexual abuse. In terms of whether sexual abuse should be categorized as an internal cause (*nei yin*) or trauma (*bu nei bu wai yin*), I believe that, in TCM terms, it must be categorized as an internal cause since trauma in TCM specifically refers to physical trauma. As with all internal damage due to the seven affects, the emotional trauma of sexual abuse causes the qi and, therefore, blood to flow contrary to norm. Most the pattern I most commonly see in patients who have suffered sexual abuse is qi stagnation and blood stasis. This may be and often is complicated by a liver-spleen disharmony and a kidney yang vacuity resulting in a heat above cold below pattern. All of this may either be caused or aggravated by the counterflow of qi initiated by the emotional trauma or internal damage.

The Mechanisms of Menstrual Disease

After discussing disease causes, some Chinese gynecology books go on to discuss disease mechanisms. Disease causes are what initially set the process of disease in motion. Disease mechanisms are the TCM description of what happens after the disease is initiated. Disease mechanisms are an important part of understanding pathological processes and are what allow us to understand why, given a particular initiating factor, a particular patient then goes on to manifest the particular signs and symptoms they do.

Disease mechanisms associated with loss of regularity in viscera & bowel function

1. Kidneys

Kidney qi insufficiency, kidney essence vacuity and debility, kidney yin vacuity detriment, and kidney yang debility may all lead to loss of regularity of the *chong* and *ren* with consequent menstrual disease, vaginal discharge disease, pre- and postpartum disease, and infertility.

A. Kidney qi insufficiency

If the former heaven is insufficient, kidney qi will not be exuberant and essence qi will not be plentiful. In that case, the *tian gui* will also be minute and the *chong* and *ren* will not be full. It is also possible for latter heaven causes to damage the kidneys. In that case, the kidney qi may become insufficient or unable to secure. This may cause blocked menstruation, painful menstruation, menstrual irregularity, or flooding and leaking, particularly leaking.

B. Kidney essence vacuity & debility

If the essence and blood become insufficient, the uterus loses its nourishment and the menses may become delayed, scanty, or blocked.

C. Kidney yin vacuity detriment

Constitutionally there may be yin insufficiency or too many births, bedroom taxation, or internal damage by the seven affects may all result in consumption of kidney yin. In addition, aging heavily damages yin essence resulting in the essence becoming deficient and the blood scanty. Thus *chong* and *ren* blood becomes vacuous and the *bao mai* loses its nourishment. In this case, there may be scanty or delayed menstruation or blocked menstruation. Also, fire and heat may scorch fluids and damage yin, or yin vacuity may give rise to internal heat with vacuity fire harassing the blood. And lastly, yin may be vacuous and yang may contend and thus kidney yin vacuity may give rise to various gynecological diseases. If vacuity heat is engendered internally, scorching the blood, the blood may be stirred, leading to early and/or profuse menstruation or flooding and leaking.

D. Kidney yang insufficiency

This may be due to constitutional yang vacuity or it may be due to some damage, such as an enduring disease damaging the kidneys. Kidney yang may thus become vacuous and weak. All these causes may lead to kidney yang vacuity and debility. If there is kidney yang vacuity, this may lead to the engenderment of vacuity cold internally. This then may hinder qi transformation and steaming and rising with the result that the engenderment of qi and blood loses its warming. Thus the flow in the vessels becomes inhibited and warming of the *chong* and *ren* is insufficient. There is *bao mai* and *bao gong* vacuity cold, and the *du mai* does not fortify. Hence various gynecological diseases occur when kidney yang is vacuous. In particular, if life gate fire is debilitated with yin cold being engendered internally, this may lead to uterine cold and thus to painful or blocked menstruation.

E. Kidney yin & yang vacuity

Detriment of yin may reach yang and yang disease may affect yin. Either kidney yin vacuity or kidney yang vacuity may eventually become kidney yin and yang dual vacuity. This then may result in the *chong* and *ren* losing their regulation or vacuity detriment causing menstrual diseases such as early menstruation, (sometimes) early, (sometimes) late, no fixed schedule menstruation, blocked menstruation, flooding and leaking, and perimenopausal syndrome.

F. Kidney qi debility & exhaustion

This may be due to the five viscera becoming vacuous with the kidney qi being wasted and suffering detriment. There may also be fulminant damage to yin blood, exuberant evils with great vacuity of righteous qi, vacuity taxation, debility and withering, or enduring disease may consume and cause detriment to the kidney qi resulting in debility and exhaustion. In that case, the menses may stop and become blocked, the hair on the head may fall, the teeth may become withered, and the facial complexion will lack luster. There will be listlessness of the essence spirit and the reproductive organs may be atrophied. In sum, one will experience premature aging. If the essence and blood are greatly consumed and original qi greatly damaged, yin and yang may definitely part and this may endanger the life destiny with such conditions as great loss of blood from profuse uterine bleeding.

2. Liver

The liver controls the storage of the blood on the one hand and coursing and discharge on the other. Most liver patterns negatively affecting menstruation begin with liver depression qi stagnation. The function of a viscus is dependent on obtaining sufficient blood to nourish that viscus. If blood does not nourish, emolliate, and harmonize the liver, then liver depression becomes more likely or worsens. Since premenstrually much of the body's blood gathers in the uterus, this may cause or worsen liver blood vacuity and, therefore, liver depression premenstrually. This is why liver depression either crops up or worsens in women premenstrually. In addition, the liver's coursing and discharge are also dependent on the life gate fire's warming and steaming the liver. Since kidney vacuity usually occurs or worsens in the late 30s and through the 40s, liver depression may also be caused or aggravated by this factor as well.

A. Liver wood invading stomach earth

Anger damages the liver and causes the qi to rise. If anger causes the liver to be effulgent, it may counterflow horizontally onto the stomach. In that case, the stomach may lose its harmony and downbearing. The stomach qi counterflows upward along with the liver qi. This may lead to pre- or perimenstrual nausea and vomiting and/or breast distention and pain.

B. Liver depression qi stagnation

If, due to emotional depression, liver qi becomes depressed and bound, the qi mechanism may become inhibited, the *chong* and *ren* may lose their regulation, and amassing and spilling may lose their proper limits. In addition, all kinds of depression may give rise to qi stagnation and blood stasis. The *chong* and *ren* may then suffer obstruction causing *chong* and *ren* obstruction and stagnation. Thus liver depression qi stagnation may result in delayed, scanty, and/or painful menstruation, premenstrual breast distention and pain, (sometimes) early, (sometimes) late, no fixed schedule menstruation, or blocked menstruation.

C. Liver depression transforming into heat

If emotional depression is not resolved for a long time, depression may transform into heat. This heat may then damage the *chong* and *ren* and may force the blood to move frenetically, thus resulting in gynecological bleeding disorders. Depressive heat may also damage yin and give rise to yin vacuity with internal heat or yin vacuity with yang hyperactivity. Further, depression leads to qi and blood irregularity which can lead to pain disorders and menstruation becoming chaotic.

D. Liver blood insufficiency, yin vacuity-yang hyperactivity, liver wind internally stirring

Constitutional blood vacuity, repeated damage to the blood, insufficient engenderment and transformation of blood, or internal damage by the affects may all damage and consume liver blood. It is also possible that, if kidney yin is deficient and vacuous, it may not be able to enrich and nourish liver yin. This may cause the onset of diseases due to liver blood insufficiency. If liver blood is vacuous, this may lead to the sea of blood not being exuberant but rather vacuous and empty. In that case, the menses may be late, menstruation may be scanty, or there may be blocked menstruation. If blood is vacuous but the liver is effulgent, this may result in menstrual movement headache. If wind is engendered and transforms dryness, this may cause itching of the genital region. If kidney yin becomes insufficient, liver yin may become vacuous and deficient. This then may lead to lower yang becoming relatively hyperactive or internal stirring of liver wind. This may easily result in premenstrual and perimenopausal syndromes.

E. Liver channel damp heat

Liver depression may transform into heat at the same time as it counterflows onto the spleen, causing the spleen to become vacuous and weak. If the spleen loses its control over movement and transformation, fluids may accumulate and transform into dampness. Since dampness is turbid and heavy, it tends to pour downward to the lower burner. If this dampness mixes with liver depressive heat or if damp depression causes qi depression and transformative heat, damp heat in the liver channel may be engendered. This damp heat in the liver channel may then give rise to premenstrual abnormal vaginal discharge, vaginal itching, and vaginal sores. If dampness and heat obstruct the free flow of the qi and blood, this may cause damp heat stasis and stagnation manifesting as profuse, prolonged, or painful menstruation.

3. Heart

A. Heart fire

If the heart is overtaxed by fatigue and exhaustion, heart yin (blood) may be consumed leading to heart fire becoming relatively hyperactive. This may then lead to stirring of ministerial fire. This may, in turn, cause chaos in the sea of blood with early and/or profuse menstruation or flooding and leaking.

B. Heart blood & yin insufficiency

During the menses, the body's yin and blood may be insufficient. If the heart contracts disease, this may lead to heart blood or yin vacuity. This then may cause menstrual period heart vexation, insomnia, etc. If heart yin is vacuous, the *bao mai* loses its nourishment. On the other hand, yin vacuity may give rise to heart fire being relatively hyperactive. This then may harass and stir the sea of blood, resulting in menstrual irregularities, blocked menstruation, or premenstrual visceral agitation.

C. Heart qi vacuity

If heart qi becomes insufficient, the qi may not be able to flow freely downward and the *bao mai* may thus be blocked. This may lead to the menses not coming. In addition, if heart qi is vacuous, the heart spirit may not be tranquil. This may then result in menstrual period lack of tranquility of the heart spirit, insomnia, and other abnormalities in the essence spirit.

4. Spleen (stomach)

The spleen's two main functions in terms of menstruation are to engender and transform the blood, thus insuring a sufficient amount of menstrual water, and to contain the blood. This means that the spleen qi is responsible for holding the blood within the channels until the proper time for menstruation arrives and so that not too much is discharged during menstruation.

A. Spleen & stomach detriment & damage

If, due to faulty diet, overtaxation, excessive thought and worry, enduring disease, or simply aging, the spleen becomes vacuous, the source of engenderment and transformation will become insufficient. The constructive and blood will thus also become vacuous and scanty and the *chong* and *ren* will be vacuous of blood. The sea of blood being empty and not exuberant, this may manifest as delayed, scanty, or blocked menstruation.

B. Spleen vacuity not able to restrain & contain the blood

If the spleen is vacuous to the point where it is not able to restrain and contain the blood, the blood will not return to its channels and will flow chaotically. This may lead to profuse menstruation or flooding and leaking.

C. Spleen qi insufficiency

If spleen qi becomes insufficient, central qi may fall, leading to the uterus not being able to secure. This then may result in uterine prolapse or perimenstrual hemorrhoids and/or dizziness.

D. Spleen yang not transporting

If spleen yang fails to transport, water and dampness will stop or gather internally. This will tend to percolate downward to the lower burner where it may cause premenstrual abnormal vaginal discharge and/or water swelling. If dampness endures and congeals into phlegm, this may result in blocked menstruation.

E. Stomach heat

Overeating acrid, peppery hot, or fatty foods or drinking too much alcohol may engender heat, and replete heat then may gather and stagnate in the stomach channel. This heat may damage stomach yin. When not during the menstruation, this may not be apparent, but during menstruation, stomach vacuity fire flaring upward may cause menstrual movement mouth sores.

5. Lungs

A. Lung qi loss of diffusion

Due to detriment from overtaxation, enduring disease, or possibly enduring cough damaging the lungs, lung qi may lose its diffusion. In that case, the water passageways may lose their regulation. This may give rise to premenstrual water swelling and non-free flowing urination. Further, if lung qi cannot move freely downward, it may not be able to link together with the heart vessel in order to move the blood. This may then result in blocked menstruation.

B. Lung yin vacuity

If lung yin is damaged, this may lead to yin vacuity with lung dryness. This condition may then result in menstrual movement epistaxis and hemoptysis. In addition, such yin vacuity may also result in blocked menstruation.

Disease mechanisms associated with loss of regularity of the qi & blood

Loss of regulation of the qi and blood can easily result in gynecological disease. Because of women's physiology, in their bodies, blood tends to be insufficient, while qi tends to be surplus. This then easily causes loss of regulation (or loss of balance) of the qi and blood. Further, since qi and blood have their source in the viscera and bowels and the channels and network vessels are the free-flowing pathways for the transportation and movement of the qi and blood, if either the viscera and bowels or the channels and network vessels contract disease, this will affect the qi and blood as well. Thus it is said in the chapter on regulating the menses in the *Ne Jing Su Wen (Inner Classic Simple Questions)*, "If qi and blood are not harmonious, the hundreds of diseases may transmute and be engendered."

Loss of regulation or balance of the qi and blood may be due to many causes. Among the six environmental excesses, heat disperses the blood, while cold congeals the blood. Dampness stagnates the blood, while wind dries it. Fire toxin pestilence plagues the blood.

Heat causes qi to be discharged, cold causes qi to contract. Dampness leads to obstruction and stagnation of the qi mechanism. If the seven affects damage the qi, this can lead to ascension of qi, descension of qi, retardation of qi, scattering of qi, qi chaos, qi binding, and qi consumption. If the seven affects damage the blood, this may cause blood deficiency, blood astingency, and blood binding. If detriment and damage of the viscera and bowels reaches the qi, this may cause qi counterflow, qi fall, qi vacuity, qi exhaustion, and qi stagnation. If it reaches the blood, it may cause blood vacuity, blood withering, blood stagnation, and blood stasis. If viscera and bowel disease is hot or is cold, the blood will be hot or cold as will the qi be hot or cold. All these pathological changes in the qi and blood can result in gynecological disease.

Because qi and blood are interdependent, damage to the qi leads to damage of the blood. Disease of the qi leads to disease of the blood. If qi moves, the blood moves. If qi stagnates, the blood stagnates. If qi becomes hot, the blood will also become hot and flow and spill over. If qi is cold, the blood will be cold and will congeal and constrict. If qi counterflows, the blood will counterflow. If qi falls, the blood will fall. Conversely, disease in the blood aspect will eventually reach the qi aspect. Thus blood vacuity will lead to qi vacuity. Blood stasis can result in qi stagnation. Blood heat can result in qi heat. Blood cold can result in obstruction and stagnation of the qi mechanism. Further, disease may be engendered in the qi division[7], in the blood division, or in both simultaneously.

1. Blood

A. Blood vacuity

If the source of blood transformation becomes insufficient, if enduring disease consumes the constructive and blood, if there is acute or chronic bleeding, such as profuse menstruation, flooding and leaking, bleeding during pregnancy or postpartum, or if prolonged breast-feeding disperses and consumes the qi and blood, any of these may lead to blood vacuity. In case of blood vacuity, the *chong* and *ren* will be insufficient, and unable to transform the breast milk above or cause the sea of blood to be exuberant below. Thus the sea of blood will be empty and vacuous and the transformation and engenderment of menstrual blood insufficient. If there is blood vacuity, this may give rise to delayed menstruation, scanty menstruation, blocked menstruation, or possible vacuity pain or vacuity heat.

---

[7] Wiseman translates *fen* as aspect. The Chinese character for *fen* shows a knife dividing something. The word *fen* can be used as a verb to mean divide. As a noun, it means a segment, level, phase, or aspect. Since the Englsih word division can also be used in exactly this way, I prefer the word division over aspect since it more closely captures all the Chinese usages and etymology of the word *fen*.

B. Blood heat

Evil heat may enter internally. Therefore the *chong* and *ren* may have deep-lying heat. This heat may then distress (or force) blood movement and hence result in gynecological bleeding disorders. Heat evils may also enter the constructive and blood, in which case the blood chamber may accumulate heat. This heat may then burn high during menstruation or postpartum. This is referred to as heat entering the blood chamber. If heat is exuberant, it may scorch yin. First it will scorch, then it will turn into stasis. This may result in static heat aching and pain. Or heat evils may be retained in the lower burner and give rise to gynecological sores and welling abscess toxins.[8]

It is also possible for qi depression to transform into heat. This depressive fire may harass the *chong* and *ren*. Depression also leads to blood stasis as well as fire and heat forcing the blood to move recklessly. Such depressive heat may consequently result in gynecological bleeding disorders and pain conditions. Static heat cooking and steaming can also give rise to blocked menstruation and abdominal masses.

Damp heat may harass the blood and may be retained in the sea of blood, uterus, or genital region. Dampness trapping may lead to qi and blood being inhibited, while heat harassing may lead to the blood being forced to move frenetically. Thus damp heat can cause both blood stasis and heat forcing frenetic movement of the blood. Hence damp heat easily gives rise to bleeding and pain as well as to genital itching and abnormal vaginal discharge.

If the body suffers repeated damage to the blood, yin and blood will become insufficient. This may give rise to vacuity heat being engendered internally and from there to various gynecological blood heat diseases. Yin vacuity blood heat associated with kidney yin vacuity, liver yin vacuity, heart yin vacuity, lung yin vacuity, or stomach yin vacuity producing blood heat are not all the same. Kidney yin vacuity leads to yin vacuity with yang contending and from thence to profuse flooding and leaking. It is also possible for yin vacuity with scanty essence to become blocked menstruation. In addition, yin vacuity may be associated with perimenopausal syndrome. Liver yin vacuity leads to yin vacuity with yang hyperactivity and menstrual movement headache. Heart yin vacuity leads to yin vacuity with fire blazing and insomnia during the menstrual period and/or oral ulcers. Lung yin vacuity leads to yin vacuity and lung dryness and thus to menstrual movement cough, epistaxis, and hemoptysis, or blocked menstruation. While stomach yin vacuity manifests during the menstrual period as stomach fire flaming upward with oral ulcers, vexatious thirst, and nausea.

---

[8] Welling abscess is Wiseman's new term for *yong*.

C. Blood cold

Cold evils may assail internally or the constitution may be yang vacuous and vacuity cold may be engendered internally. In either case, the *chong* and *ren* may suffer from cold. In this case, the blood becomes cold and congealed and the channels and vessels obstructed and stagnant. Thus blood cold leads to painful menstruation, delayed menstruation, scanty menstruation, and blocked menstruation. If cold makes a surprise attack on the uterus, this may lead to gynecological abdominal pain and abdominal masses.

D. Blood stasis

i. Qi stagnation, blood stasis

If the emotions are not uninhibited, the qi mechanism may lose its disinhibition. In that case, qi stagnation may lead to blood stagnation. The blood movement thus becomes hindered and blood stasis is created. In gynecology, usually it is liver channel depression and stagnation which result in blood stasis. In that case, the *chong* and *ren* qi and blood lose their regulation or the *bao mai* may become obstructed and stagnant. This then leads to gynecological pain conditions. This may also result in the sea of blood becoming static and stagnant, amassing and spilling lose their rightful limits, and this then results in menstrual irregularities. Liver channel qi stagnation may also manifest as premenstrual rib-side pain, breast distention, and lower abdominal pain.

ii. Cold congelation, blood stasis

If blood gets cold, it becomes static. As the *Nei Jing Su Wen (Inner Classic Simple Questions)* chapter on regulating the menses states:

> Qi and blood like warmth and are averse to cold. Cold leads to sobbing and an inability to flow. Warmth leads to dispersion and removal [of that blockage].

iii. Heat scorching, blood stasis

Heat may scorch yin blood. It cooks the blood and smelts it, turning it into stasis. If there is static heat in the interior, this may damage the *chong* and *ren*, the uterus, and the vaginal area and lead to various gynecological diseases.

iv. Qi vacuity, blood stasis

Qi vacuity may make the movement of the blood slow and relaxed[9] and thus create stagnation and stasis. Thus there may be painful menstruation and lower abdominal pain.

v. Blood vacuity, blood stasis

If the constructive and blood are vacuous and scanty, the vessels and network vessels will not be full and blood will be vacuous, while qi will be weak. Blood flow will consequently be retarded and, over time, this will create blood stasis. The *chong* and *ren* will become static and stagnant and thus lose their nourishment and moisture. This may then give rise to repletion in the midst of vacuity and thus cause painful, delayed, scanty, and/or blocked menstruation.

vi. Enduring disease becoming stasis

Enduring disease enters the network vessels. In such cases, the qi and blood are usually declining and weak and blood flow has no force. Thus it becomes static and stagnant. For instance, enduring leakage may become stasis.

vii. Bleeding becoming stasis

If the *chong* and *ren*, uterus, or genital region network vessels are damaged, blood may spill over and transform into stasis internally. Fresh blood is then not able to return to its channels and this leads to bleeding which is difficult to stop. This is seen in enduring flooding and leaking. Stasis can also make bleeding more heavy and lead to the disaster of the yin desertion.

2. Qi

A. Qi vacuity, qi fall

If the constitutional yang qi is vacuous and weak, if fatigue and taxation go beyond limit, if there is enduring or serious disease, if food and drink damage the spleen, or if damage to the blood consumes the qi, all of these causes may result in spleen qi vacuity weakness. In

---

9   The word *huan* or relaxed may be used in either a positive or negative sense in Chinese medicine. In this book, it is always used in a negative sense meaning on the verge of slow or relaxed to the point of being retarded. Thus slow means really slow and relaxed means somewhat slow but slow enough to be pathological.

that case, qi vacuity will not exercise its proper restraint and containment and the *chong* and *ren* will not secure. Thus there may be gynecological bleeding disorders.

B. Qi stagnation

If the emotions are inhibited, this may result in the qi becoming depressed and unsoothed (or unrelaxed). The qi mechanism may then lose its regulation and qi and blood become disharmonious. Or there may be damp heat, cold evils retained and stagnating, or the qi mechanism may be unable to orderly reach. In any of these cases, the *chong* and *ren* may be inhibited or the *bao mai* obstructed and thus give rise to various menstrual diseases, such as delayed, scanty, painful, or blocked menstruation.

C. Qi counterflow

If depression and anger damage the liver, coursing may be greatly excessive and this may give rise to liver qi counterflowing upward.[10] Premenstrually, this results in breast distention and pain, headache, and other such symptoms in the upper body.

Disease mechanisms associated with damage to the *chong, ren, du, dai*, & uterus

1. Detriment & damage of the *chong & ren*

A. Former heaven insufficiency

If there is former heaven insufficiency, enduring disease with loss of nourishment, or excessive births or bedroom taxation, the kidney qi may suffer damage and lose command over its treasuring. This may lead to the *chong* and *ren* not securing. Also, if kidney qi is not exuberant, this may lead to the *chong* and *ren* being insufficient.

B. Latter heaven insufficiency

If there is latter heaven insufficiency due to worry and anxiety, fatigue and taxation beyond limit, or undisciplined food and drink, the spleen may suffer damage and restraining and

---

[10] Within the Chinese literature, there seems to be some disagreement over the effect of anger on the liver. Some Chinese sources say that anger leads to liver depression. If liver depression endures and qi stagnation accumulates, eventually that qi stagnation and accumulation must vent itself or counterflow. Qin Bo-wei, on the other hand, says that anger causes excessive liver coursing and this excessive coursing then results in liver qi counterflowing upward. Qin Bo-wei gives different medicinals for these two different disease mechanisms. However, most Chinese practitioners do not make this distinction clinically.

containing may not exercise their proper authority. This may lead to the *chong* and *ren* losing their securing or engenderment and transformation losing their normalcy. If the source of transformation becomes vacuous, the *chong* and *ren* will become insufficient.

C. Inhibited emotions

If the emotions are inhibited, liver qi may suffer disease. Treasuring of blood may lose its duty and coursing and discharge may lose their normalcy. This may lead to the *chong* and *ren* becoming unregulated. Liver qi counterflow upward leads to the *chong* qi also following and counterflowing upward.

D. Qi & blood insufficiency

If qi and blood are insufficient, this may also lead to *chong* and *ren* vacuity and, therefore, to their loss of regulation and securing.

E. Damp heat, damp toxins, heat evils, etc.

If damp heat, damp toxins, or heat evils attack the *chong* and *ren*, this may lead to deeplying heat and smoldering dampness in the *chong* and *ren*. Wind chill evils contracted during menstruation or postpartum may also attack the *chong* and *ren*. This may lead to the accumulation of cold in the *chong* and *ren*. Or external injury, surgery, or parasites and toxins may cause detriment and damage to the *chong* and *ren*.

2. Detriment & damage of the *dai mai*

If the *dai mai* loses its securing, this will result in the onset of abnormal vaginal discharge disease.

3. Detriment & damage of the *du mai*

If the *ren mai* and *du mai*, *i.e.*, yin and yang, lose their regulation, this can lead to vacuity cold with cold congelation menstrual pain, delayed, scanty menstruation, or blocked menstruation.

4. Detriment & damage to the uterus

A. Kidney & central qi and the uterus

If the uterus receives kidney qi and central qi secures it, then its normalcy is maintained. However, if either central qi falls or kidney qi does not secure, this may lead to early and/or profuse menstruation or flooding and leaking.

B. The *chong* & *ren* and the uterus

The *chong* and *ren* pour into the uterus in order to move the menses and govern fetal conception. If the *chong* and *ren* and, therefore, the uterus suffer disease, then the menses will not be able to move normally.

C. Heat, cold & damp evils and the uterus

Cold, heat, and damp evils may all damage the uterus. If heat accumulates in the uterus or damp heat smolders and binds, the *bao luo* suffers damage and this may result in bleeding from the uterus. If damp turbidity flows and spills over, this may become abnormal vaginal discharge. Cold may stagnate in the uterus, the *bao mai* may become obstructed and stagnant, and the qi and blood lose their regulation. In that case, there may be aching and pain in the lower abdomen. If the uterus amasses blood, this may give rise to blood concretions. If blood stasis lasts for many days, this may give rise to stone concretions. And if there is vacuity cold in the uterus, this may lead to uterine cold delayed, painful, or blocked menstruation.

Disease mechanisms associated with various ages in women

The idea that different viscera are primary in terms of the disease mechanisms of gynecological diseases at different ages on a woman's life is an old one in Chinese medicine. Thus there is the saying:

In pubescent women, blame the kidneys,
In middle-aged women, blame the liver,
And in elderly women, blame the spleen.

1. Puberty

During this time, the kidneys begin to be exuberant. If the kidneys are not full, the *chong, ren, du*, and *dai* will be vacuous and deficient. This then may easily lead to menstrual irregularities, blocked menstruation, painful menstruation, or flooding and leaking.

Therefore, during puberty, supplementing the kidneys and nourishing the essence should be given priority.

2. Reproductive years

Because of menstruation, gestation and birthing, and lactation, yin blood is easily damaged. Damage to the blood leads to the liver is loss of nourishment, and this then results in menstrual irregularities, scanty menstruation, and even eventually in blocked menstruation. If the blood is damaged and qi becomes, therefore, surplus, the emotions may easily become excited and thus lead to liver qi depression and stagnation. This may then lead to qi binding, qi counterflow, qi chaos and thus to menstrual irregularities, premenstrual tension, painful menstruation, and premenstrual breast distention and pain. Hence, in young adult and middle-aged women, regulating the liver should be given priority.

3. Old age

Before and after the menses are cut off (at menopause), the kidney qi declines and the *chong* and *ren* are vacuous and exhausted. Therefore, kidney yin and yang may lose their regulation (or balance), and this easily leads to menopausal syndrome and flooding and leaking. In terms of treatment, it is essential that one regulate yin and yang. However, in clinical practice, although one can alleviate the symptoms, it is difficult to support the former heaven kidney qi. But one can rely on the finest essence of water and grain from the latter heaven spleen to enrich and transform the origin. Thus at this stage of life, fortifying the spleen should be given priority.

In actuality, the spleen begins to weaken long before menopause, and it is first spleen vacuity that typically leads to eventual kidney vacuity and menopause. As the *Nei Jing (Inner Classic)* states, the *yang ming, i.e.*, in this case the spleen, begins to weaken at 35 years of age in women. This then results in wrinkles on the face, in turn due to dry skin resulting from an insufficiency of blood. Because of the pervasive ill effects of faulty diet, too much thought and worry, overtaxation, and insufficient exercise, most Western women exhibit definite signs and symptoms of spleen vacuity by their late 30s at least.

The six depressions

In terms of menstrual disease mechanisms, I find that there are three further theories which must be discussed. These are not usually discussed by Chinese TCM gynecology texts since, strictly speaking, they are not gynecological theories. However, these three theories are extremely important when dealing with gynecological problems and are not as well known by Western TCM practitioners as they should be. The first is Zhu Dan-xi's enumeration of the six depressions (depression here being synonymous with stagnation).

Basically there are only four broad categories of disease mechanisms relating to menstrual disorders. These are 1) insufficient blood to allow for a normal arrival and volume of menstruate; 2) blood heat causing the blood to run frenetically outside its pathways; 3) insufficient qi failing to hold the blood within its vessels; and 4) obstruction to the free flow of the menstruate due to stagnation and accumulation. This fourth disease mechanism is a very commonly encountered one in women either as the main pattern of imbalance or as a complicating pattern. Therefore, it is important to know as much about stagnation-depression as possible since it is so often involved in menstrual complaints.

According to Zhu Dan-xi, one of the four great masters of internal medicine of the Jin-Yuan dynasties, there are six depressions. These are depression of:

1. Qi	4. Food
2. Blood	5. Phlegm
3. Dampness	6. Fire

Of these six, the qi is responsible for moving and transforming the blood, dampness, food, and phlegm. These latter four are all accumulations of yin substance. If the qi becomes stagnant and depressed, it may result in any of these four not being moved and transformed properly and thus they may accumulate. *Vice versa*, any of these four yin depressions or accumulations may also impede the free flow of yang qi, thus giving rise to the complication of qi stagnation. To understand stagnant fire, it is best to go on to the second disease mechanism theory discussed below.

Similar transformation

Liu Wan-su, another of the four great masters of internal medicine of the Jin-Yuan, recognized that the host or ruling qi of the organism is yang and, therefore, intrinsically warm. When we are alive, we are warm. When we are dead, we are "stone cold". Thus life is qi and qi is warm. According to Chinese astrology, cosmology, and etiquette, guest qi tends to transform similar to host qi. In other words, in terms of human pathophysiology, any evil qi accumulatng in the body, whether externally invading or internally engendered, will tend to become hot over time because the basic host or ruling qi of the body is hot. Thus, even if a disease is caused by an initial cold evil, there is the tendency for this disease to transform into a hot pathology if the host yang qi is sufficiently strong. This is called similar transformation since the disease tends to transform into a hot disease similar to the yang host or background qi.

Zhu Dan-xi's sixth depression is fire. If qi becomes stagnant and depressed and backs up and accumulates, this accumulation of yang qi may transform into evil heat or fire. In the same way, because all of the four yin or material depressions mentioned above obstruct the free flow of qi, qi tends to become stuck behind or entangled with these material depressions and accumulations. Therefore, these depressions and accumulations also tend to transform into hot depressions. Dampness thus tends to become damp heat. Stagnant food tends to become complicated by heat. Phlegm tends to transform into phlegm heat. And static blood also often becomes heat stasis.

When one understands the interpromoting relationship between the qi and the other five depressions and the tendency for any accumulation of evil qi to become hot, one begins to see why stagnation and heat are such often recurring disease mechanisms in Chinese medicine in general and in TCM gynecology in particular.

Yin fire

Li Dong-yuan was yet another and perhaps the greatest of the four great masters of internal medicine of the Jin-Yuan dynasties. He is primarily remembered as the founder of the school of supplementing earth and the author of the *Pi Wei Lun (Treatise on the Spleen & Stomach)*. However, if practitioners think that Li was only interested in treating diarrhea or indigestion, they are seriously mistaken. In fact, Li began by agreeing with Liu Wan-su that most disease is hot in nature. However, he did not agree that this heat should simply be cleared and cooled with the typically bitter, cold medicinals Liu primarily advocated. Instead, Li called this heat yin fire.

Yin fire (*yin huo*) should not be confused with vacuity heat (*xu re*). Vacuity heat is a type of yin fire, but the concept of yin fire is bigger and more complex than vacuity heat alone. If one looks at what Li has to say about the causes of yin fire in his *Pi Wei Lun (Treatise on the Spleen & Stomach)*, one can identify five basic mechanisms associated with the production of yin fire.

The first of these and what Li considered the root is spleen vacuity. If the spleen becomes vacuous due to faulty diet, excessive thinking and worry, overtaxation, and lack of exercise, then it will lose control over the movement and transformation of fluids. Fluids will hence gather and transform into evil dampness. This dampness will pour downward, becoming damp heat in the lower burner. Although this damp heat may be located in the lower burner, the heat also wafts up, further disturbing and damaging the spleen and harassing the heart and lungs above.

Secondly, if the spleen becomes damaged and vacuous, it will fail to hold the liver in check. According to the *Nei Jing (Inner Classic)*, when the liver becomes diseased, the spleen is the first viscus to subsequently become damaged because of the liver and spleen's relationship via the five phase control cycle. It is said that when the liver becomes diseased, one should first treat the spleen. Therefore, if the spleen becomes vacuous, this may cause or aggravate liver depression. (We have seen above that if the spleen becomes vacuous the blood may also become vacuous and such blood vacuity may fail to emolliate and harmonize the liver.) If the liver becomes depressed, this depression may transform into heat because of Liu's theory of similar transformation. Hence spleen vacuity is intimately connected with liver depression-depressive heat. Since liver yang partakes in the larger concept of life gate fire, depressive heat originating in the liver not only harasses the spleen, stomach, lungs, and heart above, it also causes stirring of ministerial fire below.

As mentioned above, if the spleen becomes vacuous and weak, it may lose control over its engenderment and transformation of blood. In that case, blood vacuity may eventually affect kidney yin since the blood and essence share a common source and the liver and kidneys share a common source. Therefore, a liver blood-kidney yin vacuity may engender vacuity heat. This is a yin fire because its source is in the lower burner or yin part of the body. Such vacuity heat also counterflows upward, disturbing and harassing the liver, spleen, stomach, lungs, and heart.

Further, sexual desire, overactivity, or overstimulation (all referred to as types of stirring in Chinese) may stir and inflame ministerial fire which then harasses and damages the self-same viscera and bowels above it. Thus there are five mechanisms giving rise to yin fire posited by Li Dong-yuan: 1) spleen vacuity, 2) damp heat , 3) liver depression, 4) blood (yin vacuity), and 5) stirring of ministerial fire, with spleen vacuity being the central and primary cause. The name, yin fire, therefore is an allusion to heat stemming from the *tai yin* spleen, heat associated with yin dampness, heat coming from the yin or lower part of the body, and heat which is pathological or yin as opposed to healthy heat or yang. However, in real life patients, the creation of yin fire is typically not due to only one or another of these mechanisms. Rather, it commonly is due to a combination of two, three, four or even all five of these mechanisms all mutually engendering and mutually promoting each other.

For instance, damp heat in the large intestine damages the source of engenderment of the kidneys (*i.e.*, the large intestine), and leads to liver-kidney dual vacuity. Stirring and upward flaring of ministerial fire leaves the lower source vacuous and cold and damages the spleen. Since spleen and kidney yang are mutually promoting, this gives rise to a hot above but cold below pattern with dual spleen-kidney vacuity.

Li's theory of yin fire is extremely important in clinical practice because it allows practitioners to see and to treat complex, multifaceted patterns as a coherent whole. It is a statistical fact that the main generation of Western patients making use of Chinese medicine is the so-called Baby Boom generation. This generation is aging and most members of this generation are already over 35 years of age. This generation has been brought up on a diet loaded with sugars and sweets, fats and oils, raw, chilled foods, and other overly nutritious and, therefore, slimy, spleen-damaging foods. This generation has indulged in sex, drugs, and rock 'n roll. This generation has had to work harder and longer than their parent's generation to pay for a lifestyle which is not as relaxed as their parents. And this generation has also had their spleen's damaged by overuse of antibiotics. In my experience treating Western women, whose complaints tend to be enduring or chronic, it is this theory which makes sense of the mixture of patterns my patients present, and it is this theory which allows me to treat my patients effectively for these mixed patterns, typically using supplementing and draining, hot and cold, drying and moistening medicinals in a single formula.

The Prevention of Menstrual Disease

One of my favorite contemporary Chinese gynecology authors is Han Bai-ling. Dr. Han was a professor of gynecology at the Heilongjiang College of Chinese Medicine in Harbin until his retirement some years ago. In his book, *Bai Ling Fu Ke (Bai Ling's Gynecology)*, Dr. Han gives seven pieces of advice for preventing menstrual diseases.

First, Dr. Han suggests avoiding fear, anger, or excessive emotions in general. According to Dr. Han, these may cause perimenstrual hemoptysis and epistaxis, profuse menstruation, and abnormal vaginal discharge. In other words, due to unrestraint of the seven affects, blood and fluids may counterflow or, due to transformative heat, may be forced to move outside their pathways.

Secondly, Dr. Han suggests avoiding excessive fatigue prior to or during menstruation so as to prevent damage to the *chong* and *ren* which may result in excessive bleeding, abnormal vaginal discharge, and uterine prolapse. Here the implication is that fatigue is associated with qi vacuity which then results in the qi's being unable to restrain and contain the blood and fluids within the body.

Third, Han Bai-ling suggests that women not dwell on negative thoughts or their frustrations. These can cause liver depression and qi stagnation which may eventually lead to blood stasis, flooding and leaking, painful menstruation, or blocked menstruation.

Fourth, Dr. Han suggests that women avoid eating chilled and uncooked foods prior to or during their menses and to also take care not to catch any external cold disease. He says that

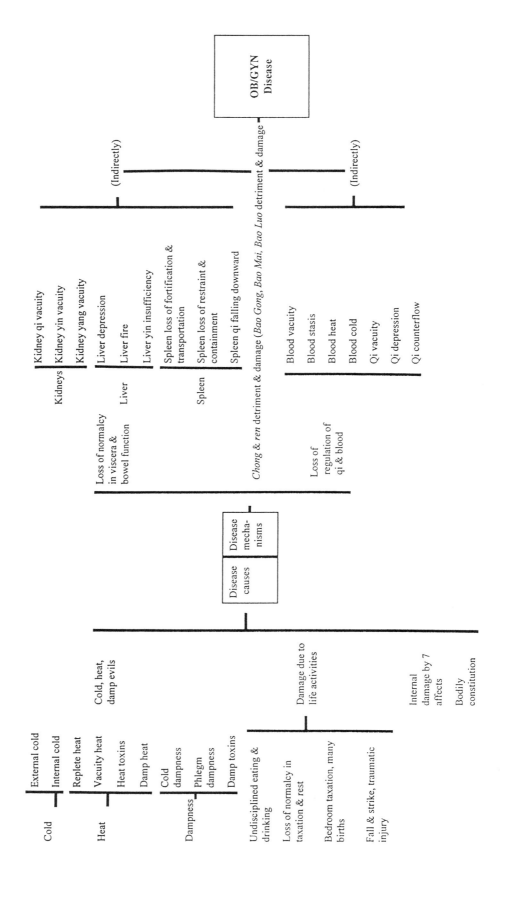

(From *Zhong Yi Fu Ke Xue* [*A Study of Chinese Medical Gynecology*] by Luo Yuan-qi et al., Shanghai Science & Technology Press, Shanghai, 1986)
DISEASE CAUSES & DISEASE MECHANISMS OF OB/GYN DISEASES

OB/GYN Disease

Disease causes

Disease mechanisms

Cold
External cold
Internal cold

Replete heat

Heat
Vacuity heat
Heat toxins
Damp heat

Dampness
Cold dampness
Phlegm dampness
Damp toxins

Cold, heat, damp evils

Undisciplined eating & drinking
Loss of normalcy in taxation & rest
Bedroom taxation, many births
Fall & strike, traumatic injury

Damage due to life activities

Internal damage by 7 affects

Bodily constitution

Loss of normalcy in viscera & bowel function

Kidneys
Kidney qi vacuity
Kidney yin vacuity
Kidney yang vacuity

Liver
Liver depression
Liver fire
Liver yin insufficiency

Spleen
Spleen loss of fortification & transportation
Spleen loss of restraint & containment
Spleen qi falling downward

(Indirectly)

Chong & ren detriment & damage (*Bao Gong, Bao Mai, Bao Luo* detriment & damage)

Loss of regulation of qi & blood
Blood vacuity
Blood stasis
Blood heat
Blood cold
Qi vacuity
Qi depression
Qi counterflow

(Indirectly)

this will prevent the blood from being congealed by cold which will, in turn, cause painful menstruation, blocked menstruation, or congealed lumps in the lower abdomen.

Fifth, Han Bai-ling suggests that women avoid having sex during their menses. According to him, this may damage the *chong* and *ren* and can lead to flooding and leaking, abnormal vaginal discharge, painful menstruation, blocked menstruation, and congealed lumps in the lower abdomen. We have discussed above the TCM disease mechanisms responsible for these stagnations and congelations due to sex during one's menses.

Sixth, Han Bai-ling suggests avoiding strong, vigorous movements or exercise during menstruation so as to prevent the qi and blood from leaving their paths. Such erratic qi flow may result in excessive bleeding, perimenstrual hemoptysis and epistaxis, and flooding and leaking. Similar prohibitions against heavy exercise during menstruation were common in the West up until 50-60 years ago.

Seventh and finally, Dr. Han suggests that women eat and drink moderately, maintain regular waking and sleeping hours, avoid eating stimulating foods, and try to be happy in order to prevent the occurrence of all gynecological problems. This is Chinese medicine's general prescription for avoiding all health problems and is not just applicable to menstrual diseases.

Liu Min-ru, author of *Zhong Yi Fu Ke Xue (A Study of Chinese Medical Gynecology)*, sums up the same basic advice by saying:

> During menstruation, the blood chamber is correctly open. Because of this, evil qi may easily invade. Therefore, it is appropriate to pay attention to taking care [of one's health]. One should maintain suitable cold and warmth, discipline their drinking and eating, regulate their emotions, and get suitable labor and rest.

The authors of *Zhong Yi Fu Chan Ke Xue (A Study of Chinese Medical Gynecology & Obstetrics)* add that during menstruation, "One should take care to insure that their genital region is clear and clean."

3

TCM Methodology

TCM as a Style of Chinese Medicine

TCM is a specific style of Chinese medicine. Its definition is the administration of treatment based on an individualized pattern discrimination.[11] This is called *bian zheng lun zhi* in Chinese. However, like all styles of Chinese medicine, TCM does also use treatment based on disease discrimination diagnosis as well, or *bian bing lun zhi*. Thus TCM diagnosis is, in actuality, dual diagnosis or both *bian bing* and *bian zheng*. As such, TCM is a combination of rational and empirical medicines.

Bian bing & bian zheng

Treatment based on pattern discrimination is individualized treatment addressed at the total constellation of a patient's signs and symptoms as well as their constitution. It is treatment of the whole person and takes into account signs and symptoms beyond those which are pathognomonic of the major complaint. Treatment based on pattern discrimination is, therefore, holistic treatment. It sees and treats the field or ground as well as the specific disease which is the figure within the ground. Once the pattern discrimination is established, the practitioner formulates theoretical treatment principles which logically redress the imbalance implied in the terminology of the pattern identification. For instance, a heat pattern is cooled or cleared, whereas a cold pattern is warmed. A vacuity pattern is supplemented, while a replete pattern is drained. The erection of such a logically deduced treatment plan is a rational process.

---

[11] Wiseman translates *bian zheng* as pattern identification. However, the character for *bian* clearly shows two things being divided. In other words, the word *bian* means to tell one thing from another or to discriminate. In fact, the words *bian* and *fen*, to divide, are often used interchangeably. The word identify in English comes from the Latin *idem*, which means the same. Thus the term pattern identification loses the idea of discriminating one pattern from another inherent in the Chinese *bian zheng*.

Treatment based on disease diagnosis is, on the other hand, empirical medicine. Based on more than 100 generations of past medical practitioners, certain discreet diseases or pathologies have been identified and certain treatments have been found to be empirically more effective than others for the treatment of specific diseases. Treatment aimed at specific diseases or at specific symptoms addresses the figure or major complaint within the total field or ground of the patient's being.

Therefore, when treatment is given based both on pattern discrimination and disease diagnosis, both figure and ground are equally taken into account. One makes equal use of the foregoing generations' recorded clinical experience as well as their own logic and reasoning abilities. Recorded experience tells the practitioner what has actually been proven to work in the past. Whereas a discriminating and individualized pattern appraisal of the unique individual allows for the idiosyncratic modification of empirical formulas to fit the exact exigencies of the case. In addition, the rational approach explains why a patient has become ill and, based on this, the practitioner can make suggestions on how to avoid a relapse or recurrence in the future. Empirical treatment treats, but rational pattern discrimination explains and thus empowers.

In terms of TCM menstrual diseases, disease discrimination is quite simple and does not need any laboratory analysis or diagnostic apparatus. Knowing whether the menses are early or late, profuse or scanty, painful or absent is simply accomplished by questioning the patient. TCM pattern discrimination, on the other hand, is not so easily accomplished. Although it likewise does not require any special apparatus, it does require three uncommon abilities: 1) more than commonly acute sense perception able to catch fine nuances in color, tone, and feeling; 2) a more than common ability to mentally manipulate Chinese technical medical terms and theories; and 3) a more than common ability to reason logically and clearly. It is no wonder that TCM as a style developed out of Confucian scholars' practice of medicine as an expression of filial piety nor that, prior to so-called Liberation in 1949, probably only a minority of all Chinese doctors practiced such a rational, *bian zheng lun zhi* style.

The 10 types of TCM pattern discrimination

In TCM as a particular style of Chinese medicine, there are 10 different ways or systems of pattern discrimination. These are:

1. Five phase pattern discrimination
2. Eight principles pattern discrimination
3. Viscera & bowel pattern discrimination
4. Qi & blood pattern discrimination
5. Fluids & humors pattern discrimination
6. Channel & network vessels pattern discrimination
7. Disease cause pattern discrimination
8. Six divisions pattern discrimination

 9. Four divisions pattern discrimination
10. Three burners pattern discrimination

Although one can identify the above 10 types of pattern discrimination within TCM, in actual clinical practice, most patient's patterns are a combination of more than a single type of pattern. For instance, if one says liver blood vacuity, one is using three types of pattern discrimination together. First, by saying liver and not heart, spleen, lungs, or large intestine, one has used viscera and bowel pattern discrimination. Secondly, by saying blood and not qi, one has used qi and blood pattern discrimination. And third, by saying vacuity, one has used eight principles pattern discrimination. If one says that their patient is suffering from a wind cold exterior pattern with lung loss of diffusion and downbearing, one is also using three types of pattern discrimination combined together. By saying wind cold, one is using disease cause pattern discrimination. By saying that the pattern is an exterior one, one is using eight principle pattern discrimination. And by saying the lungs, one is using viscera and bowel discrimination.

In TCM as a style, no one of these methods of pattern discrimination is considered superior or more correct than any other. All are accorded equal status and correctness. The issue is to use those methods of pattern discrimination which most closely and completely describe the totality of the patient's signs and symptoms. In theory, six division and four division pattern discrimination seem mutually exclusive since they both cover much of the same signs and symptoms. However, in TCM, these two methods of pattern discrimination are not seen as contradictory but as complementary. In some cases, four division pattern discrimination renders a better match between the patient's signs and symptoms and the pattern, while in other cases, six division pattern discrimination offers a closer fit. Therefore, to call, as some Westerners do, TCM "eight principle Chinese medicine" as opposed to "five element Chinese medicine" is a misnomer. If we were to put another name on TCM as a style, it can be nothing other than "treatment based on pattern discrimination Chinese medicine."

The difference between textbooks & clinical practice

Textbooks such as this typically present a number of patterns under each disease category. Each pattern is defined by a series of signs and symptoms, including and especially tongue and pulse signs, which differentiate it from the other patterns which may also account for or be associated with the disease at hand. TCM neophytes often naively assume that their job is to compare their patient's signs and symptoms with those of the discreet patterns listed. Whichever listing of signs and symptoms most closely matches their patient's thus becomes their pattern discrimination. Although this is true on paper, in clinical practice, it is more often the case that one's real-life patient displays a combination of signs and symptoms of more than a single textbook pattern. Such textbook patterns are presented for maximum resolution and contrast and are circumscribed by the limitations of the linear nature of the print medium. Therefore, although TCM textbooks make it seem that all one has to do is pigeonhole their patient in the right pattern and then use the textbook indicated formula or treatment, that is seldom the case.

Rather, one more typically must analyze their patient's signs and symptoms and parse out a complex diagnosis made up of more than a single pattern. Because this is the case more often than not, it becomes all the more important that the practitioner be sure to take the intermediary step of formulating the theoretically requisite therapeutic principles necessary to redress the imbalance at hand. If one knows that their patient exhibits both liver depression qi stagnation *and* transformative heat of the liver and stomach and then states for themselves that, in order to correct this imbalance, one must course the liver and rectify the qi, resolve depression and clear both the liver and stomach, one can then analyze the ingredients in various formulas to see which comes closest to accomplishing all of these therapeutic principles.

The importance of treatment principles

In Chinese TCM texts, it is said that the treatment principles are the link between the pattern discrimination and the guiding formula. If one describes a patient's pattern as liver depression qi stagnation with an element of spleen vacuity tinged with dampness and blood vacuity, then the correct TCM treatment principles for remedying this imbalance are to course the liver and rectify the qi, fortify the spleen and nourish the blood while also eliminating dampness. As stated, these principles both lead to and require one to choose a guiding formula from the harmonizing category of formulas. To choose a formula from any other category would be categorically incorrect. The harmonizing category of formulas contain formulas for harmonizing the constructuve and defensive. However, it also contains formulas for harmonizing the liver and spleen. By saying that the liver needs to be coursed while the spleen needs to be rectified, this implies a disharmony between the liver and spleen which needs to be harmonized. Then, within this category of formulas, one must find a formula which also nourishes the blood and eliminates dampness. In this case, one is led by the above treatment principles to *Xiao Yao San* (Rambling Powder) as one's guiding formula. The last step in this process is to make sure that the formula chosen is empirically known to treat the disease and the signs and symptoms that one's patient does suffer from. Once all of these elements are a match, then this is the correct treatment according to TCM methodology.

Thus the treatment principles funnel one to the correct treatment plan. They lead one to the correct chapter in one's *fang ji xue* or formulas and prescriptions book. Then, within that chapter, they lead one to the correct formula. Further, the secondary treatment principles lead one to the correct chapter of their *ben cao xue* or materia medica in order to choose the best modifying medicinals.

This is a very rational and precise methodology which makes it easy to go from the patient's signs and symptoms to a pattern discrimination and from the pattern discrimination to the erection of an individually tailored treatment plan. In order to get the benefits of this precise, step-by-step methodology insuring the correct choice of treatment methods and formulas, one must follow the following steps without deviation:

1. One must collect all necessary signs and symptoms, tongue and pulse signs.
2. One must analyse these signs and symptoms according to the statements of fact of Chinese medicine.
3. One must state a disease diagnosis (whether that be a modern Western or traditional Chinese disease diagnosis).
4. One must state a pattern discrimination.
5. One must state the relevant treatment principles to match the pattern discrimination.
6. One must then erect a treatment plan that embodies all of the stated treatment principles, neither more nor less.

Typically, Chinese treatment principles are stated in pairs. These are actually combinations of four words in Chinese. For instance: supplement the spleen and boost the qi, nourish the liver and enrich the kidneys, clear heat and resolve toxins, clear heat and eliminate dampness, transform phlegm and scatter nodulation. In clinical practice, the first pair of principles stated are considered the main ones governing the choice of formulas or protocols. For example, if one says clear heat and resolve toxins, quicken the blood and transform stasis, then one must choose a guiding formula from the heat-clearing, toxin-resolving chapter. Secondarily, one must then insure that the formula already does contain medicinals for quickening the blood and transforming stasis or one must add some. Conversely, if one first says quicken the blood and transform stasis, clear heat and resolve toxins, one must pick a formula from the blood-quickening category of formulas and then secondarily modify it with the addition of heat-clearing, toxin-resolving medicinals. Thus the order in which one states one's treatment principles determines under which category of formulas one is going to find their guiding prescription.

Guiding formulas & their modification

Commonly, no textbook formula may address completely and exactly all and only those treatment principles written in the patient's chart. A formula may fulfill most of the required therapeutic functions and may also address others that are not indicated. Therefore, one picks a *guiding* formula which comes as close as possible to matching the treatment principles and then modifies it to fit the patient's exact, individualized pattern and their signs and symptoms. One may delete those ingredients which are unnecessary to the case at hand and add others necessary to comprehensively and completely address the patient's entire and unique condition. Although one may start with a standard formula, one ends with a unique modification of it. If only additional ingredients are added to a formula, the words *jia wei* or added flavors are all that is appended to the formula's standard name. If, however, some ingredients are added and others deleted, then the words *jia jian* are added which mean additions (and) subtractions. This is an extremely important point, since in TCM clinical practice, the overwhelming majority of formulas are prescribed either *jia wei* or *jia jian*. Qin Bo-wei, a famous mid-century TCM practitioner and theoretician, wrote that, when saying to use *Liu Wei Di Huang Wan* (Six Flavor Rehmannia Pills), he did not mean that one should actually use the exact ingredients of that formula but rather the *idea* of *Liu Wei Di Huang Wan*.

Root & branch

Further, when writing a TCM prescription, one must take into account both the root and the branch. The root is either the underlying, fundamental, root imbalance or a chronic disease or condition. The branch is either the branch signs and symptoms or an acute disease. Theoretically, in chronic conditions, one emphasizes the treatment of the root imbalance over branch symptoms and, in acute situations, one emphasizes the branch symptoms over the root imbalance. However, in actual TCM clinical practice, most practitioners address both root and branch simultaneously. This is essentially the same as addressing both the pattern and the disease at the same time.

There are, however, certain outflows of pure substance which are considered branches requiring priority treatment in TCM. These are excessive sweating, diarrhea, seminal emission, vomiting, polyuria, and bleeding. Since all of these are a loss of both pure substance and qi, if left unchecked, they will result in the patient's constitution becoming vacuous and weak. In addition, any pain is considered a branch which requires definite and specific treatment. This is because pain affects the spirit and the health of the spirit directly affects the course and outcome of the disease.

That being said, it is important to understand that the body is not like an onion from the TCM point of view. When treating an acute infectious disease, we distinguish and treat individual divisions such as the *yang ming* or *shao yang*, the qi or the constructive. In chronic diseases, with multifaceted patterns, it is my experience that one must treat the entire pattern as a single *gestalt*. This is because yin and yang, viscera and bowels, and qi and blood all function synergistically and interdependently. Some practitioners think that treatment should proceed like peeling away the layers of an onion, first treating the spleen and then treating the kidneys when spleen and kidney vacuity exist simultaneously, or first treating the liver and then the spleen when there is simultaneous liver depression and spleen dampness. In my experience, when one takes such an approach, one may see some improvement in the patient's signs and symptoms for a few days or a couple of weeks, but then the whole constellation of symptoms return again full force. In such situations, some practitioners then separate some other viscus or so-called layer of the pattern and try treating for that. Again, some or all of the symptoms may improve or disappear, only to return again after a short while. Again the treatment strategy may be switched to some other viscus or bowel, and again the same thing may happen. In such cases, it is my experience that one must see the various aspects of such a complex pattern as a whole and treat them as a whole all at the same time. This is where Li Dong-yuan's theory on yin fire helps make the seeing and treating of such complex, multifaceted patterns easier.

Making this methodology work in clinical practice

The actual doing of TCM cannot be taught by a textbook such as this. Such textbooks only supply the armature or framework which must be fleshed out by case histories and clinical experience. In order to make TCM style gynecology work, one must have mastered a number of other disciplines within TCM. These include basic TCM physiology and pathophysiology, pattern discrimination, the materia medica, the processing of individual ingredients in order to achieve specific effects, and the composing of prescriptions. All of these are beyond the scope of a book such as this. Only those with such prior training and knowledge are suggested to attempt to put the information contained in this book into use, since, in clinical practice, the information contained herein is not employed simply and exactly as it appears.

4

The Logic Inherent in the TCM Discussion of *Yue Jing Bing*

If one compares the list of diseases in this and similar Chinese TCM gynecology books with the table of contents of the gynecology section of *The Merck Manual*[12], one will notice a striking difference. The disease categories of TCM gynecology are not the disease categories of modern Western gynecology. At first glance, it looks as if the Chinese have left out altogether many diseases. However, if one thinks thus, one has not penetrated the logic of the Chinese categorization and discussion of menstrual diseases.

As described herein, the TCM discussion of menstrual diseases does cover, in a logically complete and inclusive way, everything that can go wrong with menstruation. Since the foundation of Chinese medicine is yin and yang, the Chinese categorization of menstrual diseases is arranged as yin-yang pairs.

First we have early and late menstruation. The Chinese is *yue jing xian qi* or menstruation ahead of schedule and *yue jing hou qi* or menstruation behind schedule. Next comes the category *yue jing xian hou wu ding qi*. Literally, this means (sometimes) early, (sometimes) late, no fixed schedule menstruation. It describes a menstrual cycle which is sometimes early, sometimes late, and which has lost its regular periodicity altogether. If early and late form a yin-yang pair, (sometimes) early, (sometimes) late, no fixed schedule menstruation seems, at first glance, to stand alone or to form a tripartite group with early and late menstruation. However, the horn of this dilemma is implied and left unspoken. The logical opposite to an erratically scheduled period is a regularly scheduled one. Since this book is about menstrual diseases and a regular menstrual cycle is not pathological, it is not mentioned. However, when one takes into account that the menses can be either early, late, erratic, or regular in schedule, one sees that all of the logical possibilities concerning the periodicity of the menstruation have been covered by this scheme.

---

[12] *The Merck Manual* is the most commonly used diagnostic and treatment reference of Western MDs in the United States.

Next come the categories of *yue jing guo duo* and *yue jing guo shao*. *Yue jing guo duo* means menstruation which is excessively profuse. *Yue jing guo shao* means menstruation which is excessively scanty. These are also the two logical possibilities of the volume of the period being anything other than normal. If the menses are sometimes profuse and sometimes scanty, this is ultimately not different than the alternation between these two disease categories and is not usually seen in TCM gynecology as a third or separate disease category.

Then comes *tong jing* and a group of complaints all prefaced by the words *jing xing*. *Tong jing* means painful menstruation. As mentioned in a preceding chapter, in Chinese medicine there is the basic dictum that if there is free flow there is no pain, while if there is pain there is no free flow. Since the word for pain (*tong*) is the same both in painful menstruation and in pain in the above saying, *tong jing* implies a lack of free flow of the menstruate. This is then logically juxtaposed to those complaints which are due to inappropriate flow. These include *jing xing tu nu* (menstrual movement epistaxis & hemoptysis), *jing xing fa re* (menstrual movement fever), *jing xing xie xie* (menstrual movement diarrhea), *jing xing shen tong* (menstrual movement body pain), *jing xing fu zhong* (menstrual movement abdominal distention), *jing xing fu tong* (menstrual movement abdominal pain), *jing xing tou tong* (menstrual movement headache), *jing xing ru fang zhang tong* (menstrual movement breast swelling & pain), *jing xing nao xue* (menstrual movement hematuria), and *jing xing da bian xue* (menstrual movement hemafecia).

In the above disease category names, the words *jing xing* appear over and over again. *Jing* means the menstrual flow. *Xing* means to move or go. Its original writing showed a crossroads. To modern Chinese, this word only means to go, move, or walk. But looking at the ancient character, we see that it implied a juncture at which movement could go in a different or new and possibly even wrong direction. In the case of the above disease categories, each is an instance where the menstruate is supposed to flow down to and out of the uterus. However, either the entire or some part of the flow has taken a wrong turn, thus flowing to some unwarranted part of the body. If it flows up to the head, it may manifest as headache, bloody nose, or spitting blood. If it flows downward to the intestines, it may manifest as diarrhea or hemafecia. If it flows into the body, it may manifest as edema, fever, or aches and pains. In the preceding category of painful menstruation, the flow, *jing*, is *tong*, painful. This implies that, for some reason, the menses are not flowing freely. In the case of all the menstrual movement diseases, the flow is *xing*, moving, but moving in an inappropriate direction or counterflowing (*ni*). Thus this yin-yang dichotomy has to do with free and normal flow.

Then comes blocked menstruation and flooding and leaking. In Chinese, blocked menstruation is *jing bi* or sometimes *bi jing*. This *jing* once again means flow and this *bi* means obstructed or shut. The Chinese character shows a door which has been shut. This is then logically juxtaposed with flooding and leaking. *Beng* means avalanche or flood. *Lou* means trickle or leak. Together, flooding and leaking as a compound term means pathological bleeding like either an avalanche or a leak. In the case of *jing bi*, the picture implied is one of a shut door. In the case of *beng lou*, the picture is of a dam which either gives way or has, in any case, sprung a leak.

If one translates these Chinese disease categories as, for instance, menorrhagia and hypomenorrhea, or dysmenorrhea and vicarious menstruation, or amenorrhea and uterine bleeding, the symmetry and yin-yang logic of the Chinese scheme is obscured and the listing of menstrual diseases merely seems quaint and unscientific. However, once one sees the internal logic inherent in this presentation, one sees that it is anything but unsophisticated. Rather, it comprehensively and with great logic covers all the things that could go wrong with menstruation: its periodicity, its volume, and its free or erratic flow. Abnormal colors or clots within the menstruate are not considered disease categories within their own right, but are rather signs which help discriminate the various patterns of the foregoing menstrual diseases. (Nevertheless, I have added a discussion of various abnormal colors and consistencies and their treatment in Appendix 1.) In the 16 years I have been a TCM gynecology specialist, I have never come across a menstrual disorder which could not be categorized as one or a combination of these menstrual disease categories.

Because of the influence of modern Western medicine, the purity of this logical presentation has been tampered with a bit in order to conform to what is perceived as a more scientific and up-to-date standard. Some modern Chinese TCM gynecology texts, such as Song and Yu's *Zhong Yi Fu Ke Shou Ce (A Handbook of Chinese Medical Gynecology)*, simply include *jing xing ru fang zhang tong* or menstrual movement distention and pain in the breasts as a catch-all category for premenstrual syndrome. Others abandon such traditional terminology altogether and introduce the category *yue jing qian qi zhu zheng*. This translates literally as various complaints before the menstruation or PMS. Likewise, there is now the category of *jing duan qian hou zhu zheng*. This literally means various complaints before or after the cutting off of the menstruation or perimenopausal syndrome. Personally, I find the older, more traditional terminology and order of presentation of menstrual diseases logically preferable and, in fact, more comprehensively inclusive once one understands how to apply this logic to modern Western patients.

5

Western Disease Diagnosis & TCM Menstrual Diseases

As stated above, the TCM scheme for the categorization of menstrual complaints is a complete and comprehensive one. However, in the West, patients typically enter the office with an already established Western medical diagnosis. This may be endometriosis, an ovarian cyst, PID, or some other such named Western disease category. As a teacher and lecturer on TCM, one of the most frequent and persistent questions I am asked is how does TCM treat this Western disease or that. The answer to that question is deceptively simple. One does both a Chinese disease diagnosis and a pattern discrimination and treats the patient accordingly.

If a patient has dyspareunia or poking pain with intercourse, painful menstruation with large, dark clots, a dark tongue, and a deep, wiry pulse in the cubit position, this patient is categorized as suffering from painful menstruation due to blood stasis regardless of their Western disease diagnosis which very probably is endometriosis.

Similarly, if a patient comes with a diagnosis of chronic pelvic inflammatory disease (PID) after having gone through one or more courses of antibiotic therapy and their major complaint is a dragging pain in their uterus which gets worse after menstruation, their TCM diagnosis is again painful menstruation, but this time due to central qi fall regardless of *and* in addition to their Western medical diagnosis of PID.

In other words, there is no tit for tat identity between either traditional Chinese and modern Western disease categories or modern Western disease categories and TCM patterns. Although modern Chinese and Western authors are, more and more, replacing the traditional Chinese disease categories with modern Western ones and then giving the TCM differential pattern discrimination under these Western disease categories, this unfortunately obscures the logic behind the traditional Chinese disease categorization which does offer a certain symmetry, simplicity, and comprehensiveness.

In Chinese there is the saying:

Tong bing yi zhi,	Different diseases, one treatment;
Yi bing tong zhi.	One disease, different treatments.

This saying clearly underscores the fact that, in the TCM style of Chinese medicine, treatment is primarily based on pattern discrimination as opposed to disease categorization. Two patients may both suffer from the same named disease, whether Chinese or Western, and receive two different treatments because their pattern discrimination is different. Likewise, two patients may suffer from different named diseases and yet receive the same treatment because their TCM pattern discrimination is the same. Therefore, when doing TCM, the most important thing is the pattern discrimination and treatment predicated upon that pattern discrimination. Because of this, practitioners need not run thither and yon trying to find out how to treat this or that named Western disease. Rather, using the four methods of examination and the logic of TCM pattern discrimination, they should parse out their patient's TCM pattern of disharmony and base their treatment on the treatment principles TCM posits as the remedy for that pattern or combination of patterns.

Many Western practitioners are attracted to Chinese medicine because, in general, Chinese medicine is perceived as being safe and non-iatrogenic. What makes TCM safe and without side effects is treatment based on pattern discrimination. It is the TCM practitioner's ability to decide what combination of medicinals a specific patient with a specific disease and specific pattern should receive which makes this style of medicine both safe and effective. How the TCM practitioner decides what individualized combinations a particular patient should receive is based on that patient's individualized pattern of disharmony. There is nothing inherently safe about the Chinese medicinals themselves. Many of them are just as toxic and fraught with the potential for side effects as Western medicinals. Therefore, it is of utmost importance that, no matter what the Western medical diagnosis, TCM treatment be based on a TCM pattern discrimination.

6

Key Points in the TCM Diagnosis of Menstrual Disease

The TCM diagnosis of menstrual disease is based on none other than the four examinations. These are inspection, listening and smelling, inquiry, and palpation. Because TCM pattern discrimination is based on the concept of seeing the entire body or organism as a whole (*zheng ti guan nian*), the diagnosis of menstrual diseases is not radically different from the TCM diagnosis generally employed in *nei ke* or internal medicine. However, due to the distinctive characteristics of female physiology and pathophysiology regarding menstruation, there are certain particular signs and symptoms under each of the four diagnoses of which the practitioner should be aware.

Inspection

1. Form & color

In both discussions of the four examinations and their clinical application, inspection comes first. The first thing the practitioner inspects is the patient's bodily form and the second is their facial color or complexion. Typically, if the body is fat, this is mostly due to spleen-kidney yang vacuity with phlegm dampness internally stagnant. If the body is thin and the facial color is flushed red, this is mostly due to yin vacuity with fire effulgence. If the face is a lusterless, somber white, this is mostly due to qi and blood vacuity weakness. If the facial color is greenish bluish white, this mostly pertains to yang vacuity internal cold. If the face is greenish bluish purple, this mostly pertains to liver channel qi stagnation and blood stasis. If the face is red, this mostly pertains to heart fire internally blazing and blood division replete heat. If there is blood vacuity, mostly one sees a sallow yellow facial complexion. If there is qi vacuity, this mostly manifests in an ashen or somber white facial color or superficial edema. If there is blood stasis, there is mostly a greenish bluish, dark facial color. If this is recent in development, the facial color may only be slightly greenish blue. If the eyelids above and below are enclosed by sooty, dark circles, such patients have liver qi depression and binding with qi and blood stagnation and stasis. If both cheeks are flushed red, this is due to yin vacuity fire effulgence or yin vacuity with internal heat manifesting on the outside. A facial color which is greyish black with red cheeks is due to kidney yin insufficiency with vacuity fire flaring upward and manifesting on the exterior. In kidney qi decline and weakness, the facial color is mostly dark, dull, and lusterless. After pregnancy or with age, the face may exhibit yellow, brown or dark macules, often called age or liver spots. Locally, these are due to blood stasis in the grandchild network vessels. This stasis may be due to qi and blood vacuity, qi stagnation and blood stasis, or several other causes.

2. Tongue & lip color

A. Lips

Deep or crimson red lips indicate blood heat. Fresh or bright red lips suggest yin vacuity and effulgent fire. Pale lips indicate spleen vacuity and blood vacuity. Whereas, bluish green and pale lips suggest yang vacuity and cold. Cyanotic lips indicate cold congelation and blood stasis.

B. Tongue body

A bright or dark red tongue suggests blood heat which often presents as early or profuse menstruation and flooding and leaking. A light red tongue or slightly red tongue suggests yin and blood vacuity which typically manifests as delayed and/or scanty menstruation, blocked menstruation, or enduring but scanty blood leakage. This can also manifest as alternating flooding and leaking. There may also be a pale tongue with red tip which often indicates qi and blood dual vacuity with heart fire effulgence resulting in early menstruation and flooding and leaking.

A pale tongue suggests qi and blood vacuity. This may manifest menstrually as either scanty or blocked menstruation or prolonged uterine bleeding. A swollen, pale tongue suggests even more serious qi and blood vacuity with the same sort of menstrual manifestations.

A dry, purple tongue suggests consumption and exhaustion of fluids by blood heat. This typically manifests as early menstruation with a scanty flow. A dark, purple tongue or a tongue with purple, static macules suggests blood stasis. This most often manifests as painful menstruation, delayed menstruation, blocked menstruation, and flooding and leaking. A light purple, glossy tongue suggests vacuity cold and usually manifests menstrually as delayed menstruation or even as concretions and conglomerations.

If the sides of the tongue are swollen, this suggests liver depression with depressive heat. Since heat may make the blood move frenetically outside its pathways, such a tongue shape may indicate early or profuse menstruation or flooding and leaking. However, since liver depression is associated with non-free flow of the qi, there may be depressive heat without profuse bleeding. If the tongue surface is cracked all over, this may indicate yin vacuity, especially if the tongue color is bright red. However, it can also mean enduring spleen vacuity. If the tongue has a centerline crack running longitudinally off of which there are horizontal cracks, this definitely means serious spleen vacuity. Likewise, if there are horizontal cracks on the sides of the tongue, this also means serious spleen vacuity. Spleen vacuity often manifests as early or profuse menstruation or flooding and leaking. If the tongue is swollen and fat with the indentations of the teeth along its edges, this indicates spleen qi vacuity with accumulation of dampness. If the tongue is pale, then this suggests concomitant blood vacuity. If it is red, this suggests spleen vacuity and damp heat.

C. Tongue fur

When assessing the tongue fur diagnostically, one discriminates between thick and thin and moist and dry in combination with its color.

Thin fur suggests a light disease which has yet to affect the stomach qi. Thick fur, on the other hand, indicates a more serious disease and/or an enduring disease which has affected stomach and intestinal function and which typically is associated with the generation or accumulation of yin evils, such as damp heat, parasites, stagnant food, or phlegm dampness.

Dry tongue fur indicates damage of the fluids and humors, while moist or wet tongue fur often indicates, in terms of menstrual diseases, cold stagnation. Thin, white, dry fur means that disease has led to damage of the fluids. Thick, white, dry fur suggests that damp depression has transformed into heat, thus damaging fluids and humors. Pale, white, moist fur usually means internal cold and dampness.

Yellow fur mainly means heat. Thin, slightly yellow fur suggests a disease of recent origin. Thick, yellow fur, on the other hand, means internal heat stagnating and accumulating. Thick, yellow, slimy fur indicates damp heat obstruction and accumulation. If tongue fur is thick and brownish yellow or yellowish brown, this means that heat, typically damp heat, has scorched fluids.

Black, moist, glossy tongue fur means yang vacuity and cold. Whereas, black, dry fur means depressed fire and consumption of fluids and humors. This is an evolution from the yellowish brown tongue fur described above.

3. Color, consistency & volume of the menstruate

A bright red menstruate suggests blood heat and often causes early or profuse menstruation or flooding and leaking. If the blood is excessive in amount, the heat is replete. If the blood is scanty in amount, the heat is vacuous. If the blood begins dark red and becomes bright red or is bright red mixed with some darkish clots, this suggests depressive heat or stasis heat.

A pale red, thin, or watery menstruate suggests qi and blood dual vacuity. If it is copious, this further suggests that qi is more vacuous than blood. If it is not copious, this suggests that blood is more vacuous than qi. In the former case, this typically manifests menstrually as early and/or profuse menstruation or flooding and leaking. In the latter case, this typically manifests as delayed and scanty menstruation possibly evolving into blocked menstraution.

A dark colored menstruate always suggests stagnation and stasis. If the flow is thick and viscous and contains only some clots, this suggests mostly qi stagnation. If there are larger and more clots, this suggests relatively more serious blood stasis.

A dark or dull, thin, dilute menstrual discharge suggests vacuity cold which often manifests as delayed menstruation. A scanty, dull, dark flow with congealed lumps suggests replete cold which often manifests as painful and/or delayed menstruation which may evolve into blocked menstruation.

If the menstruate contains white, mucousy matter, this suggests accumulation of phlegm dampness which is often associated with delayed menstruation, profuse menstruation, and flooding and leaking. If the flow contains yellow matter mixed with red, is thick and viscous, and excessive in volume, this suggests damp heat. This may manifest as early menstruation. If there are clots mixed in as well, this suggests damp heat mutually entangled with and causing stasis and stagnation of the qi and blood. This may manifest as painful menstruation. If heat predominates, it may also manifest as flooding and leaking.

Neophytes should try to keep in mind the simple, yin-yang discriminations from Guo Yuan's *Shi Yong Zhong Xi Yi Jie He Fu Chan Ke Zheng Zhi (Proven Treatments in Practical Integrated Chinese-Western Obstetrics & Gynecology)* given below:

> If the menses are excessive, colored deep red, and lumpy, this is mostly categorized as blood heat.
>
> If their amount is excessive but pale in color and thin and watery, this is mostly categorized as qi emptiness.
>
> If their amount is scanty, dark, and lumpy, this is mostly categorized as blood stasis.

If their amount is scanty but pale in color and clear and watery, this is mostly categorized as spleen vacuity and scanty blood.

Listening & smelling

1. Listening

Speaking feebly or disinclination to speak due to not having enough energy suggests qi vacuity. In terms of menstrual disease, this may manifest as early and/or profuse menstruation or flooding and leaking. Sighing on the other hand, indicates stagnation of qi. It is frequently encountered in cases of liver depression qi stagnation. This may manifest as any of a number of menstrual diseases including early or delayed menstruation, painful menstruation, profuse menstruation, blocked menstruation, various premenstrual complaints, flooding and leaking, and various perimenopausal complaints.

2. Smelling

A menstruate with a foul odor suggests heat. Whereas an insipid odor suggests cold. A fishy odor is mostly associated with cold dampness. If there is a putrid, rotten odor which is difficult to stand the smell of suggests damp heat and accumulated toxins.

Inquiry

1. Age

The patient's age should be ascertained on the first visit. Because Chinese medical theory posits certain physiological changes at certain ages, it is important to factor these into the patient's diagnosis. Some diseases and patterns are more commonly encountered in younger women, such as painful menstruation delayed menstruation, and blocked menstruation. Other diseases are more commonly encountered in middle-aged women, such as various premenstrual complaints and early menstruation. Yet other diseases are more characteristic of older women, such as perimenopausal complaints and flooding and leaking. It is also true that a single disease in young women in their late 20s and early 30s, such as premenstrual breast distention, may have one disease mechanism (*i.e.*, liver qi) and that same disease in women in their late 30s and 40s may have another disease mechanism (loss of balance between the *chong* and *ren*). Failure to make this discrimination based on age may lead to unsatisfactory therapy or a tendency to relapse as soon as therapy is suspended. In addition, premature menarche in adolescents and premature menopause in women in their late 30s and early 40s must be assessed in terms of the patient's chronological age.

2. Major complaint

The patients major complaint should be ascertained. If this is stated by the patient in terms of a Western disease diagnosis, the TCM practitioner must continue questioning the patient until they ascertain the Chinese disease diagnosis, such as early or late menstruation, painful menstruation, etc. The practitioner should remember that a single Western disease may be covered by more than one Chinese menstrual disease. Often patients will be suffering from more than a single Chinese menstrual disease category.

The practitioner should ask questions and write down in the patient's chart the patient's answers regarding their major complaint's current signs and symptoms as well as its history of onset, duration, any change in signs and symptoms, and any previous treatment and the patient's response to that treatment. The practitioner should then analyze these responses in terms of the various catalogued disease mechanisms TCM posits for each of the patient's menstrual diseases. The practitioner must take care to avoid ascribing a single meaning or indication to any single sign or symptom. The actual meaning of any given sign or symptom only becomes clear when seen in relation to the entire constellation of the patient's signs and symptoms. Also, the practitioner must assess the relative necessities of treating root and branch.

3. History

A disease is part of the continuum of the patient's entire life. It is rarely an isolated event without precursor or antecedent. The relevant histories which should be taken into account when making a comprehensive TCM diagnosis include menstrual history, history of previous gynecological treatment, history of conception and pregnancy, and family history with particular attention to close, female relatives.

A. General past medical history

Because the menstruation is connected to all parts and functions of a woman's body through the qi and blood, viscera and bowels, and channels and network vessels, the practitioner should take care to record as full and complete a medical history as possible. Various Western medications taken for nonmenstrual diseases, such as Valium, may negatively affect Chinese liver function thus contributing to or aggravating any menstrual disease associated with liver qi. A history of varicose veins in the legs or hemorrhoids suggests a tendency to blood stasis. And a history of a hiatal hernia with burping and belching suggests a tendency to liver qi and with stomach qi counterflow. In other words, any past disease or its treatment may have its impact or repercussions on a woman's present menstruation.

B. Menstrual history

When the major complaint is a menstrual disease, it is extremely important that the practitioner query the patient about menarche, the timing and regularity of their cycles, the quantity and quality of their menstruate, the presence of any lower abdominal, low back, or menstrual pain, and the date of their last menses. Since both diagnosis and the planning of treatment of menstrual diseases are dependent upon the phase of the patient's menstrual cycle, it is important to ascertain what day in the woman's cycle it is. The menstrual cycle should *always* be counted beginning at day one, the onset of the last period.

(Some women spot or leak premenstrually, and, therefore, there may be some confusion on which day is the first day of the new cycle. If the woman begins spotting on day 24 and then the flow comes in more normally on day 29, then day 29 is day one of the new cycle and the previous bleeding is categorized as premenstrual spotting.)

If a woman has a history of delayed and painful menstruation accompanied by a dark, clotty discharge and now complains of blocked menstruation, TCM theory suggests that this woman's disease mechanism is an evolution of stagnant qi and blood stasis. Whereas, if a woman has a history of early, bright red but scanty menses which then become delayed and eventually evolve into blocked menstruation, TCM theory suggests that the most likely disease mechanism involved is vacuity heat eventually consuming the essence and blood. Given each patient's menstrual history, TCM disease mechanism theory can help in the development of a diagnostic hypothesis which can then be corroborated or denied by comparison to current signs, symptoms, tongue, and pulse.

C. History of previous gynecological treatment

Because of modern Western medicine's common cause of iatrogenic complaints and complications and because few Western women will not have had some previous modern Western medical treatment, it is important to query the patient regarding her past treatment and use of contraceptives. As discussed above under the cause of menstrual disease, oral contraceptives may cause consumption and stasis of the blood. IUD's and abortions often also cause blood stasis. And antibiotics tend to cause spleen vacuity and dampness, while failing to dispel blood stasis. Therefore, if a woman complains of steadily worsening painful menstruation after having an abortion, blood stasis should be suspected which can then be corroborated by other signs and symptoms.

D. History of conception & pregnancy

Each female patient should be queried on how many pregnancies and how many births she has had. If not every pregnancy has resulted in birth, then further questions regarding abortions and miscarriages are indicated. Above we have discussed the implications of abortions in terms of disease causes and mechanisms.

If a woman has had one or more miscarriages, as complete a description of the signs and symptoms of these should be gathered as possible so that a tentative retrospective TCM pattern discrimination of these may be made. For instance, if a 23 year-old woman had a miscarriage preceded by extreme mental and emotional stress, abdominal cramping, and fetal leakage of dark red blood, one may suspect that the miscarriage was due to liver depression-depressive heat. If the patient now complains of early menstruation, the most likely cause of this would be a continuation of this depressive heat complicated by blood stasis which is so often the sequela of an abortion or miscarriage. This line of reasoning would then be corroborated by other signs and symptoms.

Numerous pregnancies and births damage and cause detriment to the *chong* and *ren*. Although most contemporary Western women only have one or two children, pregnancy in one's late 30s and into their 40s also tends to weaken and cause detriment the *chong* and *ren*. Therefore, a woman who has given birth to two children, once in her late 30s and again in her early 40s, and who now suffers from flooding and leaking and insomnia should be suspected of *chong* and *ren* detriment damage, *chong* and *ren* not securing, and flaring of vacuity heat due to yin vacuity.

It is also important to query women who have given birth as to their postpartum care and recuperation. Women who have suffered from postpartum abdominal pain with fever who were treated with antibiotics and dilation and curettage may still retain unexpelled static blood. Whereas, women who experienced postpartum insomnia, night sweats, and scanty lactation may still suffer from blood and yin vacuity. These should be searched for and taken into account in terms of any current menstrual disease.

E. Family history

I am unaware of any Chinese TCM gynecology texts recommending the practitioner questioning their patient's regarding family history of gynecological complaints. However, it is a well known fact that certain gynecological complaints run in families, such as breast cancer, endometriosis, and uterine myomas. In some cases, there is a genetic basis for the complaint. In other cases, shared diet and lifestyle, including mental/emotional coping patterns, engender similar disease mechanisms in members of a single family.

Questioning the patient about their mothers', grandmothers', aunts', and sisters' gynecological history may not help establish the patient's TCM pattern, but it may help in determining the patient's prognosis. Further, gathering such information may help in developing the theory and diagnosis of TCM in the future in light of modern Western medicine. Familial factors are an area TCM has paid scant attention to so far and yet they are relevant to clinical practice.

4. Diet

A great deal of disease in the West is due to unhealthy eating habits. In particular, eating uncooked, chilled, and fluid-engendering foods, including white sugar and dairy products, citrus fruits and juices, and ice cream and frozen yogurt, tends to damage the spleen and cause the accumulation of phlegm dampness. If this phlegm and dampness percolate downward, as they typically do, they obstruct the free flow of the *chong* and *ren* resulting in painful menstruation, profuse menstruation, and flooding and leaking.

Drinking coffee and black tea and eating excessively spicy foods tends to dry and damage the blood, out-thrust and scatter the qi, and cause internal heat. This may then cause early menstruation, premenstrual breast distention and pain and various other premenstrual complaints, scanty or profuse menstruation, painful menstruation, flooding and leaking, and perimenopausal complaints.

Drinking alcohol tends to cause damp heat. In terms of menstrual disease, this may manifest as or complicate early and profuse menstruation, painful menstruation, and flooding and leaking. Likewise, eating excessively greasy foods, such as fried and deep-fried foods, greasy meats, butter, oils, and fats, may also cause damp heat with the same negative effects on the menstruation.

Simply overeating may also cause food stagnation. As discussed above under the six depressions, food stagnation tends to lead to or aggravate qi stagnation and can transform into heat or fire. Although food stagnation *per se* does not typically result in any menstrual disease, food stagnation may aggravate and complicate any disease due to liver depression, spleen qi vacuity, stomach qi counterflow, or dampness and phlegm.

5. Lifestyle

Questions about lifestyle may include questions about one's emotional stress, one's job, marriage, social affairs, physical activity and exercise, and rest and relaxation. Any or all of these may potentially play a part in the cause and disease mechanisms of menstrual disease. Especially in the West, we tend to work too much, be under too much stress, exercise too little, and get too little rest and relaxation.

A. Emotional stress

As mentioned under disease causes, stress has a profound negative effect on the liver, and the liver is one of the most important viscera in menstrual pathophysiology. Almost always among Western female patients, stress plays its part in menstrual complaints. If it is not too excessive, stress tends to cause qi stagnation. However, if it is more excessive, this qi stagnation may transform into depressive heat. If this heat is strong enough or persists over a protracted period of time, it may consume and damage yin, blood, and fluids, resulting in vacuity heat. Liver depression qi stagnation is associated with delayed menstruation, premenstrual complaints, painful menstruation, scanty menstruation, and perimenopausal complaints. Depressive heat is associated with early and/or profuse and painful menstruation, premenstrual complaints, flooding and leaking, and perimenopausal complaints. Vacuity heat is associated with early and/or scanty menstruation, blocked menstruation, protracted uterine bleeding, premenstrual and perimenopausal complaints.

B. Job stress

One's work may also affect one's menstruation. If one stands all day or lifts heavy objects, this will tend to cause or aggravate qi vacuity and central qi fall. This may manifest as early and/or profuse menstruation, flooding and leaking, or painful menstruation. If one sits all day, this may tend to cause retardation of the flow of qi and blood and also inhibition of the movement and transformation of fluids. In the first case, this may result in or cause aggravation to any menstrual disease due to qi stagnation and blood stasis. In the second case, this may cause or complicate any menstrual disease due to dampness and phlegm.

C. Marital & social stress

One's marriage and social affairs may also impact a woman's menstrual cycle. As discussed above, any negative emotions, such as anger, frustration, melancholy, and grief, may cause irregularity in the flow of qi and, therefore, blood and thus cause or contribute to menstrual disease. It is important for the practitioner to have as complete a picture of all the contributory causes and factors in a woman's menstrual disease not only in order to make a correct pattern discrimination but also in order to erect a comprehensive treatment plan that remedies the causes of the imbalance at its root.

D. Physical exercise & activity

Modern Westerners tend to be too sedentary for our own good health. Although there has been some rise in societal consciousness about the importance of regular exercise, still, far too many of us are either too busy or too lazy to get regular, adequate exercise. Insufficient exercise results in retardation in the circulation of the qi and blood, weakening of digestion and elimination, weakening of the nervous system, and accumulation of dampness and phlegm. Retardation of qi and blood may adversely affect any and all menstrual diseases having to do with qi and blood stasis and stagnation. Weakening of the digestion and elimination affects both the regularity of the qi mechanism and the flow of qi, thus contributing to or aggravating qi stagnation, depression, and counterflow. It also inhibits the spleen's engenderment and transformation of the qi and blood and may contribute to any menstrual disease due to vacuity of the qi and blood. Because lack of physical exercise contributes to weakening of the nervous system, it likewise exacerbates any condition due to emotional stress. And finally, because lack of adequate physical exercise tends to foster the gathering of dampness and the congelation of phlegm, it aggravates any menstrual disease due in any part to dampness, fluid accumulation and stagnation, or phlegm.

E. Rest & relaxation

Almost paradoxically, although we Westerners fail to get adequate physical exercise, we are far from well rested. Because we work so compulsively, at least mentally, many of us do not get the rest and relaxation we should. Therefore, it is important to query the patient regarding this issue. Insufficient physical rest and sleep results in consumption and damage of both the qi and blood, ultimately leading to yin and essence vacuity. If it is only qi and blood vacuity, this may manifest as either a tendency to bleed too frequently or too much (qi vacuity) or to bleed too scantily and too seldom (blood vacuity). If it is yin and essence vacuity, this may manifest as early and/or scanty menstruation, blocked menstrauation, flooding and leaking, and premature menopause.

Relaxation is different than sleep. Although we tend to recoup our qi by both, we store acquired essence during sleep. However, relaxation does allow the free and unimpeded flow of qi and, when left to flow freely and without constraint, the qi tends to normalize itself. Failure to relax, therefore, tends to cause or aggravate liver depression qi stagnation, and this can cause or aggravate early or late menstruation, scanty menstruation, painful menstruation, various premenstrual complaints, and various perimenopausal complaints.

6. Pain

A. Abdominal & lumbar pain

In particular, the practitioner should take great care in querying their patient regarding any pain the patient may experience either before, during, or after menstruation or any lower abdominal pain at any time during her cycle. Pain which precedes menstruation and is relieved once the menses are flowing freely tends to be due to qi stagnation. Pain which is associated with or relieved by the passing of clots, tends to be due to blood stasis. Pain which is associated with distention and bloating and is diffuse and crampy tends to suggest qi stagnation. Whereas pain which is fixed in location, is sharp, piercing, or lancinating tends to suggest blood stasis. Pain which resists pressure is indicative of repletion. Pain which feels better with pressure is indicative of vacuity. Pain which is ameliorated by heat suggests stagnation due to or accompanied by coldness. However, since warmth in general promotes the flow of qi and blood, this is not always an accurate indication. Pain which is dull, dragging, heavy, and insidious and which gets worse towards the end of menstruation or as more and more blood is lost suggests qi vacuity. Although it is typically said that vacuity pain occurs at the end of or after menstruation, liver-kidney yin vacuity painful menstruation typically occurs at the onset of menstruation and is characterized by the cramping, pulling feeling in the tops and insides of the thighs corresponding to the area traversed by the sinews channels of the liver.

Low back or sacral pain may be due either to accumulation of dampness and heat or to kidney vacuity. If it is due to kidney vacuity, it is typically a weak, achy sort of pain which is worse on first movement or when changing positions. Whereas, if it is associated with dampness and heat, it is more likely to be continuous and unrelieved by movement. In addition, there may be localized heat, redness, and/or swelling and the pain definitely feels better when it obtains coolness.

Poking pain with intercourse suggests blood stasis. It is a common symptom in women suffering from painful menstruation or endometriosis and infertility.

One must also take care in being sure exactly where the pain is felt. The practitioner should ask the patient to place their hands directly over the area of pain. Simply saying the lower abdomen is not enough. The pain may be either centralized in the middle of the lower abdomen or may be more over the ovarian region. Further, it may be unilateral or bilateral. If the patient says she has dysmenorrhea, one must even make sure that the pain is either in the front, in the back, in the thighs and upper legs, or stretches from the back to the front. Not only do these differences clarify which channels are involved, but they are vitally important to the correct selection of medicinals and acupuncture points for the treatment of the pain.

Other questions regarding pain which should be asked include whether the pain is better or worse on movement or lack of movement, whether the pain is accompanied by nausea, vomiting, sweating, fever, or chills, whether the pain is felt on defecation or urination, and at what time of the day or night the pain is better or worse. All of these questions can help clarify the disease mechanism at work and help in pattern discrimination.

The practitioner should take care to ask their questions in such a way that they receive only those answers that are relevant to a TCM pattern discrimination. Western patients often comment on how they think their pain is intestinal or uterine or ovarian. These distinctions are typically not germane to a TCM pattern discrimination and may lead the practitioner astray. Rather the practitioner should take care to ask their patient questions whose answers fit into the diagnostic logic and methodology of TCM. Channel discrimination of pain is more important in TCM than is a Western anatomical discrimination. Lower abdominal pain may be hard to distinguish between intestinal pain and ovarian pain, but rarely does this affect the TCM pattern diagnosis and treatment.

B. Vaginal pain

Vaginal sores, external injury to the genitalia, or urinary strangury and pain may all manifest vaginal pain. Mostly this is due to qi and blood obstruction and stagnation.

C. Breast pain

Breast welling abscess (*i.e.*, mastitis) is associated with redness, aching and pain, and hardness. This is usually due to depressive heat. Following along with the menstrual period, there may be nipple pain or breast distention, nodulations, and lumps. After menstruation these disappear. These pertain to liver depression qi stagnation. In particular, nipple pain is associated with depressive heat and/or blood stasis while nipple itching is due to liver wind.

D. Rib-side pain[13]

This symptom commonly manifests in gynecological conditions associated with liver qi depression and stagnation.

E. Headache

Menstrual movement headache is mostly due to yin vacuity-yang hyperactivity. Headaches occurring at the end of or after menstruation are mostly due to blood vacuity not nourishing the brain.

7. The menses

As stated in the Preface, I believe it is easier to diagnose women than men *because* they menstruate. If one knows how to question about and analyze the cyclicity, color, volume,

---

[13] Wiseman formerly translated this as lateral costal pain.

and consistency of the menses, this gives the practitioner a monthly report card corroborating the pattern discrimination and indicating how and if treatment is progressing. Therefore, questioning carefully about the menses is one of the single most important aspects of questioning gynecological patients.

A. Menstruation ahead of schedule

The menstruation may come seven or more days before schedule. If severe, it may come like a tide two to three times in one month. This is called menstruation ahead of schedule. Menstruation ahead of schedule can be either vacuity or repletion. Typically, it is mainly due to replete heat patterns. In older women, it is more often due to spleen-kidney vacuity possibly complicated by depressive or vacuity heat. If the menses are profuse in amount, purple in color, and thick in consistency, this is a blood division replete heat pattern. If the menses are scanty in amount, red in color, and thick in consistency, this is a blood division vacuity heat pattern. If the menses are sometimes profuse and sometimes scanty, their color is red or purple, and there simultaneously appears chest and rib-side pain and fullness, this is a liver depression transforming heat pattern. There may also be qi vacuity not restraining and containing menstruation ahead of schedule. In this pattern, the amount is excessive, its color is pale, and it is watery and thin in consistency.

B. Menstruation behind schedule

The menstruation may come seven or more days after schedule. If severe, it may be more than 10 days overdue. This is called menstruation behind schedule. Menstruation behind schedule is mainly either a cold pattern, a vacuity pattern, or a qi stagnation pattern. If the color of the menstruate is dull red, its amount is scanty, and it is accompanied by chilly pain in the lower abdomen, this is a replete cold pattern. If the color of the menstruate is pale, its amount scanty, and its consistency is clear and watery, this is a vacuity cold pattern. If the color of the menstruate is pale red, its amount is scanty, and it is accompanied by dizziness and vertigo, this is a blood vacuity pattern. If the menses come with clots and lower abdominal distention and pain, this is a liver depression and binding pattern.

C. Menstruation early, late, at no fixed schedule

The menstruation may lack a regular schedule. Sometimes it may come early and sometimes it may come late. This is called menstruation (sometimes) early, (sometimes) late, at no fixed schedule. If the menstruation is (sometimes) early, (sometimes) late, and not fixed in schedule, if its amount is sometimes profuse and sometimes scanty, if the menstrual movement is not normally flowing, and if before or during its movement there are chest, rib-side, breast, and/or lower abdominal pain, this a liver qi depression and binding pattern. If the menses come (sometimes) early and (sometimes) late, the amount is scanty, the color is pale, and this is accompanied by low back soreness as if it would snap, this is a kidney qi vacuity weakness pattern.

D. Profuse menstruation

If the menstrual cycle is normal but the amount of the menstruate is more than normal, this is profuse menstruation. It has the two types of patterns of qi vacuity and blood heat. If the menses are colored pale red and are thin like water, this is a qi not containing the blood pattern. If the color of the menses is purplish red and its consistency is thick and mixed with clots, this is a heart-liver blood heat pattern.

E. Scanty menstruation

If the menstrual cycle is normal but the amount of the menstruate is less than normal, this is scanty menstruation. In clinical practice, there are three types: blood vacuity, kidney vacuity, and blood stasis. In the blood vacuity pattern, the amount of the menstruate is scanty, its color is pale, and it spots and dribbles as it approaches. (This spotting and dribbling prior to the onset of menstruation is actually a symptom of qi vacuity not containing the blood, remembering that the qi and blood are mutually interdependent.) In the kidney vacuity pattern, the amount of the menstruate is scanty, its color is fresh, and it is accompanied by low back and knee soreness and weakness. In the blood stasis pattern, the amount of the menstruate is scanty, its color is purple, its consistency is thick, and it is mixed with clots. It is also accompanied by lower abdominal pain which refuses pressure and other such symptoms.

F. Menstrual movement hemoptysis and epistaxis

If, one or two days before the menstrual movement comes like a tide or during the menstrual movement itself, there is hemoptysis or epistaxis and this occurs with each successive menstrual cycle, seemingly as if the menstruation were moving upward counterflow, this is called menstrual movement spontaneous ejection of blood. It is also called vicarious menstruation and counterflow menstruation. The occurence of menstrual movement spontaneous ejection of blood is mainly due to blood heat and qi counterflow. If there is spitting blood or epistaxis whose amount is excessive and color is reddish purple, this is mostly due to liver channel depressive fire counterflowing upward. If qi upbears, blood is upborne. Blood being upborne thus leads to hemoptysis and epistaxis. If the amount of the hemoptysis and epistaxis is scanty and its color is a dark or dull red, this is mostly due to lung and kidney yin vacuity. In this case, vacuity fire flames upward, damaging and causing detriment to the blood network vessels. This then results in hemoptysis and epistaxis.

G. Blocked menstruation:

If the menstruation ceases for three whole months or more or if the woman is over 18 years of age and her menses have never come like a tide, this is called blocked menstruation. This disease has vacuity and it has repletion. If the amount of menstruation gradually becomes more scanty and eventully becomes blocked menstruation, this is mostly a qi and blood dual vacuity pattern. If the menses were initially quite late in coming or even with menarche were scanty and then gradually became blocked, this is mostly a liver-kidney insufficiency pattern. If the menses have not moved for several months and this is accompanied by chest and rib-side distention and fullness and lower abdominal distention and pain, this is mostly a qi stagnation blood stasis pattern. If a fat person has blocked menstruation and stoppage which does not move, this is mostly a phlegm damp obstruction and stagnation pattern.

H. Flooding & leaking:

If a woman precipitates a large amount of blood between her menstruation or if there is continuous dribbling and dripping of precipitated blood, this is called flooding and leaking. As the ancients said, "Sudden great precipitation of blood is flooding." This saying refers to an excessive amount of discharged blood. They also said, "Dribbling and dripping without cease is leaking." This saying refers to a continuous discharge which does not stop.

Flooding and leaking are divided into vacuity and repletion. In vacuity pattern flooding and leaking, the pattern seen is one of sudden precipitation of blood which does not stop or dribbling and dripping which does not cease. Its color is pale and its consistency is watery. This is due to spleen vacuity not containing the blood. Thus the blood does not return to its channels. If there is kidney yang vacuity, there simultaneously appears a cold body and chilled limbs and a dark, dull face. Repletion pattern flooding and leaking is divided into blood heat and blood stasis. In blood heat flooding and leaking, the blood is colored reddish purple, is excessive in amount, and there are no clots. In blood stasis flooding and leaking, the amount of blood is possibly excessive and possibly scanty. However it *must* be mixed with blood clots. It is also accompanied by abdominal pain which refuses pressure.

8. Vaginal discharge

It is essential to ask about the quantity, color, consistency, and any odor of vaginal discharge. In addition, one should ask if there is any itching. Typically, profuse, white colored discharge which is like mucus without any offensive odor is mostly due to spleen vacuity with dampness percolating downward. If the discharge is profuse and yellow in color, is thick or pussy, and has an abominable smell, this is mostly due to damp heat percolating downward or damp toxic environmental excesses assailing. If abnormal vaginal discharge is yellowish white, is foamy in consistency, and has a raw meat or fishy odor, this is due to trichomoniasis vaginitis. If the discharge is milky white in color, excessive in amount, and congealed into lumps, this is mostly due to hemophilus vaginitis. If the discharge is five colored with obvious filaments of blood or blood lumps and a foul odor which is difficult to smell, this suggests cervical cancer.

Key discriminating questions recapitulated

One should be especially sure to ascertain the following basic yin-yang, hot-cold, vacuity-repletion discriminations:

Does the patient desire warmth or detest warmth?
Does the patient desire cold or fear cold?

Is there counterflow inversion of the four extremities?
Is there heat in the five centers?

Is the body cold to the touch?
Is the body hot to the touch?

Is there a chilled or cold feeling inside the abdomen?
Is there a hot feeling inside the abdomen?

Does the patient desire cold food and drinks?
Does the patient desire warm or hot food and drinks?

Does the patient have a great thirst and desire to drink?
Does the patient have a dry mouth but no desire to drink?

Does the patient desire pressure on her abdomen?
Does the patient refuse or detest pressure on her abdomen?

In addition, because most menstrual diseases are due to dysfunction of the kidneys, spleen, and/or liver, one should constantly keep in mind that:

Low back and knee soreness and weakness, cold feet, decreased libido, and nocturia suggest the kidneys.

Fatigue, lack of physical strength, decreased appetite, and diarrhea or loose stools suggest the spleen.

And irritability, chest oppression, breast distention and pain, rib-side pain, and lower abdominal distention suggest the liver.

Developing one's inquiry skills

As a teacher of TCM, I get to read a lot of my students' case histories and get to question them about their cases. Although many Western practitioners worry over their pulse reading skills, I find that the biggest problem in Western practitioners making a correct TCM pattern discrimination is a lack of inquiry skills. In thinking about this, I have identified three skills which can help Western practitioners improve their inquiry examination.

A. Reframing

Because Western practitioners are doing TCM in a language other than Chinese, the first skill for improving one's questioning is reframing. By this I mean reframing our patients' answers to our questions until we get the same or technically equivalent answer that a Chinese patient would give. TCM patterns are defined by only certain specific signs and symptoms. If a patient does not have the Chinese signs and symptoms of a particular pattern, then, *ipso facto*, they are not manifesting that pattern. If a Chinese doctor in China asks a Chinese patient if they are suffering from chest oppression, the Chinese patient knows what the doctor means and can answer yes or no. In the West or at least in English, we have no common shared concept of chest oppression. Therefore, if we ask our patients, "Do you have chest oppression?", they will not know how to answer us. Likewise, if we ask our patients if they have heart vexation, they will probably not give us the technically precise answer the Chinese doctor would suspect. Heart vexation means an irritating feeling of dry or baked heat in the precordial region. In other words, it is not just a general sense of irritability but a definite physical sensation. This means that we may have to ask our patients more questions in order to clarify if they do or do not have the specific signs and symptoms which add up to a particular TCM pattern.

This is not the same as putting words in our patients' mouths. It is merely a process of verbal clarification. Typically, reframing is done by repeating what the patient said and then asking, "Do you mean by that...?" Until or unless we elicit the exact same words or their technical equivalent that a Chinese doctor in China would elicit, we cannot make a correct TCM pattern discrimination. There are definite standards of what signs and symptoms do add up to a particular pattern, and we need to be careful that we do not lose the precision of these pattern definitions. Basically, the necessity of reframing in developing good inquiry skills is due to a problem in translating from one language to another.

B. Asking proper follow-up questions

If a patient tells us they have a headache, by itself that means nothing at all, except that we know there is a lack of free flow in the head. But we do not yet know why there is this lack of free flow. Chinese medical theory has a lot to say about headaches. Therefore, if a patient tells us they have headaches, then we need to know where on the head those headaches are since we know that the different regions of the head are traversed by different channels. If the headache is one-sided, we need to find out which side. One side pertains to qi and the other to blood. We need to find out what the pain feels like and how severe it is, how long it lasts, what causes it, and what makes it go away. Until or unless we ask all these follow-up questions, headache by itself means nothing. Likewise, if a patient says they have loose stools, cough, nausea, fatigue, or any of the other complaints which go to make up the so-called miscellaneous diseases of internal medicine, there are all sorts of follow-up questions which need to be asked systematically. It is this kind of follow-up questioning which really nails down the disease mechanisms at work and, therefore, the patient's pattern.

C. Questioning to confirm or deny a working hypothesis

As soon as the patient tells us their major complaint, based on our past study of Chinese medicine, we should form some working hypothesis about their pattern. If the patient says she has painful menstruation, then we need to be able to scroll up in front of our mind's eye the basic patterns and their signs and symptoms defining those patterns. Then we should deliberately and systematically ask our patient if she does or does not have the symptoms of the pattern we think is the most likely candidate based on her age, facial complexion, bodily form, and demeanor or what, in Chinese, is called her essence spirit. If, we find that the patient does not have the signs or symptoms we expected based on our working hypothesis about her pattern, then we need to decide on the next most likely pattern and systematically ask questions confirming or denying the presence of that pattern.

In other words, our questioning should not be just a random collection of everything possible we can think to ask our patients. Gathering too much information can be just as misleading as gathering too little. In this sense, our questioning should be like a lawyer's in court (however with a good bedside manner). A lawyer has an opinion about how they think the person on the stand is going to answer every question they ask. There is a definite line of reasoning behind why a lawyer asks the questions they do in the order they ask them. Efficient TCM questioning has exactly that same quality.

The prerequisites for developing these skills

There are two prerequisites for developing the above three skills. The first is a firm grasp of the basic TCM statements of theoretical fact. If we do not know what areas of the head correspond to what channels and, by extension, which viscera and bowels, then we cannot ask these questions. If we do not know which side of the body pertains to qi and which to blood, then we cannot ask those questions. Therefore, before we can ask good questions, we need to really know our basic TCM theory. Secondly, we must have a very good knowledge of 1) what TCM patterns there are, 2) what are their professionally agreed upon, standard signs and symptoms, and 3) what patterns correspond to what diseases, whether they be the traditional diseases of Chinese medicine or the diseases of modern Western medicine. If this knowledge is lacking, then one cannot reframe, one cannot ask the correct follow-up questions, and one cannot develop a cogent line of reasoning.

Palpation

1. Palpation of the pulse

A. The normal female pulse

A woman's pulse compared to a man's is weaker, slightly deep, and her right pulses are larger than her left. These characteristics are considered normal pulse signs.

B. The pulses of menstruation

During the premenstruum and the menstruation itself, the normal female pulse is large and slippery, especially on the left side. This corresponds to the abundance of yin, blood, and fluids. The largeness is indicative of the volume. The slipperiness is indicative that the large volume is of blood and fluids. It is also suggestive of an increase in heat. This is the theoretically normal or healthy premenstrual and menstrual pulse. However, most women coming to the TCM gynecological specialist have some abnormality in their menses. Therefore, one must take care to distinguish a healthy large, slippery pulse from an unhealthy surging, slippery pulse. Some authorities consider a bowstring[14] and slippery or bowstring and rapid pulse also normal during the menses, but, since these are also characteristic of various menstrual diseases, I read these as at least a tendency towards certain disease mechanisms.

In terms of pathological pulses, the following are the most commonly seen pulse images and their menstrual disease indications:

---

[14] Wiseman translates *xian mai* currently as string-like. He makes the point that wire was not invented at the time this term was coined. However, the character *xian* contains the bow radical. Therefore, I believe bowstring is preferable since this also conveys the idea of tautness implied in this pulse image.

1. Floating pulse (*fu mai*): If the pulse is floating, rapid, and forceful at both inch positions and if there is no external invasion or exterior pattern, this is categorized as a normal pulse of menstruation. If the pulse is floating and forceless, this is due to qi and blood dual vacuity or blood and yin vacuity. This can be seen in flooding and leaking which has endured for days.

2. Deep pulse (*chen mai*): One may find a deep pulse if there is water dampness gathering and retention, qi and blood vacuity weakness, yang qi insufficiency, or qi stagnation and lack of movement. Mostly it is seen after menstruation or in case of blocked or painful menstruation.

3. Slow pulse (*chi mai*): This is mostly due to cold exuberance. It can be seen in cases of painful menstruation and blocked menstruation.

4. Rapid pulse (*shu mai*): Typically, this is mainly associated with heat. If the pulse is rapid and forceful, this is due to repletion. This can be seen in case of early menstruation with excessive amount and flooding and leaking in the initial stage. If the pulse is rapid and forceless, this is due to vacuity. This can be seen in early menstruation with scanty amount and flooding and leaking in its middle and latter stages.

5. Surging pulse (*hong mai*): This is mainly due to heat and yang exuberance. It can be seen in case of early menstruation with excessive amount or flooding and leaking in its initial stage.

6. Slippery pulse (*hua mai*): If the left inch is slippery and uninhibited or both cubit pulses are slippery and uninhibited and the menses have been stopped and blocked for two to three months or more, this is a normal pulse of pregnancy. This pulse image is also commonly due to damp exuberance and is frequently seen in vaginal discharge diseases.

7. Bowstring pulse (*xian mai*): This is mainly due to qi stagnation and is mainly associated with aching and pain. It is mostly seen in case of menstrual irregularity, painful menstruation, blocked menstruation, and concretions and conglomerations.

8. Tight pulse (*jin mai*): This is mainly due to cold and is mainly associated with pain. It can be seen in cases of delayed and/or scanty menstruation, blocked menstruation, or painful menstruation.

9. Fine pulse (*xi mai*): This is mainly due to yin vacuity and scanty blood. It can be seen in case of delayed and/or scanty menstruation.

10. Weak pulse (*ruo mai*): This is mainly due to qi and blood dual vacuity. Mostly it can be seen in case of delayed menstruation, scanty menstruation or blocked menstruation. It can also be seen in flooding and leaking which has endured for days.

11. Scallion stalk pulse (*kou mai*): This is mainly due to sudden desertion of yin and blood. This is mostly seen in case of flooding and leaking precipitation of blood and excessively great loss of blood postpartum.

12. Choppy pulse (*se mai*): A choppy pulse without force is due to blood vacuity. A choppy pulse with force is mainly due to blood stasis. It is mostly seen in delayed menstruation with scanty amount and blocked menstruation.

A fine, bowstring pulse, perhaps the most commonly encountered pulse amongst Western females, suggests blood vacuity and liver qi. In this case, the fine quality indicates the blood vacuity and the bowstring quality indicates the liver qi. This combined pulse quality is often encountered in women suffering from PMS, delayed menstruation, scanty menstruation, no fixed schedule menstruation, and blocked menstruation. If the pulse is also rapid or fast, this suggests depressive liver heat as well. This typically manifests in terms of menstrual disease such as PMS, early and/or profuse menstruation, painful menstruation, and flooding and leaking. If the bowstring quality is more prominent in the right bar position, this suggests liver-spleen or liver-stomach disharmony. Another commonly encountered, related pulse pattern is for the right bar to be bowstring and forceful but floating. This suggests liver/stomach transformative heat and spleen vacuity. Further, if one or both cubit positions feels deep and bowstring, this suggests an element of blood stasis as well.

A fine, weak pulse indicates spleen-kidney qi vacuity. This often manifests menstrually as profuse menstruation and flooding and leaking.

A deep, forceless pulse often indicates spleen dampness if the patient tends to be obese. This may manifest menstrually as excessive menstrual bleeding and flooding and leaking, delayed or painful menstruation. A slippery, rapid pulse suggests damp heat or phlegm heat and is often encountered in early menstruation.

According to Zhang Xue-wen, author of *Yu Xue Zheng Zhi (Static Blood Patterns & Treatments)*, in clinical practice, the commonly encountered pulses associated with blood stasis include the deep, bowstring, choppy, bound, intermittent, and fine pulses or their combinations. Menstrually, such blood stasis may manifest as a delayed, scanty, painful, or absent menstruation. Blood stasis may also complicate early menstruation, profuse menstruation, and flooding and leaking.

A deep, slippery, forceful pulse in the right cubit position with a fine, floating left cubit pulse often suggests kidney yin and yang vacuity, possibly complicated by damp heat. This compound pulse image is often seen in perimenopausal women. If the pulse is also bowstring, there is typically concomitant stasis and stagnation.

Again, the key pulse discriminations to be kept in mind are:

A floating, big, slippery pulse signifies hidden heat in the *chong* and *ren* which mostly leads to early and profuse menstruation.

A deep, slow, or fine pulse signifies yang vacuity, internal cold, or insufficiency of the sea of blood which mostly leads to delayed or scanty menstruations and blocked menstruation.

A fine, rapid pulse signifies blood heat damaging yin fluids, yin vacuity, and diminished blood leading to blocked menstruation.

In the beginning of flooding, the pulse will most often be vacuous, big, bowstring, and/or rapid.

If flooding will not stop, the pulse typically will be vacuous, big, or scallion stalk.

If leakage will not stop, the pulse typically will be fine and weak.

C. Abnormal vaginal discharge pulses

If the abnormal vaginal discharge or *dai xia* is profuse, white or yellow in color, and the pulse is bowstring and rapid, this typically indicates damp heat pouring downward. If the *dai xia* is white, thick, and pasty or like curds, and the pulse is relaxed (*i.e.*, retarded) and slippery, this mostly means spleen vacuity and accumulation of dampness. If the *dai xia* is white, watery, clear, and chilly and both cubit positions are deep, slow, minute, and weak, this is mostly due to kidney yang vacuity and debility.

D. The pulses of pregnancy

In women whose menses are late, it is important to rule out the possibility of their being pregnant before unwarrantedly administering qi-moving, and blood-quickening medicinals to promote menstruation. The pulse of pregnancy is slippery and may be a bit rapid. If a woman with delayed menstruation presents with a slippery pulse, she should be counselled to first do a pregnancy test before making a final TCM diagnosis and administering medicine.

If the menses have ceased for two to three months, the woman has a craving for sour foods which then make her vomit, and her six pulses are 1) even and harmonious, 2) both cubit positions are slippery, or 3) her left inch position is slippery, all these are considered pulses of pregnancy.

2. Abdominal palpation

If a woman complains of either blocked menstruation or painful menstruation, it is important to palpate the lower abdomen in order to ascertain the presence of any abdominal masses. If such are found, it is best if the woman is referred to a Western gynecologist for a bimanual exam and an ultrasound. Depending upon the outcome of those and other tests, TCM therapy may be given or used in combination with other Western therapies.

Hard, immovable palpable masses which are not dispersed by and are painful to pressure suggest, in TCM terms, blood stasis. Whereas, palpable masses which tend to come and go, move about the lower abdomen, and which can be dispersed by massage are categorized as accumulations of stagnant qi. Asymptomatic palpable masses are often phlegm nodulation.

It is extremely important that all masses, those recognized by modern Western medicine and those by TCM, be treated according to further TCM pattern discrimination and not all just treated as blood stasis. The most common gynecological abdominal masses seen in Western practice are uterine myomas or so-called fibroids. These are most prevalent in women in their 40s. Since most Western women in their 40s suffer from elements of spleen and kidney vacuity, it is important to take these disease mechanisms into account along with any other recognizable repletions, such as qi stagnation, blood stasis, and phlegm nodulation. Although concretion and conglomerations, accumulations and gatherings are a miscella-neous disease according to TCM gynecology, practitioners must be clear about their TCM categorization, diagnosis, and treatment according to the logic of TCM. Attacking any and every mass as a species of blood stasis leads to a lack of therapeutic result at best and damage of the blood and yin at worst.

7

Key Patterns in Menstrual Diseases

Pattern discrimination is the single, key skill lying at the very heart of TCM as a specific style of Chinese medicine. Therefore, one should go over and over the signs and symptoms, tongue and pulse until they can recite the defining signs and symptoms under each pattern as readily as their name, address, postal code, and telephone number. In addition and to help with this process of learning the signs and symptoms of all the important patterns, one should try to understand the disease mechanisms which are responsible for the production of each and every sign and symptom under a pattern.

Viscera & Bowel Pattern Discrimination

1. Kidney disease pattern discrimination

A. Kidney qi vacuity

Main symptoms: Menarche coming at more than 18 years of age, blocked menstruation, menstrual irregularities, menses colored dullish and pale, menstrual substance thin, habitual miscarriage, infertility, uterine prolapse, possible genital atrophy, lumbar pain and lower leg weakness, possible dizziness or tinnitus, possibly a darkish, blackish facial complexion lacking luster, lack of luxuriance in the hair and easy falling out, a possibly chilly, heavy lower abdomen, frequent and/or nighttime urination, loose stools, a pale red tongue with a thin, white coating, and a deep and weak or deep and slow, forceless pulse

Although these are the textbook signs and symptoms of kidney qi vacuity especially in terms of menstrual diseases, few Western women will manifest all or even a large proportion of these. Since most women entering their 40s typically suffer from some element of kidney vacuity, it is enough if they have lumbar pain, lower leg or knee aching or weakness, decreased libido, and frequent or nighttime urination. Because kidney vacuity only complicates other concomitant patterns, rarely will Western patients have the textbook tongue and pulse signs of kidney vacuity.

B. Kidney yang vacuity

Main symptoms: Blocked menstruation, scanty mesntruation, menses colored darkish and substance thin, menstrual movement diarrhea, edema, excessive abnormal vaginal discharge, its substance thin like water, infertility, lower and upper back aching and chill, possible fear of cold, chilling and heaviness in the lower abdomen, cold feet, decreased libido, excessive urination at night, possible cock-crow diarrhea, a pale, darkish, tender tongue with a thin, white coating, and a deep, slow pulse with both cubit positions weak

Again, because kidney vacuity typically only complicates other patterns, in women in their late 30s and throughout their 40s, one may make a pattern discrimination of kidney yang vacuity if there is only lumbar pain, cold feet, decreased libido, and nocturia.

C. Kidney yin vacuity

Main symptoms: Early menstruation, menses scanty or profuse, flooding and leaking, thick, purplish menses, perimenopausal syndrome, profuse vaginal discharge either greenish yellow or blood-tinged in color, infertility, possible vexatious heat in the five hearts, red cheeks, a dry, red throat, possible dizziness or tinnitus, possible insomnia or night sweats, possible pain of the feet, legs, lower or upper back, scanty, yellowish urine or dry, bound stools, a red tongue, possibly having small cracks with scanty fluids and scanty, thin, yellow or no fur, possibly a flowery, stripped coating, and a fine, rapid, forceless pulse

Although many Western women will show more and more obvious signs and symptoms of kidney yin vacuity than kidney yang vacuity, one should not expect the woman to have all of these symptoms. In addition, if there is a red tongue or a red-tipped tongue, this only means that heat is counterflowing upward. There still may be yang vacuity below. Therefore, even if there are yin vacuity-vacuity heat signs and symptoms in the upper body, one should nevertheless check for yang vacuity signs and symptoms below.

D. Kidney yin & yang vacuity

Main symptoms: A combination of kidney yang and kidney yin vacuity signs and symptoms as above

E. Kidney qi exhaustion

Main symptoms: Blocked menstruation after enduring disease, genital atrophy, premature debility, falling hair, withered teeth, essence spirit debility and dullness, a wan, sallow facial complexion, possible postpartum great loss of blood with the menses not returning or the appearance of other signs of debility associated with aging, in enduring disease, a darkish, fluidless tongue, in diseases associated with loss of essence or blood, a pale, white tongue with scanty fluids, and no specific fur, a deep, weak pulse, vacuous, rapid pulse, or a racing pulse as if about to expire

2. Liver disease pattern discrimination

A. Liver depression qi stagnation

Main symptoms: Menstruation early, late, and at no fixed time, menstruation behind schedule or scanty in amount, a darkish colored menstruate or possibly containing lumps, painful menstruation, blocked menstruation, premenstrual breast distention, a tendency to sigh, emotional depression, rib-side pain, lower abdominal distention and pain, a darkish red tongue with thin fur, and a bowstring pulse

Liver depression qi stagnation is an extremely common pattern in clinical practice. This pattern is at the root of a number of pathological transformations, such as depressive heat, depressive heat damaging and consuming yin, liver yang hyperactivity, liver fire engendering liver wind, etc. In all these cases, there will typically be the signs and symptoms of liver depression qi stagnation *plus* the signs and symptoms of the further disease mechanisms and patterns. Therefore, one must be careful to treat the whole pattern. On the one hand, one may overlook liver depression. On the other, one may overlook other concomitant patterns. This is an important point in clinical practice.

B. Liver depression transforming into heat

Main symptoms: Early menstruation, profuse menstruation, lengthened menstruation, midcycle bleeding, flooding and leaking, painful menstruation, purplish red menses containing thick blood lumps, menstrual movement epistaxis and hemoptysis, possible spontaneous discharge of breast fluids, dizziness, headache, vertigo, possible swelling and pain of the eyeballs, a bitter taste in the mouth, a dry throat, possible heart vexation and easy anger, a red tongue with thin, yellow fur, and a bowstring, rapid pulse

C. Liver qi counterflowing upward

Main symptoms: Menstrual movement epistaxis or hemoptysis, menstrual movement breast distention, possible spontaneous discharge of breast fluids, easy anger, vomiting, rib-side aching and pain, possible dizziness, normal tongue fur or thick, slimy fur if the spleen and stomach are involved, and a bowstring pulse

D. Liver channel damp heat

Main symptoms: Profuse menstruation, lengthened menstruation, painful menstruation, flooding and leaking, purplish dark menses with a foul odor, profuse vaginal discharge with an abnormal color and a foul odor, vaginal itching, urinary strangury and pain, possible abdominal pain or possible chest and rib-side fullness and oppression, heart vexation, a bitter taste in the mouth, possible loose stools or dry binding, a red tongue with thick, slimy, yellow fur, and a bowstring, rapid or slippery, rapid forceful pulse

E. Liver blood insufficiency

Main symptoms: Delayed menstruation, scanty menstruation, blocked menstruation, menstrual movement headache, menstrual movement addictive papules, vaginal itching, and/or menopause accompanied by dizziness, blurred vision, easy emotional upsetment, etc., a pale or darkish and pale tongue with thin fur, and a bowstring, fine, not very forceful pulse

Liver blood insufficiency or vacuity often goes along with liver depression qi stagnation. In some sense, these two patterns are the two sides of a single coin due to the interdependence of the qi and blood. The liver blood is what nourishes, emolliates, and harmonizes the liver, thus allowing the liver to function correctly *vis à vis* coursing and discharge.

F. Liver yang ascendant hyperactivity

Main symptoms: Menstrual movement headache, menstrual movement epistaxis or hemoptysis, perimenopausal syndrome, headache, blurred vision, nausea, vomiting, possibly a red face and red eyes, insomnia, vertigo and dizziness, a darkish, red tongue with thin, yellow fur, and a bowstring, forceful pulse

G. Liver wind internally stirring

Main symptoms: Muscular spasms, twitching facial muscles, dizziness and vertigo, a red or crimson tongue with yellow or no fur, and a bowstring, rapid pulse if due to fire stirring wind, while a pale tongue and fine, wiry pulse if blood vacuity is engendering wind

3. Spleen (& stomach) disease pattern discrimination

A. Spleen vacuity, blood scanty

Main symptoms: Delayed menstruation, scanty menstruation, blocked menstruation, a pale colored menstruate with thin substance, a sallow yellow facial complexion, possible dizziness or heart palpitations, lassitude of the spirit, diminished appetite, a fat, teeth-marked, pale tongue with thin, white fur, and a relaxed, weak pulse

This pattern may also be called heart blood-spleen qi vacuity or simply heart-spleen dual vacuity.

B. Spleen vacuity, damp encumberance

Main symptoms: Menstrual movement diarrhea, menstrual movement water swelling, abnormal vaginal discharge, chest and epigastric glomus and oppression, scanty appetite, a bland taste in the mouth, profuse phlegm, loose stools, a pale or normal tongue with white, slimy fur, and a soggy, relaxed pulse

C. Spleen vacuity not containing

Main symptoms: Early menstruation, profuse menstruation, lengthened menstruation, flooding and leaking, possible spontaneous discharge of breast fluids, shortness of breath, feeble voice, lower abdominal downward heaviness, an ashen white facial complexion, a pale tongue with thin, white fur, and a deep, relaxed, forceless pulse

D. Spleen vacuity qi fall

Main symptoms: Flooding and leaking, miscarriage, uterine or rectal prolapse, enduring hemorrhoids, shortness of breath, feeble voice, fatigue and exhaustion, desire to lie down, lower abdominal heaviness, a pale tongue with thin, white fur, and a deep, weak pulse

Personally, I often see this pattern without a deep, weak pulse. The pulse may be short, not reaching the inch position, but most commonly, it is fine and wiry. This is because, in clinical practice, it is commonly associated with liver depression and blood vacuity due to profuse bleeding. Orthostatic hypotension is an important symptom to help confirm this pattern as is worsening of symptoms after standing for a long time.

E. Stomach vacuity

Main symptoms: Menstrual movement vomiting and nausea accompanied by scanty appetite, fullness and oppression, a pale tongue with scanty fur, and a weak pulse

F. Stomach heat

Main symptoms: Menstrual movement oral cavity sores and ulcers, galactorrhea, possible breast abscess, a dry, thirsty mouth, hunger, dry, bound stools, a red tongue with scanty fluids and thin, yellow fur, and a fine, rapid, or simply rapid pulse

I commonly see more stomach heat in my Western patients than stomach vacuity even if there is concomitant spleen vacuity. Frequently, as the above signs and symptoms suggest, this heat, which tends to be enduring, damages yin fluids as well. When there is both spleen vacuity with stomach heat, the tongue may not be red.

4. Heart disease pattern discrimination

A. Heart yin vacuity

Main symptoms: Menstrual irregularity, menstrual movement oral ulcers, perimenopausal syndrome, heart vexation, heart palpitations and racing heart, insomnia, short, yellow urination, a red tongue tip with thin, yellow fur and scanty fluids, and a fine, rapid pulse

Many students use this pattern to over-diagnose. Kidney yin vacuity can also manifest a number of the same signs and symptoms, such as heart palpitations and insomnia with a red tongue tip and scanty, possibly yellow fur. In the above pattern, however, there are no signs and symptoms of kidney vacuity. This is an important distinction. If one over-diagnoses and sees this pattern where it is actually not, one will either choose the wrong guiding formula or add too many unnecessary medicinals.

B. Heart qi vacuity

Main symptoms: Blocked menstruation, menstrual movement insomnia, menstrual movement essence spirit abnormality, heart palpitations on exertion, a pale tongue with thin, white fur, and a deep, weak pulse

This pattern is not that commonly seen in clinical practice. More commonly, one sees either heart blood and spleen qi vacuity or great qi vacuity. Great qi vacuity, also called a chest qi vacuity, is a combination of heart and lung qi vacuity. Further, in both these cases, the heart and lungs fail to receive sufficient qi due to spleen vacuity not upbearing the clear.

5. Lung disease pattern discrimination

A. Lung qi not diffusing

Main symptoms: Water swelling accompanied by chest oppression, possible rapid breathing, inhibited urination, a pale colored yet dark hued tongue with thin, white fur, and a floating, slippery pulse

B. Yin vacuity lung dryness

Main symptoms: Menstrual movement epistaxis and hemoptysis, blocked menstruation, cough, tidal fever, red cheeks, a red tongue with scanty fluids and scanty fur, and a fine, rapid pulse

Qi & Blood Pattern Discrimination

1. Qi disease pattern discrimination

A. Qi vacuity, qi fall

Main symptoms: Profuse menstruation, early menstruation, lengthened menstruation, flooding and leaking, pale colored menses which are thin in substance, miscarriage, galactorrhea, and/or uterine prolapse accompanied by shortness of breath and feeble voice, fatigue and desire to lie down, possible spontaneous sweating, a pale tongue with thin, white fur, and a vacuous, forceless pulse

B. Qi stagnation

Main symptoms: Scanty menstruation, delayed menstruation, blocked menstruation, menstrual movement breast distention, leaking which dribbles and drips, a dark colored menstruate containing lumps, lower abdominal distention and pain, possible rib-side distention and pain, and possibly a normal tongue and fur but a bowstring pulse

C. Qi counterflow

Main symptoms: Menstrual movement epistaxis and hemoptysis, vomiting, spontaneous discharge of breast fluids, headache, hiccup, rib-side pain and chest oppression, a pale tongue with thin fur, and a bowstring or slippery pulse

It is important to understand that if qi stagnation either endures or becomes more severe, it may transform pathologically into two other patterns. One is depressive heat and the other is counterflow. When qi becomes depressed and stagnant, it backs up and accumulates.

Eventually, this accumulating qi has to vent itself or go somewhere. Most commonly, it counterflows upward. However, it can also counterflow horizontally. Nevertheless, when there is qi counterflow, there are still signs and symptoms of qi stagnation, such as a bowstring pulse and irritability.

2. Blood disease pattern discrimination

A. Blood vacuity

Main symptoms: Menstrual irregularity, menses colored pale and substance thin, menstrual movement headache, menstrual movement addictive papules, painful menstruation, vaginal itching, infertility, a somber white or sallow yellow facial complexion, pale, whitish lips, dizziness, blurred vision, heart palpitations, insomnia, numbness of the hands and feet, a pale tongue with thin fur, and a fine, forceless pulse

B. Blood heat

Main symptoms: Early menstruation, profuse menstruation, lengthened menstruation, menstrual movement epistaxis and hemoptysis, flooding and leaking, painful menstruation, purplish red menses which are thick in substance, heat entering the blood chamber, heart vexation, a dry mouth, vacuity heat, tidal fever, thirst with desire to drink, if severe, vexation and agitation and delirious speech, subdermal bleeding. If there is aching and pain, it is hot pain and refuses pressure. There are dry, bound stools, short, yellow urination, a red, crimson tongue and yellow fur if it is replete heat along with a surging, large, slippery, rapid pulse. There is scanty or no fur and a fine, rapid pulse if it is vacuity heat.

C. Blood cold

Main symptoms: Delayed menstruation, scanty menstruation, painful menstruation, menses colored dark blackish and containing lumps, blocked menstruation, abdominal masses, possible infertility. If it is vacuity cold, the body is cold with chilled limbs and there is aching and pain which desires warmth, while the urination is clear and long. If it is replete cold, the lower abdomen is chilly and cold and refuses pressure. The tongue is dark with thin, white fur or white, moist fur. If it is vacuity cold, the pulse is deep, slow, and choppy. If it is replete cold, the pulse is deep and tight.

D. Blood stasis

i. Qi stagnation blood stasis

Main symptoms: Delayed menstruation or menstruation which is (sometimes) early, (sometimes) late, and comes at no fixed schedule, scanty menstruation, flooding and leaking, dark colored menses containing lumps, painful menstruation, aching and pain commonly preceding menstruation, blocked menstruation, premenstrual syndrome, infertility, abdominal masses, perimenopausal syndrome, rib-side pain, lower abdominal pain, breast distention and pain, distention and pain where there is more distention than pain, emotional binding, tension, and agitation, a purplish, dark tongue or one having static spots or macules with normal tongue fur, and a bowstring and/or choppy pulse

ii. Cold congelation blood stasis

Main symptoms: The same blood cold symptoms described above plus painful menstruation seen mostly before the menses which is diminished by heat, a greenish bluish white facial complexion, a darkish tongue or static spots on the edges of the tongue with white or thick, white fur, and a deep, tight pulse

iii. Heat scorching blood stasis

Main symptoms: The same blood heat symptoms described above accompanied by aching and pain, pain which mostly refuses pressure, a scorching hot body or the affected area colored red, gynecological bleeding colored purple and bright, sticky and thick, and containing lumps, a red, crimson tongue or possibly static spots on the edges of the tongue with thick, yellow or slimy fur, and a surging, rapid or slippery, rapid pulse

iv. Qi & blood vacuity blood stasis

Main symptoms: The same symptoms as described above under qi stagnation blood stasis plus insidious pain, aching and pain which desires rubbing and pressure. If there is painful menstruation, the pain mostly occurs after menstruation. A pale, darkish tongue with thin, white fur, and a choppy pulse

v. Bleeding becoming stasis

Main symptoms: External injury to the reproductive organs leading to blood swelling, falling fetus, non-descension of the placenta, difficult delivery, etc., accompanied by aching and pain, if severe, postpartum fainting and inversion, a darkish or pale yet darkish tongue with thin fur, and a vacuous, rapid pulse. If postpartum, the pulse may be faint, rapid, and on the verge of expiry.

3. Combined qi & blood disease pattern discrimination

A. Qi & blood dual vacuity

Main symptoms: Blocked menstruation, flooding and leaking, spontaneous discharge of breast fluids, etc. accompanied by other typical qi and blood symptoms, a pale, tender tongue with thin, white fur, and a deep, slow pulse

B. Qi & blood dual depletion

Main symptoms: Flooding and leaking or profuse menstruation which is fresh red in color and clear, thin, and watery in consistency, dry throat, vexatious heat in the five hearts, shortness of breath, fainting and dizziness, a red tongue with scanty fur or pale tongue with no fur, and a vacuous, rapid, forceless pulse

Chong, Ren, Du & *Dai* Pattern Discrimination

1. *Chong* & *ren* insufficiency

Main symptoms: Delayed menstruation, scanty menstruation, blocked menstruation, habitual miscarriage, infertility, etc., accompanied by liver-kidney insufficiency or qi and blood vacuity weakness symptoms

2. *Chong* & *ren* not securing

Main symptoms: Flooding and leaking, profuse menstruation, early menstruation, lengthened menstruation, midcycle bleeding, abnormal vaginal discharge, habitual miscarriage, uterine prolapse, etc., accompanied by kidney vacuity or qi vacuity weakness symptoms of not securing and containing

3. *Chong* & *ren* loss of regularity

Main symptoms: Menstruation comes (sometimes) early, (sometimes) late, and at no fixed schedule, flooding and leaking, various possible symptoms of menstrual irregularity, etc., accompanied by kidney qi vacuity, and/or spleen qi vacuity, and/or liver depression symptoms

4. *Chong* & *ren* obstructed & stagnant

Main symptoms: Scanty menstruation, delayed menstruation, painful menstruation, blocked menstruation, flooding and, leaking, etc., accompanied by liver depression, qi stagnation, blood stasis symptoms

5. *Ren mai* not securing, *dai mai* lack of constraint

Main symptoms: Habitual miscarriage, abnormal vaginal discharge diseases, uterine prolapse

6. *Du mai* not fortifying

Main symptoms: Infertility, lumbar pain

Triple Burner Pattern Discrimination

1. Lower burner damp heat

Main symptoms: Profuse abnormal vaginal discharge which is colored yellow or is possibly pussy or streaked with blood and smells foul, vaginal itching, vaginal sores, vaginal flatulence, flooding and leaking, painful menstruation, lower abdominal aching, pain, and distention, possible loose stools and yellow urine, a red tongue with slimy, yellow fur, and a soggy, rapid pulse

2. Lower burner vacuity cold

Main symptoms: The same symptoms as described above under kidney yang vacuity or blood cold of the vacuity category

The chart below outlines some of the main pattern discriminations in the analysis of signs and symptoms associated with menstruation. In TCM pattern discrimination, it is important not to ascribe a single, absolute meaning to any given sign or symptom. The final meaning of any sign or symptom is only revealed by the entire pattern or constellation of simultaneously presenting signs and symptoms. Almost all symptoms may be produced by more than a single disease mechanism. Therefore, in developing one's skill in TCM pattern discrimination, it is important to understand all the possible disease mechanisms for a given symptom beyond just memorizing indications. When one understands the mechanisms by which symptoms are produced, one can then more easily search for the common disease mechanism behind any constellation or group of symptoms.

| | | Menstruation | | | | Abnormal vaginal discharge | Abdominal pain |
		Color	Quantity	Quality	Cycle		
Vacuity Patterns	Blood Vacuity	pale red	scanty	thin, dilute	lengthened or shortened	white, excessive, thin and dilute	dragging lower abdominal pain
	Qi Vacuity	pale red or yellow fluid	excessive metrorrhagia, menorrhagia, or continuous spotting	thin, dilute	lengthened or absent		post-menstrual pain, relieved by pressure
Repletion Patterns	Qi Stagnation	purple red	scanty, uneven flow	thick, viscous, with clots	irregular, lengthened or shortened	yellowish, white, thick and viscous	pre- or menstrual distention & pain, may refer to the subcostal region
	Blood Stasis	purple black	scanty	blood clots	lengthened or absent		pre- or post-menstrual distention, pain; localized; resists pressure; mass may be felt with deep palpation
	Phlegm Dampness	pale red	large or small in amount	thick and viscous	lengthened or absent	excessive, clear discharge	
Cold Patterns	Vacuity Cold	pale or purple black	scanty & uneven flow	thin & dilute	lengthened	clear, dilute, fishy smell	cold pain of lower abdomen; desires heat & pressure
	Replete Cold	dull black	scanty	thick, viscous, gelatinous lumps	lengthened or absent	excessive	cold pain of lower abdomen, resists palpation, relieved by warmth
Heat Patterns	Vacuity Heat	pale red	scanty or incessant spotting	clear, dilute, no clots	shortened	yellow, thick, viscous or streaked with blood	warm pain in lower abdomen
	Replete Heat	deep red or purple red	excessive like an avalanche	thick, viscous, turbid; often with blood clots	shortened		abdominal pain resisting palpation
	Damp Heat	yellow in the midst of red	excessive	thick, viscous	often shortened	yellow-white excessive with fetid odor	continuous or intermittent pain worsening with period

VISCERA & BOWEL PATTERN DISCRIMINATION

Pattern	Gynecological Condition	Generalized Symptoms	Tongue	Pulse
Kidney Qi Vacuity	Menses early, late, erratic, amount excessive or scanty, flooding & leaking, blocked menstruation, fetal stirring & restlessness, slippery fetus, infertility, uterine prolapse	low back soreness & knee weakness, dizziness, tinnitus, polyuria, devitalized essence spirit, dark, dull complexion	pale red with thin, white coating	deep fine
Kidney Yin Vacuity	early menstruation, amount scanty, color red, blocked menstruation, flooding & leaking, fetal stirring restlessness, menopausal syndrome, infertility, heart vexation during pregnancy	dizziness, tinnitus, dry mouth, parched throat, red cheeks, hands, feet, heart hot, insomnia, night sweats, dry stools, short, yellow urine, leg and foot pain	red tongue with scant or no coating	fine, rapid, forceless
Kidney Yang Vacuity	menstrual movement diarrhea, *dai xia*, amount excessive, clear, and watery, edema during pregnancy, fetal stirring restlessness, uterine cold infertility, flooding & leaking	lower & upper back aching & pain or low back pain as if about to snap, abdominal chill, fear of cold, devitalized essence spirit, dizziness, tinnitus, diminished sexual desire, clear, long urination, excessive nocturia, diarrhea	pale tongue with thin, white, moist coating	deep, slow, minute, weak; *shi* pulse particularly so
Liver Qi Depression	menses early, late, or erratic, amount excessive, scanty, unstable, color dark w/ clots, menstrual movement not smooth, painful menstruation, blocked menstruation, infertility, premenstrual breast distention, scanty lactation	chest, lateral costal, and breast distention & pain, chest oppression & discomfort, lower abdominal distention & pain, occasional sighing, essence spirit depression, burping, diminished appetite	normal tongue with a thin, white coating	bowstring
Liver Depression Transformative Heat	early menstruation, amount excessive, color purple red, flooding & leaking, menstrual movement hemoptysis & epistaxis, spontaneous discharge of breast milk	headache, vertigo, dizziness, tinnitus, red, swollen, painful eyes, bitter mouth, dry throat, lateral costal pain, vexation, agitation, easy anger	red tongue w/ thin, yellow coating	bowstring, rapid
Liver Channel Damp Heat	*dai xia*, color yellow or yellow & white simultaneously, amount excessive, thick, foul odor, vaginal itching, vaginal sores	chest oppression, torpid intake, heart vexation, bitter mouth, yellow, astringent, painful urination, dry, parched stools	red tongue w/ slimy, yellow coating	bowstring, rapid, forceful or slippery, rapid

Liver Yang Hyperactive Above	menopausal syndrome, vertigo & dizziness during pregnancy, pre-eclampsia	headache, dizziness, vertigo, red face, tinnitus, deafness, insomnia, excessive dreams, numbness & insensitivity of the limbs, trembling	red tongue w/ thin, yellow or scanty coating	bow-string, fine
Liver Wind Internally Stirring	fetal epilepsy, postpartum tetany	headache, dizziness, blurred vision, sudden clouding inversion, loss of consciousness of human affairs, hands and feet convulsive spasms, arched back rigidity	red or scarlet tongue w/ no or flowery, peeled coating	bow-string, fine, rapid
Spleen Qi Vacuity	early menstruation, excessive menstruation, blood color pale, flooding & leaking, *dai xia,* uterine prolapse, morning sickness, spontaneous flow of breast milk	face color pale yellow or vacuous edema, spiritual fatigue, lack of strength, shortness of breath, disinclination to speak, bland mouth w/ no taste, no thought for food or drink or after eating epigastric & abdominal distention	pale tongue w/ teeth indentations and a thin, white coating	relaxed, weak, forceless
Spleen Yang Vacuity	menstrual movement diarrhea, edema during pregnancy, *dai xia,* infertility	somber white facial color, fatigue, lack of strength, fear of cold, chilled limbs; if severe, superficial edema, devitalized eating & drinking, epigastric oppression, abdominal distention, loose stools or diarrhea	pale, fat tongue w/ glossy, white coating	vacuous, weak or relaxed, slippery, forceless
Phlegm Damp Blockage & Obstruction	blocked menstruation, morning sickness, *dai xia,* infertility	fat body, heavy head, vertigo & dizziness, chest & epigastric glomus & oppression, heart palpitations, shortness of breath, bland & slimy inside mouth, nausea, diminshed eating	pale w/ slimy white coating	slippery or deep, relaxed
Heart/Spleen Dual Vacuity	early menstruation, amount excessive, color pale, or late menstruation, amount scanty, clear & watery, flooding & leaking, agitated viscera	somber white facial color or sallow yellow, dizziness, vertigo, heart palpitations, shortness of breath, insomnia, excessive dreams, fatigue, diminished appetite	pale w/ thin white coating	fine, weak
Heart & Kidneys Not Joined	menopausal syndrom, agitated viscera	palpitations, poor memory, vacuity vexation, excessive dreams, dizziness, tinnitus, low back pain & knee weakness	red w/ thin or no coating	fine, rapid
Yin Vacuity Lung Dryness	blocked menstruation, menstrual movement epistaxis, cough during pregnancy	both cheeks tidal red, tidal fever, night sweats, cough w/ scanty phlegm, dry throat, parched mouth, hands, feet, heart heat	red or scarlet w/ flowery, peeled, or no coating	fine, rapid

Liver-Kidney Yin Vacuity	flooding & leaking, vertigo & dizziness during pregnancy, agitated viscera, vaginal itching	same as kidney yin vacuity plus liver yang hyperactive above	red, dry	bow-string, fine, rapid
Spleen-Kidney Yang Vacuity	menstrual movement diarrhea, *dai xia*, fetal swelling	same as kidney yang vacuity plus spleen yang vacuity	pale w/ moist, white or slimy, white coating	deep, slow or deep, weak

QI & BLOOD PATTERN DISCRIMINATION

Pattern	Gynecological Condition	Generalized Symptoms	Tongue	Pulse
Qi Vacuity	early menstruation, amount excessive, color pale, watery, flooding & leaking, lochia does not stop, spontaneous discharge of breast milk, uterus prolapse	somber white facial color, cold body, chilled limbs, heart palpitations, shortness of breath, spiritual fatigue, disinclination to speak, dizziness, vertigo, lower abdominal emptiness & sagging, spontaneous perspiration	pale w/ thin white coating	relaxed, weak
Qi Stagnation	late menstruation, menstrual movement not smooth, painful menstruation, blocked menstruation, concretions & conglomerations, scanty lactation	chest, lateral costal, lower abdominal distention & pain, pain not constant, abdominal region lumps, pushing can move them, pressure can scatter, essence spirit depression	normal tongue or darkish w/ a thin, white coating	bowstring
Blood Vacuity	late menstruation, amount scanty, color pale, watery, blocked menstruation, abdominal pain after menstruation, fetal stirring restlessness, insufficient lactation	sallow yellow facial color, lips & nails pale white, dizziness, blurred vision, heart palpitations, scanty sleep, numbness of the hands & feet, dry, bound stools	pale, w/ scant, white coating	fine, weak
Blood Stasis	delayed menstruation or lack of stability, color purple, clots, movement not smooth, painful menstruation, blocked menstruation, flooding & leaking, postpartum abdominal pain, lochia does not stop, placenta does not descend	lower abdominal aching & pain, pain is fixed, feels like piercing or pricking, if severe, accumulations & binding produce lumps, pressure aggravates pain, pushing cannot move, after blood clots precipitated, pain lessened, skin scaly & rough	purple & dark, edges have static spots	deep, bowstring, or deep, choppy
Blood Cold	Replete Cold: late menstruation, amount scanty, Color dark, clots, painful menstruation, blocked menstruation, concretions & conglomerations, infertility	lower abdominal tugging pain, better w/ heat, facial color bluish white, body cold, limbs chilled	dark w/ white coating	deep, tight
	Vacuity Cold: late menstruation, amount scanty, color pale, painful menstruation, *dai xia* clear & chilly like water	insidious abdominal pain, likes warmth & pressure, lower abdomen emits coolness, scant luster to facial color, dizziness, low back soreness, torpid intake, clear, long urination, loose stools	pale w/ moist, white coating	deep, slow, forceless

Blood Heat	Replete Heat: early menstruation, amount excessive, color purple red, sticky & thick, menstrual movement hematemesis, epitaxis, flooding & leaking, fetal leakage, lochia does not stop	red face, dry mouth, fever, thirst, liking for chilled drinks, heart vexation, heart palpitations, yellow-red urine, dry, bound stools	red w/ yellow coating	slippery, rapid, forceful
	Vacuity Heat: early menstruation, color fresh red, leakage does not stop, fetal stirring restlessness, menopausal syndrome	face color tidal red, low fever or tidal fever, vexatious heat in the 5 hearts, night sweats, scanty sleep, excessive dreams, dry mouth, parched throat, dry, parched skin, heart palpitations, dizziness	red w/ no or scanty coating	fine rapid
Cold Damp Congealing & Stagnating	late menstruation, amount scanty, color dark, clots, or like black bean juice, painful menstruation, blocked menstruation	lower abdominal chilly pain lessened w/ heat, chest oppression, nausea, face color bluish white, body cold, chilled limbs	dark w/ slimy, white coating	deep, tight, or soggy, relaxed
Damp Heat Congealing & Stagnating	early menstruation, amount excessive, color purple red, thick sticky & foul odor, *dai xia*, vaginal itching	chest oppression, heat vexation, bitter mouth, dry throat, yellow-red urine	red w/ slimy, yellow coating	slippery, rapid
Qi & Blood Dual Vacuity	painful periods, agalactia	same as qi vacuity plus blood vacuity	pale w/ thin, moist coating	vacuous, fine
Qi Stagnation, Blood Stasis	late menstruation, amount scanty, painful menstruation, blocked menstruation, concretions & conglomerations	same as qi stagnation plus blood stasis	purple, dark, w/ static spots	deep, bowstring, or bowstring, choppy

8

Treatment Principles & Chinese Medicinals

Essential Treatment Principles for Menstrual Diseases

As discussed above, in TCM methodology, the statement of treatment principles is the necessary intermediary step between formulating the pattern discrimination and erecting the treatment plan. If the treatment principles funnel the practitioner to the right chapters of their formulas and prescriptions and materia medica texts, they can only do this job if the practitioner knows what treatment principles go with what patterns. Below is a selection of the most commonly used treatment principles for the most commonly seen patterns in menstrual diseases.

1. Regulating & rectifying the qi & blood

Women's menstruation, vaginal discharge, gestation, and birthing can all easily consume the qi and damage the blood. If qi and blood loss their regulation, this may give rise to various gynecological diseases. Therefore, regulating and rectifying the qi and blood is an extremely important treatment method for the treatment of menstrual diseases.

A. If disease exists in the blood division, one should treat the blood as the root assisted by rectifying the qi. In case of blood vacuity, one should supplement and nourish the blood. In case of blood cold, one should warm the channels (or menses) and scatter cold. In case of blood heat, one should clear heat and cool the blood. In case of blood stagnation and blood stasis, one should quicken the blood and transform stasis. In case of excessive discharge of blood, one must urgently secure, astringe, and stop bleeding.

B. If disease exists in the qi division, one should mainly treat the qi assisted by rectifying the blood. In case of qi vacuity, one should supplement the qi. In case of qi fall, one should upbear and lift. In case of qi desertion, one must urgently secure the qi and stem desertion. If qi is stagnant, one should move the qi. If qi is depressed, one should resolve depression. If qi counterflows, one should downbear and normalize the flow of qi.

C. If qi and blood are both diseased, it is appropriate to treat both the qi and blood. If there is qi and blood dual vacuity, one should supplement both the qi and blood. If the qi is vacuous when the blood is stagnant, one should supplement the qi assisted by quickening the blood and scattering stasis. If blood is vacuous when the qi is stagnant, one should supplement the blood assisted by moving the qi.

2. Harmonizing the spleen & stomach

The spleen and stomach move and transform the finest essence and harmonize water dampness. They also function to restrain and contain blood and fluids. If a woman's spleen and stomach are fortified and transporting, qi and blood are full and exuberant, the sea of blood is full and exuberant, and the menstruation is on time and gestation and fertility are normal. If the spleen and stomach lose their regulation, the source of engenderment and transformation will be insufficient and will eventually affect the menses, vaginal discharge, gestation, birthing, and lactation. If the spleen and stomach are vacuous and weak, one should supplement and fortify the spleen. If the spleen and stomach are vacuous and cold, one should warm the center and scatter cold. If the spleen and stomach are damp and hot, one should clear heat and eliminate dampness. And if phlegm dampness obstructs and stagnates, one should eliminate dampness and transform phlegm.

3. Coursing liver qi

The liver rules coursing and discharge, it treasures the blood, and its nature likes orderly reaching. The *chong* is the sea of blood and is commanded by the liver. As mentioned above, menstruation, vaginal discharge, gestation, birthing, and breast-feeding may all damage the blood. If the qi division is exuberant, the emotions are easily stirred and upset. In that case, the liver may lose its orderly reaching and coursing and discharge may be excessive. The *chong* and *ren* may thus become irregular and this may cause the onset of various gynecological diseases. If liver depression is not soothed, one should course the liver and resolve depression assisted by fortifying the spleen. If liver yin is insufficient, one should nourish and foster liver yin assisted by enriching the kidneys. If liver fire is effulgent and exuberant, one should clear heat and drain the liver. If liver yang ascends hyperactively, one should foster yin and subdue yang, settle, restrain, and level the liver.

4. Supplementing kidney qi

The kidneys rule treasuring of the essence qi and the engenderment and growth of the human body. They are also the root of development and reproduction. As girls get older, their kidney qi becomes effulgent and exuberant and their *tian gui* becomes hot. Their *chong* and *ren* become free-flowing and exuberant and thus they are able to menstruate and conceive. If kidney qi is insufficient, the *chong* and *ren* will be deficient and subject to detriment. This then may affect the menstruation, vaginal discharge, gestation, and birthing, causing a variety of diseases. If kidney yin is insufficient or yin is vacuous and has suffered detriment, one should enrich the kidneys and nourish yin assisted by bone and meat types of ingredients. If kidney qi is insufficient or kidney yang is vacuous and in decline, one should supplement and boost the kidneys and invigorate yang. If yin is vacuous and yang is hyperactive, one should enrich yin and subdue yang. If yin and yang are both vacuous, one should supplement both yin and yang.

Commonly Used Chinese Medicinals in Gynecology

1. Regulating & rectifying the qi & blood

A. Qi division medicinals

i. Commonly used medicinals for supplementing the qi: Radix Panacis Ginseng (*Ren Shen*), Radix Astragali Membranacei (*Huang Qi*), Rhizoma Atractylodis Macrocephalae (*Bai Zhu*)

ii. Commonly used medicinals for moving the qi and scattering nodulation: Rhizoma Cyperi Rotundi (*Xiang Fu*), Fructus Citri Aurantii (*Zhi Ke*), Radix Auklandiae Lappae (*Mu Xiang*), Radix Linderae Strychnifoliae (*Wu Yao*), Fructus Meliae Toosendan (*Chuan Lian Zi*), Pericarpium Citri Reticulatae Viride (*Qing Pi*), Cortex Magnoliae Officinalis (*Hou Po*), Semen Citri Reticulatae (*Ju He*), Semen Litchi Sinensis (*Li Zhi He*), Calyx Diospyri Khaki (*Shi Di*)

B. Blood division medicinals

i. Commonly used medicinals to supplement & nourish the blood: Radix Angelicae Sinensis (*Dang Gui*), cooked Radix Rehmanniae (*Shu Di*), processed Radix Polygoni Multiflori (*He Shou Wu*), Gelatinum Corii Asini (*E Jiao*), Plastrum Testudinis (*Gui Ban*), Fructus Lycii Chinensis (*Gou Qi Zi*)

ii. Commonly used medicinals for quickening the blood and dispelling stasis: Flos Carthami Tinctorii (*Hong Hua*), Semen Pruni Persicae (*Tao Ren*), Radix Ligustici Wallichii (*Chuan Xiong*), Radix Salviae Miltiorrhizae (*Dan Shen*), Herba Leonuri Heterophylli (*Yi Mu Cao*), Resina Olibani (*Ru Xiang*), Resina Myrrhae (*Mo Yao*), Radix Pseudoginseng (*San Qi*), Herba Lycopi Lucidi (*Ze Lan*), Rhizoma Sparganii (*San Leng*), Rhizoma Curcumae Zedoariae (*E Zhu*), Semen Vaccariae Segetalis (*Wang Bu Liu Xing*), Radix Cyathulae Officinalis (*Chuan Niu Xi*), Fructus Crataegi (*Shan Zha*), Rhizoma Corydalis Yanhusuo (*Yan Hu Suo*), Pollen Typhae (*Pu Huang*), Feces Trogopterori Seu Pteromi (*Wu Ling Zhi*)

iii. Commonly used medicinals for clearing heat and cooling the blood: Uncooked Radix Rehmanniae (*Sheng Di*), Cortex Radicis Moutan (*Dan Pi*), Radix Rubrus Paeoniae Lactiflorae (*Chi Shao*)

iv. Commonly used medicinals for securing, astringing & stopping bleeding: Herba Agrimoniae Pilosae (*Xian He Cao*), Crinis Carbonisatus (*Xue Yu Tan*), Radix Rubiae Cordifoliae (*Qian Cao Gen*), Radix Sanguisorbae (*Di Yu*), carbonized Herba Schizonepetae Tenuifoliae (*Jing Jie*), carbonized Rhizoma Zingiberis (*Jiang Tan*), Nodus Nelumbinis Nuciferae (*Ou Jie*), Cacumen Biotae Orientalis (*Ce Bai Ye*), calcined Concha Ostreae (*Mu Li*), Os Sepiae Seu Sepiellae (*Wu Zei Gu*), carbonized Fructus Gardeniae Jasminoidis (*Zhi Zi*), Gelatinum Corii Asini (*E Jiao*), carbonized Petriolus Et Folium Trachycarpi (*Zong Lu Tan*)

2. Fortifying the spleen & harmonizing the stomach

A. Commonly used medicinals for supplementing the spleen and fortifying the stomach: Radix Astragali Membranacei (*Huang Qi*), Radix Codonopsitis Pilosulae (*Dang Shen*), Rhizoma Atractylodis (*Cang Zhu*), Rhizoma Atractylodis Macrocephalae (*Bai Zhu*), Radix Dioscoreae Oppositae (*Shan Yao*), Semen Dolichoris Lablab (*Bian Dou*), Sclerotium Poriae Cocos (*Fu Ling*), Semen Nelumbinis Nuciferae (*Lian Zi*), Semen Euryalis Ferocis (*Qian Shi*), mix-fried Radix Glycyrrhizae (*Gan Cao*), Pericarpium Citri Reticulatae (*Chen Pi*), Endothelium Corneum Gigeriae Galli (*Ji Nei Jin*), Fructus Germinatus Oryzae Sativae (*Gu Ya*), Fructus Zizyphi Jujubae (*Da Zao*)

B. Commonly used medicinals for clearing heat and harmonizing the stomach: Caulis Bambusae In Taeniis (*Zhu Ru*), Radix Scutellariae Baicalensis (*Huang Qin*), Rhizoma Coptidis Chinensis (*Huang Lian*), Rhizoma Phragmitis Communis (*Lu Gen*)

C. Commonly used medicinals for boosting the stomach and nourishing yin: Herba Dendrobii (*Shi Hu*), Radix Pseudostellariae (*Tai Zi Shen*), Radix Glehniae Littoralis (*Sha Shen*), Rhizoma Polygonati Odorati (*Yu Zhu*), Tuber Ophiopogonis Japonici (*Mai Dong*)

D. Commonly used medicinals for warming the stomach and harmonizing the center: Dry Rhizoma Zingiberis (*Gan Jiang*), Fructus Amomi (*Sha Ren*), uncooked Rhizoma Zingiberis (*Sheng Jiang*), Fructus Cardamomi (*Kou Ren*), Flos Caryophylli (*Ding Xiang*), Herba Agastachis Seu Pogostemi (*Huo Xiang*), lime-processed Rhizoma Pinelliae Ternatae (*Fa Xia*)

3. Coursing the liver & nourishing the liver

A. Commonly used medicinals for coursing the liver and resolving depression: Radix Bupleuri (*Chai Hu*), Fructus Meliae Toosendan (*Chuan Lian Zi*), Tuber Curcumae (*Yu Jin*), Rhizoma Cyperi Rotundi (*Xiang Fu*)

B. Commonly used medicinals for clearing heat and draining the liver: Radix Gentianae Scabrae (*Long Dan Cao*), Fructus Gardeniae Jasminoidis (*Zhi Ren*)

C. Commonly used medicinals for nourishing & fostering liver yin: Fructus Ligustri Lucidi (*Nu Zhen Zi*), Radix Albus Paeoniae Lactiflorae (*Bai Shao*), Fructus Mori Albi (*Sang Shen Zi*), Herba Ecliptae Prostratae (*Han Lian Cao*), Fructus Lycii Chinensis (*Gou Qi Zi*)

D. Commonly used medicinals for settling, subduing & leveling[15] the liver: Concha Haliotidis (*Shi Jue Ming*), Ramulus Uncariae Cum Uncis (*Gou Teng*), Os Draconis (*Long Gu*), Concha Ostreae (*Mu Li*), Plastrum Testudinis (*Gui Ban*)

4. Enriching & supplementing the kidneys

A. Commonly used medicinals for enriching the kidneys and nourishing yin: Cooked Radix Rehmanniae (*Shu Di*), Plastrum Testudinis (*Gui Ban*), Gelatinum Corii Asini (*E Jiao*), Rhizoma Polygonati (*Huang Jing*), Fructus Corni Officinalis (*Shan Zhu Rou*), Fructus Lycii Chinensis (*Gou Qi Zi*), Ramulus Loranthi Seu Visci (*Sang Ji Sheng*), Cordyceps Chinensis (*Dong Chong Xia Cao*)

B. Commonly used medicinals for securing the kidneys and supplementing the qi, warming the kidneys and strengthening yang: Gelatinum Cornu Cervi (*Lu Jiao*), Cornu Cervi Degelatinum (*Lu Jiao Shuang*), Semen Cuscutae Chinensis (*Tu Si Zi*), Radix Morindae Officinalis (*Ba Ji Tian*), Cortex Eucommiae Ulmoidis (*Du Zhong*), Herba Epimedii (*Yin Yang Huo*), Rhizoma Curculiginis Orchioidis (*Xian Mao*), Fructus Psoraleae Corylifoliae (*Bu Gu Zhi*), Fructus Alpiniae Oxyphyllae (*Yi Zhi Ren*), Herba Cynomorii Songarici (*Suo Yang*), Cortex Cinnamomi Cassiae (*Rou Gui*), Herba Cistanchis Deserticolae (*Rou Cong Rong*), Ootheca Mantidis (*Sang Piao Xiao*), Placenta Hominis (*Zi He Che*)

C. Commonly used medicinals for enriching yin and subduing yang: Os Draconis (*Long Gu*), Concha Ostreae (*Mu Li*), Plastrum Testudinis (*Gui Ban*), Carapax Amydae Sinensis (*Bie Jia*)

5. Seeping & disinhibiting water & dampness

A. Commonly used medicinals for fortifying the spleen and seeping dampness: Sclerotium Poriae Cocos (*Fu Ling*), Cortex Sclerotii Poriae Cocos (*Fu Ling Pi*), Sichuan Rhizoma Dioscoreae Hypoglaucae (*Chuan Bie Xie*), Semen Coicis Lachryma-jobi (*Yi Yi Ren*), Semen

---

[15] Wiseman translates the Chinese *ping gan* as calming the liver. Although *ping* does mean peaceful or calm, its character describes something horizontally level. Since levelling the liver is specifically used when liver ascends hyperactively or liver wind counterflows upward, this spatial connotation is, I believe, important for understanding what calming or levelling the liver really means and helps clarify the necessity of using heavy, subduing, and repressing medicinals.

Plantaginis (*Che Qian Zi*), Sclerotium Polypori Umbellati (*Zhu Ling*), Rhizoma Alismatis (*Ze Xie*), earth stir-fried Rhizoma Atractylodis Macrocephalae (*Bai Zhu*), Rhizoma Atractylodis (*Cang Zhu*), Semen Dolichoris Lablab (*Bian Dou*)

B. Commonly used medicinals for disinhibiting dampness and clearing heat: Herba Artemisiae Capillaris (*Yin Chen*), Rhizoma Smilacis Glabrae (*Tu Fu Ling*), Herba Patrinae Heterophyllae Cum Radice (*Bai Jiang Cao*), Cortex Phellodendri (*Huang Bai*), Flos Lonicerae Japonicae (*Jin Yin Hua*), Herba Taraxaci Mongolici Cum Radice (*Pu Gong Ying*), Herba Violae Yedoensitis Cum Radice (*Zi Hua Di Ding*), Herba Oldenlandiae Diffusae (*Bai Hua She She Cao*), Radix Sophorae Flavescentis (*Ku Shen*), Semen Plantaginis (*Che Qian Zi*), Fructus Kochiae Scopariae (*Di Fu Zi*)

6. Warming the channels (or menses) and scattering cold

Commonly used medicinals for warming the channels and scattering cold: Fructus Evodiae Rutecarpae (*Wu Zhu Yu*), Folium Artemisiae Argyii (*Ai Ye*), Ramulus Cinnamomi Cassiae (*Gui Zhi*), Radix Ligustici Wallichii (*Chuan Xiong*), Fructus Foeniculi Vulgaris (*Xiao Hui Xiang*), dry Rhizoma Zingiberis (*Gan Jiang*), Radix Angelicae Dahuricae (*Bai Zhi*), Fructus Psoraleae Corylifoliae (*Bu Gu Zhi*), Radix Lateralis Praeparatus Aconiti Carmichaeli (*Fu Pian*)

Commonly used treatment principles & methods for regulating the liver in menstrual disease

Because liver depression is such a commonly seen disease mechanism and pattern in Western women, it is especially important for Western practitioners to have as good an idea as possible about treating liver depression. When there is liver depression qi stagnation, it is almost universally in combination with one or more other disease mechanisms. Therefore, it is important to know how to course the liver and resolve depression at the same time as treating other aspects of the total pattern.

1. Liver qi depression & binding

The liver holds the office of general. Its nature likes orderly reaching and is averse to restraint and depression. Anything that leads to one's essence spirit emotions stirring excessively may lead to a loss of normalcy in the liver's coursing and discharge. This then results in the liver channel qi becoming depressed. In women, this may manifest in liver qi depression diseases such as menstrual irregularities, premenstrual breast distention, breast nodules and lumps, infertility, and even visceral agitation.

Treatment principles: Use aromatic, penetrating density and depression ingredients to course the liver, rectify the qi, and resolve depression

Guiding formula: Fructus Akebiae Trifoliatae (*Ba Yue Zha*), Rhizoma Cyperi Rotundi (*Xiang Fu*), Tuber Curcumae (*Yu Jin*), Cortex Albizziae Julibrissin (*He Huan Pi*), Folium Citri Reticulatae (*Ju Ye*), Radix Linderae Strychnifoliae (*Wu Yao*), Fructus Liquidambaris Taiwaniae (*Lu Lu Tong*), Radix Ligustici Wallichii (*Chuan Xiong*), Radix Bupleuri (*Chai Hu*), Flos Rosae Rugosae (*Mei Gui Hua*), Flos Pruni Mume (*Lu Mei Hua*)

2. Liver depression with simultaneous dampness

If there is liver qi depression and binding and its functions of coursing and discharge are obstructed, spleen and stomach qi will not transport and the spleen is checked and overwhelmed. In that case, the movement of water dampness loses its normal condition. Then dampness and turbidity may obstruct the center or phlegm fat may pour downwards. The manifestation of this in terms of gynecological disease are continuous vaginal discharge, scanty menstruation, blocked menstruation, and infertility.

Treatment principles: Diffuse depression and move stagnation, fortify the spleen and transform dampness

Guiding formula: Rhizoma Cyperi Rotundi (*Xiang Fu*), Pericarpium Arecae Catechu (*Da Fu Pi*), Fructus Citri Aurantii (*Zhi Ke*), Fructus Amomi (*Sha Ren*), Rhizoma Atractylodis (*Cang Zhu*), Rhizoma Atractylodis Macrocephalae (*Bai Zhu*), uncooked Fructus Crataegi (*Shan Zha*), Semen Phaseoli Calcarati (*Chi Xiao Dou*), Cortex Sclerotii Poriae Cocos (*Fu Ling Pi*), uncooked Cortex Rhizomatis Zingiberis (*Sheng Jiang Pi*), ginger-processed Rhizoma Pinelliae Ternatae (*Ban Xia*), Flos Dolichoris Lablab (*Bian Dou Hua*), Rhizoma Alismatis (*Ze Xie*), Rhizoma Acori Graminei (*Shi Chang Pu*), Tuber Curcumae (*Yu Jin*)

3. Qi depression & food stagnation

In the above pattern, liver depression overwhelms the spleen and water dampness is then difficult to transport. This pattern may also lead to liver wood invading the stomach in which case, accumulated food is not transformed. Most cases of this occur in persons whose body is vacuous and weak, for instance postpartum or after disease when one is still not feeling well. This may also occur if one is not careful in their food and drink which then results in their epigastrium and abdomen becoming full, distended, and oppressed. In that case, one may have hiccup, acid regurgitation, diminished appetite, nausea, etc. In women, this pattern is also seen due to disharmony of the liver and stomach after artificial abortion. In that case, there is diminished appetite and abdominal distention.

Treatment principles: Open depression and harmonize the stomach assisted by dispersing the food

Guiding formula: Rhizoma Pinelliae Ternatae (*Xian Ban Xia*), northern Semen Panici Italici (*Bei Shu Mi*), Pericarpium Citri Reticulatae (*Ju Pi*), Retinervus Fasicularis Citri Reticulatae (*Ju Luo*), Tuber Curcumae (*Yu Jin*), Flos Pruni Mume (*Lu Mei Hua*), Flos Rosae Rugosae (*Mei Gui Hua*), Sclerotium Poriae Cocos (*Fu Ling*), Corneum Endothelium Gigeriae Galli (*Ji Nei Jin*), Radix Pseudostellariae (*Tai Zi Shen*), Herba Dendrobii (*Shi Hu*), carbonized Fructus Crataegi (*Shan Zha*), Rhizoma Acori Graminei (*Shi Chang Pu*)

4. Liver channel damp heat

If the seven emotions are beyond limit, liver qi may counterflow, and depressive wood heat becomes ablaze. The five emotions transform into fire. Therefore, tension, agitation, and easy anger may easily lead to liver fire flaring upward. If there is fire and heat in the liver channel, blood may counterflow and qi become chaotic. In women, this mostly leads to early menstruation and profuse menstruation whose color is purple. It is also possible to see menstrual movement epistaxis and hemoptysis, dizziness and headache, red eyes, tinnitus, vexation and agitation, and insomnia. If depressive fire binds internally and simultaneously damp toxins invade from outside, internal fire and external toxins may mutually wrestle, causing steaming sores in the lower burner. In women, this mostly manifests as menstrual irregularity, yellowish red vaginal discharge, and lower abdominal burning pain associated with either acute or chronic pelvic inflammatory disease.

Treatment principles: Treat counterflow by levelling it; treat heat by clearing it

Guiding formula: *Long Dan Xie Gan Tang* (Gentiana Drain the Liver Decoction) or Cortex Phellodendri (*Huang Bai*), Rhizoma Coptidis Chinensis (*Huang Lian*), processed Radix Et Rhizoma Rhei (*Da Huang*), Radix Rubrus Paeoniae Lactiflorae (*Chi Shao*), Herba Patriniae Heterophyllae Cum Radice (*Bai Jiang Cao*), Radix Linderae Strychnifoliae (*Wu Yao*), processed Resina Myrrhae (*Mo Yao*), and other ingredients depending upon the symptoms

5. Cold congelation in the liver channel

Most liver diseases are hot patterns. However, if liver qi is insufficient and liver function loses command, cold damp evils may congeal and stagnate in the liver channel. In men this can cause cold *shan* abdominal pain, while in women it causes cold congelation menstrual pain and lower abdominal qi surging. In women, infertility is commonly due to liver-kidney cold dampness retention and stagnation. This may be due to overtaxation, fatigue, and lack of strength, constitutional insufficiency of qi, or possible lack of care during menstruation and birthing, in which case wind cold enters the lower body. This then congeals in the *jue yin* in the lower abdomen.

Treatment principles: Warm the liver, warm the channels (or menses), and scatter cold

Guiding formula: Fructus Foeniculi Vulgaris (*Xiao Hui Xiang*), scalded Fructus Evodiae Rutecarpae (*Wu Zhu Yu*), Cortex Cinnamomi Cassiae (*Rou Gui*), Folium Artemisiae Argyii (*Ai Ye*), Semen Litchi Sinensis (*Li Zhi He*), Semen Citri Reticulatae (*Ju He*), Radix Linderae Strychnifoliae (*Wu Yao*). While using this formula, do not use yin, cold, enriching, slimy ingredients. However, after the symptoms are relieved, it is appropriate to nourish the blood and warmly open, assisted by quickening the network vessels.

6. Yin vacuity, liver effulgence

In this pattern, liver form (*i.e.*, yin) is insufficient. Women have a tendency toward liver-kidney dual vacuity. It is also possible during menstruation for constructive blood to precipitate and desert. During pregnancy, the constructive blood flows downward to the uterus to gather and nourish the fetal origin. And during old age, water and blood may be withered and water no longer moistens wood. In any of these cases, the liver form loses its nourishment. Hence liver yang may become hyperactive and rise up. In that case, one may see dizziness and vertigo, heart palpitations, loss of sleep, vexation and agitation, etc. In addition, there may be premenstrual headache, visceral agitation, or even perimenopausal syndrome.

Treatment principles: Nourish yin and subdue yang, foster yin and clear the liver

Guiding formula: Fructus Lycii Chinensis (*Qi Zi*), mix-fried Radix Glycyrrhizae (*Gan Cao*), uncooked Radix Albus Paeoniae Lactiflorae (*Bai Shao*), Semen Zizyphi Spinosae (*Suan Zao Ren*), uncooked Radix Rehmanniae (*Sheng Di*), Radix Polygoni Multiflori (*Shou Wu*), Bulbus Lilii (*Bai He*), Tuber Ophiopogonis Japonici (*Mai Dong*), Radix Angelicae Sinensis (*Dang Gui*), Fructus Tribuli Terrestris (*Bai Ji Li*), Fructus Tritici Aestivi (*Huai Xiao Mai*), Fructus Zizyphi Jujubae (*Hong Zao*)

7. Blood vacuity, wind stirring

In this pattern, liver form is also insufficient. The liver stores the blood and rules the sinews. If yin blood suddenly becomes exhausted, the liver loses its nourishment and the sinews are moistened by scanty blood and thus become nonfunctional. The commonly seen manifestations of this condition are arched back rigidity, clenched teeth, convulsive spasms, etc. In women, postpartum blood loss may be excessive. It is also possible for wind to make a surprise attack postpartum. This easily leads to this pattern.

Treatment principles: Enrich yin and nourish blood, emolliate the liver and track down wind

Guiding formula: Uncooked Radix Rehmanniae (*Sheng Di*), cooked Radix Rehmanniae (*Shu Di*), Radix Albus Paeoniae Lactiflorae (*Bai Shao*), Fructus Corni Officinalis (*Zhu Rou*), Fructus Lycii Chinensis (*Qi Zi*), Fructus Tribuli Terrestris (*Ji Li*), Cortex Radicis Moutan (*Dan Pi*), Gelatinum Corii Asini (*E Jiao*), Ramulus Uncariae Cum Uncis (*Gou Teng*), sweet Flos Chrysanthemi Morifolii (*Gan Ju Hua*), uncooked Concha Ostreae (*Mu Li*), Plastrum Testudinis (*Gui Ban*), Carapax Amydae Sinensis (*Bie Jia*)

8. Liver reversal[16]

If liver yin and yang lose their regulation (or balance), qi and blood may counterflow and become chaotic. Clinically, one may see the manifestations of liver reversal pattern. Liver reversal is also called qi reversal. The lungs command respiration and rule all the external qi of the body. The liver rules coursing and discharge and commands all the internal qi of the body. Liver reversal is mostly due to counterflow due to the emotions. Anger leads to ascent of qi. Thus qi and blood simultaneously rush upward, obstructing and blocking the clear portals. Therefore there is dimness reversal (*i.e.*, syncope) and falling down. In women, emotional frustration, jealousy and anger, vexation and agitation, and restlessness and depression may lead to yin and yang qi becoming chaotic. This results in dizziness and vertigo, falling down, and even loss of consciousness of human affairs with convulsive spasms of the four limbs.

Treatment pinciples: Settle the liver, clear and soothe, wash away phlegm and open depression

Guiding formula: Powdered Margarita (*Zhen Zhu Fen*) or Concha Margaritiferae (*Zhen Zhu Mu*), Magnetitum (*Ling Ci Shi*), Tuber Curcumae (*Yu Jin*), Rhizoma Acori Graminei (*Shi Chang Pu*), Cortex Albizziae Julibrissin (*He Huan Pi*), uncooked Radix Albus Paeoniae Lactiflorae (*Bai Shao*), Fructus Ligustri Lucidi (*Nu Zhen Zi*), Concretio Silicea Bambusae (*Tian Zhu Huang*), Succus Lophatheri Gracilis (*Dan Zhu Li*), cinnabar-processed Medulla Junci Effusi (*Deng Xin*)

Supporting the righteous while resolving depression in gynecology

Most Western women with liver depression qi stagnation suffer from some simulataneous vacuity. Therefore, in clinical practice it is typically necessary to course the liver and resolve depression at the same time as supporting the righteous.

1. Fostering yin & resolving depression

The liver viscus in form is yin but in function is yang. If liver depression is enduring and is not

---

[16] Wiseman's previous term for reversal was inversion.

healed by coursing or if the condition is severe, liver form will lose its nature of being moist and soft. In that case, constructive yin will become insufficient and form or physical yin will become deficient and subject to detriment. If liver qi depression and stagnation or enduring depression has transformed into fire and damaged yin, clinically this may manifest as early menstruation, profuse menstruation, premenstrual breast distention, chest oppression and vexation, possible vexatious heat in the five hearts, restless sleep at night, possible dry, bound stools, a tongue with a red tip, and a bowstring, fine pulse which may also be rapid. These may occur with premenstrual tension or perimenopausal syndrome.

Treatment principles: Nourish the form of liver yin, course the function of liver wood

Guiding formula: Uncooked Radix Rehmanniae (*Sheng Di*), uncooked Radix Albus Paeoniae Lactiflorae (*Bai Shao*), Cortex Radicis Lycii (*Di Gu Pi*), cinnabar-processed Tuber Ophiopogonis Japonici (*Mai Dong*), Cortex Albizziae Julibrissin (*He Huan Pi*), Radix Glehniae Littoralis (*Bei Sha Shen*), Rhizoma Polygonati Odorati (*Yu Zhu*), Fructus Akebiae Trifoliatae (*Ba Yue Zha*), Fructus Meliae Toosendan (*Chuan Lian Zi*), Flos Pruni Mume (*Lu Mei Hua*), Fructus Levis Tritici (*Huai Xiao Mai*), etc. based on the patient's signs and symptoms

2. Supporting the spleen & resolving depression

In case of enduring liver depression, constructive yin may not be damaged but spleen earth may be invaded. Liver disease commonly affects the spleen or overwhelms the stomach. According to Fu Qing-zhu:

> If with the stools there is precipitated excessive blood, the essence spirit is short and scanty, and the person is emaciated, this is related to liver qi not being soothed. Enduring depression thus damages the spleen. If the spleen is damaged, it is not able to contain the blood...

In this case, postpartum and after miscarriage, the muscles and body may be vacuous and weak, the essence spirit may not be clear, the patient may be subject to fright and worry, and one may also see irregularity in stomach and intestinal function, premenstrual tension, menstrual movement diarrhea, and other such symptoms due to spleen vacuity and liver depression.

Treatment principles: Nourish the blood and support the spleen, rectify the qi and resolve depression

Guiding formula: Radix Pseudostellariae (*Tai Zi Shen*), Radix Albus Paeoniae Lactiflorae (*Bai Shao*), cinnabar-processed Tuber Ophiopogonis Japonici (*Mai Dong*), cinnabar-processed Sclerotium Poriae Cocos (*Fu Ling*), Fructus Akebiae Trifoliatae (*Ba Yue Zha*), Flos Dolichoris Lablab (*Bian Dou Hua*), Fructus Piperis Cubebae (*Bi Cheng Qie*), Rhizoma Pinelliae Ternatae (*Xian Ban Xia*), Flos Rosae Rugosae (*Mei Gui Hua*), Pericarpium Citri Reticulatae (*Ju Pi*),

Retinervus Fasicularis Citri Reticulatae (*Ju Luo*), etc. according to the patient's signs and symptoms

3. Boosting the kidneys & resolving depression

Liver wood and kidney water have a mother-son mutual relationship and *bing* and *gui* share a common source.[17] The liver's coursing, discharge, and orderly reaching and its function of regulating and disciplining blood flow depend upon the kidneys' self-restraint. The kidneys receive the essence of the five viscera snd six bowels, including liver-gallbladder essence blood, and then treasures these. This results in kidney essence being full and sufficient. In liver depression pattern, if liver yin has been vacuous and subject to detriment for a long time, eventually this will also affect the kidneys, leading to liver-kidney insufficiency. In women, the liver and kidneys are the root of the *chong* and *ren*. Therefore, liver-kidney disease will also affect the *chong* and *ren*. If the kidneys are vacuous and the liver qi is not regulated, this will mostly manifest as blocked menstruation, infertility, and pre- and postmenstrual symptoms.

Treatment principles: Boost the kidneys and resolve depression. Boosting the kidneys mostly means filling and supplementing kidney essence and enriching and nourishing the liver and kidneys.

Guiding formula: Cooked Radix Rehmanniae (*Shu Di*), Herba Dendrobii (*Shi Hu Ye*), Herba Epimedii (*Xian Ling Pi*), Semen Cuscutae Chinensis (*Tu Si Zi*), Cornu Cervi (*Lu Jiao Pian*), Radix Angelicae Sinensis (*Dang Gui*), Radix Albus Paeoniae Lactiflorae (*Bai Shao*), etc. depending on the patient's signs and symptoms. In order to course liver qi, use Fructus Akebiae Trifoliatae (*Ba Yue Zha*), Fructus Liquidambaris Taiwaniae (*Lu Lu Tong*), small Pericarpium Citri Reticulatae Viride (*Qing Pi*), uncooked Fructus Germinatus Hordei Vulgaris (*Mai Ya*), etc.

Important points in using fragrant, aromatic, coursing the liver & rectifying the qi medicinals in menstrual diseases

The medicinals used for rectifying the qi and resolving depression are all windy, upbearing, drying, and aromatic ones. Because these medicinals are almost the same in nature to exterior-resolving medicinals, they easily damage yin used inappropriately or unwarrantedly. For instance, Radix Bupleuri (*Chai Hu*) is one of the most commonly used Chinese medicinals for coursing the liver and rectifying the qi. However, this medicinal is not categorized as a qi-rectifying medicinal but as an exterior-resolver. Below are some guidelines on using liver-coursing, qi-rectifying medicinals safely and effectively.

---

[17] *Bing* is the heavenly stem corresponding to liver wood, while *gui* is the heavenly stem corresponding to kidney water.

1. Fragrant, aromatic medicinal substances are very aromatic and dry and thus easily damage yin. Therefore, in order to prevent liver form vacuity and weakness, one should combine such medicinals with one or two ingredients which are emolliating and moistening, such as Radix Albus Paeoniae Lactiflorae (*Bai Shao*) and Radix Angelicae Sinensis (*Dang Gui*). It is also important not to use fragrant, aromatic medicinals for prolonged periods of time and to stop them as soon as they are no longer needed.

2. Liver depression easily transforms into heat. If the tongue has yellow, slimy fur and the pulse is bowstring and rapid, depression is not resolved and heat is exuberant internally. In that case, it is appropriate to resolve depression and move the qi accompanied by medicinals which clear the liver and discharge heat. For instance, in *Yue Ju Wan* (Escape Restraint Pills), there is both Rhizoma Cyperi Rotundi (*Xiang Fu*) and Fructus Gardeniae Jasminoidis (*Zhi Zi*).

3. If, in depression patterns, there is a red tongue tip and scanty fur, the yin division has also been damaged. In that case, it is appropriate to first use ingredients which enrich yin and nourish the blood. If depression is not resolved, it is OK to add a small amount of qi-moving medicinals. For instance, in the treatment of depressive heat, withered blood blocked menstruation with *Yi Guan Qian* (One Link Decoction), there is the single flavor, Fructus Meliae Toosendan (*Chuan Lian Zi*).[18]

4. Fragrant, aromatic, qi-moving medicinals should not be used in too great amounts. For instance, Flos Pruni Mume (*Lu Mei Hua*), Fructus Citri Medicae (*Xiang Yuan*), Fructus Citri Sacrodactylis (*Fo Shou*), Fructus Amomi (*Sha Ren*), and Radix Linderae Strychnifoliae (*Wu Yao*) should all be prescribed at between 3-6g. Flos Citri Aurantii (*Dai Dai Hua*), Fructus Piperis Longi (*Bi Ba*), and Rhizoma Nardostachytis (*Gan Song*) should each be 1.5-3g.

5. The fragrant, aromatic medicinals Flos Rosae Rugosae (*Mei Gui Hua*) and Flos Et Fructus Rosae Chinensis (*Yue Ji Hua*) can both be used to resolve depression. However, their use is not exactly the same. Flos Rosae Rugosae is suitable for use when the menstruation is excessive or when there is diarrhea since it has a stopping, and astringing ability. Conversely, Flos Et Fructus Rosae Chinensis is suitable for use in blocked menstruation and dry, bound stools.

6. When decocting such medicinals, Flos Rosae Rugosae (*Mei Gui Hua*), Flos Citri Aurantii (*Dai Dai Hua*), and Fructus Amomi (*Sha Ren*) should be added at the end of the decocting process. It is not appropriate for these to be cooked for a long period of time. Prolonged cooking of fragrant, aromatic medicinals scatters their qi and flavor thus losing and weakening their medicinal benefits.

---

[18] In the Chinese medical literature, medicinals are either referred to as medicinals (*yao*), materials (*wu*), or flavors (*wei*).

Commonly used treatment methods & principles for quickening the blood & transforming stasis in menstrual diseases

Blood stasis is a very commonly seen disease mechanism and pattern in women's menstrual disease. It may be either the main mechanism and pattern or a concomitant mechanism and pattern. Therefore it is important for TCM gynecology practitioners to know how to treat blood stasis both when it occurs alone and when it occurs in combination with other disease mechanisms and patterns. Below are treatment methods all having to do with blood stasis.

1. Stopping bleeding & transforming stasis method

This method is used in the treatment of uterine bleeding which has gone on for a long time, is dribbling and dripping, and will not be cut off or has only recently been stopped. The color of the blood is purple and dark, there is lower abdominal distention and pain, and the tongue is purplish. In this case, static blood is not finished, the qi mechanism is not disinhibited, and new blood is not being engendered. In this case, one should use medicinals such as: Radix Pseudoginseng (*San Qi*), Radix Rubiae Cordifoliae (*Qian Cao*), Herba Leonuri Heterophylli (*Yi Mu Cao*), Pollen Typhae (*Pu Huang*), Sanguis Draconis (*Xue Jie*), and Herba Chenopodii Hybridi (*Xue Jian Chou*).

2. Rectifying the qi & transforming stasis method

This method is used when there are lower abdominal concretions and conglomerations, accumulations and gatherings with pain which does not move or alter or there may also be pressure pain. In addition, there may be breast swelling and lumps with distention and pain. In this case, there is qi stagnation and blood stasis, the qi mechanism is obstructed, and, because there is no free flow, there is pain. The commonly used medicinals are: Fructus Immaturus Citri Aurantii (*Zhi Shi*), Pericarpium Citri Reticulatae Viride (*Qing Pi*), Radix Linderae Strychnifoliae (*Wu Yao*), Guangdong Radix Auklandiae Lappae (*Guang Mu Xiang*), Fructus Citri Sacrodactylis (*Fo Shou*), Rhizoma Corydalis Yanhusuo (*Yan Hu Suo*), Radix Ligustici Wallichii (*Chuan Xiong*), Tuber Curcumae (*Yu Jin*), Radix Platycodi Grandiflori (*Jie Geng*), Semen Citri Reticulatae (*Ju He*), Rhizoma Cyperi Rotundi (*Xiang Fu*), Rhizoma Curcumae Zedoariae (*E Zhu*), Retinervus Fascicularis Luffae (*Si Gua Luo*), Feces Trogopterori Seu Pteromi (*Wu Ling Zhi*), Pollen Typhae (*Pu Huang*), Radix Angelicae Sinensis (*Dang Gui*), Radix Rubrus Paeoniae Lactiflorae (*Chi Shao*), Flos Carthami Tinctorii (*Hong Hua*), and Semen Pruni Persicae (*Tao Ren*).

3. Percolating, seeping & transforming stasis method

This method is used when there is damp heat in the lower burner with continuous abnormal vaginal discharge, lurking lower abdominal pain, low back soreness and upper back distention and possible fallopian tube inflammation or water swelling and accumulated fluids. The affected area usually has distention, pain, and pressure pain. The commonly used medicinals are: Herba Lycopi Lucidi (*Ze Lan*), Herba Verbenae Officinalis (*Ma Bian Cao*), Herba Patrinae Hetero-phyllae Cum Radice (*Bai Jiang Cao*), Succinum (*Hu Po*), Semen Coicis Lachryma-jobi (*Yi Yi Ren*), Semen Benincasae Hispidae (*Dong Gua Ren*), Rhizoma Atractylodis Macrocephalae (*Bai Zhu*), Sclerotium Poriae Cocos (*Fu Ling*), Semen Plantaginis (*Che Qian Zi*), Semen Pruni Persicae (*Tao Ren*), Radix Angelicae Sinensis (*Dang Gui*), Radix Rubrus Paeoniae Lactiflorae (*Chi Shao*), and Cortex Radicis Moutan (*Dan Pi*).

4. Scattering cold & transforming stasis method

This method is used when there are deep-lying cold evils internally which have become mutually bound with the blood causing lower abdominal concretions and bindings which have not been dispersed for many days. In this case, qi and blood flow dawdles. There is fear of cold, chilled limbs, and the affected area desires warmth. There may be breast swelling and lumps, enduring binding which is not transformed, and neither pain nor heat. The commonly used medicinals are: Radix Lateralis Praeparatus Aconiti Carmichaeli (*Fu Zi*), Ramulus Cinnamomi Cassiae (*Gui Zhi*), Cortex Cinnamomi Cassiae (*Rou Gui*), dry Rhizoma Zingiberis (*Gan Jiang*), Fructus Evodiae Rutecarpae (*Wu Zhu Yu*), Gelatinum Cornu Cervi (*Lu Jiao Jiao*), Herba Ephedrae (*Ma Huang*), Radix Clematidis Chinensis (*Wei Ling Xian*), Rhizoma Curcumae Zedoariae (*E Zhu*), Rhizoma Sparganii (*San Leng*), Radix Salviae Miltiorrhizae (*Dan Shen*), Hirudo (*Shui Zhi*), Radix Angelicae Sinensis (*Dang Gui*), Radix Ligustici Wallichii (*Chuan Xiong*), Semen Pruni Persicae (*Tao Ren*), and Radix Astragali Membranacei (*Huang Qi*).

5. Freeing the stools & transforming stasis method

This method is used in cases of acute pelvic inflammation or chronic pelvic inflammation which has become acute again, acute stage fallopian tube inflammation, etc. accompanied by constipation. The commonly used medicinals are: Radix Et Rhizoma Rhei (*Da Huang*), and Mirabilitum (*Mang Xiao*) to free the stools, plus Cortex Radicis Moutan (*Dan Pi*), Radix Salviae Miltiorrhizae (*Dan Shen*), Semen Pruni Persicae (*Tao Ren*), Radix Rubrus Paeoniae Lactiflorae (*Chi Shao*), Herba Patriniae Heterophyllae Cum Radice (*Bai Jiang Cao*), Radix Angelicae Sinensis (*Dang Gui*), Radix Angelicae Dahuricae (*Bai Zhi*), Caulis Sargentodoxae (*Hong Teng*), Herba Taraxaci Mongolici Cum Radice (*Pu Gong Ying*), and Hirudo (*Shui Zhi*) to clear heat and resolve toxins, quicken the blood and transform stasis.

6. Dispersing swelling & transforming stasis method

This method is used for the treatment of mastitis and acute reproductive tract infections when the affected area has pressure pain or rebound pain and there is fever. The commonly used

129

medicinals are: Radix Rubrus Paeoniae Lactilforae (*Chi Shao*), Cortex Radicis Moutan (*Dan Pi*), Radix Angelicae Dahuricae (*Bai Zhi*), Spina Gleditschiae Chinensis (*Zao Jiao Ci*), Squama Manitis Pentadactylis (*Chuan Shan Jia*), Fructus Trichosanthis Kirlowii (*Quan Gua Lou*), Resina Olibani (*Ru Xiang*), Resina Myrrhae (*Mo Yao*), Radix Trichosanthis Kirlowii (*Hua Fen*), and Radix Angelicae Sinensis (*Dang Gui*).

7. Supporting the righteous & transforming stasis method

If qi has been stagnant and blood static for a prolonged time, the body will eventually become weak and qi and blood will become insufficient. Yin and yang both become vacuous. Thus, in the midst of repletion there is vacuity. Hence supplementation should take priority or one should attack and supplement at the same time. In any case, it is important to attack without damaging the righteous. The commonly used medicinals in this situation are: Radix Astragali Membranacei (*Huang Qi*), Radix Angelicae Sinensis (*Dang Gui*), Radix Codonopsitis Pilosuale (*Dang Shen*), Caulis Milletiae Seu Spatholobi (*Ji Xue Teng*), Radix Salviae Miltiorrhizae (*Dan Shen*), Radix Rubrus Paeoniae Lactiflorae (*Chi Shao*), Radix Ligustici Wallichii (*Chuan Xiong*), cooked Radix Rehmanniae (*Shu Di*), and Gelatinum Cornu Cervi (*Lu Jiao Jiao*).

8. Opening the channels (or menses) & transforming stasis method

This method is used in cases of blocked menstruation or painful menstruation when the transportation and movement of qi and blood is inhibited and the color of the menstruate is puplish black and contains lumps. There is fixed pain in the lower abdomen. If severe, the whole body may be overcome. The commonly used medicinals are: Herba Leonuri Heterophylli (*Yi Mu Cao*), Radix Angelicae Sinensis (*Dang Gui*), Flos Carthami Tinctorii (*Hong Hua*), Radix Ligustici Wallichii (*Chuan Xiong*), Feces Trogopterori Seu Pteromi (*Wu Ling Zhi*), Radix Cyathulae Officinalis (*Chuan Niu Xi*), Rhizoma Cyperi Rotundi (*Xiang Fu*), Herba Lycopi Lucidi (*Ze Lan*), and Cortex Radicis Moutan (*Dan Pi*).

9. Softening the hard & transforming stasis method

The breasts may have swellings and lumps or there may be uterine myomas or fibroids. If one has used the typical qi-rectifying and blood-quickening medicinals but without full success, one may then consider using softening the hard and nodulation-scattering medicinals. Some of the commonly used medicinals in this case are: Carapax Amydae Sinensis (*Bie Jia*), Concha Ostreae (*Mu Li*), Spica Prunellae Vulgaris (*Xia Ku Cao*), Herba Sargassii (*Hai Zao*), Sal Ammoniac (*Nao Sha*), Potassium Nitrate (*Xiao Shi*), Semen Polygoni Orientalis (*Shui Hong Hua Zi*), Squama Manitis Pentadactylis (*Chuan Shan Jia*), Spina Gleditschiae Chinensis (*Zao Jiao Ci*), Radix Salviae Miltiorrhizae (*Dan Shen*), Radix Clematidis Chinensis (*Wei Ling Xian*), and Semen Vaccariae Segetalis (*Wang Bu Liu Xing*).

When it comes to eliminating blood stasis, one can *huo xue hua yu* or quicken the blood and transform stasis, *qu yu huo xue* or dispel stasis and quicken the blood, *po yu* or break stasis, or *po yu xiao zheng*, break stasis and disperse concretions. Each of these is a stronger, more forceful attacking therapy. Their use depends upon the relative seriousness of the blood stasis ranging from insubstantial to substantial stagnation. If too strong a method is employed or is employed too long, this will result in damage to the blood. It is also possible to *qu yu sheng xin*. This means to dispel stasis in order to promote the engenderment and transformation of new (blood). If a woman suffers from both blood stasis and blood emptiness, it is necessary to eliminate stasis at the same time as attempting to supplement and enrich the blood. If one attempts to supplement the blood without first eliminating the stasis, this may result in a worsening of the stasis and will not result in the engenderment of new blood.

In addition, it is said:

> New diseases are in the channels. Enduring diseases enter the network vessels.

The clinical implication of this saying is that, if blood stasis endures over a long time, this stasis will enter the network vessels. When stasis enters the network vessels. Specific medicinals must be used based on the principles of quickening the blood and freeing the flow of the network vessels. Such medicinals may be divided into three main categories: 1) resins, 2) "insects", and 3) network vessel like medicinals.

Resinous medicinals which enter the network vessels and quicken the blood and free the flow of the network vessels include: Resina Olibani (*Ru Xiang*), Resina Myrrhae (*Mo Yao*), Sanguis Draconis (*Xue Jie*), Succinum (*Hu Po*), and Resina Liquidambaris Taiwaniae (*Feng Xiang Zhi* or *Bai Jiao Xiang*). These medicinals are able to enter the network vessels the same way as tree sap is able to permeate and wend its way through all the reticular nooks and crannies of a tree.

The Chinese word *chong* is very difficult to translate. Wiseman gives both worms and insects but also agrees that this word may be left in Pinyin. This is because the word *chong* covers insects and worms, but it also covers reptiles and amphibians, such as snakes, lizards, and frogs. In English, there really is no one word that covers all these animals. In any case, there are a number of *chong* medicinals which enter the network vessels the same way that insects can insinuate themselves into the smallest cracks as they hunt their prey. Those "insect" medicinals which quicken the blood and free the flow of the network vessels include: Eupolyphaga Seu Opisthoplatia (*Di Bie Chong*), Lumbricus (*Di Long*), Buthus Martensis (*Quan Xie*), Scolopendra Subspinipes (*Wu Gong*), Hirudo (*Shui Zhi*), Tabanus (*Meng Chong*), and Squama Manitis Pentadactylis (*Chuan Shan Jia*). These last are the scales of the scaley anteater which shows how difficult it is to find an English equivalent of the Chinese concept *chong*.

The last main category of medicinals which enter and free the flow of the network vessels are medicinals whose shape is that of a network. These include: Retinervus Fascicularis Luffae Cylindricae (*Si Gua Luo*) and Retinervus Fascicularis Citri Reticulatae (*Ju Luo*). Another medicinal with a pronounced ability to enter the network vessels but which does not fit into any of the above three categories is Lignum Sappan (*Su Mu*). It is said that if one makes a strong decoction of this medicinal and leaves it overnight in a glass jar that, in the morning, some of this liquid will have migrated through the porosities of the glass. In any case, this medicinal is clinically effective for treating patterns characterized by stasis in the network vessels.

When there is both qi stagnation and blood stasis, it is not uncommon for the blood stasis to resolve first and then the stagnant qi. In terms of painful menstruation, this often means that a patient who experienced both sharp, stabbing, localized pain as well as diffuse, colicky, cramping pain may, in the first months after initiation of therapy, experience the disappearance of the sharp pain but the colicky, cramping pain may continue. In such cases, it is important that the practitioner up-date the patient's pattern discriminaton and alter their treatment principles accordingly. In such a case, the emphasis should change from dispelling stasis to rectifying the qi. If such a change in therapeutic strategy is not made, the practitioner will iatrogenically damage the blood.

Because the menstruation itself is a discharge of blood, patients with blood stasis should be treated more intensively just prior to and during the first couple of days of the menses in order to quicken the blood and dispel stasis. This stasis can then be discharged from the body during the menses. Such intensive treatment may include both internal medicine, externally applied plasters, poultices, and compresses, and acupuncture and moxibustion.

As mentioned above, each menstruation is a report card and this is especially the case with blood stasis. However, sometimes the report may be misleading to the neophyte practitioner. The first menstruation after initiating therapy may actually be more painful than before. This may frighten both the unknowing practitioner and the patient. If, however, the pattern discrimination was correct and the therapy administered based on that diagnosis was appropriate, such a seeming aggravation is a sign that the body is attempting to break down and discharge the static blood. In this case, one should feel confident that the next menstruation will be markedly better than before initiating therapy both in terms of pain and the color and quality of the menstruate.

Similarly, during the first menses or so after initiating blood stasis eliminating therapy, the patient's clots may be either bigger or smaller, or more or less numerous. In all these cases, if the therapy has been correctly chosen and applied, these are potentially good signs. If the clots are bigger, it means the blood stasis is being expelled *en masse*. If they are smaller, it means the blood stasis has been broken or cracked before being expelled. If there are more clots, this also suggests the body is discharging the blood stasis. Whereas if there are markedly less clots, one may feel confident that quickening of the blood has resulted in transformation of the stasis.

Commonly used treatment principles & methods for clearing heat & eliminating dampness in menstrual diseases

It is not uncommon to find damp heat complicating the treatment of Western gynecological patients. In large part this has to do with our Western diet which tends to damage the spleen and engender dampness. Then, either dampness causes or aggravates qi depression which transforms into heat, resulting in damp heat, or overeating hot, acrid, peppery foods and drinking alcohol helps transform dampness into heat. Therefore, it is especially important for Western practitioners to have a good grasp of treating damp heat as a concomitant disease mechanism and pattern.

1. Clearing heat & eliminating dampness method

If the spleen is vacuous, dampness may pour downward causing depression and stagnation in the lower burner. If this dampness is removed, heat cannot remain. The commonly seen manifestations of this mechanism are white colored vaginal discharge which is thin in consistency and without foul odor. In addition, the appetite may be lessened and the stools loose. There may be fatigue and lack of strength, a sallow yellow facial complexion, scanty menstruation, delayed menstruation, or early menstruation which is profuse in amount. The commonly used medicinals in this case are: Rhizoma Atractylodis Macrocephalae (*Bai Zhu*), Rhizoma Atractylodis (*Cang Zhu*), Sclerotium Poriae Cocos (*Fu Ling*), Semen Plantaginis (*Che Qian Zi*), Radix Dioscoreae Oppositae (*Shan Yao*), Radix Codonopsitis Pilosulae (*Dang Shen*), Semen Coicis Lachryma-jobi (*Yi Yi Ren*), Semen Euryalis Ferocis (*Qian Shi*), Rhizoma Cimicifugae (*Sheng Ma*), and Radix Angelicae Dahuricae (*Bai Zhi*).

2. Clearing heat & resolving toxins method

This method is used for treating damp toxic evils depressed and stagnating in the lower burner. There is profuse vaginal discharge which is sticky and thick and colored yellow. Or it may be pussy or bloody, has an odor, and is accompanied by lower abdominal sagging pain. There may be uterine bleeding simultaneously with abnormal vaginal discharge, alternating cold and hot, a red tongue with yellow fur, and a slippery, rapid, large pulse. The commonly used medicinals are: Herba Patriniae Heterophyllae Cum Radice (*Bai Jiang Cao*), Herba Senecionis (*Qian Li Guang*), Cortex Phellodendri (*Huang Bai*), Radix Scutellariae Baicalensis (*Huang Qin*), Rhizoma Coptidis Chinensis (*Huang Lian*), Cortex Radicis Moutan (*Dan Pi*), Radix Rubrus Paeoniae Lactiflorae (*Chi Shao*), Herba Oldenlandiae Diffusae (*Bai Hua She She Cao*), Flos Lonicerae Japonicae (*Yin Hua*), Fructus Forsythiae Suspensae (*Lian Qiao*), Herba Taraxaci Mongolici Cum Radice (*Pu Gong Ying*), Herba Violae Yedoensitis Cum Radice (*Zi Hua Di Ding*), Semen Coicis Lachryma-jobi (*Yi Yi Ren*), Semen Plantaginis (*Che Qian Zi*), Semen Benincasae Hispidae (*Dong Gua Ren*), Radix Angelicae Dahuricae (*Bai Zhi*), Rhizoma Atractylodis Macrocephalae (*Bai Zhu*), and Rhizoma Atractylodis (*Cang Zhu*).

3. Nourishing yin & eliminating dampness method

Damp heat may smolder and soar. If it remains for a prolonged period of time, it will consume kidney yin and give rise to vexatious heat in the five hearts. This will be accompanied by low back and buttock soreness and pain. The mouth will be dry and the tongue red. And the pulse will be fine and rapid. The commonly used medicinals are: Radix Dipsaci (*Xu Duan*), Ramulus Loranthi Seu Visci (*Sang Ji Sheng*), Radix Albus Paeoniae Lactiflorae (*Bai Shao*), uncooked Radix Rehmanniae (*Sheng Di*), cooked Radix Rehmanniae (*Shu Di*), Rhizoma Anemarrhenae Aspheloidis (*Zhi Mu*), Radix Scrophulariae Ningpoensis (*Xuan Shen*), Tuber Ophiopogonis Japonici (*Mai Men Dong*), Tuber Asparagi Cochinensis (*Tian Men Dong*), Fructus Ligustri Lucidi (*Nu Zhen Zi*), and Herba Ecliptae Prostratae (*Han Lian Cao*) to mainly nourish yin, plus Rhizoma Dioscoreae Hypoglaucae (*Bie Xie*), Cortex Toonae Sinensis (*Chun Gen Pi*), Semen Coicis Lachryma-jobi (*Yi Yi Ren*), Semen Benincasae Hispidae (*Dong Gua Ren*), Radix Ampelopsis (*Bai Lian*), Herba Senecionis (*Qian Li Guang*), and Herba Andrographidis (*Chuan Xin Lian*).

4. Warming yang & disinhibiting dampness method

If there has been flooding and leaking and vaginal discharge for many days, the *chong* and *ren* may be vacuous and have suffered detriment and the lower source may be vacuous and exhausted. In that case, kidney yang will be insufficient and abnormal vaginal discharge will be excessive. It will dribble and drip without cease and its color will be white like water. There will be lumbar soreness and chilled limbs. At night there will be polyuria. The tongue will be white and the pulse will be slow. In that case, the commonly used medicinals consist of: Radix Lateralis Praeparatus Aconiti Carmichaeli (*Fu Zi*), Cortex Cinnamomi Cassiae (*Rou Gui*), Gelatinum Cornu Cervi (*Lu Jiao Jiao*), Semen Cuscutae (*Tu Si Zi*), Herba Cistanchis Deseticolae (*Rou Cong Rong*), and Ootheca Mantidis (*Sang Piao Xiao*) to mainly supplement the kidneys and support yang, plus Rhizoma Atractylodis Macrocephalae (*Bai Zhu*), Radix Dioscoreae Oppositae (*Shan Yao*), Semen Gingkonis Bilobae (*Bai Guo*), Hallyositum Rubrum (*Chi Shi Zhi*), Cornu Degelatinum Cervi (*Lu Jiao Shuang*), Os Sepiae Seu Sepiellae (*Wu Zei Gu*), Os Draconis (*Long Gu*), and Radix Rubiae Cordifoliae (*Qian Cao*) to secure and astringe, eliminate dampness, and stop abnormal vaginal discharge.

5. Dispersing stasis & disinhibiting dampness method

If there is damp heat in the lower burner which has accumulated and is exuberant and this is combined with static blood which has stopped and been retained, there will be lower abdominal aching and pain, sagging and distention that is not comfortable. There may also be obvious pressure pain and fishy or meaty smelling abnormal vaginal discharge and even fever. The commonly used medicinals in that case are: Cortex Radicis Moutan (*Dan Pi*), Radix Rubrus Paeoniae Lactiflorae (*Chi Shao*), Radix Angelicae Sinensis (*Dang Gui*), Semen Pruni Persicae

(*Tao Ren*), and Rhizoma Corydalis Yanhusuo (*Yan Hu Suo*) to mainly quicken the blood and transform stasis, plus Cortex Phellodendri (*Huang Bai*), Rhizoma Atractylodis (*Cang Zhu*), Herba Senecionis (*Qian Li Guang*), Semen Coicis Lachryma-jobi (*Bai Jiang Cao*), and Herba Patriniae Heterophyllae Cum Radice (*Bai Jiang Cao*) to clear heat and disinhibit dampness.

Ten Important Points in Using Chinese Medicinals in Gynecology

1. When treating the qi, do not neglect the blood.

2. When treating the blood, do not neglect the qi.

3. When coursing the liver, do not neglect the spleen.

4. When supplementing yang, do not neglect yin.

5. When enriching and supplementing, do not neglect stagnation of qi and blood.

6. When rectifying the qi, do not overuse acrid, scattering medicinals.

7. During the menstrual period, it is not appropriate to overuse cold and cool medicinal substances.

8. During the menstrual period, be careful in using blood-breaking and urine-disinhibiting medicinals.

9. During pregnancy, if fetal fire is effulgent and exuberant, it is appropriate to use cooling medicinals.

10. If postpartum the qi and blood have been excessively consumed and damaged, it is appropriate to use warm supplementing medicinals.

9

Treatment Strategies & Expectations

Staging treatment

When treating various menstrual diseases, it is important to erect one's treatment plan in coordination with the woman's cycle. For instance, since qi and blood are at their maximum from midcycle to the onset of menstruation, this is the most necessary and appropriate time to rectify the qi and quicken the blood so as to prevent their stasis and stagnation or counterflow. Because this is also the time that the woman is the warmest, one should also take care to clear both depressive and replete heat as appropriate. After menstruation, because the woman's blood is relatively vacuous and empty, it is appropriate to nourish and enrich the blood at the same time that the body itself is engaged in replenishing these. If the woman suffers from yin vacuity, this is the time to nourish and enrich that as well.

Along the same lines, unless the patient has painful menstruation or one is attempting to discharge blood stasis, it is best not to continue internal therapy during menstruation itself. Although typically contemporary Chinese gynecologists using the so-called man-made or artificial method of regulating the menstrual cycle say that the appropriate treatment principles during menstruation are to regulate the menses, this only means to regulate the menses *if they are irregular*. Menstrual irregularites include painful menstraution, profuse menstruation, menstruation which stops and starts, lengthened menstruation, and scanty menstruation (especially that due to stasis and stagnation). In other words, if there is not a pathology requiring treatment during the menses, it is best not to treat. This is in order to avoid the risk of damaging the blood, causing excessive bleeding, or inadvertently stopping the healthy discharge of the menstruate.

Of course, even if a woman's menses are not irregular, she can be treated during menstruation for any sign or symptom or disease which continues to present during menstruation. In that case, treatment is only actually restoring balance to the body and, therefore, should in no way negatively impact the menstruation. Therefore, although it is a general principle of not treating during menstruation if there is no problem with menstruation, one can treat a woman for any other chronic or acute disease. The fact of the matter is that most acute and/or chronic diseases will cause menstrual irregularities in any case due to the interconnections and interdependence of the uterus and menstruation with all the other viscera and bowels, channels and network vessels, and qi and blood.

When treating premenstrual complaints, one should commence therapy as soon as the very first signs and symptoms appear. If the therapy is correct, the onset of these signs and symptoms should appear later and later each month as well as be lighter and lighter. Most symptoms of PMS can be treated in three to four menstrual cycles.

In fact, most menstrual diseases can be treated in three to five menstrual cycles. During the first cycle, one formulates their initial diagnosis or working hypothesis and initiates therapy based on that hypothesis. In many cases, the patient comes too soon before the onset of their next menstruation for the therapy to have much chance to work. In such instances, one must wait till the next menstruation before one gets a clear indication of whether their initial diagnosis and treatment plan is correct. In any case, either the first or second menstruation should show signs of improvement if the diagnosis and treatment are correct. During the next couple of menses, one may have to adjust their diagnosis and treatment plan either to account for aspects of the case that were missed in the initial diagnosis or to deal with the changing diagnosis of the patient in response to treatment.

Seeming complications encountered during therapy

There are some seeming anomalies that may be encountered during treatment of menstrual diseases which must be either learned from experience or from the guidance of a senior practitioner. For instance, if a woman is diagnosed as suffering from blood and/or yin vacuity, although she may also have some stagnation of qi, this may not be readily apparent. In this case, when one supplements the blood and yin, the volume of qi and blood increase. If the lumena of the channels and network vessels are constricted, this increased volume of qi and blood will suddenly manifest symptoms of stagnation and even depressive or static heat. The patient and the novice practitioner may both assume this is a serious setback in recuperation. However, although it may not be the most elegant of treatment strategies, it does show that, in terms of the patient's righteous qi and blood, improvement has been made. Now one must switch from supplementation to regulation and elimination of stagnation.

Using the menstrual cycle in the treatment of other complaints

When treating females, many other complaints tend to crop up at certain segments of the cycle due to the rise and fall of qi, the growth and decline of blood and yin, the increase and decrease in host warmth, and fluctuations in the patency of the flow of qi and blood. Such complaints or accompanying signs and symptoms can either be diagnosed more accurately in relationship to menstruation or may help to diagnose disease mechanisms causing menstrual diseases.

For example, a woman's major complaint may be premenstrual acne. TCM theory posits that acne is often due to heat from the stomach wafting up to accumulate in the lungs. This steams the blood in the lungs and causes the eruption of red, inflamed skin lesions on the face in those areas associated with the stomach and lungs. If one understands that liver qi worsens during the premenstruum, often transforms into depressive heat, and that this transformative heat often causes mutual overheating of the stomach as well, it is easy to see why a woman's acne may worsen or be associated with her premenstruum. In such a case, one needs to course and clear the liver as well as clear the stomach and lungs in order to affect any real, lasting change in this woman's acne.

On the other hand, if this same woman's major complaint was sore, swollen breasts during her premenstruum, her premenstrual acne helps explain the disease mechanism at work. Knowing that acne typically involves stomach heat steaming the lungs, one may then also know that the soreness of the breasts is not just an accumulation of liver qi but of heat in the foot *yang ming* as well. Therefore, appropriate medicinals which clear heat from the stomach can be added to a formula for breast distention otherwise based on coursing the liver and rectifying the qi.

Similarly, if a woman's major complaint is herpes genitalia, when she has an outbreak in relationship to her menstruation each month helps to establish the pattern discrimination of her herpes. If the herpes lesions tend to erupt before the menses, one may surmise that this is due to the increase in heat and dampness in the lower burner prior to menstruation, in turn based on basic TCM theory concerning the menstrual cycle. Whereas, if the herpes appear after each menstruation, one may surmise that they are due more to vacuity heat because of the relative vacuity of blood and yin at the end of the menses. Although the disease category is the same in both cases, the pattern discrimination is quite different and, therefore, each patient must be treated according to different therapeutic principles and with different treatment methods.

OVULATION & BASAL BODY TEMPERATURE CHART

DATE	Month																																
	Day																																
Sexual Intercourse																																	
	Menses																																
	Day of Cycle	1	2	3	4	5	6	7	8	9	10	11	12	13	14	15	16	17	18	19	20	21	22	23	24	25	26	27	28	29	30	31	32

Temperature rows: 99.0°, .8, .6, .4, .2, 98.0°, .8, .6, .4, .2, 97.0°

Mucus Discharge						
	Egg White					
	Wet					
	Dry					
	Thick Yellow					

Ovulation & the onset of the menses

Western biological science says that a woman's menses can typically be expected 14 days after ovulation as long as there is no luteal phase defect. This fact should be taken into account when erecting a TCM treatment plan for either early menstruation (if there is early ovulation) or delayed menstruation. If one is treating for irregularity in the cyclicity of the menses and the patient is able to tell when she ovulates, whether by *mittelschmerz*, increase and change in consistency of vaginal mucous, or basal body temperature, this information can increase the practitioner's ability to prognosticate about the onset of the menses. If a woman is being treated for early menstruation and, after a couple of months, her cycle has lengthened out to 26-27 days, and if this month she experiences ovulation on day 10, the practitioner can assume that her menses will come 14 days later or on day 24. In such a case, the practitioner will need to reconsider their current formula and also query the patient about her diet and lifestyle. If the premature ovulation can be explained due to some indiscretion in the patient's diet or some excess of stress in her life, this can be pointed out to the patient and may prove extremely useful educationally. In addition, knowing that, in all probability, the menses are going to come early that month can help deflect and assuage the disappointment that might otherwise come if the menstruation comes too early unexpectedly. In this case, foreknowledge can be used to both instruct the patient and keep them with the treatment program.

As discussed above under introductory theory, modern practitioners of TCM in China are beginning to use BBT or basal body temperature as an aid in their diagnosis and treatment of women with menstrual diseases. Although this methodology is most often employed in the treatment of women suffering from infertility, I personally find it useful in the treatment of early or late menstruation as well. Knowing where in the cycle the defect lies can help the practitioner apply the right medicinals at the right time. I typically furnish my menstrual disease patients with the chart on the preceding page in order to more accurately track their symptoms, progress, ovulation, and BBT. The basal body temperature is taken orally as soon as the patient awakens in the morning and before she gets up or moves around.

Adjunctive therapies

TCM *fu ke* or gynecology usually follows *nei ke* or internal medicine in Chinese texts and is usually classified along with *nei ke* as opposed to external medicine or *wai ke*. Internal medicine in TCM not only implies disease of the viscera and bowels but also the administration of internal medicine as opposed to acupuncture, moxibustion, massage, etc. Therefore, most TCM gynecology texts only describe the internal medicinal treatment of gynecological complaints. TCM acupuncture and moxibustion texts contain sections concerning the treatment of gynecological diseases, but Chinese gynecology texts *per se* tend to concentrate exclusively on internal medicine. Be that as it may, the combined use of acupuncture and moxibustion and certain other external therapies, such as poultices, plasters, compresses, and enemas as well as dietary therapy, exercise, relaxation therapy, and lifestyle modification are all useful and, in many cases, necessary in order to achieve true, lasting therapeutic results.

In this current book, similar to most Chinese gynecology texts, I have mostly concentrated on discussing the internal medical treatment of menstrual diseases. However, this does not mean or imply that such other adjunctive therapies are not also appropriate or necessary. As the great Tang dynasty physician, Sun Si-miao, said, the superior doctor should first suggest changes in the patient's diet and lifestyle and only secondarily administer herbs and acupuncture. Practitioners should also remember the Chinese saying, "Three parts medicine, seven parts nursing." In this case, nursing or recuperation implies diet, exercise, rest and relaxation, and the adoption of a healthy lifestyle.

Book Two

The Diagnosis & Treatment
of Menstrual Diseases

1

Menstruation Ahead of Schedule

Menstruation ahead of schedule or early menstruation refers to the arrival of the menses before their normally expected due date. Since this results, over the course of time, in more menses than normal, this is sometimes also referred to as polymenorrhea. Although some Chinese gynecology texts define early menstruation as one which occurs eight to nine days ahead of schedule, I consider any menstruation as early as 25 days to be early. In fact, in my clinical practice, I find many women with early menstruation coming anywhere from 22-26 days after previously having regular menses at 28-30 days. It is also my experience that early menstruation is more commonly encountered in women in their mid to late 30s and through their 40s. Very commonly, one or more years of early menstruation precedes the switch to delayed or no fixed schedule menstruation which typically precedes menopause.

Because menstruation ahead of schedule means that the woman is discharging more blood than is normal over a given length of time, such early menstruation should be treated in order to preserve and conserve yin blood and fluids and ultimately essence. Further, if chronic or enduring early menstruation is not remedied, it may also cause a weakening in kidney astringency. This is supported by the statement by Wu Ben-li quoted in the *Nu Ke Mi Jue Da Quan (A Great Compendium of Secrets of Success in Gynecology)*: "If a woman over 40 years old menstruates perhaps two to three days [early] each time, with the passage of time, surely this will turn into *lin zheng*." *Lin zheng* literally means dribbling condition and is usually applied to urinary dribbling and dripping conditions. However, it may also be applied to dribbling and dripping of the blood as well.

Disease causes, disease mechanisms

In thinking about early menstruation, one must first realize that early menses are nothing other than a species of bleeding. They are instances of bleeding when the woman should not be. Therefore, in thinking about the causes and mechanisms of early menstruation, one should first think about the TCM mechanisms of bleeding in general.

According to TCM theory, there are only four mechanisms accounting for pathological bleeding. These are: 1) heat making the blood move frenetically outside its *dao* or pathways; 2) blood stasis forcing the blood outside its *mai* or vessels; 3) insufficient qi unable to contain the blood within its vessels; and 4) physical trauma cutting or severing the channels and vessels. Heat forcing the blood to move frenetically outside its vessels can be imagined like a pot of water on a stove which boils over. Blood stasis forcing the blood outside its vessels can be imagined like a boulder in the middle of a rushing stream that forces the flowing water up over the stream banks. Qi vacuity resulting in inability to contain the qi within its vessels is like a leaky pot or container. In Chinese medicine, the qi secures the vessels, uterus, and exterior. This means the qi keeps the exterior closed together and impermeable. If the qi becomes insufficient to hold the exterior and vessels together (literally, densely packed), their contents are able to leak out through the pores or holes which result. Trauma rupturing the channels and vessels results in what might be imagined as a broken pipe. The channels and vessels channelize or canalize the qi and blood. When these channels are cut or ruptured, the blood spills out or extravasates and pools in the surrounding tissue. In terms of menstrual diseases, trauma is not a main etiological factor. The one place it is discussed *vis à vis* bleeding is when sex during menstruation causes profuse menstruation. Other than these four, TCM posits no other mechanisms accounting for pathological or inappropriate bleeding. These four mechanisms are illustrated in the diagram below.

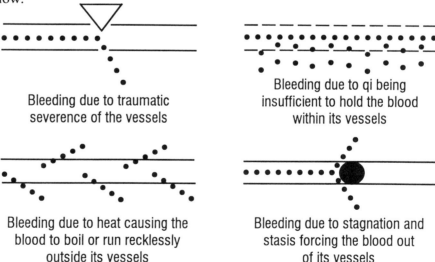

Bleeding due to traumatic
severence of the vessels

Bleeding due to qi being
insufficient to hold the blood
within its vessels

Bleeding due to heat causing the
blood to boil or run recklessly
outside its vessels

Bleeding due to stagnation and
stasis forcing the blood out
of its vessels

Figure 4. Mechanisms of Bleeding

Menstruation ahead of schedule is not due to physical trauma or severance of the channels and vessels. Therefore, its mechanisms must be none other than the remaining three. Of these three, heat and qi vacuity are the main mechanisms, with blood stasis occurring more as a complicating factor than a primary mechanism.

When one talks about heat in relationship to early menstruation, or in terms of any menstrual disease for that matter, one must understand that there are various causes and types of heat and that each of these require individualized treatment according to TCM. There are five main types of heat involved in early menstruation and each type has its own causes. The first type is replete heat. Replete heat is most often due to overeating hot, spicy, greasy foods. It may also be caused, however, by an overly hot external environment. Abnormally hot external or macrocosmic host qi may cause a woman's internal or microcosmic guest qi to become too hot. This then may cause the blood to move frenetically outside its pathways. And third, this type of heat may also been seen in young, robust women with a constitutional effulgence of heat. Nonetheless, whether due to diet, external temperature, or natural endowment, this is replete heat.

The second type of heat resulting in menstruation ahead of schedule is depressive heat. Emotional stress and frustration may result in liver depression qi stagnation. Because qi is yang and, therefore, warm, when it accumulates in any one place, it may also manifest as warmth or heat. Depressive heat transforms from accumulation of qi due to stagnation and inhibited flow. This depressive heat is primarily localized in the liver which also stores the blood. Thus, this depressive heat may easily cause the blood to boil over resulting in menstruation ahead of schedule.

The third type of heat associated with early menstruation is phlegm heat. There are two basic mechanisms which can result in the formation of phlegm heat. Heat may give rise to phlegm due to the stewing of juices and eventual congelation. This may be likened to the cooking of pudding. In some instances, heat does not just boil away fluids or evaporate them but may also result in their thickening and congelation. Phlegm may also be caused by spleen dysfunction in terms of the movement and transformation of fluids. If the spleen does not move and transform properly, fluids may gather and transform into dampness. This dampness may congeal and transform into phlegm. Phlegm then may obstruct the free flow of qi causing an accumulation of warm qi behind and within the phlegm, and thus there may arise signs and symptoms of a combination of phlegm and heat or phlegm heat. Poor spleen function may be due to worry and anxiety, lack of exercise, or overeating sweets, chilled and uncooked foods, and/or foods which strongly engender fluids. Often phlegm heat results from a combination of spleen dysfunction and depressive liver heat. However, no matter what the mechanism behind phlegm production, it is the heat which causes the blood to move frenetically outside its pathways, resulting in menstruation ahead of schedule.

The fourth type of heat is very similar to phlegm heat and, therefore, most Chinese gynecology texts do not discuss it as a separate type. However, in my clinical experience, damp heat may be associated with menstruation ahead of schedule. Just as heat may precipitate and congeal phlegm, so heat may precipitate dampness. Likewise, if dampness accumulates due to faulty diet damaging the spleen, it may result in transformative heat. Dampness being yin impedes the qi flow which is yang and warm and results in a combination of dampness and heat. Because dampness is heavy and turbid, it tends to pour down to the lower burner. Damp heat can also be due to external invasion by sexually transmitted evils and may also be complicated by *chong* or parasites and, in particular, overgrowth of *Candida albicans*.

The fifth type of heat involved with menstruation ahead of schedule is vacuity heat. If yin becomes vacuous due to damage by excessive or prolonged heat or due to consumption in turn caused by overactivity, poor nutrition and digestion, or constitutional insufficiency, it can no longer control and restrain yang. Yang becomes effulgent and this effulgence may manifest as heat. This evil heat is due to vacuity and insufficiency of yin and so is called vacuity heat. Any activity may cause consumption of yin since all activity entails a transformation of yin by and into yang. In particular, vacuity heat is easily caused by overthinking, continuous fear, too much sex, stimulants and recreational drugs, and lack of adequate or restful sleep. Because the aging process is the process of yang activity transforming and consuming yin, including kidney essence, the tendency to yin vacuity and vacuity heat increases as one ages and often manifests in women its first signs and symptoms in the mid to late 30s.

Insufficient qi failing to contain the blood within its vessels can be due to overthinking, worry, lack of adequate exercise, and overeating sweets, chilled and uncooked foods, and foods which strongly engender fluids. In other words, this qi vacuity is mostly described in Chinese gynecology texts as vacuity of spleen qi. It is the spleen qi which is responsible for containing the blood within its vessels. However, if bleeding continues for a long time, due to either spleen qi vacuity or vacuity heat, this may eventually cause the kidney qi to also lose its ability to secure the *chong mai*. Since the kidneys become weak with age and since the qi is a part of yang, many women with menstruation ahead of schedule in their late 30s and 40s suffer from both spleen vacuity not containing the blood and kidney yang insufficiency failing to secure the essence.

In Chinese medicine, the structure of the body is seen as a latticework or web. It is one of the five functions of qi to hold the openings of this latticework close together so that no body fluids are allowed to leak inappropriately. Thus the body is seen as something like a woven, watertight bag. Although there are potential spaces between the weave, the weave is normally so tight, nothing leaks out. When one speaks of lack of securing, the Chinese character for *gu* describes a four-sided enclosure without any open windows or doors. Kidney qi and yang's ability to secure means that the windows and doors, *i.e.*, the two lower yin (the anus and vaginal meatus-urethra in women), are closed shut to prevent leakage.

Because kidney yang is the root of spleen qi, often these two vacuities manifest together.

Unfortunately, to make matters more confusing, such spleen-kidney dual vacuity may often be complicated by signs and symptoms of liver depression, blood stasis, damp heat, and/or yin vacuity. One of the best ways of discriminating such a complication as spleen-kidney dual vacuity is by basal body temperature. If the premenstrual temperature drops too soon, this typically means that, although there may be signs and symptoms of damp heat and/or vacuity heat, spleen and kidney qi are insufficient to contain and secure the blood within the body.

As mentioned above, blood stasis may also obstruct the channels and vessels. The blood attempting to flow through these channels and vessels (which may also be translated as menstrual vessels) may be pushed outside their vessels in their effort to continue their flow. This may result in early menstruation due to blood stasis. Such blood stasis is often due to lower abdominal trauma, prolonged stress leading to chronic liver qi leading to blood stasis, abortions, oral birth control pills, IUD's, possible sexual abuse, intercourse during menses, and the ingestion of chilled foods and liquids just before or during the menses. Blood stasis is rarely the sole cause of menstruation ahead of schedule, but is often a complicating factor, especially in cases due to depressive or chronic damp or phlegmatic heat. Therefore, many TCM gynecology texts do not describe this as a separate pattern. Nevertheless, because blood stasis is so commonly encountered in modern Western women, I think it should be included as a separate disease mechanism at least, if not as a separate pattern.

Treatment based on pattern discrimination

The hallmark of TCM as a specific style of Chinese medicine is treatment based on a discrimination of patterns. Based on the above three disease mechanisms for menstruation ahead of schedule, one can distinguish three basic categories of patterns associated with this disease. These are blood heat, qi vacuity, and blood stasis.

Blood heat

1. Replete heat

Main symptoms: Excessive menstrual volume which is either bright red or dark red in color. The blood may even be purplish and clotty with a bad or offensive odor. There may be lower abdominal pain and typically there is thirst with a preference for cold drinks, a red face, vexatious heat in the heart, and dry, knotted constipation. In severe cases, there may be red eyes, sores in the mouth, and nosebleeds. The tongue is red with yellow fur and the pulse is slippery and rapid or surging and rapid.

Treatment principles: Clear heat and cool the blood

Guiding formulas:

1. Fu Qing-zhu's *Qing Jing San* (Clear the Menses Powder)

Ingredients: Cortex Radicis Moutan (*Dan Pi*), Cortex Radicis Lycii Chinensis (*Di Gu Pi*), Radix Albus Paeoniae Lactiflorae (*Bai Shao*), Herba Artemisiae Apiaceae (*Qing Hao*), uncooked Radix Rehmanniae (*Sheng Di*), Cortex Phellodenri (*Huang Bai*), Sclerotium Poriae Cocoris (*Fu Ling*)

Additions: If the bleeding is excessive in amount, add Radix Sanguisorbae (*Di Yu*) and Herba Agrimoniae Pilosae (*Xian He Cao*). If there is lower abdominal pain which is predominantly due to qi stagnation, add Rhizoma Corydalis Yanhusuo (*Yan Hu Suo*) and Fructus Meliae Toosendan (*Chuan Lian Zi*). If there is lower abdominal pain predominantly due to blood stasis, add Feces Trogopterori Seu Pteromi (*Wu Ling Zhi*) and Sanguis Draconis (*Xue Jie*). One variation of this formula includes Herba Artemisiae Apiaceae (*Qing Hao*), Cortex Phellodendri (*Huang Bai*), uncooked Radix Rehmanniae (*Sheng Di*), Radix Scutellariae Baicalensis (*Huang Qin*), Cortex Radicis Moutan (*Dan Pi*). Another variation of this formula includes Cortex Radicis Moutan (*Dan Pi*), Cortex Radicis Lycii Chinensis (*Di Gu Pi*), Radix Albus Paeoniae Lactiflorae (*Bai Shao*), uncooked Radix Rehmanniae (*Sheng Di*), Herba Artemisiae Apiaceae (*Qing Hao*), Cortex Phellodendri (*Huang Bai*), Herba Leonuri Heterophylli (*Yi Mu Cao*), Radix Sanguisorbae (*Di Yu*).

2. *Qin Lian Si Wu Tang* (Scutellaria & Coptis Four Materials Decoction)

Ingredients: Radix Angelicae Sinensis (*Dang Gui*), uncooked Radix Rehmanniae (*Sheng Di*), Radix Albus Paeoniae Lactiflorae (*Bai Shao*), Radix Ligustici Wallichii (*Chuan Xiong*), Radix Scutellariae Baicalensis (*Huang Qin*), Rhizoma Coptidis Chinensis (*Huang Lian*)

This formula is based on Zhu Dan-xi's statement that for menstruation ahead of schedule, use *Si Wu Tang* plus Rhizoma Coptidis Chinensis.

3. *Xian Qi Tang* (Ahead of Schedule Decoction)

Ingredients: Radix Angelicae Sinensis (*Dang Gui*), uncooked Radix Rehmanniae (*Sheng Di*), Radix Albus Paeoniae Lactiflorae (*Bai Shao*), Radix Ligustici Wallichii (*Chuan Xiong*), Rhizoma Anemarrhenae Aspheloidis (*Zhi Mu*), Radix Scutellariae Baicalensis (*Huang Qin*), Cortex Phellodendri (*Huang Bai*), Rhizoma Coptidis Chinensis (*Huang Lian*), Gelatinum Corii Asini (*E Jiao*), Folium Artemisiae Argyii (*Ai Ye*), Rhizoma Cyperi Rotundi (*Xiang Fu*), Radix Glycyrrhizae (*Gan Cao*)

Additions: If bleeding is profuse in amount, one may add Herba Cephalanopoloris Segeti (*Xiao Ji*) and Radix Rubiae Cordifoliae (*Qian Cao*) to cool the blood and stop bleeding.

4. Unnamed formula from *Wan Shi Fu Ren Ke (Master Wan's Gynecology)*

Ingredients: Radix Rubrus Paeoniae Lactiflorae (*Chi Shao*), uncooked Radix Rehmanniae (*Sheng Di*), Rhizoma Anemarrhenae Aspheloidis (*Zhi Mu*), Tuber Ophiopogonis Japonici (*Mai Dong*), Cortex Radicis Lycii Chinensis (*Di Gu Pi*), Radix Angelicae Sinensis (*Dang Gui*), Radix Ligustici Wallichii (*Chuan Xiong*), Radix Glycyrrhizae (*Gan Cao*)

Wan Mi-zhai suggests this formula for blood heat menstruation ahead of schedule if the woman's personality is warm and harmonious and she has no other disease than this. This heat, Master Wan says, is merely due to the blood's exuberance.

2. Depressive heat

Main symptoms: Early menstruation which is either red or purple, profuse or scanty in amount (depending on how much the heat has damaged the blood), possible clots, the beginning of the menses inhibited or not smoothly flowing, breast, chest, rib-side, and lower abdominal distention and pain, vexation and agitation, disquietude[19], a dry mouth with a bitter taste, a red tongue with possibly dry, yellow fur or dark, red, inflated rims, and a rapid, bowstring pulse.

This is depressive heat transformed from liver depression qi stagnation. If the liver assails the stomach and the stomach thus loses its harmony, there may also be burping, belching, acid regurgitation, facial acne, and increased appetite, in which case the tongue fur is usually yellow and the right bar pulse may be either slippery or especially bowstring. If the liver assails the spleen, there may be loss of appetite, fatigue, cravings for sweets and carbohydrates, and constipation premenstrually turning into diarrhea and even nausea and vomiting when the menses arrive. The tongue fur may be yellow and the right bar pulse may be floating and bowstring.

Treatment principles: Course the liver and rectify the qi, clear heat and resolve depression

---

[19] Wiseman translated *an* as quiet. Therefore, *bu an,* not quiet, becomes disquietude as a noun. Connotatively, this means restlessness.

Guiding formulas:

1. *Dan Zhi Xiao Yao San* (Moutan & Gardenia Rambling Powder)

Ingredients: Radix Bupleuri (*Chai Hu*), Radix Angelicae Sinensis (*Dang Gui*), Radix Albus Paeoniae Lactiflorae (*Bai Shao*), Rhizoma Atractylodis Macrocephalae (*Bai Zhu*), Sclerotium Poriae Cocos (*Fu Ling*), Cortex Radicis Moutan (*Dan Pi*), Fructus Gardeniae Jasminoidis (*Zhi Zi*), Herba Menthae Haplocalycis (*Bo He*)

Additions: One may add Radix Scutellariae Baicalensis (*Huang Qin*) and uncooked Radix Rehmanniae (*Sheng Di*) to clear heat and cool the blood in case of profuse bleeding. Or one might add Radix Rubiae Cordifoliae (*Qian Cao*) to diminish profuse bleeding. If qi stagnation is pronounced, one may add Rhizoma Cyperi Rotundi (*Xiang Fu*) and Pericarpium Citri Reticulatae Viride (*Qing Pi*) to further move the qi and disperse distention. If liver assailing the stomach accompanied by vomiting is prominent, add *Zuo Jin Wan* (Left Gold Pills) which are composed of Rhizoma Coptidis Chinensis (*Huang Lian*) and Fructus Evodiae Rutecarpae (*Wu Zhu Yu*), or one may use Rhizoma Pinelliae Ternatae (*Ban Xia*) and Caulis Bambusae In Taeniis (*Zhu Ru*). If spleen vacuity is more obvious and pronounced, one may add Radix Panacis Ginseng (*Ren Shen*) or Radix Codonopsitis Pilosulae (*Dang Shen*)[20] and/or Radix Astragali Membranacei (*Huang Qi*). If there is loss of appetite, one may add Fructus Crataegi (*Shan Zha*) and Fructus Amomi (*Sha Ren*). In fact, the possible modifications of this formula are numerous. This is one of the most famous formulas in TCM gynecology.

2. *Hei Xiao Yao San Jia Wei* (Black Rambling Powder with Added Flavors)

Ingredients: Radix Bupleuri (*Chai Hu*), Radix Angelicae Sinensis (*Dang Gui*), Radix Albus Paeoniae Lactiflorae (*Bai Shao*), Rhizoma Atractylodis Macrocephalae (*Bai Zhu*), Sclerotium Poriae Cocos (*Fu Ling*), mix-fried Radix Glycyrrhizae (*Gan Cao*), Herba Menthae Haplocalycis (*Bo He*), uncooked Rhizoma Zingiberis (*Sheng Jiang*), uncooked Radix Rehmanniae (*Sheng Di*), Plastrum Testudinis (*Gui Ban*)

This formula is for the treatment of menstruation ahead of schedule with a heavy, red discharge due to blood heat and qi stagnation.

---

[20] In contemporary TCM, Ginseng and Codonopsis are used interchangeably, Codonopsis often being used as a cheaper substitute for Ginseng, which in China, is largely reserved for high officials or export. It was Dr. Chen Wei's opinion that the highest quality Codonopsis is inferior to the lowest grade of Ginseng. In my practice, I mostly prescribe Ginseng rather than Codonopsis. Unless otherwise specified, Ginseng means white or Jilin Ginseng.

3. *Qing Jing San Jia Jian* (Clear the Menses Powder with Additions & Subtractions)

Ingredients: Cortex Radicis Moutan (*Dan Pi*), Cortex Radicis Lycii Chinensis (*Di Gu Pi*), Radix Albus Paeoniae Lactiflorae (*Bai Shao*), Radix Rehmanniae (*Sheng Di*), Herba Artemisiae Apiaceae (*Qing Hao*), Radix Sanguisorbae (*Di Yu*), Fructus Gardeniae Jasminoidis (*Zhi Zi*), Radix Bupleuri (*Chai Hu*), Flos Rosae Rugosae (*Mei Gui Hua*)

This formula is for liver depression-depressive heat with premenstrual breast and lower abdominal distention, heart vexation, and a bitter taste in the mouth.

4. *Xiao Chai Hu Tang* (Minor Bupleurum Decoction)

Ingredients: Radix Bupleuri (*Chai Hu*), Radix Scutellariae Baicalensis (*Huang Qin*), Radix Panacis Ginseng (*Ren Shen*) or Radix Codonopsitis Pilosulae (*Dang Shen*), Rhizoma Pinelliae Ternatae (*Ban Xia*), Fructus Zizyphi Jujubae (*Da Zao*), uncooked Rhizoma Zingiberis (*Sheng Jiang*), mix-fried Radix Glycyrrhizae (*Gan Cao*)

Xue Li-zhai, as quoted in *Nu Ke Mi Jue Da Quan (A Great Compendium of Secrets of Success in Gynecology)*, says that if early menstruation is caused by liver stasis and stagnation, use *Jia Wei Xiao Yao San*. But if it is caused by liver channel flames of fury, use *Jia Wei Xiao Chai Hu Tang*. "Flames of fury" suggests heat travelling up and disturbing the lungs and heart. Radix Scutellariae Baicalensis (*Huang Qin*), one of the ingredients in *Xiao Chai Hu Tang*, clears heat from the upper burner. When used for premenstrual and menstrual diseases, usually Radix Angelicae Sinensis (*Dang Gui*) and Radix Albus Paeoniae Lactiflorae (*Bai Shao*) or Rhizoma Cyperi Rotundi (*Xiang Fu*) and Radix Albus Paeoniae Lactiflorae (*Bai Shao*) are added to the basic formula.

5. *Si Wu Chai Qin Tang* (Four Materials Bupleurum & Scutellaria Decoction)

Ingredients: Uncooked Radix Rehmanniae (*Sheng Di*), Radix Angelicae Sinensis (*Dang Gui*), Radix Albus Paeoniae Lactiflorae (*Bai Shao*), Radix Ligustici Wallichii (*Chuan Xiong*), stir-fried Pollen Typhae (*Pu Huang*), Gelatinum Corii Asini (*E Jiao*), stir-fried till carbonized Herba Schizonepetae Tenuifoliae (*Jing Jie*), wine stir-fried Radix Scutellariae Baicalensis (*Huang Qin*), stir-fried till carbonized Cortex Phellodendri (*Huang Bai*), Radix Bupleuri (*Chai Hu*)

Du Jie-hui, author of *Nan Nu Bing Mi Yan Liang Fang (Secret, Proven, Fine Formulas for Men's & Women's Diseases)*, recommends this formula for the treatment of liver depression, blood heat early and profuse menstruation.

6. Unnamed formula from *Wan Shi Fu Ren Ke (Master Wan's Gynecology)*

Ingredients: Radix Angelicae Sinensis (*Dang Gui*), Radix Ligustici Wallichii (*Chuan Xiong*), Radix Albus Paeoniae Lactiflorae (*Bai Shao*), uncooked Radix Rehmanniae (*Sheng Di*), stir-fried Radix Scutellariae Baicalensis (*Tiao Qin*), stir-fried Rhizoma Coptidis Chinensis (*Huang Lian*), stir-fried Rhizoma Cyperi Rotundi (*Xiang Fu*), uncooked Radix Glycyrrhizae (*Gan Cao*)

Master Wan says to use this formula for an irascible woman with excessive anger and excessive envy or jealousy. Master Wan says that, in this case, both the qi and blood are hot due to depression.

7. Unnamed formula from *Nu Ke Jing Wei (Profundities from the Gynecological Classics)*

Ingredients: Body of Radix Angelicae Sinensis (*Dang Gui Shen*), uncooked Hangzhou Radix Albus Paeoniae Lactiflorae (*Hang Shao*), vinegar-processed Radix Bupleuri (*Chai Hu*), Cortex Radicis Moutan (*Dan Pi*), uncooked Radix Astragali Membranacei (*Huang Qi*), Guangdong Radix Auklandiae Lappae (*Guang Mu Xiang*), scorched Fructus Gardeniae Jasminoidis (*Shan Zhi*), scorched Semen Zizyphi Spinosae (*Zao Ren*), earth stir-fried Rhizoma Atractylodis Macrocephalae (*Bai Zhu*), processed Rhizoma Cyperi Rotundi (*Xiang Fu*), blood-processed Radix Salviae Miltiorrhizae (*Dan Shen*), uncooked Radix Glycyrrhizae (*Gan Cao*)

Additions & subtractions: If accompanied by lower abdominal pain, add Fructus Meliae Toosendan (*Chuan Lian Zi*) and stir-fried Pericarpium Citri Reticulatae Viride (*Qing Pi*). Once liver depression has been resolved and after heat has been cleared, remove Bupleurum, Moutan, and Gardenia and add Radix Dioscoreae Oppositae (*Huai Shan Yao*), Semen Biotae Orientalis (*Bai Zi Ren*), and Cortex Radicis Lycii Chinensis (*Di Gu Pi*). If there is heart fluster and heart palpitations with difficulty going to sleep, add Dens Draconis (*Long Chi*). If there is dizziness, add Concha Margaritiferae (*Zhen Zhu Mu*).

Lu Guo-zhi and Song Shu-de, in *Nu Ke Jing Wei (Profundities from the Gynecological Classics)* give the above unnamed formula for the treatment of liver effulgence, heart-spleen vacuity. This means liver depression-depressive heat accompanied by a heart blood-spleen qi vacuity. This is a very real, complicated pattern, the type of multifaceted pattern one actually sees in clinical practice. Its signs and symptoms are dizziness, vertigo, a red face, chest and rib-side glomus and pain, heart fluster, heart palpitations, occasional vexation and agitation, sleep not replete, excessive fright, early menstruation, amount scanty, color red, no blood clots, and a pale tongue with thin, white fur and a red tongue tip. The left bar is wiry and large, the inch is soggy and vacuous, and the right pulses overall are deep, fine, weak, and/or small. This formula's composition is based on the principles of coursing the liver, boosting the spleen, and clearing heat assisted by nourishing the blood and quieting the heart

8. Unnamed formula from *Nu Ke Jing Wei* (*Profundities from the Gynecological Classics*)

Ingredients: Radix Gentianae Scabrae (*Long Dan Cao*), scorched Fructus Gardeniae Jasminoidis (*Shan Zhi*), Cortex Radicis Moutan (*Dan Pi*), stir-fried Radix Scutellariae Baicalensis (*Huang Qin*), vinegar-processed Radix Bupleuri (*Chai Hu*), uncooked Radix Albus Paeoniae Lactiflorae (*Bai Shao*), whole Radix Angelicae Sinensis (*Quan Dang Gui*), stir-fried Pericarpium Citri Reticulatae Viride (*Qing Pi*), uncooked Radix Rehmanniae (*Sheng Di*), Rhizoma Corydalis Yanhusuo (*Yan Hu Suo*), Herba Leonuri Heterophylli (*Yi Mu Cao*), uncooked Radix Glycyrrhizae (*Gan Cao*)

This formula is for depressive heat in the liver channel complicated by an element of blood stasis and with no concomitant spleen, kidney, or blood vacuities. As such, it is not, in my opinion, that useful for treating Western women who mostly do exhibit at least some signs and symptoms of righteous vacuity. When and if practitioners choose to use this formula, it should only be in a very robust patient with a completely replete pattern and it should not be used for extended periods of time. Gardenia and Gentiana Scabra are two of the coldest, bitterest medicinals in the Chinese materia medica and easily damage the spleen and stomach.

3. Phlegm heat

Main symptoms: Early menstruation with either moderate or profuse blood flow most typically in a woman who is overweight, a puffy, edematous, yellowish face, fullness in the head, heaviness of the limbs, dizziness, chest oppression, and a tendency to copious phlegm production, a fat tongue with slimy, yellow or white fur, and a slippery, rapid pulse

If spleen vacuity and damp encumbrance are more pronounced, there may be loose stools, lack of appetite, glossy or wet tongue fur, and a soggy pulse. Since this condition is often combined with liver depression qi stagnation, the pulse may also be bowstring. Since the spleen is the root of blood engenderment and transformation, the pulse may even be fine and the tongue in that case will be pale, fat, and have teeth marks along its edges.

Treatment principles: Fortify the spleen and disinhibit dampness, clear heat and transform phlegm

Guiding formulas:

1. According to Professors Song and Yu, authors of *Zhong Yi Fu Ke Shou Ce (A Handbook of Chinese Medical Gynecology)*, for remedying this pattern of early menstruation, one can use a formula found in Zhu Dan-xi's *Dan Xi Xin Fa (Dan-xi's Secret or Heart Methods)*.

Ingredients: Rhizoma Arisaematis (*Nan Xing*), Rhizoma Atractylodis Macrocephalae (*Bai Zhu*), Rhizoma Atractylodis (*Cang Zhu*), Rhizoma Coptidis Chinensis (*Huang Lian*), Rhizoma Cyperus Rotundi (*Xiang Fu*), Radix Ligustici Wallichii (*Chuan Xiong*)

According to Zhu Dan-xi, these medicinals are to be ground into powder and made into pills. However, I have used this formula in decoction with good results.

2. *Huang Lian Wen Dan Tang* (Coptis Warm the Gallbladder Decoction)

Ingredients: Rhizoma Pinelliae Ternatae (*Ban Xia*), Pericarpium Citri Reticulatae (*Chen Pi*), Sclerotium Poriae Cocos (*Fu Ling*), Fructus Immaturus Citri Aurantii (*Zhi Shi*), Caulis Bambusae In Taeniis (*Zhu Ru*), Rhizoma Coptidis Chinensis (*Huang Lian*), Fructus Zizyphi Jujubae (*Da Zao*), Radix Glycyrrhizae (*Gan Cao*)

3. *Tao Hong Er Chen Tang Jia Wei* (Persica & Carthamus Two Aged [Ingredients] Decoction with Added Flavors)

Ingredients: Rhizoma Pinelliae Ternatae (*Ban Xia*), Pericarpium Citri Reticulatae (*Chen Pi*), Sclerotium Poriae Cocos (*Fu Ling*), Semen Pruni Persicae (*Tao Ren*), Flos Carthami Tinctorii (*Hong Hua*), Rhizoma Coptidis Chinensis (*Huang Lian*), Radix Scutellariae Baicalensis (*Huang Qin*), Rhizoma Arisaematis (*Nan Xing*)

This formula is for a combination of phlegm, blood stasis, and heat. If there is qi and blood vacuity, one can add Radix Codonopsitis Pilosulae (*Dang Shen*) and Semen Zizyphi Spinosae (*Suan Zao Ren*). If there is more pronounced spleen vacuity, one can add Radix Codonopsitis Pilosulae (*Dang Shen*) and Rhizoma Atractylodis Macrocephalae (*Bai Zhu*).

4. Unnamed formula from *Wan Shi Fu Ren Ke* (Master Wan's Gynecology)

Ingredients: Radix Angelicae Sinensis (*Dang Gui*), Radix Ligustici Wallichii (*Chuan Xiong*), Pericarpium Citri Reticulatae (*Chen Pi*), Rhizoma Pinelliae Ternatae (*Ban Xia*), Sclerotium Poriae Cocos (*Bai Ling*), Radix Glycyrrhizae (*Sheng Cao*), stir-fried Radix Scutellariae Baicalensis (*Tiao Qin*), stir-fried Rhizoma Cyperi Rotundi (*Xiang Fu*), stir-fried Rhizoma Coptidis Chinensis (*Huang Lian*), uncooked Rhizoma Zingiberis (*Sheng Jiang*)

Master Wan gives this formula for the treatment of menstruation ahead of schedule in fat women who have both lots of phlegm and lots of depression. In this case, Master Wan says that their blood is vacuous but their qi is hot.

4. Damp heat

Main symptoms: Early menstruation preceded by abnormally profuse vaginal discharge or mixed with dark red, purplish discharge, possibly foul smelling, possible vaginal irritation preceding the period, low back or hip pain, sciatic pain with swelling and redness, hot to the touch, chronic lower abdominal pain worsened by the approach of the menses, a red tongue with slimy, yellow fur in the rear, and a slippery, bowstring, rapid pulse

Depending upon whether heat is causing dampness or dampness is causing heat, whether heat or dampness are more pronounced, and whether there are toxins and/or parasites, the exact signs and symptoms of this type of early menstruation may vary. Few Chinese gynecology texts give this pattern as a species of menstruation ahead of schedule because its treatment primarily relies on the same formulas or types of formulas used to treat replete heat. However, I believe there are reasons to identify this as a potential pattern. Frequently, damp heat only complicates other mechanisms, such as spleen vacuity and liver depression also involved in the causation of early menstruation. If one does not know that damp heat may be a cause of menstruation ahead of schedule, one may fail to recognize it when it does occur.

Treatment principles: Clear heat and disinhibit dampness, possibly resolve toxins and/or dispel parasites

Guiding formulas:

1. *Jia Wei Er Chen Tang* (Added Flavors Two Aged [Ingredients] Decoction)

Ingredients: Rhizoma Pinelliae Ternatae (*Ban Xia*), Pericarpium Citri Reticulatae (*Chen Pi*), Sclerotium Poriae Cocos (*Fu Ling*), Rhizoma Atractylodis (*Cang Zhu*), Radix Angelicae Dahuricae (*Bai Zhi*), Radix Scutellariae Baicalensis (*Huang Qin*), Rhizoma Coptidis Chinensis (*Huang Lian*), Cortex Phellodendri (*Huang Bai*), Radix Albus Paeoniae Lactiflorae (*Bai Shao*), Cortex Toonae Chinensis (*Chun Bai Pi*), Radix Glycyrrhizae (*Gan Cao*)

This formula treats damp heat due to spleen vacuity where dampness and heat are equal in prominence.

2. *Dang Gui Liu Huang Tang* (Dang Gui Six Yellows Decoction)

Ingredients: Radix Angelicae Sinensis (*Dang Gui*), uncooked Radix Rehmanniae (*Sheng Di*), cooked Radix Rehmanniae (*Shu Di*), Radix Astragali Membrancei (*Huang Qi*), Radix Scutellariae Baicalensis (*Huang Qin*), Rhizoma Coptidis Chinensis (*Huang Lian*), Cortex Phellodendri (*Huang Bai*)

This formula is frequently used for the treatment of night sweats and hot flashes associated with menopause. It is usually described as indicated for yin vacuity with internal heat. However, I find it very useful to treat a combination of damp heat and spleen qi vacuity where heat is more prominent than dampness. This formula is especially useful for many women with early menses and candidiasis who have been diagnosed as going through premature menopause. Often women suitable for this formula have a red, cracked tongue with either yellow, geographic fur or slimy, yellow fur to the rear.

3. *Wen Qing Yin* (Warming & Clearing Drink)

Ingredients: Radix Angelicae Sinensis (*Dang Gui*), uncooked Radix Rehmanniae (*Sheng Di*), Radix Albus Paeoniae Lactiflorae (*Bai Shao*), Radix Ligustici Wallichii (*Chuan Xiong*), Radix Scutellariae Baicalensis (*Huang Qin*), Rhizoma Coptidis Chinensis (*Huang Lian*), Cortex Phellodendri (*Huang Bai*), Fructus Gardeniae Jasminoidis (*Zhi Zi*)

This formula is a combination of *Si Wu Tang* (Four Materials Decoction) and *Huang Lian Jie Du Tang* (Coptis Resolve Toxins Decoction). It is for the treatment of blood vacuity complicated by internal or damp heat. It is very similar to the preceding formula. It treats not only early menstruation due to damp heat but also profuse menstruation, flooding and leaking, persistent vaginal discharge, ulcers of the mouth or tongue, itching, and hives or any combination of these when due to blood vacuity and damp heat. If there is spleen qi vacuity, one can add Radix Astragali Membranacei (*Huang Qi*). If there is more pronounced dampness, one can add Semen Coicis Lachryma-jobi (*Yi Yi Ren*). And in any case, one can add uncooked Radix Glycyrrhizae (*Gan Cao*) to further clear heat while harmonizing the other medicinals and protecting the stomach from damage due to the bitter, cold medicinals.

5. Vacuity heat

Main symptoms: Menstruation ahead of schedule with a scanty menstruate, red in color, possibly sticky and thick in consistency, typically a lack of abdominal pain and distention, both cheeks flushed red, heat in the centers of the hands, feet, and heart, a dry mouth but no increased tendency to drink, dizziness, heart palpitations, tidal fever, night sweats, a red tongue with thin, yellow, dry, or no fur, and a fine, rapid pulse

Treatment principles: Nourish yin and cool the blood

Guiding formulas:

1. *Liang Di Tang* (Two Di's Decoction)

Ingredients: Uncooked Radix Rehmanniae (*Sheng Di*), Cortex Radicis Lycii Chinensis (*Di Gu Pi*), Radix Scrophulariae Ningpoensis (*Yuan Shen*), Radix Albus Paeoniae Lactiflorae (*Bai Shao*), Tuber Ophiopogonis Japonici (*Mai Dong*), Gelatinum Corii Asini (*E Jiao*)

2. *Qing Jing Tang* (Clear the Menses Decoction)

Ingredients: Cortex Radicis Moutan (*Dan Pi*), Cortex Radicis Lycii Chinensis (*Di Gu Pi*), Radix Albus Paeoniae Lactiflorae (*Bai Shao*), Herba Artemisiae Apiaceae (*Qing Hao*), uncooked Radix Rehmanniae (*Sheng Di*), Cortex Phellodendri (*Huang Bai*), Sclerotium Poriae Cocos (*Fu Ling*)

This formula has been discussed above under replete heat. Han Bai-ling suggests it for the treatment of yin vacuity blood heat. Whether the heat is replete or vacuous, medicinals which clear heat from the blood division and cool the blood are in order.

Additions & subtractions: For yin vacuity blood heat early menstruation, delete Artemisia Apiacea and Phellodendron and add Radix Scrophulariae Ningpoensis (*Yuan Shen*), Gelatinum Corii Asini (*E Jiao*), Fructus Ligustri Lucidi (*Nu Zhen Zi*), and Herba Ecliptae Prostratae (*Han Lian Cao*)

3. *Di Gu Pi Yin* (Cortex Lycii Drink)

Ingredients: Radix Angelicae Sinensis (*Dang Gui*), uncooked Radix Rehmanniae (*Sheng Di*), Radix Albus Paeoniae Lactiflorae (*Bai Shao*), Radix Ligustici Wallichii (*Chuan Xiong*), Cortex Radicis Lycii Chinensis (*Di Gu Pi*), Cortex Radicis Moutan (*Dan Pi*)

Additions: Han Bai-ling says to add Tuber Ophiopogonis Japonici (*Mai Dong*) and Radix Scutellariae Baicalensis (*Huang Qin*) to further help nourish yin and clear heat.

4. Unnamed formula from *Wan Shi Fu Ren Ke (Master Wan's Gynecology)*

Ingredients: Radix Angelicae Sinensis (*Dang Gui*), Radix Albus Paeoniae Lactiflorae (*Bai Shao*), cooked Radix Rehmanniae (*Shu Di*), Radix Panacis Ginseng (*Ren Shen*), Rhizoma Anemarrhenae Aspheloidis (*Zhi Mu*), Tuber Ophiopogonis Japonici (*Mai Dong*), Radix Ligustici Wallichii (*Chuan Xiong*), mix-fried Radix Glycyrrhizae (*Zhi Cao*), Fructus

Zizyphi Jujubae (*Da Zao*), uncooked Rhizoma Zingiberis (*Sheng Jiang*)

Master Wan recommends this formula for the treatment of menstruation ahead of schedule due to heat in a person with a thin or emaciated body and heat. Master Wan says that such a woman's *chong* and *ren* have been internally damaged. This is clearly a picture of vacuity heat. Master Wan further recommends such women to constantly take *Di Huang Wan*. This is none other than *Liu Wei Di Huang Wan* (Six Flavors Rehmannia Pills) whose ingredients are: cooked Radix Rehmanniae (*Shu Di*), Fructus Corni Officinalis (*Shan Zhu Rou*), Radix Dioscoreae Oppositae (*Shan Yao*), Sclerotium Poriae Cocos (*Fu Ling*), Rhizoma Alismatis (*Ze Xie*), and Cortex Radicis Moutan (*Dan Pi*).

5. Unnamed formula from *Wan Shi Fu Ren Ke (Master Wan's Gynecology)*

Ingredients: Radix Angelicae Sinensis (*Dang Gui*), Radix Rubrus Paeoniae Lactiflorae (*Chi Shao*), Radix Ligustici Wallichii (*Chuan Xiong*), uncooked Radix Rehmanniae (*Sheng Di*), stir-fried Cortex Phellodendri (*Huang Bai*), Rhizoma Anemarrhenae Aspheloidis (*Zhi Mu*), Caulis Akebiae Mutong (*Mu Tong*)

Wan Mi-zhai suggests this formula for the treatment of menstruation ahead of schedule due to heat in turn due to erroneously using acrid, warm medicinals. Such women have hidden or deep-lying fire in their *chong* and *ren* according to Master Wan.

6. *Qin Jing Si Wu Tang* (Scutellaria & Schizonepeta Four Materials Decoction)

Ingredients: Radix Angelicae Sinensis (*Dang Gui*), cooked Radix Rehmanniae (*Shu Di*), Radix Ligustici Wallichi (*Chuan Xiong*), Radix Albus Paeoniae Lactiflorae (*Bai Shao*), Radix Scutellariae Baicalensis (*Huang Qin*), carbonized Herba Schizonepetae Tenuifoliae (*Jing Jie*)

Chen and Chen in *A Comprehensive Guide to Chinese Herbal Medicine* recommend this formula for the treatment of early menstruation due to heat and blood vacuity. By changing cooked Rehmannia to uncooked Rehmannia and white Peony to red Peony, one can also use this formula for replete heat menstruation ahead of schedule.

Additions: If there is abdominal pain due to concomitant liver depression qi stagnation, add Fructus Meliae Toosendan (*Chuan Lian Zi*) and Rhizoma Cyperi Rotundi (*Xiang Fu*) to rectify and move the qi. If there is lumbar pain, add Radix Dipsaci (*Xu Duan*) and Cortex Eucommiae Ulmoidis (*Du Zhong*) to supplement the kidneys and strengthen the low back. If there is breast distention also due to qi stagnation, add Radix Bupleuri (*Chai Hu*).

7. *Yi Guan Jian Jia Jian* (One Link Decoction with Additions & Subtractions)

Ingredients: Uncooked Radix Rehmanniae (*Sheng Di*), Cortex Radicis Lycii Chinensis (*Di Gu Pi*), Tuber Ophiopogonis Japonici (*Mai Dong*), Radix Angelicae Sinensis (*Dang Gui*), Radix Glehniae Littoralis (*Sha Shen*), Fructus Meliae Toosendan (*Chao Chuan Lian Zi*)

Professors Song and Yu, the authors of *Zhong Yi Fu Ke Shou Ce (A Handbook of Chinese Medical Gynecology)*, suggest that this formula may be used for the treatment of depressive heat menstruation due to excessive anger. In TCM, this formula is most typically indicated for the treatment of liver blood-kidney yin vacuity complicated by liver depression qi stagnation. In this case, depressive liver heat counterflows upward, accumulating in the heart and lungs and disturbing the heart's control of the blood and the lungs' dispersion of the qi. Often, patients with this scenario suffer from sore throat and flu-like symptoms consistent with yin vacuity and fluid dryness before or during their menses.

8. Unnamed formula from *Nu Ke Jing Wei (Profundities from the Gynecological Classics)*

Ingredients: Body of Radix Angelicae Sinensis (*Dang Gui Shen*), uncooked Hangzhou Radix Albus Paeoniae Lactiflorae (*Hang Shao*), large cooked Radix Rehmanniae (*Shu Di*), uncooked Plastrum Testudinis (*Gui Ban*), fat Rhizoma Anemarrhenae Aspheloidis (*Zhi Mu*), salt-processed Cortex Phellodendri (*Huang Bai*), uncooked Rhizoma Polygonati Odorati (*Yu Zhu*), Cortex Radicis Lycii Chinensis (*Di Gu Pi*), true Gelatinum Corii Asini (*E Jiao*), mix-fried Radix Glycyrrhizae (*Gan Cao*), dry Tuber Ophiopogonis Japonici (*Mai Dong*)

The authors of the book from which this formula is taken say it is for liver-kidney yin vacuity with yang effulgence. The signs and symptoms they give for this are basically the same as above. However, when it comes to the pulse, they say it is bowstring, fine, small, and rapid with both cubit positions floating and slippery. Floating and possibly slippery pulses in the cubit positions (either one or both cubits) are extremely common in Western women and should not be read as replete pulses. Specifically, they indicate yin vacuity below failing to control yang which counterflows and becomes effulgent above.

6. Qi vacuity

Main symptoms: Menstruation ahead of schedule, excessive in amount but pale red, clear, and watery in color and consistency, a lack of lower abdominal distention and pain, dizziness, heart palpitations, shortness of breath, spontaneous sweating on movement, weariness and fatigue, lack of strength in the extremities, a pale white facial complexion, a light red tongue with thin, moist or wet fur, and a vacuous, large, and forceless pulse

Treatment principles: Boost the qi and nourish the blood, secure, conserve, and lift desertion

Guiding formulas:

1. *Gui Pi Tang* (Return the Spleen Decoction)

Ingredients: Radix Panacis Ginseng (*Ren Shen*) or Radix Codonopsitis Pilosulae (*Dang Shen*), Radix Astragali Membranacei (*Huang Qi*), Radix Angelicae Sinensis (*Dang Gui*), Rhizoma Atractylodis Macrocephalae (*Bai Zhu*), Sclerotium Poriae Cocos (*Fu Ling*), Radix Auklandiae Lappae (*Mu Xiang*), Semen Zizyphi Spinosae (*Suan Zao Ren*), Radix Polygalae Tenuifoliae (*Yuan Zhi*), Arillus Euphoriae Longanae (*Long Yan Rou*), mix-fried Radix Glycyrrhizae (*Zhi Gan Cao*), Fructus Zizyphi Jujubae (*Da Zao*), uncooked Rhizoma Zingiberis (*Sheng Jiang*)

Additions & subtractions: If bleeding is profuse, add Crinis Carbonisatus (*Xue Yu Tan*), carbonized Folium Et Petriolus Trachycarpi (*Zong Lu Tan*), Os Draconis (*Long Gu*), and Concha Ostreae (*Mu Li*) to aid astringing and stop bleeding. Sun Jiu-ling, the author of *Fu Ke Zheng Zhi (Gynecological Patterns & Treatments)*, adds Radix Bupleuri (*Chai Hu*), Rhizoma Cimicifugae (*Sheng Ma*), Os Draconis (*Sheng Long Gu*), Concha Ostreae (*Sheng Mu Li*), Os Sepiae Seu Sepiellae (*Hai Piao Xiao*) and Rhizoma Cyperi Rotundi (*Xiang Fu*) while deleting Zizyphus Spinosa, Polygalae Tenuifoliae, and Auklandia. This is in order to better upbear clear yang and to aid securing and astringing. Additionally, these modifications address the liver depression qi stagnation that commonly accompanies most if not all menstrual diseases in young and middle-aged women.

2. *Ju Yuan Jian* (Lift the Origin Decoction)

Ingredients: Radix Panacis Ginseng (*Ren Shen*), Radix Astragali Membranacei (*Huang Qi*), Radix Glycyrrhizae (*Gan Cao*), Rhizoma Cimicifugae (*Sheng Ma*), Rhizoma Atractylodis Macrocephalae (*Bai Zhu*)

Original qi can refer to either kidney qi or spleen qi. In this case, this term is used the way Li Dong-yuan used it, referring to the central or qi which is the latter heaven source or origin of the engenderment and transformation of qi, blood, and essence. This formula is obviously a truncated form of the next formula below, *Bu Zhong Yi Qi Tang* (Supplement the Center & Boost the Qi Decoction). It is a good one to remember when spleen qi vacuity causing early menstruation complicates other patterns, in which case, these are the key or core medicinals from that formula to add to other guiding formulas appropriate for other patterns.

Additions: Han Bai-ling recommends adding Gelatinum Corii Asini (*E Jiao*) and Os Sepiae

Seu Sepiellae (*Hai Piao Xiao*) to lift yin and stop bleeding. Gelatinum Corii Asini nourishes the blood and stops bleeding, while Os Sepiae Seu Sepiellae astringes and secures and stops bleeding. As an astringent, this last medicinal specifically strengthens the kidneys' astring-ing and securing, and, as we will see below, in clinical practice, spleen vacuity menstruation ahead of schedule is mostly complicated by kidney vacuity as well.

3. *Bu Zhong Yi Qi Tang* (Supplement the Center & Boost the Qi Decoction)

Ingredients: Radix Astragali Membranacei (*Huang Qi*), Radix Panacis Ginseng (*Ren Shen*) or Radix Codonopsitis Pilosulae (*Dang Shen*), Rhizoma Atractylodis Macrocephalae (*Bai Zhu*), Pericarpium Citri Reticulatae (*Chen Pi*), Rhizoma Cimicifugae (*Sheng Ma*), Radix Bupleuri (*Chai Hu*), Radix Angelicae Sinensis (*Dang Gui*), mix-freid Radix Glycyrrhizae (*Gan Cao*)

This formula is indicated by Xue Li-zhai in *Nu Ke Mi Jue Da Quan (A Great Compendium of Secrets of Success in Gynecology)* for the treatment of menstruation ahead of schedule due to taxation labor fire stirring. This means qi vacuity with Li Dong-yuan's concept of yin fire. In this case, central qi falls and fails to contain the blood within its vessels. This often looks superficially like vacuity heat, but the total constellation of signs and symptoms, tongue, and pulse points to qi vacuity instead. In my practice, I use this formula more commonly as the base of my prescriptions for menstruation ahead of schedule than any other. Readers should keep in mind, that Bupleurum, aged Orange Peel, and Cimicifuga all rectify the qi. In addition, some Chinese authors argue that Astragalus, because it upbears the clear and, therefore, disinhibits the qi mechanism, also rectifies the qi and resolves depression. Thus, although this formula is the standard textbook formula for central qi fall, its ingredients do treat liver depression as well as spleen vacuity. This is a very important point to remember with this formula.

Additions: Zhang En-qin *et al.*, in *Zhong Yi Lin Chuang Ge Ke (Various Clinical Specialties in Traditional Chinese Medicine)*, adds Herba Leonuri Heterophylli (*Yi Mu Cao*) to this basic for-mula. They then suggest adding Sclerotium Pararadicis Poriae Cocos (*Fu Shen*) and Semen Zizyphi Spinosae (*Suan Zao Ren*) if there are heart palpitations and Gelatinum Cornu Cervi (*Lu Jiao Jiao*) and Cortex Eucommiae Ulmoidis (*Du Zhong*) for yang vacuity low back pain and loose stools. The first addition attests to the fact that blood stasis often complicates this pattern. Qi and blood vacuity may cause blood stasis and blood stasis prevents the engenderment of fresh or new blood. Therefore, Leonurus has the benefit of quickening the blood without damaging it. The addition of Dear Antler and Eucommia again attest to the fact that, in clinical practice, kidney yang vacuity typically complicates spleen vacuity menstruation ahead of schedule.

4. *Ba Zhen Tang* (Eight Pearls Decoction)

Ingredients: Radix Panacis Ginseng (*Ren Shen*) or Radix Codonopsitis Pilosulae (*Dang Shen*), Rhizoma Atractylodis Macrocephalae (*Bai Zhu*), Sclerotium Poriae Cocos (*Fu Ling*), mix-fried Radix Glycyrrhizae (*Gan Cao*), Radix Angelicae Sinensis (*Dang Gui*), Radix Albus Paeoniae Lactiflorae (*Bai Shao*), cooked Radix Rehmanniae (*Shu Di*), Radix Ligustici Wallichii (*Chuan Xiong*)

If there is pronounced blood vacuity accompanying qi vacuity, one may use *Ba Zhen Tang* to supplement the qi and nourish the blood.

Additions & subtractions: Because Ligusticum moves the qi and quickens the blood, its dosage should be half that of the other blood-nourishing ingredients or it may be deleted altogether. In general, one should be careful of using this medicinal if there is early menstruation uncomplicated by blood stasis. If, due to spleen vacuity, cooked Rehmannia is deemed too enriching and slimy and there is concern for its damaging the spleen, one may delete it and add Herba Ecliptae Prostratae (*Han Lian Cao*) and Fructus Ligustri Lucidi (*Nu Zhen Zi*). If there is concomitant liver depression, one can add Radix Bupleuri (*Chai Hu*), Rhizoma Cyperi Rotundi (*Xiang Fu*), and/or other such qi-rectifying medicinals depending on the exact signs and symptoms or area of the body affected by the qi stagnation. If there is kidney yang vacuity, one may add Cortex Eucommiae Ulmoidis (*Du Zhong*) and Radix Dipsaci (*Xu Duan*) if there is lumbar pain, or one may add Rhizoma Curculiginis Orchioidis (*Xian Mao*) and Herba Epimedii (*Xian Ling Pi* or *Yin Yang Huo*) if there is decreased libido.

5. *Er Xian Tang Jia Jian* (Two Immortals Decoction with Additions & Subtractions)

Ingredients: Rhizoma Curculiginis Orchioidis (*Xian Mao*), Herba Epimedii (*Xian Ling Pi*), Radix Morindae Officinalis (*Ba Ji Tian*), scorched Rhizoma Atractylodis Macrocephalae (*Bai Zhu*), Radix Codonopsitis Pilosulae (*Dang Shen*), Radix Glycyrrhizae (*Gan Cao*), uncooked Rhizoma Zingiberis (*Sheng Jiang*), Fructus Zizyphi Jujubae (*Da Zao*)

This formula is given by Guo Yuan in *Shi Yong Zhong Xi Yi Jie He Fu Chan Ke Zheng Zhi (Practical Integrated Chinese-Western Obstetrics & Gynecology Patterns & Treatments)* under the category spleen-kidney yang vacuity. In this case, Guo Yuan gives the signs and symptoms as menstruation ahead of schedule, color pale, clear, and watery, face ashen white, body cold, limbs chilled, diminished appetite, loose stools, desire for warm food and drink, a pale tongue with scanty fur, and a deep, fine, weak pulse. The therapeutic principles Guo gives are to supplement the kidneys and invigorate yang, fortify the spleen and regulate the menses.

I frequently use a slightly different variation on *Er Xian Tang* for chronically early menses where there is both spleen qi and kidney yang vacuity, blood or yin vacuity, and liver depression. Because of the yin vacuity, the tongue may be red or have a red tip and there may not be such pronounced signs of vacuity cold as described above. The ingredients in the formula which I often use are Herba Epimedii (*Xian Ling Pi*), Rhizoma Curculiginis Orchioidis (*Xian Mao*), Fructus Ligustri Lucidi (*Nu Zhen Zi*), Herba Ecliptae Prostratae (*Han Lian Cao*), Radix Angelicae Sinensis (*Dang Gui*), Radix Salviae Miltiorrhizae (*Dan Shen*), Rhizoma Cyperi Rotundi (*Xiang Fu*), Radix Linderae Strychnifoliae (*Wu Yao*), Rhizoma Alismatis (*Ze Xie*), Radix Astragali Membranacei (*Huang Qi*), Radix Codonopsitis Pilosulae (*Dang Shen*), Rhizoma Atractylodis Macrocephalae (*Bai Zhu*), Rhizoma Cimicifugae (*Sheng Ma*), and Gelatinum Corii Asini (*E Jiao*).

6. *Gui Shen Wan* (Return the Kidneys Pills)

Ingredients: Cooked Radix Rehmanniae (*Shu Di*), Radix Dioscoreae Oppositae (*Shan Yao*), Fructus Corni Officinalis (*Shan Zhu Yu*), Sclerotium Poriae Cocos (*Fu Ling*), Radix Angelicae Sinensis (*Dang Gui*), Fructus Lycii Chinensis (*Gou Qi Zi*), Cortex Eucommiae Ulmoidis (*Du Zhong*), Semen Cuscutae (*Tu Si Zi*)

Du Jie-hui, in *Nan Nu Bing Mi Yan Liang Fang (Secret, Proven, Fine Formulas for Men's & Women's Disease)*, recommends this formula for kidney qi not securing the *chong* resulting in early menstruation. This formula nourishes yin at the same time as it supplements yang. Technically, it can be said to search out yang in the midst of yin. However, in my practice, I never see kidney yang vacuity menstruation ahead of schedule without simultaneous spleen vacuity.

7. *Wen Chong Tang* (Warm the *Chong* Decoction)

Ingredients: Radix Dioscoreae Oppositae (*Shan Yao*), Radix Angelicae Sinensis (*Dang Gui*), Radix Lateralis Praeparatus Aconiti Carmichaeli (*Wu Fu Zi*), Cortex Cinnamomi Cassiae (*Rou Gui*), Fructus Psoraleae Corylifoliae (*Bu Gu Zhi*), Fructus Foeniculi Vulgaris (*Xiao Hui Xiang*), Semen Juglandis Regiae (*Hu Tao Ren*), Amethystum (*Zi Shi Ying*), Gelatinum Cornu Cervi (*Lu Jiao Jiao*)

This formula is also suggested by Du Jie-hui. It is indicated for kidney yang vacuity resulting in kidney qi not securing the *chong* and, therefore, menstruation ahead of schedule. The addition of Aconite and Cinnamon suggests pronounced symptoms of vacuity chilling. Usually, my patients do not present with such cold symptoms. In fact, one must be careful not to overlook the symptoms of kidney vacuity in the majority of early menstruation patients since this is rarely, in my experience, the main presenting pattern. Even when it is the main presenting pattern, its symptoms usually have more to do with lumbar pain, nighttime urination, and diminished libido than pronounced cold.

Blood stasis

Main symptoms: Menstruation ahead of schedule, scanty, purplish blood with clots, abdominal pain resisting pressure which diminishes with the passage of clots, a dark, purplish tongue or static spots or macules on the tongue, possibly dry, yellowish tongue fur, and a deep, fine, bowstring, and/or choppy pulse

Treatment principles: Quicken the blood and transform stasis

Guiding formula: *Tao Hong Si Wu Tang* (Persica & Carthamus Four Materials Decoction)

Ingredients: Uncooked Radix Rehmanniae (*Sheng Di*), Radix Angelicae Sinensis (*Dang Gui*), Radix Rubrus Paeoniae Lactiflorae (*Chi Shao*), Radix Ligustici Wallichii (*Chuan Xiong*), Semen Pruni Persicae (*Tao Ren*), Flos Carthami Tinctorii (*Hong Hua*)

Additions: If there is more pronounced abdominal pain, add Feces Trogopterori Seu Pteromi (*Wu Ling Zhi*) and Cortex Radicis Moutan (*Dan Pi*)

This fomula is the guiding textbook formula for blood stasis due to or complicated by blood vacuity. Although blood stasis rarely appears as the sole or even the main cause of early menstruation, when blood stasis is the most prominent aspect of a complicated pattern, this formula may be used as the guiding formula and modified as appropriate. One can temper the degree of attack by using Radix Albus Paeoniae Lactiflorae (*Bai Shao*) instead of red Peony and cooked Radix Rehmanniae (*Shu Di*) instead of uncooked Rehmannia.

Discussion

Menstruation ahead of schedule is a very commonly encountered disease category in clinical practice. Rarely do Western women come to the clinic, however, with early menstruation as their major complaint. More often, they may complain of endometriosis, PMS, cervical dysplasia, or infertility. When doing a TCM diagnosis, if a patient suffers from one of the latter three diseases and her menses are early, remedying of the early menses should be a priority in terms of her Chinese disease category. If, however, she experiences endometriosis or menstrual pain, she should first be treated for that, *i.e.*, painful menstruation. In that case, one may choose a guiding formula from under that disease category but should also take the mechanism causing early menstruation into account and modify for it.

Treating and correcting early menstruation is subsumed under the more general treatment principle of regulating the menses (*tiao jing*). Some TCM gynecology texts do not discuss the category of menstruation ahead of schedule but merely *yue jing bu tiao* or menstrual irregularities. This includes early, late, profuse, and scanty menstruation. From a Western point of view, early menstruation is typically due to a hormonal imbalance. Treating and correcting early menstruation through TCM does result in restoring balance to the endocrine system and ovarian function.

Prognosis

Replete heat menstruation ahead of schedule is usually easy to treat. If one can identify the source of the heat, usually dietary, and remove that, in many cases one only has to administer internal medication for one cycle. Once this heat is cleared, as long as the patient does not indulge in the offending food or drink and granting that the replete heat is not due to the external environment, once treated it should not come back. If due to hot macrocosmic qi, once the weather changes or the woman returns to her normal environment, the menses should regulate themselves automatically. Otherwise, treatment can be given which should be short and successful as long as the case is not complicated by other factors.

Depressive heat, on the other hand, is mostly due to emotional stress and frustration. It can be aggravated by faulty diet but is mostly a lifestyle and maladaptive stress response. When the patient encounters stress and frustration, she tenses, tightening the muscles of her body and thus constricting the flow of qi and blood through her channels and network vessels. Treatment may successfully clear heat and resolve depression, but unless the patient is able to modify their lifestyle and their reaction to stress, they will develop this same depressive heat again. Ways to cope with depressive heat due to liver qi are to exercise regularly in order to circulate and blow off or out-thrust stagnant qi and to practice deep relaxation in order to train in how to remain relaxed in the midst of one's stresses and frustrations. The bowstring pulse emblematic of liver qi is due to constriction by the sinews surrounding the vessels. The sinews are the tissue associated with the liver. Learning to keep these sinews relaxed is the key to long-term resolution of this problem. However, because this is easier said than done, this pattern has a high recidivism rate.

I do not see phlegm heat all that often since I live in a very health conscious city where obesity is the exception rather than the rule. The heat in phlegm heat is usually easy to clear, but phlegm, because it is heavy and recalcitrant to treatment, is harder to eliminate and wash away. Also, in my experience, most women with phlegm heat have a large component of liver depression qi stagnation mixed in, and this is often difficult to resolve. These women are frustrated because they are overweight. But because they are frustrated, their spleen finds it hard to recuperate due to constant over-control by liver wood. On the other hand, if the spleen could only recuperate, this would help keep their liver under better control. It is extremely important to counsel such women on the TCM theories regarding digestion and fat as phlegm stagnation. These theories must then be put into practice in terms of the woman's diet. Chinese dietary therapy has a great deal of wisdom when it comes to obesity and phlegm, and proper diet must play an important role in any treatment plan for phlegm heat.

One must also be careful not to diagnose every obese woman with early menstruation as suffering from phlegm heat. Many overweight women with early menstruation suffer from spleen qi vacuity or even kidney yang vacuity. In such cases, phlegm may complicate their scenario and vacuous yang may even counterflow upward, but emphasis in treatment should be on boosting the qi or supplementing and leading yang back down to its lower source.

Damp heat menstruation ahead of schedule is also usually relatively easy to treat. Most often, such damp heat is associated with spleen vacuity and dampness pouring downward. In that case, one must commonly fortify the spleen and boost the qi at the same time as clearing heat and resolving dampness. Also in such cases, correct diet is essential for either a complete or lasting cure.

If there is polysystemic, chronic candidiasis, as there often is in Western women, administration of bitter, cold medicinals which have pronounced fungicidal abilities, such as Cortex Phellodendri (*Huang Bai*), Radix Scutellariae Baicalensis (*Huang Qin*), and Rhizoma Coptidis Chinensis (*Huang Lian*), may cause a Herxheimer or die-off reaction. So many yeast die and begin to decompose that the body develops a histamine or allergic reaction to the foreign proteins released into the system. This can cause aggravation of all the patient's signs and symptoms or provoke diarrhea, gas, headache, body aches and pains, and even fever. In this case, this is not necessarily a bad or negative reaction to therapy. In fact, it is a sign that the goal of combatting fungus is being accomplished. At this point, one should advise the patient to drink more water, soak in a bathtub of warm water and Epsom Salts, and/or do one or two warm water enemas per day. These adjunctive therapies help to rid the body of the breakdown products of the yeast bodies and thus eliminate these reactive signs and symptoms. Such Herxheimer reaction signs and symptoms usually only last for 24-48 days and are then followed by an unmistakable, systemic improvement in the patient's condition. If loose stools, nausea, or vomiting continue for more than 48 hours, then the formula may be damaging the spleen and the patient's pattern discrimination and prescription should be re-evaluated and modified.

If damp heat is due to retained evils associated with a past and incompletely treated sexually transmitted or pelvic inflammatory disease, TCM treatment is still usually effective. In this case, however, early menstruation tends to accompany lower abdominal pain which increases as the menses come closer. Therefore, the main complaint or focus of treatment should be the pain since, in TCM, pain is considered a primary branch symptom. However, when pain is diminished due to therapy directed at that pain, the menses may still have a tendency to come early. In that case, complicating spleen and/or kidney vacuity should be suspected. If present, these vacuities should be supplemented as the main theme of therapy, with clearing heat and eliminating dampness as the minor motif.

Vacuity heat early menstruation can be difficult to treat if the woman is getting older or if she cannot or will not slow down her pace. In some cases, clearing heat and cooling the blood is not as effective as nourishing the blood and, therefore, automatically cooling it. Because of this, *Si Wu Tang* (Four Materials Decoction) often makes a very good guiding formula for the treatment of yin vacuity-vacuity heat early menstruation accompanied by kidney supplements, such as Semen Cuscutae Chinensis (*Tu Si Zi*) and Radix Dioscoreae Oppositae (*Shan Yao*) and not too many bitter, cold medicinals.

When it comes to qi vacuity types of menstruation ahead of schedule, one rarely encounters a pure qi vacuity pattern. Kidney qi vacuity menstruation usually occurs in women beginning as early as the mid-30s and increasing in incidence through the 40s until menopause. As mentioned above, kidney yang vacuity (which includes within it kidney qi vacuity) is always accompanied by spleen qi vacuity. This is due to the fact that the spleen first becomes vacuous and then the kidneys become vacuous due to the latter and former heavens' mutual relationship. Therefore, in clinical practice, the issue is which of these two factors is most important, not whether there is one or the other.

If spleen vacuity is most prominent, then the treatment principles are to fortify the spleen and boost the qi assisted by supplementing the kidneys and invigorating yang. In that case, one chooses a formula from the qi supplementing category of formulas, such as *Bu Zhong Yi Qi Tang* (Supplement the Center & Boost the Qi Decoction) and then adds medicinals that supplement the kidneys and invigorate yang, such as Radix Dipsaci (*Xu Duan*) and Cortex Eucommiae Ulmoidis (*Du Zhong*) or Rhizoma Curculiginis Orchioidis (*Xian Mao*) and Herba Epimedii (*Xian Ling Pi*). If kidney yang vacuity signs and symptoms are more prominent, then the treatment principles are to supplement the kidneys and invigorate yang assisted by fortifying the spleen and boosting the qi. In that case, one chooses from the yang-supplementing category of formulas, such as *Er Xian Tang* (Two Immortals Decoction) and then adds medicinals which fortify the spleen and boost the qi, such as the ingredients in *Ju Yuan Jian* (Lift the Origin Decoction).

However, to make matters more complicated, spleen-kidney vacuity menstruation is almost always complicated by liver depression. It may also be complicated by damp heat and/or blood stasis. However, even in such complicated cases, one simply tallies up the signs and symptoms and makes one's pattern discrimination. Depending on which element in the total pattern is most prominent, then that is the category of formulas from which one chooses their guiding formula. For instance, if there is a liver-spleen disharmony with depressive heat in the stomach and lungs as well as kidney yang vacuity, then one might choose *Xiao Chia Hu Tang* (Minor Bupleurum Decoction) as their guiding formula. This formula is a harmonizing formula which courses the liver and fortifies the spleen at the same time as it clears heat from the stomach and lungs.

Then one would modify this guiding formula. Because liver depression worsens premenstrually due to a combination of blood vacuity and spleen qi vacuity, one might add either or both Radix Angelicae Sinensis (*Dang Gui*) and Radix Albus Paeoniae Lactiflorae (*Bai Shao*) in order to nourish the blood and thus emolliate and harmonize the liver. If the patient is definitely fatigued, then one might add Radix Astragali Membranacei (*Huang Qi*) to further supplement the spleen and boost the qi. In order to also supplement the kidneys and invigorate yang, one could add Rhizoma Curculiginis Orchioidis (*Xian Mao*), Herba Epimedii (*Xian Ling Pi*), Cortex Eucommiae Ulmoidis (*Du Zhong*), Radix Morindae Officinalis (*Ba Ji Tian*), Herba Cistanchis Deserticolae (*Rou Cong Rong*) depending upon the patients exact symptoms of kidney yang vacuity.

When there is spleen qi and kidney yang vacuity, the bowstring, fine pulse and other signs and symptoms of liver depression qi stagnation and/or blood vacuity do not go away. Therefore, practitioners may easily see the prominent symptoms of liver qi and liver blood vacuity but miss the symptoms of either spleen qi or kidney yang vacuity. The likelihood of missing these is even greater if there is either depressive, damp, phelgm, or vacuity heat. Therefore, it is very important to carefully and systematically check for signs and symptoms of spleen and kidney vacuity in female patients beginning in their mid to late 30s. When there is spleen qi and kidney vacuity early menstruation and one correctly treats for this, then this condition can usually also be remedied in one to three menstrual cycles.

As mentioned above, blood stasis is usually not the main cause of menstruation ahead of schedule. It is, however, a commonly met complication. Blood stasis involved with menstruation ahead of schedule most often responds to therapy quickly and well. If the blood stasis is the result of an IUD, one or more abortions, or some other historical factor, once it is dispelled, it should not return. If blood stasis is due to long-term liver qi and this liver qi remains unresolved, then, over time, the blood stasis may return. I regard any clots in the discharge as a sign of some complicating blood stasis. A woman should not have any clots in her menstrual discharge even from a modern Western medical point of view.

Clinical tips

If a woman's early menstruation is due to vacuity heat but she also suffers from qi stagnation, the earlier the menstruation comes, typically the less PMS and menstrual pain she will

170

have. This is because there is simply not the volume of yin fluids to put pressure on the constriction and stagnation. As supplementation takes effect and the cycle lengthens out, some women will report more PMS and more menstrual pain. This should be taken as a sign that vcuity has been supplemented but now the liver should be coursed and the qi rectified more strongly. In some cases, vacuity heat when supplemented may turn into depressive heat. In that case, one must then clear heat and resolve (literally, unbind) depression.

In women from their mid-30s on, always look for spleen-kidney vacuity no matter what other patterns may be present. If present and left untreated, menstruation ahead of schedule will not be brought under control. The majority of women in their later 30s and early 40s with early menstruation suffer from a luteal phase defect due to the aging of their ovaries. Such a luteal phase defect can be confirmed by the patient's charting of her basal body temperature for one to three cycles. If she is ovulating on day 14 but her menses come on day 26 or before, then there is a luteal phase defect. Most often this is due to spleen-kidney yang vacuity. If there is premenstrual breast distention and pain, lower abdominal distention and fullness, increased irritability, and a bowstring pulse, there is also liver depression qi stagnation. If there is breast pain or nipple hypersensitivity, premenstrual acne, more pronounced irritability, and a rapid, bowstring pulse, then there is also depressive heat. This commonly manifests as a saw-toothed pattern during the hyperthermal phase. If the woman is ovulating on day 14 and there is a luteal phase defect, then treatment should be focused on the luteal phase or premenstruum. Commonly in such cases, the woman does not need to be treated throughout her cycle other than improving her stress-reduction and coping skills and improving her diet.

If, on the other hand, a woman has early ovulation or a shortened hypothermal phase as shown by her BBT chart, changes and increases in her vaginal mucus, and/or *mittleschmerz* or midcylce, ovulatory pain, then the most common pattern discriminations are depressive or vacuity heat. We have seen above that there are only three possible causes of menstruation ahead of schedule: 1) heat, 2) qi vacuity, and 3) blood stasis. We have also seen that ovulation occurs due to yin transforming into yang. Since that transformation is hampered if the qi mechanism is inhibited, then blood stasis is not likely to leads to early ovulation. Since spleen and kidney vacuity during the hypothermal phase typically lead to late or lack of ovulation, then they are also not likely candidates for causing early ovulation. This then leaves heat. This heat may, in my experience, be either depressive or vacuity heat. In theory, it might be damp heat, but I have yet to confirm this from clinical experience.

In cases of early ovulation and menstruation therefore ahead of schedule, it is important to initiate treatment either before the menses stop or immediately after their cessation. If one treats after ovulation, it is difficult to see any improvement in the length of the cycle.

However, in my experience, women with early menstruation due to early ovulation in turn due to depressive heat typically do have PMS. In that case, it is also necessary to treat during their premenstruum as well. If they also have painful menstruation, treatment may extend into the first day or two of their menses in order to stop pain. Thus charting the BBT can be a significant help in timing the treatment of menstruation ahead of schedule.

In the treatment of early menstruation, blood-stopping medicinals should not be used without due care. In some cases of menstruation ahead of schedule, blood-stopping medicinals should be used if there is also profuse bleeding or if the case is otherwise recalcitrant to treatment. However, blood-stopping medicinals can cause blood stasis if over or inappropriately used. When using Chinese blood-stopping medicinals, one should be sure that the actions of the medicinals employed also match the requisite TCM treatment principles for that case. For instance, Folium Artemisiae Argyii (*Ai Ye*) warms the womb and stops bleeding; Cacumen Biotae Orientalis (*Ce Bai Ye*) cools the blood and stops bleeding; and Receptaculum Nelumbinis Nuciferae (*Lian Fang*) dispels stasis and stops bleeding.

If a woman develops breast tenderness and other such PMS symptoms and then all of these suddenly disappear, this suggests that menstruation is about to begin within the next 24-36 hours.

Key patterns to memorize

It is important to memorize the following disease mechanisms and patterns accounting for menstruation ahead of schedule. Then, whenever any woman presents with early menstruation, one can immediately see these in their mind's eye and begin questioning and examining to confirm or deny their presence and participation.

1. Heat	A. Replete heat B. Depressive heat C. Vacuity heat D. Phlegm heat E. Damp heat
2. Qi vacuity (usually complicates)	A. Spleen qi vacuity B. Kidney qi (and yang) vacuity
3. Blood stasis (usually only complicates)	

Menstruation Ahead of Schedule, Profuse Menstruation, Menstrual Cramps, Midcycle Bleeding

Diseases→ Treatments↘ Patterns	Menstruation Ahead of Schedule Treatment Methods	Formula	Profuse Menstruation Treatment Methods	Formula	Menstrual Cramps Treatment Methods	Formula	Midcycle Bleeding Treatment Methods	Formula
Qi Vacuity	Supplement qi Contain blood Regulate menses	Bu Zhong Yi Qi Tang	Supplement qi Contain blood Secure chong	Ju Yuan Jian				
Blood Heat — Replete Heat — blood heat	Clear heat, cool blood, regulate menses	Qing Jing San	Cool blood, clear heat, stop bleeding	Pao Yin Jian Jia De Yu Huai Hua				
Blood Heat — Replete Heat — Liver depression blood heat	Clear liver, resolve depression, regulate menses	Dan Zhi Xiao Yao San						
Blood Heat — Vacuity Heat (Yin Vacuity Blood Heat)	Nourish yin, clear heat, regulate menses	Liang Di Tang	Nourish yin, clear heat, stop bleeding	Liang Di Tang plus Er Zhi Wan plus Qian Cao, Wu Zei Gu, Yi Mu Cao				
Kidney Yin Vacuity							Enrich yin, stop bleeding	Liang Di Tang plus Er Zhi Wan
Blood Stasis			Quicken blood, transform stasis, stop bleeding	Shi Xiao San Jia Xue Yu Tan, Qian Cao, Yi Mu Cao	Quicken blood, dispel stasis, stop bleeding	Tao Hong Si Wu Tang plus Shi Xiao San plus Yi Mu Cao, Qian Cao	Transform stasis, stop bleeding	Zhu Yu Zhi Xue Tang
Damp Heat							Clear & disinhibit dampness & heat	Qing Gan Zhi Lin Tang

2

Menstruation Behind Schedule

Professors Song and Yu define menstruation behind schedule or late menstruation as the occurrence of menstruation at least seven days later than its expected due date. Han Bai-ling corroborates this, saying that if the menses comes only three to five days late without any other abnormal complaints, this should not be categorized as a disease state nor should it be treated medicinally. Likewise, if the menses are only occasionally delayed, this also should not be categorized as a pathologically late menstruation. However, if there are other complaints accompanying a habitually delayed period of more than three to five days, I do find it useful and important to take this delay into account when assessing the patient's entire condition both in terms of disease discrimination and pattern discrimination.

Disease causes, disease mechanisms

Menstruation behind schedule are a species of not bleeding when one should. There are only two TCM mechanisms which may account for this. Either the body is not producing enough blood within 28 days to fill and overflow the uterus or something is obstructing the free and smooth flow of the blood. Beyond these two basic mechanisms, there are not any other causes of delayed menstruation. However, within these two general categories of disease mechanisms, there are several different subcategories.

If menstruation is delayed because of insufficient blood, this may be due in turn either to excessive blood loss, damage of the blood by heat, or failure of the body to engender sufficient fresh blood. If due to hemorrhage or other excessive loss of body fluids, such as through excessive sweating, diarrhea, or vomiting, this should be easily ascertained through questioning.

Zhu Dan-xi was also of the opinion that blood vacuity delayed menstruation can be due to heat entering the blood division, where it stews the juices and consumes the blood. This results in blood vacuity and insufficient blood to brim over as the menstruate.

If, on the other hand, the body is failing to engender sufficient fresh blood, one must look at the three viscera in charge of the engenderment and transformation of blood. These are the spleen, heart, and kidneys. Due to faulty diet, for instance not eating enough foods with sufficient *wei* or flavor, such as animal flesh, or eating too many uncooked, chilled foods, or due to faulty digestion, the spleen may not be able to separate the pure from turbid and send the pure part of the turbid upward. Faulty digestion may be due to excessive worry and anxiety and also to lack of exercise. Or, due to longing and unhappiness, the spirit residing in the heart may be disturbed and thus hinder the heart's turning the blood red. It is also possible for either yin or yang vacuity of the kidneys to result in insufficiency of blood engenderment and transformation.

Some kidney essence must be sent up to the heart to help in the engenderment and transformation of the blood. Mostly one thinks of kidney essence in terms of the blood as being yin. However, essence may be either yin or yang depending upon how it is transformed and used. If kidney yin is insufficient, there will not be the material substrate for the creation of the blood. But if kidney yang is vacuous and weak, the engenderment of the blood will not be catalyzed, nor will there be free-flowing qi flow in the lower burner. This latter mechanism may complicate insufficient blood in the lower burner by restricted movement in turn due to lack of motivating yang, remembering that kidney yang provides the motivating force for all lower burner qi and fluids. Kidney yin vacuity may be constitutional. It may also be the result of hyperactivity, excessive stress and stimulation, excessive sex, recreational drugs, enduring disease, poor sleep, and the aging process. Kidney yang vacuity with vacuity cold may also be due to age, drug use, enduring disease, overtaxation, and excessive sex.

In terms of obstruction to the flow of blood, any of four pathological accumulations may result in delayed menstruation. First, if full cold lodges in the uterus, it will constrict and congeal the menstruate. This may be due to overeating uncooked, chilled foods, swimming in cold water too near the menses, exposure to dampness and cold weather, and, in my experience, exposure to cold during lower abdominal surgery or abortions. Cold causes contraction and congelation and thus blood stasis. Secondly, if there is qi stagnation due to stress and frustration, because the qi commands and moves the blood, the blood will not be able to flow freely to and from the uterus. Third, due to trauma, iatrogenesis, or enduring qi stagnation, the blood may become static. This blood stasis then hinders or restricts the free flow and egress of the menstruate from the uterus. And fourth, due to faulty diet and digestion and lack of sufficient exercise, phlegm may accumulate in the channels and vessels, thus obstructing the free flow of blood. It should be remembered that in Chinese, the word for the menses, *jing*, is the same as for channels. When discussing phlegm accumulation, TCM theory posits that phlegm may accumulate under the skin and between the tissues, it may accumulate and block the clear orifices and the orifices of the heart, and it may accumulate and obstruct the *jing*. When enough qi and blood finally back up behind the obstruction, they eventually push their way through and the menses come even though they are late.

Treatment based on pattern discrimination

Based on the above disease mechanisms, menstruation behind schedule can be divided into replete and vacuity varieties.

Vacuity patterns

1. Vacuity cold

Main symptoms: Delayed menstruation, pale colored menstruate, scanty in amount, insidious lower abdominal pain ameliorated by warmth and pressure, dizziness, a pale white facial complexion, lack of strength in the low back and knees, a pale tongue with thin, white fur, and a deep, slow, forceless pulse

Treatment principles: Warm the channels (or menses) and scatter cold, boost the qi and nourish the blood

Guiding formulas:

1. Zhang Jing-yue's *Da Ying Jian* (Greatly Constructing Decoction)

Ingredients: Fructus Lycii Chinensis (*Gou Ji Zi*), Cortex Eucommiae Ulmoidis (*Du Zhong*), Cortex Cinnamomi Cassiae (*Rou Gui*), Radix Achyranthis Bidentatae (*Niu Xi*), Radix Angelicae Sinensis (*Dang Gui*), cooked Radix Rehmanniae (*Shu Di*), mix-fried Radix Glycyrrhizae (*Gan Cao*)

Additions: For qi vacuity, add Radix Panacis Ginseng (*Ren Shen*). For yin cold, add Radix Lateralis Praeparatus Aconiti Carmichaeli (*Fu Zi*). To warm the kidneys and invigorate yang, add Radix Morindae Officinalis (*Ba Ji Tian*) and Fructus Psoraleae Corylifoliae (*Bu Gu Zhi*).

2. *Wen Jing Tang* (Warm the Channels [or Menses] Decoction)

Ingredients: Fructus Evodiae Rutecarpae (*Wu Zhu Yu*), Ramulus Cinnamomi Cassiae (*Gui Zhi*), Radix Angelicae Sinensis (*Dang Gui*), Radix Albus Paeoniae Lactiflorae (*Bai Shao*), Cortex Radicis Moutan (*Dan Pi*), Radix Ligustici Wallichii (*Chuan Xiong*), Gelatinum Corii Asini (*E Jiao*), Tuber Ophiopogonis Japonici (*Mai Dong*), Radix Panacis Ginseng (*Ren Shen*), Rhizoma Pinelliae Ternatae (*Ban Xia*), Radix Glycyrrhizae (*Gan Cao*), uncooked Rhizoma Zingiberis (*Sheng Jiang*)

Additions & subtractions: Sun Jiu-ling suggests deleting Pinellia and adding Herba Epimedii (*Xian Ling Pi*) to supplement the kidneys and invigorate yang. Zhao Rei-ling suggests adding carbonized Folium Artemisiae Argyii (*Ai Ye*), stir-fried Feces Trogopterori Seu Pteromi (*Wu Ling Zhi*), and stir-fried Pollen Typhae (*Pu Huang*) to quicken the blood and dispel stasis at the same time as stopping bleeding if accompanied by heavy bleeding.

3. *Yi Pi Wen Shen Tang* (Boost the Spleen & Warm the Kidneys Decoction)

Ingredients: Radix Panacis Ginseng (*Ren Shen*), Rhizoma Atractylodis Macrocephalae (*Bai Zhu*), Radix Dioscoreae Oppositae (*Shan Yao*), Radix Morindae Officinalis (*Ba Ji Tian*), Semen Cuscutae (*Tu Si Zi*), Radix Angelicae Sinensis (*Dang Gui*), Radix Glycyrrhizae (*Gan Cao*)

Additions: For white vaginal discharge, add Semen Coicis Lachryma-jobi (*Yi Yi Ren)* and Fructus Psoraleae Corylifoliae (*Bu Gu Zhi*) to warm the kidneys, secure, and astringe.

4. *Wu Yao San Jia Wei* (Lindera Powder with Added Flavors)

Ingredients: Radix Linderae Strychnifoliae (*Wu Yao*), Rhizoma Cyperi Rotundi (*Xiang Fu*), Sclerotium Poriae Cocos (*Fu Ling*), Pericarpium Citri Reticulatae (*Chen Pi*), Fructus Crataegi (*Shan Zha*), Radix Angelicae Sinensis (*Dang Gui*), Radix Albus Paeoniae Lactiflorae (*Bai Shao*), Rhizoma Corydalis Yanhusuo (*Yan Hu Suo*), Ramulus Cinnamomi Cassiae (*Gui Zhi*)

Additions: If there is lumbar pain and soreness, add Cortex Eucommiae Ulmoidis (*Du Zhong*) and Radix Dipsaci (*Xu Duan*) to supplement the kidneys, invigorate yang, and strengthen the low back.

5. *Si Wu Tang Jia Wei* (Four Materials Decoction with Added Flavors)

Ingredients: Radix Angelicae Sinensis (*Dang Gui*), Radix Albus Paeoniae Lactiflorae (*Bai Shao*), cooked Radix Rehmanniae (*Shu Di*), Radix Ligustici Wallichii (*Chuan Xiong*), Folium Artemisiae Argyii (*Ai Ye*), Rhizoma Cyperi Rotundi (*Xiang Fu*), Fructus Evodiae Rutecarpae (*Wu Zhu Yu*), Ramulus Cinnamomi Cassiae (*Gui Zhi*)

6. *Gui Fu Wan Jia Wei* (Dang Gui & Cyperus Pills with Added Flavors)

Ingredients: Radix Angelicae Sinensis (*Dang Gui*), Rhizoma Cyperi Rotundi (*Xiang Fu*), Cortex Cinnamomi Cassiae (*Rou Gui*), Radix Lateralis Praeparatus Aconiti Carmichaeli (*Fu Zi*), Lignum Aquilariae Agallochae (*Chen Xiang*), Flos Caryophylli (*Ding Xiang*)

7. *Ai Jian Wan* (Mugwort Fortifying Pills)

Ingredients: Fructus Evodiae Rutecarpae (*Wu Zhu Yu*), Radix Angelicae Sinensis (*Dang Gui*), cooked Radix Rehmanniae (*Shu Di*), Radix Albus Paeoniae Lactiflorae (*Bai Shao*), Rhizoma Acori Graminei (*Shi Chang Pu*), Radix Ligustici Wallichii (*Chuan Xiong*), Radix Panacis Ginseng (*Ren Shen*), Folium Artemisiae Argyii (*Ai Ye*), Exocarpium Citri Rubri (*Ju Hong*)

8. *Ai Fu Nuan Gong Wan* (Mugwort & Aconite Warm the Uterus Pills)

Ingredients: Folium Artemisiae Argyii (*Ai Ye*), Rhizoma Cyperi Rotundi (*Xiang Fu*), Radix Angelicae Sinensis (*Dang Gui*), Radix Dipsaci (*Xu Duan*), Fructus Evodiae Rutecarpae (*Wu Zhu Yu*), Radix Ligustici Wallichii (*Chuan Xiong*), Radix Astragali Membranacei (*Huang Qi*), uncooked Radix Rehmanniae (*Sheng Di*), Cortex Tubiformis Cinnamomi Cassiae (*Guan Gui*)

Du Jie-hui recommends this formula for the treatment of vacuity cold menstruation behind schedule.

9. Unnamed formula from *Nu Ke Jing Wei (Profundities from the Gynecological Classics)*

Ingredients: Fructus Psoraleae Corylifoliae (*Bu Gu Zhi*), scorched Cortex Eucommiae Ulmoidis (*Du Zhong*), Semen Juglandis Regiae (*Hu Tao Ren*), large Radix Codonopsitis Pilosulae (*Dang Shen*), earth stir-fried Rhizoma Atractylodis Macrocephalae (*Bai Zhu*), baked-dry Rhizoma Zingiberis (*Gan Jiang*), whole Radix Angelicae Sinensis (*Quan Dang Gui*), uncooked Radix Astragali Membranacei (*Huang Qi*), Fructus Evodiae Rutecarpae (*Wu Zhu Yu*), Fructus Foeniculi Vulgaris (*Xiao Hui Xiang*), uncooked Radix Glycyrrhizae (*Gan Cao*), superior Cortex Cinnamomi Cassiae (*Rou Gui*)

This formula is for spleen-kidney yang vacuity with vacuity cold menstruation behind schedule.

Additions: If lower abdominal cold is severe with icy chill, add Fructus Foeni-graeci (*Hu Lu Ba*) and carbonized blast-fried Rhizoma Zingiberis (*Pao Jiang*). If usually there is white vaginal discharge which is clear and watery and excessive in amount, add uncooked Concha Ostreae (*Mu Li*), Os Sepiae Seu Sepiellae (*Wu Zei Gu*), and uncooked Os Draconis (*Long Gu*) to secure, astringe, and stop vaginal discharge. If the stools are watery and loose and the urine incontinent, add Fructus Alpiniae Oxyphyllae (*Yi Zhi Ren*) and Fructus Pruni Mume (*Wu Mei Rou*).

2. Blood vacuity

Main symptoms: A prolonged menstrual cycle with a scanty, dilute, pinkish flow, dizziness, heart palpitations, empty or slight lower abdominal pain desiring pressure, bodily emaciation and weakness, a sallow yellow facial complexion, dry skin, blurred vision, dry, astringent *i.e.*, scratchy eyes, a pale red tongue with no fur, and a vacuous, fine pulse

Treatment principles: Boost the qi and supplement the blood

Guiding formulas:

1. *Ren Shen Yang Rong Tang* (Ginseng Nourish the Constructive Decoction)

Ingredients: Radix Panacis Ginseng (*Ren Shen*), Radix Astragali Membranacei (*Huang Qi*), Radix Angelicae Sinensis (*Dang Gui*), Radix Albus Paeoniae Lactiflorae (*Bai Shao*), cooked Radix Rehmanniae (*Shu Di*), Cortex Cinnamomi Cassiae (*Rou Gui Xin*), Pericarpium Citri Reticulatae (*Chen Pi*), Rhizoma Atractylodis Macrocephalae (*Bai Zhu*), Sclerotium Poriae Cocos (*Fu Ling*), Fructus Schisandrae Chinensis (*Wu Wei Zi*), Radix Polygalae Tenuifoliae (*Yuan Zhi*), Radix Glycyrrhizae (*Gan Cao*), uncooked Rhizoma Zingiberis (*Sheng Jiang*), Fructus Zizyphi Jujubae (*Da Zao*)

This formula treats blood vacuity due to both spleen and heart dysfunction.

2. *Ren Shen Zi Xue Tang* (Ginseng Enrich the Blood Decoction)

Ingredients: Radix Panacis Ginseng (*Ren Shen*), Radix Dioscoreae Oppositae (*Shan Yao*), Sclerotium Poriae Cocos (*Fu Ling*), Radix Ligustici Wallichii (*Chuan Xiong*), Radix Albus Paeoniae Lactiflorae (*Bai Shao*), cooked Radix Rehmanniae (*Shu Di*), Radix Angelicae Sinensis (*Dang Gui*)

This formula treats blood vacuity due to kidney yin vacuity.

3. *Ren Shen Gu Ben Wan* (Ginseng Secure the Root Pills)

Ingredients: Radix Panacis Ginseng (*Ren Shen*), uncooked Radix Rehmanniae (*Sheng Di*), cooked Radix Rehmanniae (*Shu Di*), Tuber Asparagi Cochinensis (*Tian Men Dong*), Tuber Ophiopogonis Japonici (*Mai Men Dong*)

This formula treats blood vacuity where there is kidney yin vacuity and fluid dryness.

4. *Shi Quan Da Bu Tang Jia Jian* (Ten [Ingredients] Completely & Greatly Supplementing Decoction with Additions & Subtractions)

Ingredients: Radix Codonopsitis Pilosulae (*Dang Shen*), Radix Astragali Membranacei (*Huang Qi*), Rhizoma Atractylodis Macrocephalae (*Bai Zhu*), Sclerotium Poriae Cocos (*Fu*

Ling), Radix Angelicae Sinensis (*Dang Gui*), cooked Radix Rehmanniae (*Shu Di*), Radix Albus Paeoniae Lactiflorae (*Bai Shao*), Cortex Cinnamomi Cassiae (*Rou Gui*), Herba Leonuri Heterophylli (*Yi Mu Cao*)

This formula is indicated where there is qi and blood vacuity mixed with vacuity cold plus some blood stasis. Leonurus has the ability to open the menses. In combination with the preceding ingredients, it enables supplementation without stagnation. According to Philippe Sionneau, the Cinnamon in this formula is not to warm cold but simply to promote the more efficient engenderment and transformation of the qi and blood. Wan Mi-zhai suggests using the unmodified version of this formula. This means deleting Leonurus and adding Radix Ligustici Wallichii (*Chuan Xiong*). Master Wan recommends this formula for thin women with no other disease who suffer from insufficiency of both qi and blood.

5. Unnamed formula from Xia Gui-cheng *et al.'s Concise Traditional Chinese Gynecology*

Ingredients: Radix Angelicae Sinensis (*Dang Gui*), Radix Salviae Miltiorrhizae (*Dan Shen*), Radix Albus Paeoniae Lactiflorae (*Bai Shao*), Radix Astragali Membranacei (*Huang Qi*), Radix Codonopsitis Pilosulae (*Dang Shen*)

This formula treats blood vacuity by way of the spleen. However, it can also be used when there is an element of blood stasis, since Salvia is actually more effective for quickening than nourishing the blood.[21]

6. *Ba Zhen Tang* (Eight Pearl's Decoction)

Ingredients: Radix Codonopsitis Pilosulae (*Dang Shen*), Rhizoma Atractylodis Macrocephalae (*Bai Zhu*), Sclerotium Poriae Cocos (*Fu Ling*), mix-fried Radix Glycyrrhizae (*Gan Cao*), Radix Angelicae Sinensis (*Dang Gui*), cooked Radix Rehmanniae (*Shu Di*), Radix Albus Paeoniae Lactiflorae (*Bai Shao*), Radix Ligustici Wallichii (*Chuan Xiong*)
Xue Li-zhai and Wu Ben-li both say to use *Ba Zhen Tang* for qi and blood vacuity. Wan Mi-zhai says to use this formula if the woman has a warm, good-natured, and harmonious disposition and no other disease but this. In this case, Master Wan says the blood is just vacuous and scanty.

Additions: Wu Ben-li suggests adding Rhizoma Cyperi Rotundi (*Xiang Fu*) to move the qi.

---

[21] It is said that Salvia is as good as *Si Wu Tang (Four Materials Decoction)* in that it supplements and quickens the blood. However, this should not be taken literally. It is merely a reminder that Salvia has some ability to nourish as well as primarily quicken the blood. Therefore, it should not be taken as a major blood-nourishing ingredient.

7. *Liu Wei Di Huang Wan* (Six Flavors Rehmannia Pills)

Ingredients: Cooked Radix Rehmanniae (*Shu Di*), Radix Dioscoreae Oppositae (*Shan Yao*), Fructus Corni Officinalis (*Shan Zhu Yu*), Cortex Radicis Moutan (*Dan Pi*), Rhizoma Alismatis (*Ze Xie*), Sclerotium Poriae Cocos (*Fu Ling*)

Xue Li-zhai says to use *Liu Wei Di Huang Wan* for delayed menstruation due to liver channel blood scantiness. This means liver blood-kidney yin vacuity since this formula is classically indicated for kidney yin vacuity.

Additions: Han Bai-ling suggests adding Radix Angelicae Sinensis (*Dang Gui*) and Radix Albus Paeoniae Lactiflorae (*Bai Shao*) to more effectively address liver blood vacuity.

8. Zhang Jing-yue's *Yi Guan Jian* (One Link Decoction)

Ingredients: Uncooked Radix Rehmanniae (*Sheng Di*), cooked Radix Rehmanniae (*Shu Di*), Radix Albus Paeoniae Lactiflorae (*Bai Shao*), Tuber Ophiopogonis Japonici (*Mai Dong*), Radix Glycyrrhizae (*Gan Cao*), Radix Achyranthis Bidentatae (*Niu Xi*), Cortex Radicis Moutan (*Dan Pi*)

Additions: Han Bai-ling suggests adding Rhizoma Anemarrhenae Aspheloidis (*Zhi Mu*) and Cortex Radicis Lycii Chinensis (*Di Gu Pi*). He says this formula is to enrich yin and engender the blood. It is typically indicated for the treatment of liver blood-kidney yin vacuity. By adding Anemarrhena and Cortex Lycii, Han Bai-ling is implying that this blood and yin insufficiency is associated with vacuity heat which is further consuming the blood.

9. Zhu Dan-xi's *Si Wu Tang Jia Wei* (Four Materials Decoction with Added Flavors) for blood vacuity due to heat

Ingredients: Uncooked Radix Rehmanniae (*Sheng Di*), Radix Albus Paeoniae Lactiflorae (*Bai Shao*), Radix Angelicae Sinensis (*Dang Gui*), Radix Ligustici Wallichii (*Chuan Xiong*), Rhizoma Cyperi Rotundi (*Xiang Fu*), Rhizoma Coptidis Chinensis (*Huang Lian*)

This version of *Si Wu Tang* is for blood vacuity damaged by heat. Zhu Dan-xi says, "If [the menses] are behind schedule and purple black in color with lumps and chunks, this is blood heat and [the woman] surely feels pain."

10. Zhu Dan-xi's *Si Wu Tang Jia Wei* (Four Materials Decoction with Added Flavors) for qi & blood vacuity

Ingredients: Cooked Radix Rehmanniae (*Shu Di*), Radix Angelicae Sinensis (*Dang Gui*), Radix Albus Paeoniae Lactiflorae (*Bai Shao*), Radix Ligustici Wallichii (*Chuan Xiong*), Radix Astragali Membrancei (*Huang Qi*), Pericarpium Citri Reticulatae (*Chen Pi*), Rhizoma Cimicifugae (*Sheng Ma*)

11. *Yi Mu Sheng Jin Dan* (Leonurus Engender Fluids Elixir)

Ingredients: Radix Angelicae Sinensis (*Dang Gui*), Radix Ligustici Wallichii (*Chuan Xiong*), cooked Radix Rehmanniae (*Shu Di*), Radix Albus Paeoniae Lactiflorae (*Bai Shao*), Radix Salviae Miltiorrhizae (*Dan Shen*), Rhizoma Atractylodis Macrocephalae (*Bai Zhu*), Semen Leonuri Heterophylli (*Chong Wei Zi*), Rhizoma Cyperi Rotundi (*Xiang Fu*), Herba Leonuri Heterophylli (*Yi Mu Cao*)

Du Jie-hui recommends this formula for menstruation behind schedule due to blood vacuity complicated by blood stasis.

12. *Ze Lan Tang* (Lycopus Decoction)

Ingredients: Herba Lycopi Lucidi (*Ze Lan*), Radix Angelicae Sinensis (*Dang Gui*), Radix Albus Paeoniae Lactiflorae (*Bai Shao*), Radix Glycyrrhizae (*Gan Cao*)

This formula supplements without causing stagnation and moves without being harsh. By nourishing the blood, it frees the menses/channels. It can also be used for scanty menstruation and blocked menstruation.

13. *Tiao Jing Yang Rong Tang* (Regulate the Menses & Nourish the Constructive Decoction)

Ingredients: Radix Angelicae Sinensis (*Dang Gui*), Radix Ligustici Wallichii (*Chuan Xiong*), cooked Radix Rehmanniae (*Shu Di*), Radix Albus Paeoniae Lactiflorae (*Bai Shao*), Radix Panacis Ginseng (*Ren Shen*), Rhizoma Atractylodis Macrocephalae (*Bai Zhu*), Pericarpium Citri Reticulatae (*Chen Pi*), Rhizoma Cimicifugae (*Sheng Ma*)

This formula boosts the qi, nourishes the blood, and balances the menses in the treatment of blood vacuity delayed menstruation.

14. *Yi Gong San Jia Dang Gui Chuan Xiong Tang* (Special Achievement Powder plus Dang Gui & Ligusticum Decoction)

Ingredients: Radix Panacis Ginseng (*Ren Shen*), Rhizoma Atractylodis Macrocephalae (*Bai Zhu*), Sclerotium Poriae Cocos (*Bai Ling*), mix-fried Radix Glycyrrhizae (*Zhi Cao*), Pericarpium Citri Reticulatae (*Chen Pi*), Radix Angelicae Sinensis (*Dang Gui*), Radix Ligustici Wallichii (*Chuan Xiong*), uncooked Rhizoma Zingiberis (*Sheng Jiang*), Fructus Zizyphi Jujubae (*Da Zao*)

Wan Mi-zhai recommends this formula for the treatment of delayed menstruation in thin women who eat little because their spleen-stomachs are damaged and weak. Thus their qi and blood are vacuous and scanty.

15. *Gui Pi Tang Jia Wei* (Restore the Spleen Decoction with Added Flavors)

Ingredients: Body of Radix Angelicae Sinensis (*Dang Gui Shen*), uncooked Radix Astragali Membranacei (*Huang Qi*), earth stir-fried Rhizoma Atractylodis Macrocephalae (*Bai Zhu*), large Radix Codonopsitis Pilosulae (*Dang Shen*), large cooked Radix Rehmanniae (*Shu Di*), uncooked Radix Albus Paeoniae Lactiflorae (*Bai Shao*), Yunnan Sclerotium Poriae Cocos (*Yun Fu Ling*), scorched Semen Zizyphi Spinosae (*Zao Ren*), Guangdong Auklandiae Lappae (*Guang Mu Xiang*), Radix Polygalae Tenuifoliae (*Yuan Zhi*), true Gelatinum Corii Asini (*E Jiao*), uncooked Radix Glycyrrhizae (*Gan Cao*), processed Rhizoma Cyperi Rotundi (*Xiang Fu*), uncooked Rhizoma Zingiberis (*Sheng Jiang*), Fructus Zizyphi Jujubae (*Da Zao*)

This formula is for heart blood-spleen qi vacuity menstruation behind schedule with a minor element of qi stagnation.

Additions & subtractions: If headache and insomnia are severe, add blood-processed Radix Salviae Miltiorrhizae (*Dan Shen*), Dens Draconis (*Long Chi*), and Concha Margaritiferae (*Zhen Zhu Mu*). If there is lumbar soreness and pain, remove Poria and Auklandia and add scorched Cortex Eucommiae Ulmoidis (*Du Zhong*) and Radix Dipscai (*Chuan Xu Duan*). One can also take *Gui Pi Wan* (Restore the Spleen Pills) every day, 10g each time, three times per day washed down with warm water.

Replete patterns

1. Blood cold

Main symptoms: Menstruation behind schedule with scanty, dark, purplish, clotty flow, lower abdominal soreness and pain, preference for warmth, chilled limbs, aversion to cold, a pale or pale and purplish tongue with thin, white fur, and a deep, tight pulse or a deep, slow pulse with force

Treatment principles: Warm the channels (or menses) and scatter cold, quicken the blood and transform stasis

Guiding formulas:

1. *Shao Fu Zhu Yu Tang* (Lower Abdomen Dispel Stasis Decoction)

Ingredients: Fructus Foeniculi Vulgaris (*Xiao Hui Xiang*), dry Rhizoma Zingiberis (*Gan Jiang*), Cortex Cinnamomi Cassiae (*Rou Gui*), Radix Angelicae Sinensis (*Dang Gui*), Radix Ligustici Wallichii (*Chuan Xiong*), Radix Rubrus Paeoniae Lactiflorae (*Chi Shao*), Rhizoma Corydalis Yanhusuo (*Yan Hu Suo*), Feces Trogopterori Seu Pteromi (*Wu Ling Zhi*), uncooked Pollen Typhae (*Pu Huang*), Resina Myrrhae (*Mo Yao*)

2. *Wen Jing Tang* **(Warm the Channels [or Menses] Decoction) from the** *Fu Ren Da Quan Liang Fang (A Great Compendium of Fine Formulas for Women)*

Ingredients: Radix Panacis Ginseng (*Ren Shen*), Radix Achyranthis Bidentatae (*Niu Xi*), Radix Angelicae Sinensis (*Dang Gui*), Radix Ligustici Wallichii (*Chuan Xiong*), Radix Rubrus Paeoniae Lactiflorae (*Chi Shao*), Cortex Cinnamomi Cassiae (*Rou Gui Xin*), Rhizoma Curcumae Zedoariae (*E Zhu*), Cortex Radicis Moutan (*Dan Pi*), Radix Glycyrrhizae (*Gan Cao*)

Han Bai-ling gives this formula for the treatment of cold repletion. Its inclusion of supplementing ingredients suggests that the condition for which it is indicated is tinged with vacuity. Its main thrust, however, is towards dispelling and even breaking stasis. In this case, enduring blood stasis may be impeding the engenderment and transfomation of new or fresh blood.

3. *Dang Gui Si Ni Tang* **(Dang Gui Four Counterflows Decoction)**

Ingredients: Radix Angelicae Sinensis (*Dang Gui*), Ramulus Cinnamomi Cassiae (*Gui Zhi*), Radix Albus Paeoniae Lactiflorae (*Bai Shao*), mix-fried Radix Glycyrrhizae (*Gan Cao*), Fructus Zizyphi Jujubae (*Da Zao*), Medulla Tetrapanacis Papyriferi (*Tong Cao*), Herba Asari Cum Radice (*Xi Xin*)

This formula warms the channels (or menses) and scatters cold, nourishes the blood and stops pain. It is first found in the *Shang Han Lun (Treatise on Cold Damage)*. It is indicated for blood cold menstruation behind schedule.

2. Qi stagnation

Main symptoms: Delayed menstruation with darkish and even clotty blood, lower abdominal distention and pain, rib-side and breast distention, thin tongue fur, and a bowstring pulse. If there is concomitant spleen and blood vacuity, the tongue may be pale red and the pulse fine and bowstring. Otherwise, the tongue may be either normally colored or a little dusky.

Treatment principles: Course the liver and rectify the qi, quicken the blood and regulate the menses

Guiding formulas:

1. *Jia Wei Wu Yao Tang* **(Added Flavors Lindera Decoction)**

Ingredients: Radix Linderae Strychnifoliae (*Wu Yao*), Rhizoma Corydalis Yanhusuo (*Yan Hu Suo*), Semen Arecae Catechu (*Bing Lang*), Rhizoma Cyperi Rotundi (*Xiang Fu*), Fructus Amomi (*Sha Ren*), Radix Auklandiae Lappae (*Mu Xiang*), Radix Angelicae Sinensis (*Dang Gui*), Radix Ligustici Wallichii (*Chuan Xiong*), Radix Glycyrrhizae (*Gan Cao*)

2. *Jia Wei Xiang Fu Wan* (Added Flavors Cyperus Pills)

Ingredients: Fructus Foeniculi Vulgaris (*Xiao Hui Xiang*), Radix Scutellariae Baicalensis (*Huang Qin*), Rhizoma Cyperi Rotundi (*Xiang Fu*), Radix Angelicae Sinensis (*Dang Gui*), uncooked Radix Rehmanniae (*Sheng Di*), Pericarpium Citri Reticulatae (*Chen Pi*), Radix Albus Paeoniae Lactiflorae (*Bai Shao*), Radix Ligustici Wallichii (*Chuan Xiong*), Rhizoma Atractylodis Macrocephalae (*Bai Zhu*)

3. *Xiao Yao San* (Rambling Powder)

Ingredients: Radix Bupleuri (*Chai Hu*), Radix Angelicae Sinensis (*Dang Gui*), Radix Albus Paeoniae Lactiflorae (*Bai Shao*), Rhizoma Atractylodis Macrocephalae (*Bai Zhu*), Sclerotium Poriae Cocos (*Fu Ling*), mix-fried Radix Glycyrrhizae (*Gan Cao*), uncooked Rhizoma Zingiberis (*Sheng Jiang*), Herba Menthae Haplocalycis (*Bo He*)

Additions: Han Bai-ling suggests adding Fructus Meliae Toosendan (*Chuan Lian Zi*), Semen Pruni Persicae (*Tao Ren*), Flos Carthami Tinctorii (*Hong Hua*), and Radix Achyranthis Bidentatae (*Niu Xi*) to this formula if there is concomitant blood stasis.

4. *Qi Zhi Xiang Fu Wan* (Qi Stagnation Cyperus Pills)

Ingredients: Rhizoma Cyperi Rotundi (*Xiang Fu*), Radix Angelicae Sinensis (*Dang Gui*), Rhizoma Sparganii (*San Leng*), Rhizoma Curcumae Zedoariae (*E Zhu*), Cortex Radicis Moutan (*Dan Pi*), Folium Artemisiae Argyii (*Ai Ye*), Radix Linderae Strychnifoliae (*Wu Yao*), Radix Ligustici Wallichii (*Chuan Xiong*), Rhizoma Corydalis Yanhusuo (*Yan Hu Suo*), Radix Bupleuri (*Chai Hu*), Flos Carthami Tinctorii (*Hong Hua*)

Additions & subtractions: Sun Jiu-ling's version of this formula omits Corydales, Artemisia Argyium, and Moutan and adds Herba Leonuri Heterophylli (*Yi Mu Cao*), Radix Cyathulae Officinalis (*Chuan Niu Xi*), and Caulis Milletiae Seu Spatholobi (*Ji Xue Teng*). Sun Jiu-ling, in *Fu Ke Zheng Zhi (Gynecological Patterns & Treatments)*, prescribes this formula to open depression and move the qi, quicken the blood and regulate the menses.

5. *Chai Hu Si Wu Tang Jia Wei* (Bupleurum Four Materials Decoction with Added Flavors)

Ingredients: Uncooked Radix Rehmanniae (*Sheng Di*), Radix Ligustici Wallichii (*Chuan Xiong*), Radix Angelicae Sinensis (*Dang Gui*), Radix Albus Paeoniae Lactiflorae (*Bai Shao*), Radix Bupleuri (*Chai Hu*), Rhizoma Cyperi Rotundi (*Xiang Fu*), Tuber Curcumae (*Yu Jin*), Radix Salviae Miltiorrhizae (*Dan Shen*), Fructus Citri Sacrodactylis (*Fo Shou*), Flos Pruni Mume (*Lu O Mei*)

6. *Xiao Chai Hu Tang He Si Wu Tang Jia Jian* (Minor Bupleurum Decoction plus Four Materials Decoction with Additions & Subtractions)

Ingredients: Radix Bupleuri (*Chai Hu*), Radix Scutellariae Baicalensis (*Huang Qin*), Rhizoma Pinelliae Ternatae (*Ban Xia*), Radix Glycyrrhizae (*Gan Cao*), uncooked Rhizoma Zingiberis (*Sheng Jiang*), Radix Angelicae Sinensis (*Dang Gui*), Radix Albus Paeoniae Lactiflorae (*Bai Shao*), uncooked Radix Rehmanniae (*Sheng Di*), Radix Ligustici Wallichii (*Chuan Xiong*), Rhizoma Cyperi Rotundi (*Xiang Fu*), Tuber Curcumae (*Yu Jin*), Cortex Radicis Moutan (*Dan Pi*)

7. *Chen Xiang Jiang Qi Tang* (Aquilaria Downbear the Qi Decoction)

Ingredients: Radix Linderae Strychnifoliae (*Wu Yao*), Radix Auklandiae Lappae (*Mu Xiang*), Rhizoma Cyperi Rotundi (*Xiang Fu*), Radix Glycyrrhizae (*Gan Cao*), Fructus Amomi (*Sha Ren*)

Du Jie-hui recommends this formula for the treatment of qi stagnation delayed menstruation as well as scanty menstruation. It normalizes the qi and frees the flow of the blood vessels.

8. *Ba Zhen Jia Xiang Fu Tang* (Eight Perals Plus Cyperus Decoction)

Ingredients: Radix Ligustici Wallichii (*Chuan Xiong*), Radix Albus Paeoniae Lactiflorae (*Bai Shao*), Radix Panacis Ginseng (*Ren Shen*), Sclerotium Poriae Cocos (*Fu Ling*), Radix Angelicae Sinensis (*Dang Gui*), Radix Glycyrrhizae (*Gan Cao*), uncooked Radix Rehmanniae (*Sheng Di*), Rhizoma Atractylodis Macrocephalae (*Bai Zhu*), uncooked Rhizoma Zingiberis (*Sheng Jiang*), Fructus Zizyphi Jujubae (*Da Zao*), stir-fried Rhizoma Cyperi Rotundi (*Xiang Fu*), Pericarpium Citri Reticulatae Viride (*Qing Pi*)

Wan Mi-zhai, a.k.a. Wan Quan, suggests this formula for irascible women with lots of anger and jealousy whose menses are delayed due to qi counterflow and scanty blood.

9. Unnamed formula from *Nu Ke Jing Wei (Profundities from the Gynecological Classics)*

Ingredients: Vinegar-processed Radix Bupleuri (*Chai Hu*), Extremitas Radicis Angelicae Sinensis (*Dang Gui Wei*), uncooked Radix Albus Paeoniae Lactiflorae (*Bai Shao*), processed Rhizoma Cyperi Rotundi (*Xiang Fu*), Guangdong Radix Auklandiae Lappae (*Guang Mu Xiang*), old Radix Ligustici Wallichii (*Chuan Xiong*), uncooked Semen Pruni Persicae (*Tao Ren*), Flos Carthami Tinctorii (*Hong Hua*), Rhizoma Corydalis Yanhusuo (*Yan Hu Suo*), Fructus Meliae Toosendan (*Chuan Lian Rou*), uncooked Radix Glycyrrhizae (*Gan Cao*), Tian Tai Radix Linderae Strychnifoliae (*Tian Tai Wu*)

This formula is for qi stagnation and blood stasis menstruation behind schedule.

Additions & subtractions: If there is vexation and agitation with tinnitus, add Cortex Radicis Moutan (*Dan Pi*). If there is abdominal pain, sagging, and distention, add stir-fried Pericarpium Citri Reticulatae Viride (*Qing Pi*), Rhizoma Sparganii (*San Leng*), and Rhizoma Curcumae Zedoariae (*Peng E Zhu*). After administering, if the qi is smoothed and the blood is quickened, and after the abdominal pain disappears, remove Lindera, Persica, and Carthamus and add Herba Leonuri Heterophylli (*Yi Mu Cao*) and Herba Lycopi Lucidi (*Ze Lan Ye*) in order to engender fresh blood in the middle of dispelling static blood. If there is glomus, distention, and discomfort in both rib-side regions reaching to the stomach and epigastrium with no thought for food, add stir-fried Fructus Citri Aurantii (*Zhi Ke*) and Fructus Citri Sacrodactylis (*Fo Shou*) in order to loosen the chest and diffuse the network vessels, thus downbearing the qi.

3. Blood stasis

Main symptoms: Menstruation behind schedule, dull purple menstrual discharge with clots, pain relieved after evacuation of clots, abdominal pain resisting pressure, more pain and less distention, fixed, piercing pain, a dark, purplish tongue or static spots and macules with yellowish tongue fur, and a deep, choppy, forceful pulse

Treatment principles: Quicken the blood and transform stasis

Guiding formulas:

1. *Jia Jian Niu Xi Tang* (Additions & Subtractions Achyranthes Decoction)

Ingredients: Radix Achyranthis Bidentatae (*Niu Xi*), Extremitas Radicis Angelicae Sinensis (*Dang Gui*), wine-processed Radix Salviae Miltiorrhizae (*Dan Shen*), Semen Pruni Persicae (*Tao Ren*), Rhizoma Cyperi Rotundi (*Xiang Fu*), Radix Linderae Strychnifoliae (*Wu Yao*), Rhizoma Corydalis Yanhusuo (*Yan Hu Suo*), Lignum Santali Albi (*Tan Xiang*)

2. *Tao Hong Si Wu Tang Jia Wei* (Persica & Carthamus Four Materials Decoction with Added Flavors)

Ingredients: Cooked Radix Rehmanniae (*Shu Di*), Radix Angelicae Sinensis (*Dang Gui*), Radix Albus Paeoniae Lactiflorae (*Bai Shao*), Radix Ligustici Wallichii (*Chuan Xiong*), Semen Pruni Persicae (*Tao Ren*), Flos Carthami Tinctorii (*Hong Hua*), Rhizoma Cyperi Rotundi (*Xiang Fu*), Rhizoma Curcumae Zedoariae (*E Zhu*), Caulis Akebiae Mutong (*Mu Tong*), Cortex Cinnamomi Cassiae (*Rou Gui*), mix-fried Radix Glycyrrhizae (*Gan Cao*)

Most Chinese gynecology texts lump qi stagnation and blood stasis menstruation behind schedule together, since this, in fact, tends to form a continuum. Typically, if there is one, there is some element of the other. Therefore, the formulas listed under qi stagnation include blood stasis eliminating medicinals and the formulas given here under blood stasis also contains qi-rectifying ingredients.

4. Phlegm obstruction

Main symptoms: Retardation of the menstrual flow may vary from days to weeks and even months. The discharge is pale in color and scanty in amount. It may also be thick and pasty in consistency. There is often continuous abnormal vaginal discharge, chest oppression, rib-side distention, and profuse phlegm. The essence spirit is listless and fatigued. The facial complexion is puffy and edematous. The four limbs are heavy and there is dizziness, heart palpitations, shortness of breath, white, slimy tongue fur, and a bowstring, slippery pulse.

Because the spleen is the root of blood engenderment and transformation as well as of phlegm engenderment, in this type of delayed menstruation, not only may the channels/menses be obstructed by phlegm, but dampness may impede spleen function leading to blood vacuity as well. In such cases, there may be less phlegm but more obvious signs of qi and blood vacuity or dampness. Because phlegm is nothing other than congealed fluids, since blood and fluids share a common source and since it is the qi which moves the blood and fluids together, enduring blood stasis may become complicated by phlegm obstruction. Therefore, one must be careful to distinguish whether this obstruction is a simple repletion or a mixed repletion-vacuity pattern and treat accordingly.

Treatment principles: Fortify the spleen and transform phlegm unless there is phlegm mixed with enduring blood stasis, in which case, one should quicken the blood and transform stasis, transform and wash away phlegm.

Guiding formulas:

1. *Xiong Gui Er Chen Tang* (Ligusticum & Dang Gui Two Aged [Ingredients] Decoction)

Ingredients: Rhizoma Pinelliae Ternatae (*Ban Xia*), Sclerotium Poriae Cocos (*Fu Ling*), Pericarpium Citri Reticulatae (*Chen Pi*), Radix Glycyrrhizae (*Gan Cao*), Radix Angelicae Sinensis (*Dang Gui*), Radix Ligustici Wallichii (*Chuan Xiong*)

Additions: This formula may be used for either phlegm and blood vacuity or phlegm and blood stasis. In the latter case, one can add Rhizoma Arisaematis (*Nan Xing*) and Flos Carthami Tinctorii (*Hong Hua*) to make it more effective at washing away phlegm and dispelling stasis.

2. *Jia Wei Er Chen Tang* (Added Flavors Two Aged [Ingredients] Decoction)

Ingredients: Rhizoma Pinelliae Ternatae (*Ban Xia*), Sclerotium Poriae Cocos (*Fu Ling*), Pericarpium Citri Reticulatae (*Chen Pi*), Radix Glycyrrhizae (*Gan Cao*), Rhizoma Cyperi

Rotundi (*Xiang Fu*), uncooked Rhizoma Zingiberis (*Sheng Jiang*), Fructus Amomi (*Sha Ren*)

This formula is suggested by Wang Ken-tang. It is indicated for phlegm obstruction with little or no blood stasis but more obvious qi stagnation.

3. *Xiang Sha Liu Jun Zi Tang* (Auklandia & Amomum Six Gentlemen Decoction)

Ingredients: Radix Codonopsitis Pilosulae (*Dang Shen*), Sclerotium Poriae Cocos (*Fu Ling*), Rhizoma Atractylodis Macrocephalae (*Bai Zhu*), Pericarpium Citri Reticulatae (*Chen Pi*), mix-fried Radix Glycyrrhizae (*Gan Cao*), Rhizoma Pinelliae Ternatae (*Ban Xia*), Radix Auklandiae Lappae (*Mu Xiang*), Fructus Amomi (*Sha Ren*)

This formula is for more pronounced spleen vacuity weakness as evidenced by fatigue, loose stools, diminished appetite, etc. and also accompanied by a degree of qi stagnation. The use of this formula recognizes that the spleen is the root of phlegm engenderment.

Additions: For use in cases of delayed menstruation, this formula should be combined with either blood-nourishing ingredients, such as Radix Angelicae Sinensis (*Dang Gui*) and Radix Albus Paeoniae Lactiflorae (*Bai Shao)* or blood-quickening medicinals, such as Radix Angelicae Sinensis (*Dang Gui*) and Radix Ligustici Wallichii (*Chuan Xiong*).

4. *Gui Shao Si Jun Zi Tang* (Dang Gui & Peony Four Gentlemen Decoction)

Ingredients: Radix Angelicae Sinensis (*Dang Gui*), Radix Albus Paeoniae Lactiflorae (*Bai Shao*), Radix Codonopsitis Pilosulae (*Dang Shen*), Rhizoma Atractylodis Macrocephalae (*Bai Zhu*), Sclerotium Poriae Cocos (*Fu Ling*), mix-fried Radix Glycyrrhizae (*Gan Cao*)

This formula is somewhat similar to the above but with the addition of Radix Angelicae Sinensis (*Dang Gui*) and Radix Albus Paeoniae Lactiflorae (*Bai Shao*) in order to nourish and harmonize the liver, nourish and quicken the blood. It is indicated in cases where there is spleen vacuity and dampness plus blood vacuity. Because Radix Angelicae Sinensis (*Dang Gui*) tends to be rich and slimy, when included in formulas for phlegm and dampness, it is best used in either small amounts or stir-fried in ginger juice.

5. *Liu Jun Zi Jia Gui Xiong Tang* (Six Gentlemen Plus Dang Gui & Ligusticum Decoction)

Ingredients: Radix Panacis Ginseng (*Ren Shen*), Rhizoma Atractylodis Macrocephalae (*Bai Zhu*), Sclerotium Poriae Cocos (*Fu Ling*), mix-fried Radix Glycyrrhizae (*Gan Cao*), Pericarpium Citri Reticulatae (*Chen Pi*), Rhizoma Pinelliae Ternatae (*Ban Xia*), Radix Angelicae Sinensis (*Dang Gui*), Radix Ligustici Wallichii (*Chuan Xiong*), Rhizoma Cyperi Rotundi (*Xiang Fu*), uncooked Rhizoma Zingiberis (*Sheng Jiang*)

Wan Mi-zhai gives this formula for the treatment of obese women who eat and drink very excessively. In this case, there is damp phlegm gathering and stagnation. This is the same as formula #3 above with its additions for quickening the blood plus Rhizoma Cyperi Rotundi for moving and rectifying the qi.

6. *Shen Ling Bai Zhu San Jia Gui Xiong Di Huang Wan Jia Jian* (Ginseng, Poria & Atractylodes Powder plus Dang Gui & Ligusticum Rehmannia Pills with Additions & Subtractions)

Ingredients: Radix Panacis Ginseng (*Ren Shen*), Rhizoma Atractylodis Macrocephalae (*Bai Zhu*), Sclerotium Poriae Cocos (*Bai Ling*), Pericarpium Citri Reticulatae (*Chen Pi*), Semen Nelumbinis Nuciferae (*Lian Rou*), Radix Angelicae Sinensis (*Dang Gui*), mix-fried Radix Glycyrrhizae (*Gan Cao*), Radix Dioscoreae Oppositae (*Shan Yao*), Fructus Amomi (*Sha Ren*), Radix Ligustici Wallichii (*Chuan Xiong*), Rhizoma Acori Graminei (*Shi Chang Pu*)

Wan Mi-zhai suggests this formula for the treatment of menstruation behind schedule in women with profuse phlegm due to spleen-stomach vacuity and damage. Thus the qi and blood lose their nourishment. This is a case of both phlegm obstruction and blood vacuity with both mechanisms being due to faulty spleen function.

7. *Cang Fu Dao Tan Tang* (Atractylodes & Cyperus Abduct Phlegm Decoction)

Ingredients: Rhizoma Atractylodis (*Cang Zhu*), Rhizoma Cyperi Rotundi (*Xiang Fu*), Pericarpium Citri Reticulatae (*Chen Pi*), Rhizoma Pinelliae Ternatae (*Ban Xia*), Fructus Citri Aurantii (*Zhi Ke*), Sclerotium Poriae Cocos (*Fu Ling*), bile-processed Rhizoma Arisaematis (*Dan Nan Xing*), Radix Glycyrrhizae (*Gan Cao*), Succus Zingiberis (*Jiang Zhi*), Massa Medica Fermentata (*Shen Qu*)

Within this formula, *Dao Tan Tang* (Abduct Phlegm Decoction) and Atractylodes move the qi and dry dampness, transform phlegm and disperse fat. Cyperus is an essential medicinal in gynecology for resolving phlegm depression and moving the qi and blood. It is ok to add Radix Angelicae Sinensis (*Dang Gui*), Radix Ligustici Wallichii (*Chuan Xiong*), and Herba Leonuri Heterophylli (*Kun Cao*) in order to regulate and rectify the *chong* and *ren*, move the qi and quicken the blood.

8. *Yi Qi Tang Jia Wei* (Restrain the Qi Decoction)

Ingredients: Sclerotium Poriae Cocos (*Fu Ling*), Rhizoma Cyperi Rotundi (*Xiang Fu*), Pericarpium Citri Reticulatae (*Chen Pi*), Radix Glycyrrhizae (*Gan Cao*), Fructus Citri Aurantii (*Zhi Ke*), Radix Bupleuri (*Chai Hu*), Folium Citri Reticulatae (*Ju Ye*), Tuber Curcumae (*Yu Jin*), Herba Leonuri Heterophylli (*Yi Mu Cao*)

This formula is for liver depression and phlegm obstruction. Within this formula, Poria fortifies the spleen, transforms phlegm, and expels dampness. Orange Peel and Citrus move the qi, harmonize the stomach, and transform phlegm. Cyperus and Leonurus move the qi, quicken the blood, and regulate the menses. Bupleurum and Orange Leaf course the liver, move the qi, and resolve depression. Curcuma opens depression and transforms phlegm. If depression has been enduring and transformed into heat, it is ok to add Fructus Gardeniae Jasminoidis (*Zhi Zi*) and Cortex Radicis Moutan (*Dan Pi*) to resolve depression, clear heat, and eliminate vexation. If chest and rib-side pain are severe, add Fructus Meliae Toosendan (*Chuan Lian*) and Rhizoma Corydalis Yanhusuo (*Yuan Hu*).

9. *Liu Jun Zi Tang Jia Cang Fu Dao Tan Wan* (Six Gentlemen Decoction plus Atractylodes & Cyperus Abduct Phlegm Pills)

Ingredients: Pericarpium Citri Reticulatae (*Chen Pi*), Rhizoma Pinelliae Ternatae (*Ban Xia*), Sclerotium Poriae Cocos (*Fu Ling*), Radix Glycyrrhizae (*Gan Cao*), Radix Panacis Ginseng (*Ren Shen*), Rhizoma Atractylodis Macrocephalae (*Bai Zhu*), Rhizoma Atractylodis (*Cang Zhu*), Rhizoma Cyperi Rotundi (*Xiang Fu*), Fructus Citri Aurantii (*Zhi Ke*), bile-processed Rhizoma Arisaematis (*Dan Nan Xing*), Succus Zingiberis (*Jiang Ye*), Massa Medica Fermentata (*Shen Qu*)

This formula is for marked spleen vacuity with phlegm obstruction. If the constructive and blood are vacuous, then combine *Liu Jun Zi Tang* (Six Gentlemen Decoction) with *Ren Shen Yang Ying Tang* (Ginseng Nourish the Constructive Decoction): Radix Panacis Ginseng (*Ren Shen*), Fructus Schisandrae Chinensis (*Wu Wei Zi*), Tuber Ophiopogonis Japonici (*Mai Men Dong*), uncooked Radix Rehmanniae (*Sheng Di*), Radix Angelicae Sinensis (*Dang Gui*), Radix Albus Paeoniae Lactiflorae (*Bai Shao*), Rhizoma Anemarrhenae Aspheloidis (*Zhi Mu*), Pericarpium Citri Reticulatae (*Chen Pi*), Radix Glyycrrhizae (*Gan Cao*). This is in order to greatly boost the qi and nourish the blood.

10. *Lu Jiao Shuang Yin* (Degelatinized Deer Horn Drink)

Ingredients: Cornu Degelatinum Cervi (*Lu Jiao Shuang*), Rhizoma Atractylodis Macrocephalae (*Bai Zhu*), Fructus Citri Aurantii (*Zhi Ke*), Radix Astragali Membranacei (*Huang Qi*), Radix Angelicae Sinensis (*Dang Gui*), Radix Ligustici Wallichii (*Chuan Xiong*), Thallus Algae (*Kun Bu*), Rhizoma Pinelliae Ternatae (*Ban Xia*), Herba Leonuri Heterophylli (*Yi Mu Cao*)

This formula is for phlegm obstruction with simultaneous kidney yang vacuity. The symptoms of this are delayed menstruation, pale colored menses, watery or sticky consistency, amount possibly scanty, a relatively fat body, chest oppression, profuse phlegm, heart palpitations, shortness of breath, lumbar weakness, lack of strength, loose stools, long, clear urination, a pale tongue with white, glossy, slimy fur, and a deep, slow, weak pulse

Within this formula, degelatinized Deer Horn supplements the kidneys and fills the essence. Astragalus and Atractylodes fortify the spleen and boost the qi, dry dampness and transform phlegm. Thallus Algae, Pinellia, and Citrus move the qi and transform phlegm. Dang Gui, Ligusticum, and Leonurus nourish the blood and quicken the blood, regulate and rectify the *chong* and *ren*. If kidney vacuity cold is severe, one can add Cortex Cinnamomi Cassiae (*Rou Gui*), Radix Morindae Officinalis (*Ba Ji*), and Fructus Psoraleae Corylifoliae (*Bu Gu Zhi*) to warm the kidneys and invigorate yang.

Discussion

Menstruation behind schedule is sometimes encountered as a Western female's major complaint. However, it also often complicates a number of other complaints and conditions. Because it is a species of not bleeding when one should, it is frequently encountered with other similar conditions, for instance scanty menstruation. In some women, if left untreated, this condition may evolve into blocked menstruation. In clinical practice, I used to see more menstruation behind schedule than I do now. This is because of the aging of my main patient population, the Baby Boom generation. As women age, at least here in the West, they are more often to develop menstruation ahead of schedule than behind.

If a woman presents with delayed menstruation but has no prior history of such tardy menstruation, possible pregnancy should be ruled out before commencing therapy. In the West, reliable home pregnancy test kits are widely available and relatively inexpensive. Use of such a test need only delay possible therapy a single day.

Prognosis

In general, I would say that most varieties of delayed menstruation respond well to Chinese medicinal therapy. Of these, I find replete cold and qi stagnation and blood stasis varieties the easiest to treat. With replete cold, if one scatters the cold and dispels blood stasis, the menses should quickly return to normal with little, if any, recidivism. Likewise, qi stagnation and blood stasis also respond well to TCM treatment. The more blood stasis there is due to a past historical event, the easier I find the case to treat, since once this blood stasis is eliminated, it plays no further role in the case. If there is more pronounced qi stagnation due to emotional stress and frustration, the case can be more difficult to treat, but, if the woman understands the use of exercise and deep relaxation, even this type of delayed menstruation can usually be remedied. However, depending upon how well the woman maintains her lifestyle and stress management, this condition may relapse.

Blood vacuity due to spleen dysfunction in turn due to lack of exercise and faulty diet is usually also easily treated. If blood vacuity has persisted for some time and the heart has also become vacuous or if the heart spirit is disturbed by longing or sadness, the case may be recalcitrant to treatment until the emotional situation is resolved. If there is liver blood-kidney yin vacuity, this can usually be remedied but takes time and persistence. This is especially the case in women in their mid to late 30s and on into their 40s in whom yin is becoming progressively vacuous due to aging. Therefore, treatment of this pattern in these women is uphill and requires even more persistance. If there is also vacuous heat, the case may be more difficult, since this makes a patient jittery and restless, and such patients have trouble sticking to a single, protracted regime.

I rarely see vacuity cold as the sole mechanism at work in my gynecological patients. However, because of the progressive decline of the spleen and kidneys after the mid-30s, many of my patients' cases are complicated by vacuity cold. Happily, Chinese medicinals for supplementing the kidneys and invigorating yang are extremely effective and this pattern usually responds to treatment quite well.

I find that phlegm obstruction can sometimes be difficult and sometimes relatively easy to treat. When the engenderment of phlegm is primarily due to weak spleen function, this can be easy to treat at least in terms of delayed menstruation. Treating for this pattern, one can see success in regulating the menses, even though the patient will probably not loose significant weight. When phlegm engenderment is more due to kidney yang vacuity in turn due to an insufficiency of natural endowment, this can be more difficult to treat. In addition, when phlegm obstruction is complicated by significant liver depression qi stagantion, the phlegm may be relatively easy to treat, but the liver depression may be more recalcitrant depending on how well the patient can make changes in their essence spirit or pysche. In my experience, most women with phlegm obstruction suffer from liver qi as well and may even have some degree of blood stasis. In such women, exercise is quite important, as is proper dietary therapy.

Charting the basal body temperature can help determine when and why the ovulation is delayed. If ovulation is delayed, this means the hypothermal lasts too long and ovulation is not occurring on day 14 as it should. This may be due either to yin vacuity, yang vacuity, qi stagnation, blood stasis, or phlegm obstruction. Treatment for yin and blood vacuity should be initiated during the menses and continued through to whenever ovulation occurs. Treatment for yang vacuity should be begun after the menses cease and possibly waiting till day 10. Then it should be continued until the temperature goes up. Qi stagnation and blood stasis should primarily be treated from days 10-16 in order to free the flow of the qi mechanism. Then treatment should usually be given again during the premenstruum depending on the woman's signs and symptoms. If there is actual blood stasis, treatment should continue or be given during the first days of the menses in order to dispel and precipitate the stasis through menstruation.

Case history: The patient was a 33 year-old female whose major complaint was "menstrual irregularity." However, it turned out that her menses always came at more than 50 days. Menarche had occurred at 12 and her menses lasted five to seven days. A year or so before, her Western MD had done an intravaginal ultrasound and had found no endometrial thickening even though the patient had not menstruated for over five months. The MD referred the patient to an acupuncturist/TCM practitioner. The patient had been treated by this practitioner for one year with a combination of acupuncture and Chinese medicinals. Based on the previous practitioner's formulas, it seemed that that practitioner's diagnosis was primarily liver-kidney yin vacuity. During the time that this patient was receiving treatment from this other practitioner, her menses came regularly at three month intervals. When she moved and had to discontinue treatment with this other practitioner, her menstrual cycle had lengthened back out again.

At the time of our initial examination, the patient had a pale face with a light red flush. She was medium thin in build with relatively unpronounced secondary sexual characteristics. She had very few other signs or symptoms other than that her hands always tended to be cold. Currently, she was at day 57 in her cycle. She had been doing BBT charting for several months, and the current chart suggested that she had ovulated on day 52. Since then, her breasts had become a little sore and distended, she was a little irritable, and she was a little fatigued. She had one to two bowel movements per day, usually two. When she menstruated, she did experience some lower abdominal cramping. The blood began dark red and then became bright red. The flow always contained some clots. The cramps extended to the insides and tops of her thighs. When she was younger, she had had severe menstrual pain, but that had lessened with age (not necessarily with treatment). Her tongue was light red with a redder tip and was cracked over its entire surface. The fur was thin. Her pulse was rapid, fine, and bowstring. My diagnosis was menstruation behind schedule due to constitutional yin vacuity complicated by liver depression, spleen vacuity, and some blood stasis.

Since this patient had already ovulated, I expected her menses to come on day 66. Therefore, because I knew that the menses were already coming, my treatment focused on relieving her premenstrual swollen and painful breasts and menstrual pain. My treatment principles were to supplement the kidneys and spleen, nourish the liver, rectify the qi and quicken the blood. Therefore, I chose a formula from the painful menstruation chapter under liver-kidney vacuity detriment and modified this for spleen vacuity, liver depression, and blood stasis. The formula was *Xue Beng Fang Jia Jian* (Blood Flooding Formula with Additions & Subtractions): Radix Angelicae Sinensis (*Dang Gui*), 9g, Pollen Typhae (*Pu Huang*), 9g, Radix Achyranthis Bidentatae (*Niu Xi*), 9g, Radix Rubrus Paeoniae Lactiflorae

(*Chi Shao*), 9g, Radix Albus Paeoniae Lactiflorae (*Bai Shao*), 18g, Rhizoma Cyperi Rotundi (*Xiang Fu*), 9g, Radix Linderae Strychnifoliae (*Wu Yao*), 9g, Fructus Meliae Toosendan (*Chuan Lian Zi*), 9g, Radix Codonopsitis Pilosulae (*Dang Shen*), 9g, Radix Dioscoreae Oppositae (*Shan Yao*), 9g, Radix Dipsaci (*Xu Duan*), 9g, Sclerotium Poriae Cocos (*Fu Ling*), 9g, mix-fried Radix Glycyrrhizae (*Gan Cao*), 6g.

The patient took this formula for four days as a trial. She then reported no side effects and that she felt a bit more energetic. Her breasts had not gotten worse and her abdomen did not feel bloated or crampy as it usually did at that point before her menses. I again prescribed four days of the same formula. On day 65, she reported that her temperature had gone down that AM. Therefore, it did look like her menses would come on day 66 as predicted. I prescribed the same formula again for two more days to help with her menstrual cramps. I also prescribed eight days of a formula for delayed menstruation due to liver-kidney yin vacuity which I modified for spleen vacuity, qi stagnation, and a very minor element of blood stasis. The formula was *Liu Wei Di Huang Wan Jia Wei* (Six Flavors Rehmannia Pills with Added Flavors): Cooked Radix Rehmanniae (*Shu Di*), 12g, Radix Albus Paeoniae Lactiflorae (*Bai Shao*), 9g, Radix Angelicae Sinensis (*Dang Gui*), 9g, Fructus Lycii Chinensis (*Gou Qi Zi*), 9g, Fructus Corni Officinalis (*Shan Zhu Yu*), 18g, Radix Dioscoreae Oppositae (*Shan Yao*), 9g, Radix Astragali Membranacei (*Huang Qi*), 9g, Radix Panacis Ginseng (*Ren Shen*), 6g, Rhizoma Atractylodis Macrocephalae (*Bai Zhu*), 9g, Sclerotium Poriae Cocos (*Fu Ling*), 9g, Radix Auklandiae Lappae (*Mu Xiang*), 6g, Fructus Amomi (*Sha Ren*), 4.5g, Cortex Radicis Moutan (*Dan Pi*), 9g, Semen Leonuri Heterophylli (*Chong Wei Zi*), 9g, Rhizoma Alismatis (*Ze Xie*), 9g.

I instructed the patient to begin taking this latter formula beginning on day two of her menses. The purpose of this formula was primarily to supplement yin in order to shorten the hypothermal phase and promote an earlier ovulation. This case shows how charting and using the BBT can help make the TCM pattern discrimination and help determine what treatment principles to emphasize when during the cycle.

Acupuncture-moxibustion, compresses & other adjunctive therapies

If there is either replete or vacuity cold, I recommend using some form of direct warming method to the lower burner/uterus. This can be ginger compresses nightly in the week before the menses and/or moxibustion. For replete cold, indirect moxa warming the entire lower abdomen and also the *Ba Liao* points (Bl 31-34) on the sacrum is generally sufficient. For vacuity cold, one should warm the kidneys and invigorate yang by doing direct, non-scarring, thread moxa with supplementation at *Guan Yuan* (CV 4), *Qi Hai* (CV 6), *Shen Shu*

(Bl 23), and *Ming Men* (GV 4), choosing several points each treatment and treating especially from days 10-16 in order to promote ovulation.

If there is pronounced blood stasis, acupuncture can be very effective when done every day from days 10-16 in order to also promote ovulation. In that case, one can choose *San Yin Jiao* (Sp 6), *Xue Hai* (Sp 10), *Tai Chong* (Liv 3), *Shui Dao* (St 28), *Gui Lai* (St 29), and/or *Zi Gong Xue* (M-CA-18). If the patient wants and there is no concomitant heat, the patient can also be instucted how to do indirect moxa at home on their lower abdomen daily with a moxa pole during these same days. Heat makes the qi and blood move more freely and smoothly whether or not there is actual cold.

Another possibility for all types of delayed menstruation where there is no concomitant heat is to use ginger compresses nightly on the lower abdomen from days 10-16. This type of compress should be left in place for 20 minutes once each day. And further, the woman can soak her feet and lower legs up to the level of *San Yin Jiao* (Sp 6) in hot water every night from days 10-16 for 20 minutes each time. During this same phase in her menstrual cycle, the woman should not walk around on cold floors with bare feet and should not swim or bathe in cold water. Why all these treatments should be given from days 10-16 is in order to promote the transformation of yin into yang. The acupuncture seeks to move the qi and free the network vessels, while the moxibustion and ginger compresses seek to warm yang and scatter cold. Soaking one's feet and lower legs in warm water is in order to warm the qi and blood in the three leg yin channels which all connect with the uterus.

Key patterns to memorize	
1. Vacuity	**A. Vacuity cold** **B. Blood vacuity**
2. Repletion	**A. Blood cold** **B. Qi stagnation** **C. Blood stasis** **D. Phlegm obstruction**

LATE MENSTRUATION, SCANTY MENSTRUATION, BLOCKED MENSTRUATION

Pattern	Menstruation Behind Schedule		Scanty Menstruation		Blocked Menstruation	
	Treatment Method	Formula	Treatment Method	Formula	Treatment Method	Formula
Blood Cold	warm menses scatter cold regulate menses	*Wen Jing Tang*				
Vacuity Cold	support yang dispel cold regulate menses	*Ai Fu Huan Gong Tang*				
Blood Vacuity	nourish blood regulate menses	*Ren Shen Yang Ying Wan*	nourish blood regulate menses	*Bu Xue Tang*		
Qi Stagnation	rectify qi regulate menses	*Wu Yao Tang*				
Kidney Vacuity	supplement kidneys nourish blood regulate menses	*Gui Shen Wan*	supplement kidneys, nourish blood, regulate menses	*Gui Shen Wan*		
Blood Stasis			quicken blood transform stasis regulate menses	*Tao Ren Si Wu Tang*	quicken blood dispel stasis rectify qi open menses	*Xue Fu Zhu Yu Tang*
Phlegm Dampness			transform phlegm dry dampness regulate menses	*Cang Fu Dao Tan Wan*	break phlegm, eliminate damp, quicken blood, open menses	*Cang Fu Dao Tan Wan plus Fo Shou San*
Liver/ Kidney Insufficiency					supplement kidneys, nourish liver	*Gui Shen Wan Jia Wei*
Qi & Blood Vacuity Weakness					supplement qi, boost blood	*Ren Shen Yang Rong Wan*
Yin Vacuity, Blood Dryness					nourish yin, clear heat	*Jia Jian Yi Guan Jian*

3

(Sometimes) Early, (Sometimes) Late, Menstruation At No Fixed Schedule

This disease category might be called irregular menstruation in English except that the Chinese term *yue jing bu tiao* or menstrual irregularities is not the equivalent of *yue jing xian hou wu ding qi*. As mentioned above, *yue jing bu tiao* is a more generic term covering early or late or profuse or scanty mesntruation. Therefore, it is important to translate this disease category's name in full. Otherwise, practitioners may not understand its actual definition. In this disease, sometimes the menses come ahead of schedule and sometimes they come behind schedule. Since there is no telling when they are going to come in any given month, they come at no fixed schedule. If the menses are erratic but always come behind schedule, that is not this disease category. Likewise, if the menses are erratic but always come before schedule, then this is also not this disease. The definition of this disease requires that sometimes the menses come before schedule and sometimes they come behind schedule. This is a very important point for making this menstrual disease diagnosis.

Disease causes, disease mechanisms

This disease category is a little difficult to write about because, in fact, it is made up of both the preceding categories and their mechanisms. Although Chinese gynecology texts talk about the mechanisms of this category as if it were a single category, women suffering from this condition have nothing other than sometimes early and sometimes late menstruations. In other words, there is not some whole other set of mechanisms at work here, only those discussed already above. One can say, as Professors Song and Yu do, that menstruation at no fixed time is due to disharmony between qi and blood, *chong* and *ren,* liver and spleen, and yin and yang. However, this does not necessarily tell one much.

Basically, there are three viscera involved in (sometimes) early, (sometimes) late, no fixed schedule menstruation. These are the liver, spleen, and kidneys. The liver controls coursing and discharge. It maintains the smooth and free flow of the qi which moves the blood. It also stores the blood. The spleen is both the latter heaven root of blood engenderment and transformation and contains the blood within its vessels. And the kidneys are the former heaven source of blood engenderment and transformation and the source of movement and securing in the lower burner.

Therefore, the disease causes of (sometimes) early, (sometimes) late, no fixed schedule menstruation pertaining to the liver are, once again, emotional stress and frustration. Those pertaining to the spleen are overthinking, worry, lack of adequate exercise, and faulty diet. And those pertaining to the kidneys are insufficiency of natural endowment, enduring disease, overstimulation, enduring or excessive stress and anxiety, excessive sex, drug use, prolonged or persistent lack of sleep, and the aging process itself.

If (sometimes) early, (sometimes) late, no fixed schedule menstruation is mainly due to liver qi, then when the qi is mostly just stagnant, the menses come behind schedule. If there is more stagnation which transforms into depressive heat, this transformative heat may cause the menses to come early. If (sometimes) early, (sometimes) late, no fixed schedule menstruation is due to spleen vacuity and the menses come early, this is due to spleen qi insufficiency unable to contain the blood within its vessels. If the menses come late, this is due to the spleen not engendering and transforming the blood. In this case, the tardiness of the menses is due to insufficiency of blood. If the kidneys are at the root of a woman's (sometimes) early, (sometimes) late, no fixed schedule menstruation, one must further discriminate between yin and yang vacuities. If there is kidney yin vacuity, insufficiency of yin blood may cause delayed menstruation, but flaring of vacuity fire may cause the menses to come early. On the other hand, if there is kidney yang vacuity, vacuity cold may cause delayed menstruation, but loss of kidney astringency and securing may cause early menstruation.

In actual clinical fact, these three viscera are not discreet and independent. Due to their various normal physiological and pathophysiological relationships, these three viscera may jointly form complicated disease mechanisms involving more than a single viscus. For instance, because of the tendency for the liver and spleen to come out of harmony together, delayed menstruation may be due to a combination of both liver qi and spleen vacuity causing blood vacuity. In this case, there is both an insufficiency of blood and stagnation of qi. But, if the liver becomes even more depressed and bound up and this stagnation transforms into fire, this fire may then cause menstruation ahead of schedule. If this fire persists, it may also consume kidney yin and transform into vacuity fire which then may result in either early or late menstruation depending upon what is most prominent during a given cycle, vacuity heat or insufficiency of yin blood and fluids and humors.

Yang Yi-ya, in *Gynecology*, Volume 11 of *Zhong Yi Xue Cong Shu (The Chinese Medicine Self-study Series)*, also gives blood stasis as a possible disease mechanism of (sometimes) early, (sometimes) late, no fixed schedule menstruation. According to Yang, qi stagnation enduring for days may result in depression, binding, and non-movement, while invasion by cold and suffering chill during menstruation or postpartum may result in cold congelation. Either cause leads to static blood obstructing and stagnating. Thus the menses come behind schedule. However, static blood may prevent fresh blood from returning to the channels. Hence the menses may also come before schedule. Although I have not personally seen this (or perhaps I should say identified this) in clinical practice, I am including it here for sake of completeness in terms of the Chinese gynecological literature. Like blood stasis in other menstrual diseases, my opinion is that this is really only a complicating factor.

Hou Tian-yin and Wang Chun-hua, in *Tan Zheng Lun (Treatise on Phelgm Conditions)* published by the Peoples' Army Medical Press, Beijing, 1989, also say that phlegm can cause (sometimes) early, (sometimes) late, no fixed schedule menstruation. They say this condition is mostly seen in women with obese, fat bodies and phlegm dampness. It is due to loss of regulation of the emotions with depression and anger damaging the liver. It may also be possible that if phlegm dampness is exuberant internally, earth becomes congested and wood becomes depressed. Liver qi thus becomes depressed and stagnant and coursing and discharge lose their command. The *chong* and *ren* become irregular and the filling and spilling over of the sea of blood loses its normalcy. If, due to wood depression, coursing and discharge are excessive, then the menses come before schedule. If, due to phlegm congestion, coursing and discharge do not reach, then the menstruation comes late. Hence the menstrual cycle has no fixed schedule. If this condition persists for a long time without being cured, due to the close relationship between the spleen and kidneys, it will lead to a more serious disease state or undergo transformation. That being said, I regard this pattern as nothing other than one of liver depression, spleen vacuity, and phlegm and dampness.

Treatment based on pattern discrimination

Liver depression qi stagnation

Main symptoms: The menses may sometimes come early and sometimes come late. The volume of the menstruate tends to be astringent and scanty and has difficulty descending. Its color is purple and dark. There is chest and rib-side distention and oppression, breast distention, and lower abdominal aching and pain. There tends to be excessive irritability, even irascibility. The facial complexion is dark and stagnant, the tongue fur is thin and white or slightly yellow, and the pulse is bowstring and forceful.

Treatment principles: Regulate the liver, rectify the qi, and harmonize the blood

Guiding formulas:

1. *Xiao Yao San* (Rambling Powder)

Ingredients: Radix Bupleuri (*Chai Hu*), Radix Angelicae Sinensis (*Dang Gui*), Radix Albus Paeoniae Lactiflorae (*Bai Shao*), Rhizoma Atractylodis Macrocephalae (*Bai Zhu*), Sclerotium Poriae Cocos (*Fu Ling*), mix-fried Radix Glycyrrhizae (*Zhi Gan Cao*), uncooked Rhizoma Zingiberis (*Sheng Jiang*), Herba Menthae Haplocalycis (*Bo He*)

Additions & subtractions: Professors Song and Yu suggest deleting uncooked Ginger and Mentha and adding Tuber Curcumae (*Yu Jin*), Radix Ligustici Wallichii (*Chuan Xiong*), Rhizoma Cyperi Rotundi (*Xiang Fu*), Fructus Meliae Toosendan (*Chuan Lian Zi*), and Fructus Citri Sacrodactylis (*Fo Shou*). However, because Curcuma and Citrus Sacrodactylis both move the blood downward, I would only add these medicinals if mostly the menses are late. Han Bai-ling says to add Fructus Meliae Toosendan (*Chuan Lian Zi*) to further rectify the qi. To clear heat, add Radix Scutellariae Baicalensis (*Huang Qin*), Cortex Radicis Moutan (*Dan Pi*), and Fructus Gardeniae Jasminoidis (*Zhi Zi*) and delete uncooked Ginger. Sun Jiu-ling says that, if there is abdominal pain when the menses come, add Rhizoma Cyperi Rotundi (*Xiang Fu*), Flos Carthami Tinctorii (*Hong Hua*), and Radix Achyranthis Bidentatae (*Chuan Niu Xi*). For lumbar pain, add Radix Dipsaci (*Xu Duan*) and Semen Cuscutae (*Tu Si Zi*). Another set of additions for (sometimes) early, (sometimes) late, no fixed schedule menstruation with distention and pain in the lower abdomen and a sensation of heat due to qi stagnation and blood stasis is Rhizoma Cyperi Rotundi (*Xiang Fu*), Tuber Curcumae (*Yu Jin*), and Herba Schizonepetae Tenuifoliae (*Jing Jie Sui*).

2. *Xiao Yao San Jia Wei* (Rambling Powder with Added Flavors)

Radix Bupleuri (*Chai Hu*), Radix Angelicae Sinensis (*Dang Gui*), Radix Albus Paeoniae Lactiflorae (*Bai Shao*), Rhizoma Atractylodis Macrocephalae (*Bai Zhu*), Sclerotium Poriae Cocos (*Fu Ling*), mix-fried Radix Glycyrrhizae (*Zhi Gan Cao*), roasted Rhizoma Zingiberis (*Wei Jiang*), Herba Menthae Haplocalycis (*Bo He*), Pericarpium Citri Reticulatae (*Chen Pi*), Rhizoma Pinelliae Ternatae (*Ban Xia*), Rhizoma Atractylodis (*Cang Zhu*), Fructus Citri Aurantii (*Zhi Ke*)

In this formula, Bupleurum courses the liver and resolves depression. Dang Gui and Peony supplement the blood and regulate the menses. Poria, Atractylodes Macrocephala, Pinellia, and Atractylodes dry dampness and transform phlegm, fortify the spleen and supplement the middle. Orange Peel and Citrus move the qi and transform phlegm and with Dang Gui and Peony are used to regulate and harmonize the qi and blood. When used together, these medicinals have the ability to resolve depression and transform phlegm, course the liver and fortify the spleen, regulate and harmonize the qi and blood.

If this condition endures for a long time, eventually it will affect the kidneys. If dizziness and tinnitus, lumbar soreness as if about to break, emptiness and falling of the urination, excessive nocturia, and loose stools appear, treatment should mainly supplement the kidneys and regulate the *chong* and *ren*, assisted by transforming phlegm. The formula to use is *Ding Jing Tang* (Stabilize the Menses Decoction): Radix Angelicae Sinensis (*Dang Gui*), cooked Radix Rehmanniae (*Shu Di*), Radix Albus Paeoniae Lactiflorae (*Bai Shao*), Semen Cuscutae (*Tu Si Zi*), Radix Dioscoreae Oppositae (*Shan Yao*), Radix Bupleuri (*Chai Hu*), Herba Schizonepetae Tenuifoliae (*Jing Jie*), Sclerotium Poriae Cocos (*Fu Ling*) plus Rhizoma Atractylodis (*Cang Zhu*) and Rhizoma Arisaematis (*Nan Xing*).

3. *Shen Ling Bai Zhu San* (Ginseng, Poria & Atractylodes Powder)

Ingredients: Radix Panacis Ginseng (*Ren Shen*), Rhizoma Atractylodis Macrocephalae (*Bai Zhu*), Sclerotium Poriae Cocos (*Fu Ling*), mix-fried Radix Glycyrrhizae (*Zhi Gan Cao*), Radix Dioscoreae Oppositae (*Shan Yao*), Semen Dolichoris Lablab (*Bai Bian Dou*), Semen Coicis Lachryma-jobi (*Yi Yi Ren*), Semen Nelumbinis Nuciferae (*Lian Zi*), Fructus Amomi (*Sha Ren*), Radix Platycodi Grandiflori (*Jie Geng*)

The authors of *Zhong Yi Fu Ke Xue (A Study of Chinese Medical Gynecology)* suggest that one use this formula in the case of (sometimes) early, (sometimes) late, no fixed schedule menstruation due to liver qi stagnation when spleen vacuity is more prominent. Other authors simply suggest it for spleen vacuity no fixed schedule menstruation.

4. *Wu Yao Tang Jia Jian* (Lindera Decoction with Additions & Subtractions)

Ingredients: Radix Linderae Strychnifoliae (*Wu Yao*), Rhizoma Cyperi Rotundi (*Xiang Fu*), Radix Auklandiae Lappae (*Mu Xiang*), Fructus Amomi (*Sha Ren*), Rhizoma Corydalis Yanhusuo (*Yan Hu Suo*), Radix Glycyrrhizae (*Gan Cao*)

5. Unnamed formula from *Nu Ke Jing Wei (Profundities from the Gynecological Classics)*

Ingredients: Vinegar-processed Radix Bupleuri (*Chai Hu*), body of Radix Angelicae Sinensis (*Dang Gui Shen*), uncooked Radix Albus Paeoniae Lactiflorae (*Bai Shao*), processed Rhizoma Cyperi Rotundi (*Xiang Fu*), stir-fried Pericarpium Citri Reticulatae Viride (*Qing Pi*), Guangdong Radix Auklandiae Lappae (*Guang Mu Xiang*), Yunnan Sclerotium Poriae Cocos (*Yun Fu Ling*), Rhizoma Corydalis Yanhusuo (*Yan Hu Suo*), blood-processed Radix Salviae Miltiorrhizae (*Dan Shen*), Radix Polygalae Tenuifoliae (*Yuan Zhi*), scorched Semen Zizyphi

Spinosae (*Zao Ren*), Semen Biotae Orientalis (*Bai Zi Ren*), scorched Fructus Gardeniae Jasminoidis (*Shan Zhi*), Cortex Radicis Moutan (*Dan Pi*), uncooked Radix Glycyrrhizae (*Gan Cao*)

This formula is for liver depression-depressive heat with heart-spleen qi binding. This means that there is liver depression with depressive heat complicated by heart blood and spleen qi vacuity. This formula is a modification of *Dan Zhi Xiao Yao San* (Moutan & Gardenia Rambling Powder) with elements of *Gu Pi Tang* (Restore the Spleen Decoction).

Additions & subtractions: If the menses come early and are profuse in amount, liver depressive heat is severe. In that case, remove Salvia and Poria from this formula and add Cortex Radicis Lycii Chinensis (*Di Gu Pi*), Herba Agrimoniae Pilosae (*Xian He Cao*), and carbonized Herba Schizonepetae Tenuifoliae (*Jie Sui*). If the menses are late and the amount is scanty and color is pale, then remove the Moutan and Gardenia and add earth stir-fried Rhizoma Atractylodis Macrocephalae (*Bai Zhu*), Guangdong Pericarpium Citri Reticulatae (*Guang Chen Pi*), and uncooked Radix Astragali Membranacei (*Huang Qi*). If there is rib-side and abdominal distention and pain and no desire for food, add Sichuan Cortex Magnoliae Officinalis (*Chuan Hou Po*) and old Radix Ligustici Wallichii (*Chuan Xiong*).

Spleen vacuity

Main symptoms: The menses may come either early or late, are scanty in volume or drip continually without stopping. Their color is pale red. There is shortness of breath, lack of strength, dizziness and heart palpitations, reduced appetite, and the stools may be flimsy and loose. The tongue fur is white and slimy and the pulse is vacuous, relaxed (retarded), and without force.

Treatment principles: Fortify the spleen and warm the stomach

Guiding formulas:

1. *Wen Wei Yin* (Warm the Stomach Drink)

Ingredients: Radix Panacis Ginseng (*Ren Shen*), Rhizoma Atractylodis Macrocephalae (*Bai Zhu*), Semen Dolichoris Lablab (*Bai Bian Dou*), Pericarpium Citri Reticulatae (*Chen Pi*), uncooked Rhizoma Zingiberis (*Sheng Jiang*), mix-fried Radix Glycyrrhizae (*Gan Cao*), Radix Angelicae Sinensis (*Dang Gui*)

2. *Jia Jian Ba Zhen Tang* (Additions & Subtractions Eight Pearls Decoction)

Ingredients: Radix Panacis Ginseng (*Ren Shen*), Rhizoma Atractylodis Macrocephalae (*Bai Zhu*), Sclerotium Poriae Cocos (*Fu Ling*), mix-fried Radix Glycyrrhizae (*Gan Cao*), Radix

Albus Paeoniae Lactiflorae (*Bai Shao*), Radix Angelicae Sinensis (*Dang Gui*), Pericarpium Citri Reticulatae (*Chen Pi*), Rhizoma Cyperi Rotundi (*Xiang Fu*), Cortex Radicis Moutan (*Mu Dan Pi*)

Wan Mi-zhai recommends *Ba Zhen Tang* for dual qi and blood vacuity (sometimes) early, (sometimes) late, no fixed schedule menstruation. It was one of his favorite gynecological formulas.

3. *Tiao Jing Wu Ji Wan* (Regulate the Menses Black Chicken Pills)

Ingredients: Black Chicken (*Wu Ji*), Radix Panacis Ginseng (*Ren Shen*), Herba Cistanchis Deserticolae (*Rou Cong Rong*), Fructus Psoraleae Corylifoliae (*Po Gu Zhi*), amomum-processed Radix Angelicae Sinensis (*Dang Gui*), Rhizoma Atractylodis Macrocephalae (*Bai Zhu*), Radix Ligustici Wallichii (*Chuan Xiong*), Radix Salviae Miltiorrhizae (*Dan Shen*), Sclerotium Poriae Cocos (*Fu Ling*), Radix Glycyrrhizae (*Gan Cao*), Cortex Eucommiae Ulmoidis (*Du Zhong*), Rhizoma Cyperi Rotundi (*Xiang Fu*)

Kidney qi vacuity, *chong* & *ren* lose their regulation

Main symptoms: The menses come early, late, and at no fixed time. Their amount is scanty and their consistency is watery, thin, and slack. There is dizziness, impaired memory, tinnitus, lumbar aching and weakness in the knees, the lower abdomen is heavy and distended, stools are loose, and urination is clear and copious. The four extremities are not warm and the facial complexion is darkish and dull. The tongue is pale and moist and the pulse is deep and weak. This condition is most often encountered in women in their 40s who are either experiencing premature or normal menopause.

Treatment principles: Warm the kidneys, support yang, and secure the *chong*

Guiding formulas:

1. *Wen Shen Fu Yang Tang* (Warm the Kidneys & Support Yang Decoction)

Ingredients: Radix Panacis Ginseng (*Ren Shen*), cooked Radix Rehmanniae (*Shu Di*), Radix Dioscoreae Oppositae (*Shan Yao*), Fructus Corni Officinalis (*Shan Zhu Yu*), Semen Cuscutae (*Tu Si Zi*), Radix Polygalae Tenuifoliae (*Yuan Zhi*), Fructus Schisandrae Chinensis (*Wu Wei Zi*), mix-fried Radix Glycyrrhizae (*Gan Cao*), Radix Lateralis Praeparatus Aconiti Carmichaeli (*Fu Zi*), Cortex Cinnamomi Cassiae (*Rou Gui*), Fructus Psoraleae Corylifoliae (*Bu Gu Zhi*)

2. *Er Xian Tang* (Two Immortals Decoction)

Ingredients: Rhizoma Curculiginis Orchioidis (*Xian Mao*), Herba Epimedii (*Xian Ling Pi*), Radix Morindae Officinalis (*Ba Ji Tian*), Radix Angelicae Sinensis (*Dang Gui*), Cortex Phellodendri (*Huang Bai*), Rhizoma Anemarrhenae (*Zhi Mu*)

This formula is for the somewhat complicated pattern of liver blood-kidney yin vacuity with kidney yang vacuity and vacuity heat flaring upward. It is an extremely important formula for the treatment of menstrual diseases in women in their late 30s and older. Although its standard ingredients are relatively few, it is a very sophisticated and profound formula. It was developed originally for the treatment of menopausal hypertension at the Shu Guang Hospital in Shanghai. Its two main ingredients are Curculigo and Epimedium. If one only uses these two medicinals, one can still say they are prescribing the Two Immortals.

Additions & subtractions: If there is no yin vacuity with vacuity heat, delete the Phellodendron and Anemarrhena. For enduring breast lumps in women more than 35 years old with no fixed schedule menstruation, add Radix Scrophulariae Ningpoensis (*Yuan Shen*), Concha Ostreae (*Mu Li*), Bulbus Fritillariae Thunbergii (*Bei Mu*), Semen Citri Reticulatae (*Ju He*), Spica Prunellae Vulgaris (*Xia Gu Cao*), and Semen Vaccariae Segetalis (*Wang Bu Liu Xing*). For chilly pain in the lumbar region, add Radix Linderae Strychnifoliae (*Wu Yao*), Radix Achyranthis Bidentatae (*Niu Xi*), Cortex Eucommiae Ulmoidis (*Du Zhong*), and blast-fried Rhizoma Zingiberis (*Pao Jiang*). For oppression and fullness in the chest and rib-sides along with dry stools, add Radix Bupleuri (*Chai Hu*), Tuber Curcumae (*Yu Jin*), Fructus Meliae Toosendan (*Chuan Lian Zi*), Radix Albus Paeoniae Lactiflorae (*Bai Shao*), and Fructus Trichosanthis Kirlowii (*Gua Lou*). In some women or during hot seasons, this formula may be too hot and cause mouth sores, sore throat, dry mouth, etc. In this case, delete Radix Morindae Officinalis (*Ba Ji Tian*).

3. *Gu Yin Jian Jia Wei* (Secure Yin Decoction with Added Flavors)

Ingredients: Radix Panacis Ginseng (*Ren Shen*), cooked Radix Rehmanniae (*Shu Di*), Radix Dioscoreae Oppositae (*Shan Yao*), Fructus Corni Officinalis (*Shan Zhu Yu*), Semen Cuscutae (*Tu Si Zi*), Radix Polygalae Tenuifoliae (*Yuan Zhi*), Fructus Schisandrae Chinensis (*Wu Wei Zi*), mix-fried Radix Glycyrrhizae (*Gan Cao*), Radix Lateralis Praeparatus Aconiti Carmichaeli (*Fu Zi*), Cortex Cinnamomi Cassiae (*Rou Gui*), Fructus Psoraleae Corylifoliae (*Bu Gu Zhi*)

This formula, found in Zhang Jing-yue's *Jing Yue Quan Shu ([Zhang] Jing-yue's Complete Book)*, is suggested by the authors of *Zhong Yi Fu Ke Xue (A Study of Chinese Medical Gynecology)* for the treatment of kidney vacuity (sometimes) early, (sometimes) late, no fixed schedule menstruation. It is for the treatment of both yin and yang vacuity where all three viscera which engender and transform the blood are involved. In particular, Polygala helps insure the free communication or interaction between the heart and kidneys.

4. *Tiao Yin Jian* (Regulate Yin Decoction)

Ingredients: Radix Codonopsitis Pilosulae (*Dang Shen*), cooked Radix Rehmanniae (*Shu Di*), stir-fried Radix Dioscoreae Oppositae (*Shan Yao*), Fructus Corni Officinalis (*Shan Zhu Yu*), Semen Cuscutae (*Tu Si Zi*), Radix Polygalae Tenuifoliae (*Yuan Zhi*), Fructus Schisandrae Chinensis (*Wu Wei Zi*), mix-fried Radix Glycyrrhizae (*Gan Cao*)

This formula is basically the same as the preceding one but without the warming-yang medicinals.

Kidney yin vacuity, *chong* & *ren* not securing/secured

Main symptoms: Menses scanty in amount and fresh red in color, dizziness, blurred vision, tidal fever, night sweats, lumbar pain, lower limb and heel pain, a red facial complexion, cheeks flushed, tongue dry, red, and without fur, heat in the center of the hands, feet, and heart, stools held back, and a fine, rapid pulse

Treatment principles: Nourish yin, supplement the kidneys, and secure the *chong*

Guiding formulas:

1. *Zhi Bai Di Huang Wan* (Anemarrhena & Phellodendron Rehmannia Pills)

Ingredients: Cooked Radix Rehmanniae (*Shu Di*), Fructus Corni Officinalis (*Shan Zhu Yu*), Radix Dioscoreae Oppositae (*Shan Yao*), Cortex Radicis Moutan (*Dan Pi*), Rhizoma Alismatis (*Ze Xie*), Sclerotium Poriae Cocos (*Fu Ling*), Rhizoma Anemarrhenae Aspheloidis (*Zhi Mu*), Cortex Phellodendri (*Huang Bai*)

This formula nourishes yin, supplements the kidneys, and clears vacuity heat.

2. *Liu Wei Di Huang Wan Jia Wei* (Six Flavors Rehmannia Pills with Added Flavors)

Ingredients: Cooked Radix Rehmanniae (*Shu Di*), Radix Dioscoreae Oppositae (*Shan Yao*), Fructus Corni Officinalis (*Shan Zhu Yu*), Cortex Radicis Moutan (*Dan Pi*), Sclerotium Poriae Cocos (*Fu Ling*), Rhizoma Alismatis (*Ze Xie*), Rhizoma Anemarrhenae Aspheloidis (*Zhi Mu*), Cortex Radicis Lycii Chinensis (*Di Gu Pi*)

Additions & subtractions: Han Bai-ling gives this variation of the first formula, substituting Cortex Lycii for Phellodendron. This makes this formula more effective for clearing vacuity heat which is flushing upward and causing night sweats, hot flashes, and malar flushing. Also, Cortex

Lycii clears heat and cools the blood. The combination of it and Moutan stops unwanted bleeding, including irregular menstrual bleeding.

3. *Gu Yin Jian* (Secure Yin Decoction)

Ingredients: Radix Panacis Ginseng (*Ren Shen*), Radix Dioscoreae Oppositae (*Shan Yao*), cooked Radix Rehmanniae (*Shu Di*), Fructus Corni Officinalis (*Shan Zhu Yu*), Radix Polygalae Tenuifoliae (*Yuan Zhi*), mix-fried Radix Glycyrrhizae (*Gan Cao*), Fructus Schisandrae Chinensis (*Wu Wei Zi*), Semen Cuscutae (*Tu Si Zi*)

4. Fu Qing-zhu's *Ding Jing Tang* (Stabilize the Menses Decoction)

Ingredients: Semen Cuscutae (*Tu Si Zi*), Radix Albus Paeoniae Lactiflorae (*Bai Shao*), Radix Angelicae Sinensis (*Dang Gui*), cooked Radix Rehmanniae (*Shu Di*), Radix Dioscoreae Oppositae (*Shan Yao*), Sclerotium Poriae Cocos (*Fu Ling*), Herba Schizo-nepetae Tenuifoliae (*Jing Jie*), Radix Bupleuri (*Chai Hu*)

This formula is very useful in cases where there is liver blood and kidney yin vacuity with pronounced liver depression qi stagnation. Such women may have (sometimes) early, (sometimes) late, no fixed schedules menstruation, all the usual liver qi signs and symptoms, *and* soreness and weakness of the low back and knees.

5. Unnamed formula from *Nu Ke Jing Wei (Profundities from the Gynecological Classics)*

Ingredients: Large cooked Radix Rehmanniae (*Shu Di*), uncooked Hangzhou Radix Albus Paeoniae Lactiflorae (*Hang Shao*), Radix Dioscoreae Oppositae (*Huai Shan Yao*), Fructus Corni Officinalis (*Shan Zhu Rou*), uncooked Plastrum Testudinis (*Gui Ban*), scorched Cortex Eucommiae Ulmoidis (*Du Zhong*), whole Radix Angelicae Sinensis (*Quan Dang Gui*), true Gelatinum Corii Asini (*E Jiao*), fat Rhizoma Anemarrhenae (*Zhi Mu*), salt-processed Cortex Phellodendri (*Huang Bai*), mix-fried Radix Glycyrrhizae (*Gan Cao*), processed Rhizoma Cyperi Rotundi (*Xiang Fu*), Rhizoma Alismatis (*Ze Xie*)

Additions: If the menses come like a tide and are excessive in amount, add carbonized Herba Schizonepetae Tenuifoliae (*Jie Sui*) and carbonized Petiolus Et Folium Trachycarpi (*Zong Lu Tan*). If there is vexatious heat in the five hearts and thief (*i.e.*, night) sweats, substitute fine uncooked Radix Rehmanniae (*Sheng Di*) for cooked Rehmannia, add uncooked Concha Ostreae (*Mu Li*), Cortex Radicis Lycii Chinensis (*Di Gu Pi*), and Herba Artemisiae Apiaceae (*Qing Hao*), and remove Phellodendron. If lumbar pain is severe as if about to break, add Ramulus Loranthi Seu Visci (*Sang Ji Sheng*) and Sichuan Radix Dipsaci (*Chuan Xu Duan*).

Blood stasis

Main symptoms: The menstrual cycle is unstable. The amount of the menstuate may be profuse or may be scanty. The color of the menses is purplish and dark and contains clots or it may be fresh red. There is lower abdominal aching and pain which refuses pressure. The tongue is purple and dark, and the pulse is deep and choppy.

Treatment principles: Quicken the blood, transform stasis, and regulate the menses

Guiding formula: *Tao Hong Si Wu Tang Jia Xiang Fu Wu Yao* **(Persica & Carthamus Four Materials Decoction plus Cyperus & Lindera)**

Ingredients: Semen Pruni Persicae (*Tao Ren*), Flos Carthami Tinctorii (*Hong Hua*), Radix Angelicae Sinensis (*Dang Gui*), cooked Radix Rehmanniae (*Shu Di*), Radix Albus Paeoniae Lactiflorae (*Bai Shao*), Radix Ligustici Wallichii (*Chuan Xiong*), Radix Linderae Strychnifoliae (*Wu Yao*), Rhizoma Cyperi Rotundi (*Xiang Fu*)

Additions: If there is lower abdominal aching and pain with chest oppression and discomfort and other signs of obvious qi depression, add Radix Bupleuri (*Chai Hu*), Fructus Meliae Toosendan (*Chuan Lian Zi*), and Pericarpium Citri Reticulatae Viride (*Qing Pi*) to course the liver and out-thrust depression. If there is lower abdominal chilly pain with a bland taste in the mouth and dark tongue due to cold qi being relatively exuberant, add Fructus Evodiae Rutecarpae (*Wu Zhu Yu*) and Radix Auklandiae Lappae (*Mu Xiang*) to scatter cold and move stagnation.

Discussion

Menstruation at no fixed time is usually best treated over a period of several months with not too many adjustments in the formulas. By this, I mean that one need not necessarily try to discriminate each month the exact mechanism which is dominant. Such precise discriminaton sounds good in theory but may be difficult and frustrating to achieve in practice. Therefore, I prefer to identify the key mechanism at work and then give the same formula consistently over not less than three cycles.

Because there is a swing or shift in the disease mechanism in (sometimes) early, (sometimes) late, no fixed schedule menstrauton accounting for their sometimes coming early and sometimes late, both mechanisms are not constantly present. In the case of liver qi transforming into depressive heat, the foundation of depressive heat is stagnant qi. If this stagnant qi is addressed, it will undercut the transformative disease mechanism of depressive heat without necessarily having to include ingredients which clear heat and resolve depression. Such ingredients would only have to be included if the heat and depression are fairly constant. When the heat and depression are not present, if one courses the liver and rectifies the qi, there is no basis for the arisal of depressive heat. If such heat-clearing medicinals were included in the patient's formula even when she did not need them, one would run the risk of damaging a spleen which is very likely vacuous to begin with.

(Sometimes) early, (sometimes) late, no fixed schedule menstruation is not usually a patient's main complaint, but they are a part of many women's total disease diagnosis. For instance, a woman may complain of lower abdominal menstrual pain and, when one does a thorough questioning about the woman's menses, finds out that her menses are also sometimes early, sometimes late, and come at no fixed schedule. In this case, the woman's TCM disease diagnosis is (sometimes) early, (sometimes) late, no fixed schedule menstruation and painful menstruation.

When questioning Western women, one must be careful to find out exactly what a woman means if she says her menses are irregular. Many women will say their menses are irregular, but what they mean is that they are always late. The exact date of their arrival may fluctuate even widely, but as long as it is after 30 days, this is not (sometimes) early, (sometimes) late, no fixed schedule menstruation but rather menstruation behind schedule and it should be treated as such.

Prognosis

Most (sometimes) early, (sometimes) late, no fixed schedule menstruation occurring in younger women is due to liver-spleen disharmony. Liver depression causes the menses to come late coupled with blood vacuity, or depressive liver heat causes the menses to come early coupled with spleen qi vacuity. Although women with such erratic menstruation are very sensitive to emotional fluctuations, their cycles can usually be evened out without too much difficulty.

As a woman moves into her mid-30s, most (sometimes) early, (sometimes) late, no fixed schedule menstruation continues to be due to liver qi but now typically becomes complicated by kidney vacuity as well. If the menses have been coming early and then switch to late in a woman in her late 30s or early 40s, premature menopause should be suspected and headed off.

(Sometimes) early, (sometimes) late, no fixed schedule menstruation complicated by either blood stasis or phlegm dampness presents no special difficulties. When these two disease mechanisms play a part in this disease, they are only as complicating factors, with the main issues usually being liver depression, spleen, and/or kidney vacuity. Therefore, one will pick one's guiding formula based on those mechanisms and then modify those formulas with the inclusion of blood quickening and stasis-dispelling or phlegm transforming and damp-eliminating medicinals.

By charting the BBT, one can often get a better idea about when ovulation is occurring and what the pattern or combination of patterns is. However, this charting must be carried out for at least three cycles.

Key patterns to memorize:	
1. Repletion patterns	A. Qi stagnation B. Blood stasis

2. Vacuity patterns	A. Spleen qi vacuity
	B. Kidney vacuity
	    i. Kidney yin vacuity
	    ii. Kidney yang vacuity

3. Mixed vacuity-repletion pattern	Phlegm Obstruction

4

Profuse Menstruation

Yue jing guo duo refers to a menstrual discharge which is excessive in volume. The menses come on schedule, but the volume of blood discharged is abnormally profuse. As with many other Chinese menstrual diseases, profuse menstruation may be either the main complaint or part of a woman's total TCM disease diagnosis. Not only may the menses be excessive in volume, but the flow may also be prolonged. As long as this excessive and prolonged bleeding occurs at the regular scheduled time of menstruation, it is classified as profuse menstruation. This disease category corresponds to menorrhagia in Western medicine, *i.e.*, excessive flow occurring during the regularly scheduled menses, as distinct from metrorrhagia which we will cover below under flooding and leaking.

Disease causes, disease mechanisms

Profuse menstruation is none other than a species of abnormal bleeding. Therefore, like menstruation ahead of schedule, its disease mechanisms cannot be anything but heat forcing the blood to move frenetically outside its pathways, qi vacuity not containing the blood within its vessels, blood stasis preventing fresh blood to return to its channels, or trauma causing a rupture in the channels and network vessels. While trauma is not usually discussed as an etiological factor in terms of menstruation ahead of schedule, sex during menstruation can result in damage of the blood vessels resulting in profuse menstruation.

Of these possible disease mechanisms, most Chinese gynecology texts only discuss heat and qi vacuity. These are undoubtedly the main mechanisms at work. However, blood stasis can contribute to profuse menstruation.

Heat in the blood making it move frenetically outside its pathways may be due to either depressive heat or liver fire. Either depression transforms into heat or extreme anger and irritation causes effulgence of liver fire. It is also said that all excessive emotions may transform into fire and this fire may accumulate in the heart, the fire viscus. Such heat or fire in the heart may also cause profuse menstruation. In either case, heat makes it impossible for the liver to store the blood and for the heart to participate normally in its control of the blood. Profuse menstruation may also be due to replete heat derived from overeating hot, spicy foods, greasy, oily foods, or drinking alcohol. It is even possible for vacuity heat due to kidney yin vacuity to also result in profuse menstruation. The causes of yin vacuity have been discussed above. Although vacuity heat generally does not cause profuse menstruation all at once, it does cause prolonged menstruation. Therefore, the total volume of blood discharged is profuse.

Qi vacuity failing to restrain the blood within its vessels may involve the spleen and heart. Spleen qi may become too weak to contain the blood due to faulty diet, lack of exercise, excessive fatigue, and excessive worry and anxiety. Excessive worry, anxiety, or longing and grief can also affect the heart and thence the spleen via the five phase engenderment cycle. Due to age, exhaustion, drug abuse, or congenital insufficiency, kidney yang may be vacuous and debilitated, in which case kidney qi may not astringe and secure the sea of blood properly.

Professors Song and Yu also list as a possible cause and species of profuse menstruation detriment suffered by the *chong* and *ren*. Song and Yu say this may be due to sex during menstruation which damages and causes detriment to the blood network vessels. This is aggravated by the collision of descending and ascending qi and aggravation of heat locally. In the Chinese literature, it is said that essence excited during sex takes the place of the blood which cannot return to the channels. This results in the blood flowing outside its channels and network vessels and thus profuse menstruation. This is one instance where damage or trauma plays a part in the creation of a menstrual disease.

Some Chinese gynecology texts also discuss blood stasis as a possible cause of excessive menstrual bleeding. Once again, this can be due to the effects of past trauma to the lower burner, IUDs, the sequelae of abortions and oral contraceptives (OCs), or enduring, persistent qi stagnation. In this case, blood stasis prevents the blood from returning to its channels.

Likewise, some Chinese gynecology texts also list phlegm dampness or phlegm rheum as possible causes of excessive menstrual bleeding. This phlegm and dampness is typically due to spleen vacuity losing its command over the movement and transformation of fluids in turn due to faulty diet, lack of exercise, and excessive thinking and worry. The reason that many other TCM gynecology texts do not list this as a separate mechanism and species of profuse menstruation is that the excessive bleeding itself is due to spleen qi vacuity, remembering that spleen dampness is a mixed repletion/vacuity pattern. When one encounters phlegm and dampness in profuse menstruation, it is not uncommon for these to be complicated by depressive heat as well, making this scenario even more of a mixed repletion and vacuity.

Treatment based on pattern discrimination

Blood heat

Main symptoms: Excessive menstrual bleeding either deep red and pasty and sticky or bright red with purplish clots, thirst, a preference for chilled drinks, heart vexation, a red facial complexion, difficulty sleeping, low back and abdominal distention and pain, urination either yellow or short and red, stools constipated and bound, a red tongue with yellow fur, and a slippery, rapid pulse

Treatment principles: Clear heat and cool the blood

Guiding formulas:

1. *Xian Qi Tang* (Before Schedule Decoction)

Ingredients: Uncooked Radix Rehmanniae (*Sheng Di*), Rhizoma Anemarrhenae Aspheloidis (*Zhi Mu*), Rhizoma Coptidis Chinensis (*Huang Lian*), Radix Angelicae Sinensis (*Dang Gui*), Radix Albus Paeoniae Lactiflorae (*Bai Shao*), Radix Ligustici Wallichii (*Chuan Xiong*), Cortex Phellodendri (*Huang Bai*), Radix Scutellariae Baicalensis (*Huang Qin*), Gelatinum Corii Asini (*E Jiao*), Herba Artemisiae Argyii (*Ai Ye*), Rhizoma Cyperi Rotundi (*Xiang Fu*), mix-fried Radix Glycyrrhizae (*Gan Cao*)

We have seen this formula above in the chapter on menstruation ahead of schedule. In fact, it is not uncommon to find profuse menstruation and menstruation ahead of schedule occurring simultaneously.

Additions & subtractions: Sun Jiu-ling says to delete Dang Gui and add Os Sepiae Seu Sepiellae (*Hai Piao Xiao*) and Radix Rubiae Cordifoliae (*Qian Cao*) in order to improve the astringing and stopping of bleeding.

2. *Bao Yin Jian Jia Wei* (Protect Yin Decoction with Added Flavors)

Ingredients: Uncooked Radix Rehmanniae (*Sheng Di*), cooked Radix Rehmanniae (*Shu Di*), Cortex Phellodendri (*Huang Bai*), Radix Dipsaci (*Xu Duan*), Radix Dioscoreae Oppositae (*Shan Yao*), Radix Scutellariae Baicalensis (*Huang Qin*), Radix Albus Paeoniae Lactiflorae (*Bai Shao*), Radix Glycyrrhizae (*Gan Cao*), Radix Sanguisorbae (*Di Yu*), Flos Immaturus Sophorae Japonicae (*Huai Hua Mi*)

This formula is for vacuity heat profuse menstruation.

3. Unnamed formula from *Concise Traditional Chinese Gynecology*

Ingredients: Mix-fried Plastrum Testudinis (*Gui Ban*), Cortex Phellodendri (*Huang Bai*), Herba Ecliptae Prostratae (*Han Lian Cao*), Radix Scutellariae Baicalensis (*Huang Qin*)

This formula is also for yin vacuity-vacuity fire profuse menstraution.

4. *Dang Gui Yin* (Dang Gui Drink)

Ingredients: Radix Angelicae Sinensis (*Dang Gui*), Radix Ligustici Wallichii (*Chuan Xiong*), Radix Albus Paeoniae Lactiflorae (*Bai Shao*), cooked Radix Rehmanniae (*Shu Di*), Rhizoma Atractylodis Macrocephalae (*Bai Zhu*), Radix Scutellariae Baicalensis (*Huang Qin*)

Professors Song and Yu suggest this guiding formula for blood heat profuse menstruation based on the treatment principles of clearing heat and banking yin, enriching the liver and nourishing blood. This means that this formula is also primarily for vacuity heat. However, they go on to say that one can add ingredients such as Gelatinum Corii Asini (*E Jiao*), stir-fried Fructus Gardeniae Jasminoidis (*Zhi Zi*), carbonized Herba Schizonepetae Tenuifoliae (*Jing Jie*), Radix Glycyrrhizae (*Gan Cao*), and the juice of Rhizoma Phragmitis Communis (*Lu Geng Zhi*) to more effectively clear heat and stop bleeding.

5. *Qing Gan Zhi Xue Tang* (Clear the Liver & Stop Bleeding Decoction)

Ingredients: Radix Bupleuri (*Chai Hu*), Radix Albus Paeoniae Lactiflorae (*Bai Shao*), Radix Rubrus Paeoniae Lactiflorae (*Chi Shao*), Cortex Radicis Moutan (*Dan Pi*), Folium Mori Albi (*Sang Ye*), Rhizoma Cyperi Rotundi (*Xiang Fu*), uncooked Radix Rehmanniae (*Sheng Di*), Radix Scutellariae Baicalensis (*Huang Qin*), Ramulus Uncariae Cum Uncis (*Gou Teng*), Radix Angelicae Sinensis (*Dang Gui*)

This formula treats liver fire profuse menstruation.

Additions & subtractions: If there is liver yin vacuity with a rapid, fine, bowstring pulse and a red tongue with scant moisture, delete Bupleurum and Cyperus and add Fructus Ligustri Lucidi (*Nu Zhen Zi*) and Herba Ecliptae Prostratae (*Han Lian Cao*).

6. *Dan Zhi Xiao Yao San Jia Jian* (Moutan & Gardenia Rambling Powder with Additions & Subtractions)

Ingredients: Radix Bupleuri (*Chai Hu*), Rhizoma Cyperi Rotundi (*Xiang Fu*), Radix Albus Paeoniae Albae (*Bai Shao*), Radix Angelicae Sinensis (*Dang Gui*), Rhizoma Atractylodis Macrocephalae (*Bai Zhu*), Sclerotium Poriae Cocos (*Fu Ling*), Cortex Radicis Moutan (*Dan*

Pi), Fructus Gardeniae Jasminoidis (*Zhi Zi*), Os Sepiae Seu Sepiellae (*Hai Piao Xiao*), Radix Rubiae Cordifoliae (*Qian Cao*), stir-fried Pollen Typhae (*Chao Pu Huang*), uncooked Concha Ostreae (*Mu Li*), Radix Glycyrrhizae (*Gan Cao*)

This formula is for depressive liver heat profuse menstruation complicated by blood vacuity and loss or lack of securing and astringing. It is chosen based on the treatment principles of coursing the liver and resolving depression, nourishing and cooling the blood, and securing, astringing, and stopping bleeding. Loss or lack of astringing and securing refers to kidney vacuity not securing and constraining. This is seen in women in their late 30s and 40s or when profuse menstruation has endured a long time and enduring disease has damaged the kidneys.

7. *Qing Hai Tang* (Clear the Sea Decoction)

Ingredients: Stir-fried Radix Albus Paeoniae Lactiflorae (*Bai Shao*), carbonized Flos Immaturus Sophorae Japonicae (*Huai Hua Mi*), Folium Mori Albi (*Sang Ye*), Herba Leonuri Heterophylli (*Yi Mu Cao*), Radix Scrophulariae Ningpoensis (*Yuan Shen*), carbonized Receptaculum Nelumbinis Nuciferae (*Lian Fang*), Cortex Radicis Moutan (*Dan Pi*), Caulis Bambusae In Taeniis (*Zhu Ru*), sweet Flos Chrysanthemi Morifolii (*Gan Ju Hua*)

This formula is for excessive menstrual bleeding due to liver fire effulgence.

8. *Jia Wei Bai Di Tang* (Added Flavors Pulsatilla & Sanguisorba/Rehmannia Decoction)

Ingredients: Radix Pulsatillae Chinensis (*Bai Tou Weng*), Radix Sanguisorbae (*Di Yu*), uncooked Radix Rehmanniae (*Sheng Di*), Saccarhum Granulorum (*Bai Tang*)

This very simple formula treats excessive menstrual bleeding due to overeating spicy, hot, greasy foods. Chinese texts comment that this condition is more often encountered in adolescent females who have a robust constitution tending towards fire effulgence.

9. *Liang Di Tang* (Two Di's Decoction)

Ingredients: Uncooked Radix Rehmanniae (*Sheng Di*), Radix Scrophulariae Ningpoensis (*Yuan Shen*), Tuber Ophiopogonis Japonici (*Mai Dong*), Radix Albus Paeoniae Lactiflorae (*Bai Shao*), Cortex Radicis Lycii Chinensis (*Di Gu Pi*), Gelatinum Corii Asini (*E Jiao*)

This formula is for yin vacuity blood heat. In this formula, nourishing yin is primary but is assisted by clearing heat. When yin is nourished, vacuity heat or yang is automatically controlled and the blood is cooled. However, by clearing heat and cooling the blood, yin can regenerate all the better.

10. *Wen Qing Yin* (Warming & Clearing Drink)

Ingredients: Uncooked Radix Rehmanniae (*Sheng Di*), Radix Rubrus Paeoniae Lactiflorae (*Chi Shao*), Radix Angelicae Sinensis (*Dang Gui*), Radix Ligustici Wallichii (*Chuan Xiong*), Radix Scutellariae Baicalensis (*Huang Qin*), Rhizoma Coptidis Chinensis (*Huang Lian*), Cortex Phellodendri (*Huang Bai*), Fructus Gardeniae Jasminoidis (*Zhi Zi*)

This formula treats profuse menstruation, flooding and leaking, and other types of bleeding, chronic skin complaints, such as pruritus, urticaria, dermatitis, eczema, and tinea, emotional disorders, and hypertension. In TCM, it is described as treating blood heat with yin and blood vacuity. This formula can be used for treating yin and blood vacuity with replete or damp heat, depressive heat or vacuity heat depending on what types of Rehmannia and Peony are used and what other additions and subtractions are made. See the chapter on menstruation ahead of schedule for modifications of this formula.

11. *Shao Ying Jian* (Scanty Constructive Decoction)

Ingredients: Cooked Radix Rehmanniae (*Di Huang*), Radix Albus Paeoniae Lactiflorae (*Shao Yao*), Radix Glycyrrhizae (*Gan Cao*), Radix Dipsaci (*Xu Duan*), Radix Sanguisorbae (*Di Yu*), Radix Scutellariae Baicalensis (*Huang Qin*), Flos Immaturus Sophorae Japonicae (*Huai Hua*), stir-fried till scorched Herba Schizonepetae Tenuifoliae (*Jing Jie Sui*), Fructus Pruni Mume (*Wu Mei*)

This formula clears heat and cools the blood, stops bleeding and secures the *chong*.

12. *An Chong Tang* (Quiet the *Chong* [*Mai*] Decoction)

Ingredients: Stir-fried Rhizoma Atractylodis Macrocephalae (*Bai Zhu*), Radix Astragali Membranacei (*Sheng Huang Qi*), uncooked Os Draconis (*Long Gu*), uncooked Concha Ostreae (*Mu Li*), large uncooked Radix Rehmanniae (*Sheng Di*), uncooked Hangzhou Radix Albus Paeoniae Lactiflorae (*Hang Shao*), Os Sepiae Seu Sepiellae (*Hai Piao Xiao*), Radix Rubiae Cordifoliae (*Qian Cao*), Radix Dipsaci (*Chuan Xu Duan*)

This formula boosts the qi and nourishes yin, cools the blood and stops bleeding. Du Jie-hui indicates it for the treatment of blood heat profuse menstruation complicated by qi vacuity as manifested by shortness of breath, weariness, fatigue, lack of strength, and reduced intake of food and drink. These last several symptoms are all associated with spleen qi vacuity. However, because of the additions of astringents, such as Oyster Shell and Cuttlebone, and kidney-supplements like Dipsacus, I would say it also treats an element of kidney vacuity not securing and astringing as well.

13. *Liang Xu Gu Zhen Tang* (Dual Vacuity Secure the True Decoction)

Ingredients: Radix Angelicae Sinensis (*Dang Gui*), Radix Ligustici Wallichii (*Chuan Xiong*), Radix Albus Paeoniae Lactiflorae (*Bai Shao*), uncooked Radix Rehmanniae (*Sheng Di*), cooked Radix Rehmanniae (*Shu Di*), Radix Scutellariae Baicalensis (*Sheng Qin*), Rhizoma Cyperi Rotundi (*Xiang Fu*), Radix Dipsaci (*Xu Duan*), Radix Bupleuri (*Chai Hu*), Radix Salviae Miltiorrhizae (*Dan Shen*), Rhizoma Atractylodis Macrocephalae (*Bai Zhu*), Herba Schizonepetae Tenuifoliae (*Jing Jie Sui*), stir-fried Cortex Phellodendri (*Huang Bai*)

Du Jie-hui indicates this formula for the treatment of vacuity heat profuse menstruation as well as menstruation ahead of schedule. It nourishes yin and clears heat, supplements the spleen and boosts the kidneys, and rectifies the qi and stops bleeding.

Chong & Ren Suffer Detriment

Main symptoms: Excessive menstrual bleeding after sex during menstruation

Treatment principles: Nourish and quicken the blood, stop bleeding

Guiding formulas:

1. *Jiao Ai Tang* (Donkey Skin Glue & Mugwort Decoction)

Ingredients: Cooked Radix Rehmanniae (*Shu Di*), Radix Albus Paeoniae Lactiflorae (*Bai Shao*), Radix Angelicae Sinensis (*Dang Gui*), Folium Artemisiae Argyii (*Ai Ye*), Gelatinum Corii Asini (*E Jiao*), Radix Ligustici Wallichii (*Chuan Xiong*), mix-fried Radix Glycyrrhizae (*Gan Cao*)

2. *Jia Jian Si Wu Tang* (Additions & Subtractions Four Materials Decoction)

Ingredients: Cooked Radix Rehmanniae (*Shu Di Huang*), Radix Albus Paeoniae Lactiflorae (*Bai Shao*), Radix Angelicae Sinensis (*Dang Gui*), Radix Ligustici Wallichii (*Chuan Xiong*), Rhizoma Atractylodis Macrocephalae (*Bai Zhu*), blackened Herba Schizonepetae Tenuifoliae (*Jing Jie Sui*), Fructus Corni Officinalis (*Shan Zhu Yu*), Radix Dipsaci (*Chuan Xu Duan*), Radix Glycyrrhizae (*Gan Cao*)

The reader should note that the above formula contains at least two specfically kidney-supplementing medicinals, Cornus and Dipsacus. In general, the concept of detriment damage of the *chong* and *ren* includes the assumption of kidney vacuity. This is because the *chong* and *ren* both arise from the uterus which is connected to the kidneys. If detriment and damage to the blood network vessels and pentrating vessel results in profuse bleeding, this profuse bleeding then easily damages the kidneys, causing them to become vacuous.

Spleen vacuity

Main symptoms: Heavy menstrual bleeding but pale in color and thin in consistency, shortness of breath, fatigue, weakness in the extremities, a light red tongue with thin, white fur, and a fine, weak pulse

If there is central qi vacuity and fall, there will also be a heavy, dragging feeling at the bottom of the pelvis and the pulse will be short or deep. If there is blood vacuity due to loss, the tongue will be more markedly pale, the pulse may be scallion stalk if the bleeding was very massively profuse, and there may be heart palpitations, a pale facial complexion, and dry tongue fur. These symptoms indicate spleen qi and heart blood vacuity.

Treatment principles: For primarily qi vacuity, supplement the spleen and boost the qi, lift the fallen and stop bleeding. For qi and blood vacuity, boost the qi and nourish the blood, fortify the spleen and supplement the heart.

Guiding formulas:

1. *Ju Yuan Jian Jia Wei* (Lift the Source Decoction with Added Flavors)

Ingredients: Rhizoma Cimicifugae (*Sheng Ma*), Folium Artemisiae Argyii (*Ai Ye*), blast-fried till carbonized Rhizoma Zingiberis (*Pao Jiang*), mix-fried Radix Glycyrrhizae (*Gan Cao*), Radix Panacis Ginseng (*Ren Shen*), Radix Astragali Membrancei (*Huang Qi*), Gelatinum Corii Asini (*E Jiao*), Rhizoma Atractylodis Macrocephalae (*Bai Zhu*)

Additions: For heavy bleeding, add Os Sepiae Seu Sepiellae (*Hai Piao Xiao*) and carbonized Radix Rubiae Cordifoliae (*Qian Cao*).

2. *Bu Zhong Yi Qi Tang Jia Wei* (Supplement the Center & Boost the Qi Decoction with Added Flavors)

Ingredients: Radix Panacis Ginseng (*Ren Shen*) or Radix Codonopsitis Pilosulae (*Dang Shen*), Radix Astragali Memebranacei (*Huang Qi*), Rhizoma Atractylodis Macrocephalae (*Bai Zhu*), mix-fried Radix Glycyrrhizae (*Gan Cao*), Radix Angelicae Sinensis (*Dang Gui*), Rhizoma Cimicifugae (*Sheng Ma*), Radix Bupleuri (*Chai Hu*), Pericarpium Citri Reticulatae (*Chen Pi*), Radix Scutellariae Baicalensis (*Huang Qin*), Radix Albus Paeoniae Lactiflorae (*Bai Shao*)

This formula is for qi vacuity and fall combined with liver heat.

3. *Gui Pi Tang* (Restore the Spleen Decoction)

Ingredients: Radix Panacis Ginseng (*Ren Shen*) or Radix Codonopsitis Pilosulae (*Dang Shen*), Radix Astragali Membranacei (*Huang Qi*), Radix Angelicae Sinensis (*Dang Gui*), Arillus Euphoriae Longanae (*Long Yan Rou*), Rhizoma Atractylodis Macrocephalae (*Bai Zhu*), Radix Auklandiae Lappae (*Mu Xiang*), Sclerotium Poriae Cocos (*Fu Ling*), Radix Polygalae Tenuifoliae (*Yuan Zhi*), Semen Zizyphi Spinosae (*Suan Zao Ren*), mix-fried Radix Glycyrrhizae (*Gan Cao*), uncooked Rhizoma Zingiberis (*Sheng Jiang*), Fructus Zizyphi Jujubae (*Da Zao*)

This formula is for heart blood-spleen qi vacuity.

Additions: For menstruation that suddenly changes in volume and flows continuously, add Fructus Corni Officinalis (*Shan Zhu Yu*) and Fructus Schisandrae Chinensis (*Wu Wei Zi*). This is for excessive menstrual bleeding which has gone on so long that astringency and securing have been lost. For excessive blood flow which is watery in consistency and pale in color, add Gelatinum Corii Asini (*E Jiao*), Ramulus Loranthi Seu Visci (*Sang Ji Sheng*), and Radix Polygoni Multiflori (*He Shou Wu*).

4. *Jiao Ai Ba Zhen Tang* (Donkey Skin Glue & Mugwort Eight Pearls Decoction)

Ingredients: Radix Codonopsitis Pilosulae (*Dang Shen*), Rhizoma Atractylodis Macrocephalae (*Bai Zhu*), Sclerotium Poriae Cocos (*Fu Ling*), mix-fried Radix Glycyrrhizae (*Gan Cao*), cooked Radix Rehmanniae (*Shu Di*), Radix Angelicae Sinensis (*Dang Gui*), Radix Albus Paeoniae Lactiflorae (*Bai Shao*), Radix Ligustici Wallichii (*Chuan Xiong*), Gelatinum Corii Asini (*E Jiao*), Folium Artemisiae Argyii (*Ai Ye*)

This formula is for qi and blood dual vacuity.

5. *Jing Shui Guo Duo Fang* (Menstrual Water Overly Excessive Formula)

Ingredients: Rhizoma Atractylodis Macrocephalae (*Bai Zhu*), uncooked Radix Astragali Membranacei (*Huang Qi*), Pericarpium Citri Reticulatae (*Chen Pi*), Radix Panacis Ginseng (*Ren Shen*), mix-fried Radix Glycyrrhizae (*Gan Cao*)

6. *Zong Hui San* (Trachycarpus Ash Powder)

Ingredients: Stir-fried Rhizoma Cyperi Rotundi (*Xiang Fu*), stir-fried Pollen Typhae (*Pu Huang*), Radix Panacis Ginseng (*Ren Shen*), Radix Astragali Membranacei (*Huang Qi*), Radix Sanguisorbae (*Di Yu*), Rhizoma Cimicifugae (*Sheng Ma*), carbonized Petiolus Et Folium Trachycarpi (*Zong Lu Hui*), Rhizoma Atractylodis Macrocephalae (*Bai Zhu*)

Kidney yang vacuity

Main symptoms: This pattern is usually met with in premenopausal women, congenitally vacuous and insufficient women, women suffering from enduring disease, and those in whom excessive menstrual bleeding has remained unchecked for a long time. The menstrual blood is pale in color, thin in consistency, but persistent in its flow. There is lumbar pain, chilling of the lower extremities, possible thin, clear vaginal discharge or polyuria, dizziness, tinnitus, impaired memory, a pale tongue with thin, white fur, and a deep, forceless pulse.

Treatment principles: Warm the kidneys and invigorate yang, secure the *chong* and stop bleeding

Guiding formulas:

1. *Fu Fang Shi Hui San* (Compound Ten Ashes Powder)

Ingredients: Radix Codonopsitis Pilosulae (*Dang Shen*), cooked Radix Rehmanniae (*Shu Di*), Cortex Eucommiae Ulmoidis (*Du Zhong*), Radix Dipsaci (*Xu Duan*), dry Rhizoma Zingiberis (*Gan Jiang*), Gelatinum Cornu Cervi (*Lu Jiao Jiao*) plus 1 1/2 grams of *Shi Hui San* (Ten Ashes Powder) with each dose

The ingredients of *Shi Hui San* are: Herba Cirsii Japonicae (*Da Ji*), Folium Nelumbinis Nuciferae (*He Ye*), Rhizoma Imperatae Cylindricae (*Ban Mao Geng*), Radix Et Rhizoma Rhei (*Da Huang*), Folium Et Petriolus Trachycarpi (*Chen Zong*), Herba Cephalanopoloris Segeti (*Xiao Ji*), Cacumen Biotae Orientalis (*Ce Bai Ye*), Radix Rubiae Cordifoliae (*Qian Cao*), Fructus Gardeniae Jasminoidis (*Zhi Zi*), Cortex Radicis Moutan (*Dan Pi*). All of these ingredients are carbonized, powdered, and mixed together. This is a combination of styptics and hemostatics which can be used to stop bleeding due to a number of causes. In this case, a small amount of this powder is taken with a decoction of the preceding qi and kidney-supplementing medicinals.

2. *Bu Shen Gu Jing Tang* (Supplement the Kidneys & Secure the Essence Decoction)

Ingredients: Hallyositum Rubrum (*Chi Shi Zhi*), Fructus Psoraleae Corylifoliae (*Po Gu Zhi*)

This simple formula supplements the kidneys and secures and astringes. It is indicated for the treatment of kidney vacuity not securing profuse menstruation. These two medicinals can be added to other formulas when other patterns of profuse menstruation are complicated by kidney yang vacuity.

Blood stasis

Main symptoms: Spotting or sudden discharge with clots, fixed pain worse in the evening or at night, a purplish tongue or static spots or macules on the tongue, often yellowish tongue fur, and a deep, bowstring, choppy, or bound pulse

This mechanism of bleeding is rarely encountered as the sole or main cause of profuse menstruation. Most Chinese gynecology texts do not list it, although some do. No matter what other patterns or mechanisms blood stasis is mixed with, the stasis should still be transformed and dispelled. Some practitioners may hesitate to quicken the blood during excessive bleeding. However, blood stasis can be a mechanism for bleeding, and, when it is, *it must be quickened and dispelled*. This is called opening in the face of openness in TCM. This is a very important treatment principle to know and understand. Otherwise one will not be able to completely control excessive menstrual bleeding associated with blood stasis by employing only other treatment principles and methods.

Treatment principles: Quicken the blood and transform stasis

Guiding formula: *Shi Xiao San* (Loose a Smile Powder)

Ingredients: Feces Trogopterori Seu Pteromi (*Wu Ling Zhi*), Pollen Typhae (*Pu Huang*)

The ingredients of this small formula may be added to other formulas when blood stasis plays a part in excessive menstrual bleeding.

Phlegm rheum

Main symptoms: Large volume of discharge, pale, thick, and viscous, profuse vaginal discharge, obesity and/or profuse phlegm, tastelessness in the mouth, chest oppression and epigastric fullness, a pale tongue with slimy fur, and a slippery pulse

Treatment principles: Fortify the spleen, eliminate dampness, and transform phlegm

Guiding formula: *Liu Jun Zi Tang Jia Wei* (Six Gentlemen Decoction with Added Flavors)

Ingredients: Radix Codonopsitis Pilosulae (*Dang Shen*), Rhizoma Atractylodis Macrocephalae (*Bai Zhu*), Sclerotium Poriae Cocos (*Fu Ling*), Pericarpium Citri Reticulatae (*Chen Pi*), Rhizoma Pinelliae Ternatae (*Ban Xia*), mix-fried Radix Glycyrrhizae (*Gan Cao*), Rhizoma Atractylodis (*Cang Zhu*), Radix Angelicae Sinensis (*Dang Gui*), Radix Albus Paeoniae Lactiflorae (*Bai Shao*), Rhizoma Arisaematis (*Tian Nan Xing*)

Discussion

Profuse menstruation is very similar to flooding and leaking. The difference between these is that flooding and leaking covers abnormal vaginal bleeding at times other than the normally scheduled menses. Thus, in Western medical terms, profuse menstruation corresponds specifically to menorrhagia and flooding and leaking corresponds to metrorrhagia or functional uterine bleeding. The disease mechanisms of both these Chinese categories are basically the same. Han Bai-ling, in *Bai Ling Fu Ke (Bai-ling's Gynecology)*, does not discuss either profuse menstruation or scanty menstruation. Rather, he discusses flooding and leaking and blocked menstruation or amenorrhea, since, in a sense, these are but the most extreme manifestations of profuse and scanty menstruation.

When preparing this book, I struggled with whether to include both categories, *i.e.*, profuse menstruation and flooding and leaking, since the pattern discrimination is basically the same, as are the treatment principles and guiding formulas. I have decided to include both categories since profuse and scanty menstruation and flooding and leaking and blocked menstruation are yin-yang dichotomies. To leave out any of these categories, it seems to me, would blur the logic of the Chinese categorization and description of menstrual diseases. If one understands the relationship between early and late menses, profuse and scanty, and flooding and leaking and blocked menstruation, one can then categorize and treat any woman whose menstruation is irregular no matter what her Western gynecological disease diagnosis. It is very important for practitioners to understand this principle.

Root & branch

As discussed in the first section on theory, bleeding is an outflow of pure substance which is given priority in treatment. Therefore, during the menses itself, if it is too heavy and voluminous, one should emphasize stopping bleeding. This means that, in acute situations, one should emphasize treating the branch. But, after the bleeding is under control, one should then emphasize the root disease mechanism so as to prevent bleeding in the future. This means to treat the root in chronic situations. When stopping bleeding, one may use hemostatic and styptic medicinals. One should be careful, however, not to use these excessively or for too prolonged a period so as to avoid creating blood stasis iatrogenically.

Acupuncture & moxibustion

Because excessive bleeding is a branch condition which should be addressed immediately and forcefully, one may choose to not only administer internal medicine but to also do acupuncture and/or moxibustion. For qi vacuity failing to contain the blood, moxa indirectly with a moxa pole at *Bai Hui* (GV 20) to upbear yang and lift the fallen. Another treatment is to moxa directly *Yin Bai* (Sp 1) and *Da Dun* (Liv 1). If there is blood stasis, drain *Xue Hai* (Sp 10) and use so-called even needling at *San Yin Jiao* (Sp 6). And if there is lack of kidney securing, moxa directly *Guan Yuan* (CV 4).

Prognosis

TCM treats profuse menstruation quite effectively. In general, all the patterns of profuse menstruation respond favorably to treatment. In particular, spleen qi vacuity typically responds almost immediately to great supplementation. When excessive bleeding is difficult to bring under control, it is most often because one has not perceived and treated for complicating blood stasis or kidney qi not securing.

Even in the phlegm rheum variety of profuse menstruation, one can usually quickly bring the heavy bleeding under control. This is because the mechanism at work causing the excessive bleeding is none other than spleen qi vacuity. Although phlegm and dampness may be difficult to eliminate, one can usually supplement the qi enough to stop the bleeding. Simple qi vacuity profuse menstruation is mostly due to fatigue and exhaustion. Whereas, phlegm dampness is more due to constitutional spleen/stomach weakness and chronically faulty diet. Because of these differences in etiology, spleen qi vacuity profuse menstraution does not usually recur chronically, but phlegm rheum profuse menstruation does tend to recur.

Nursing

Some women with profuse menstruation may lose so much blood that they become faint or dizzy. In such cases, they should lie down with their feet elevated and rest and relax. They should not attempt to get up and move around or work. If there is great blood loss, women should also be instructed to drink more fluids. If blood loss leads to night or spontaneous sweating, one should replace electrolytes as well. In some few cases, a woman may lose so much blood that she needs to be hospitalized and receive intravenous support. This, however, is not commonly encountered.

Tips on clinical practice

TCM textbooks such as this describe each individual pattern as if each patient belonged to only one or another of these discreet categories. In the case of profuse menstruation, this is usually not the case. In my experience, most women with profuse menstruation suffer from more than a single mechanism and, unless both or even the three or four mechanisms are addressed, treatment will usually not be 100% satisfactory. Therefore, the guiding formulas given above must be modified accordingly.

Since many women with profuse menstruation in their late 30s and 40s have uterine myomas or so-called fibroids, it is important for such women to receive a modern Western medical diagnosis. Chinese medicine can sometimes stop the heavy bleeding associated with myomas and sometimes not depending on the size of the myoma and what tissue it is located within. If a myoma is larger than a robin's egg and excessive bleeding is not brought under control within two or three cycles, the woman should be advised to consider a myomectomy if she is a candidate for one. However, since women with myomas often have small, "seed" fibroids which cannot be seen during surgery, 50% of women treated surgically for myomas do go on to see one or more of these seed myomas develop into a larger myoma. Therefore, even if there is a myoma causing the profuse menstruation and this myoma is surgically removed, the woman should still be advised to continue TCM treatment for the underlying disease mechanisms causing the growth of her fibroids. The TCM diagnosis and treatment of fibroids is discussed as an addendum of flooding and leaking. So-called functional uteirne bleeding due to hormonal imbalance is better and more easily treated with TCM.

Addendum: Prolonged menstruation

Guo Yuan gives, as a subcategory or addendum to profuse menstruation, the category of prolonged menstruation. Guo defines this as a menstrual flow in excess of seven days. Although one does not really need to list this as a separate menstrual disease, I have discussed it below as such in order to make its diagnosis and treatment all the easier for Western practitioners.

Disease causes, disease mechanisms

The *Fu Ren Liang Fang (Fine Formulas for Women)* says:

> A woman's menses does not cease. There is dribbling and dripping and abdominal pain. This is possibly due to taxation damaging the qi and blood and damaging the *chong* and *ren*. Or it is caused by union of yin and yang during the menstrual water. This results in external evils settling inside the uterus. Thus there is stagnation of the sea of blood.

Based on the above cite, prolonged menstruation is believed to be due to three disease mechanisms. First, taxation and fatigue may exhaust the qi's ability to contain the blood within its vessels. Secondly, heat may force the blood to move recklessly outside its pathways. This heat is either vacuity heat due to fatigue, enduring disease, age, excessive sex, drugs, etc., or damp heat. Third, blood stasis due to any of a number of causes, including sexual intercourse during menstruation, may prevent the fresh blood from returning to its channels.

Treatment according to pattern discrimination

Qi vacuity

Main symptoms: Prolonged menstruation, color pale, amount scanty, a yellowish white facial complexion, diminished qi, four limbs sunken, *i.e.*, emaciated, movement leads to shortness of breath and heart palpitations, a pale tongue with thin, white fur, and an empty or fine, weak pulse

Treatment principles: Supplement the qi and nourish the blood, secure the *chong* and *ren*

Guiding formulas:

1. *Gui Pi Tang* (Restore the Spleen Decoction)

Ingredients: Radix Panacis Ginseng (*Ren Shen*), Radix Astragali Membranacei (*Huang Qi*), Radix Angelicae Sinensis (*Dang Gui*), Rhizoma Atractylodis Macrocephalae (*Bai Zhu*), Sclerotium Poriae Cocos (*Fu Ling*), Arillus Euphoriae Longanae (*Long Yan Rou*), Radix Polygalae Tenuifoliae (*Yuan Zhi*), Fructus Zizyphi Jujubae (*Da Zao*), Radix Auklandiae Lappae (*Mu Xiang*), Radix Glycyrrhizae (*Gan Cao*)

Additions: Yang Yi-ya suggests adding Os Sepiae Seu Sepiellae (*Wu Zei Gu*), Concha Ostreae (*Mu Li*), and carbonized Petiolus Et Folium Trachycarpi (*Zong Lu*) to this formula to increase its ability to secure and astringe and thus stop bleeding.

2. *Bu Zhong Yi Qi Tang Jia Wei* (Supplement the Center & Boost the Qi Decoction with Added Flavors)

Ingredients: Radix Astragali Membranacei (*Huang Qi*), Radix Panacis Ginseng (*Ren Shen*), Rhizoma Atractylodis Macrocephalae (*Bai Zhu*), mix-fried Radix Glycyrrhizae (*Gan Cao*), Radix Angelicae Sinensis (*Dang Gui*), Radix Bupleuri (*Chai Hu*), Rhizoma Cimicifugae (*Sheng Ma*), Pericarpium Citri Reticulatae (*Chen Pi*), Radix Rubiae Cordifoliae (*Qian Cao*), Os Sepiae Seu Sepiellae (*Hai Piao Xiao*), Crinis Carbonisatus (*Xue Yu Tan*)

Additions: If qi vacuity is severe, add Radix Dioscoreae Oppositae (*Shan Yao*). If blood vacuity is severe, add Fructus Lycii Chinensis (*Gou Qi Zi*), Arillus Euphoriae Longanae (*Long Yan Rou*), and Gelatinum Corii Asini (*E Jiao*).

3. Unnamed formula from *Zhong Yi Fu Ke Zhi Liao Shou Ce (A Handbook of Chinese Medical Gynecology Treatments)*

Ingredients: Radix Bupleuri (*Chai Hu*), carbonized Folium Artemisiae Argyii (*Ai Ye*), carbonized Radix Schisandrae Chinensis (*Wu Wei Zi Gen*), carbonized Rhizoma Dryopteridis (*Guan Zhong*), carbonized Radix Sanguisorbae (*Di Yu*), mix-fried Radix Astragali Membranacei (*Huang Qi*), Gelatinum Corii Asini (*E Jiao*)

This formula treats qi vacuity with simultaneous blood heat lengthened menstruation whether due to liver depression or damp heat.

4. Unnamed formula from *Zhong Yi Fu Ke Zhi Liao Shou Ce (A Handbook of Chinese Medical Gynecology Treatments)*

Ingredients: Herba Leonouri Heterophylli (*Yi Mu Cao*), Cacumen Biotae Orientalis (*Ce Bai Ye*), Radix Salviae Miltiorrhizae (*Dan Shen*), Crinis Carbonisatus (*Xue Yu Tan*), Rhizoma Atractylodis Macrocephalae (*Bai Zhu*), Radix Dioscoreae Oppositae (*San Yao*)

This formula treats qi vacuity with simultaneous blood stasis lengthened menstruation.

Blood heat

A. Vacuity heat

Main symptoms: Prolonged menstruation, scanty amount, color red, a yellow facial complexion, cheeks red, heat in the five hearts, dry mouth, red lips, a red tongue with scanty fur, and a fine, rapid pulse

Treatment principles: Enrich yin and cool the blood, nourish the blood and regulate the menses

Guiding formulas:

1. *Liang Di Tang* (Two Di's Decoction)

Ingredients: Radix Scrophulariae Ningpoensis (*Yuan Shen*), uncooked Radix Rehmanniae (*Sheng Di Huang*), Tuber Ophiopogonis Japonici (*Mai Dong*), Cortex Radicis Lycii Chinensis (*Di Gu Pi*), Radix Albus Paeoniae Lactiflorae (*Bai Shao*), Gelatinum Corii Asini (*E Jiao*)

2. *Er Huang Xiao Yao San* (Two Yellows Rambling Powder)

Ingredients: Radix Bupleuri (*Chai Hu*), Radix Angelicae Sinensis (*Dang Gui*), Radix Albus Paeoniae Lactiflorae (*Bai Shao*), Rhizoma Atractylodis Macrocephalae (*Bai Zhu*), Sclerotium Poriae Cocos (*Fu Ling*), uncooked Rhizoma Zingiberis (*Sheng Jiang*), Herba Menthae Haplocalycis (*Bo He*), mix-fried Radix Glycyrrhizae (*Gan Cao*), Radix Scutellariae Baicalensis (*Huang Qin*), Cortex Phellodendri (*Huang Bai*)

This formula is for continuous spotting and dribbling with distention and lower abdominal discomfort due to heat drying liver blood and exhausting kidney yin. In this formula, the heat is due to liver depression qi stagnation transforming into heat. Although this formula courses the liver, rectifies the qi, and clears heat, the difference between it and *Dan Zhi Xiao Yao San* (Moutan & Gardenia Rambling Powder) is that Phellodendron specifically clears vacuity heat arising from insufficiency of kidney yin.

3. *Di Shao Liang Xue Tang Jia Wei* (Rehmannia & Peony Cool the Blood Decoction with Added Flavors)

Ingredients: Uncooked Radix Rehmanniae (*Sheng Di*), Radix Albus Paeoniae Lactiflorae (*Bai Shao*), Tuber Ophiopogonis Japonici (*Mai Dong*), Radix Dioscoreae Oppositae (*Shan Yao*), Gelatinum Corii Asini (*E Jiao*), Fructus Ligustri Lucidi (*Nu Zhen Zi*), Herba Ecliptae Prostratae (*Han Lian Cao*)

Additions & subtractions: Yang Shi-xing and Qi Cheng-lin, authors of *Zhong Yi Fu Ke Zhi Liao Shou Ce (A Handbook of Chinese Medical Gynecology Treatments)*, say to add Radix Cynanchi Atrati (*Bai Wei*) instead of the Donkey Skin Glue. If the amount of the menstrual blood is excessive in amount and fresh red in color due to heat harassing the *chong* and *ren* with instability of the sea of blood, then add carbonized Nodus Nelumbinis Nuciferae (*Ou Jie*) and Cortex Radicis Moutan (*Dan Pi*) to cool the blood and secure the *chong*.

4. Unnamed formula from *Zhong Yi Fu Ke Zhi Liao Shou Ce (A Handbook of Chinese Medical Gynecology Treatments)*

Ingredients: Cooked Radix Rehmanniae (*Shu Di*), Cortex Radicis Moutan (*Dan Pi*), Cortex Radicis Lycii Chinensis (*Di Gu Pi*), Herba Artemisiae Apiaceae (*Qing Hao*), Cortex Pehllodendri (*Huang Bai*), Sclerotium Poriae Cocos (*Fu Ling*), Herba Agrimoniae Pilosae (*He Xian Cao*), Crinis Carbonisatus (*Xue Yu Tan*)

5. *Liu Wei Di Huang Wan Jia Jian* (Six Flavors Rehmannia Pills with Additions & Subtractions)

Ingredients: Cooked Radix Rehmnniae (*Shu Di*), Fructus Corni Officinalis (*Shan Zhu*), Radix Dioscoreae Oppositae (*Shan Yao*), Cortex Radicis Moutan (*Dan Pi*), Yunnan Sclerotium Poriae Cocos (*Yun Ling*), Cortex Radicis Lycii Chinensis (*Di Gu Pi*), mix-fried Carapax Amydae Sinensis (*Bie Jia*), Gelatinum Corii Asini (*E Jiao*), Fructus Schisandrae Chinensis (*Wu Wei Zi*)

6. *Gu Jing Wan Jia Jian* (Secure the Essence Pills with Additions & Subtractions)

Ingredients: Radix Albus Paeoniae Lactiflorae (*Bai Shao*), Plastrum Testudinis (*Gui Ban*), Radix Scutellariae Baicalensis (*Huang Qin*), Cortex Ailanthi Altissimi (*Chu Gen Pi*), cooked Radix Rehmanniae (*Shu Di*), Cortex Radicis Lycii Chinensis (*Di Gu Pi*)

This formula is given by Liu Lan-fang and Liu Dian-gong, the authors of *Fu Ke San Bai Zheng (Three Hundred Gynecological Conditions)*, for yin vacuity-vacuity heat profuse menstruation. Because Ailanthus clears heat and eliminates dampness, this formula may be used especially when damp heat complicates vacuity heat.

B. Damp heat

Main symptoms: The menstrual water does not cease but dribbles and drips for days. Its color is purplish black or it may be accompanied by yellow vaginal discharge. There is yellow, slimy tongue fur, and a slippery, rapid pulse.

Treatment principles: Clear heat, secure the menses, and stop bleeding

Guiding formulas:

1. *Jie Du Si Wu Tang* (Resolve Toxins Four Materials Decoction)

Ingredients: Radix Angelicae Sinensis (*Dang Gui*), Radix Ligustici Wallichii (*Chuan Xiong*), Radix Paeoniae Lactiflorae (*Shao Yao*), Radix Rehmanniae (*Di Huang*), Radix Scutellariae Baicalensis (*Huang Qin*), Rhizoma Coptidis Chinensis (*Huang Lian*), Cortex Phellodendri (*Huang Bai*), Fructus Gardeniae Jasminoidis (*Shan Zhi*)

2. Unnamed formula from *Zhong Yi Fu Ke Zhi Liao Shou Ce (A Handbook of Chinese Medical Gynecology Treatments)*

Ingredients: Uncooked Radix Rehmanniae (*Sheng Di*), Radix Angelicae Sinensis (*Dang Gui*), Radix Albus Paeoniae Lactiflorae (*Bai Shao*), Cortex Pehllodendri (*Huang Bai*),

Rhizoma Anemarrhenae Aspheloidis (*Zhi Mu*), Herba Artemisiae Capillaris (*Yin Chen*), Fructus Forsythiae Suspensae (*Lian Qiao*), carbonized Cacumen Biotae Orientalis (*Ce Bai Ye*)

3. *Si Wu Kan Li Wan Jia Wei* (Four Materials Bank the Hole Pills plus Added Flavors)

Ingredients: Uncooked Radix Rehmanniae (*Sheng Di*), Radix Angelicae Sinensis (*Dang Gui*), Radix Albus Paeoniae Lactiflorae (*Bai Shao*), Cortex Phellodendri (*Huang Bai*), Rhizoma Anemarrhenae Aspheloidis (*Zhi Mu*), Fructus Immaturus Sophorae Japonicae (*Huai Zi*), Fructus Forsythiae Suspensae (*Lian Qiao*), Semen Phaseoli Calcarati (*Chi Xiao Dou*), Sclerotium Rubrum Poriae Cocos (*Chi Fu Ling*)

Blood stasis

Main symptoms: Some patients may have blood stasis, stoppage, and stagnation. The blood does not return to the channels and causes the menses to be prolonged. The amount can be more or less and is not fixed. Its color is blackish with clots or lumps. There is lower abdominal pain or discomfort. The tongue has static spots or macules and the pulse is bowstring, fine, and/or choppy.

Treatment principles: Quicken the blood and transform stasis, regulate the *chong* and *ren*

Guiding formulas:

1. *Shi Xiao San Jia Wei* (Loose a Smile Powder with Added Flavors)

Ingredients: Half uncooked and half stir-fried Pollen Typhae (*Pu Huang*), stir-fried Feces Trogopterori Seu Pteromi (*Wu Ling Zhi*), Radix Angelicae Sinensis (*Dang Gui*), Radix Ligustici Wallichii (*Chuan Xiong*), Herba Leonuri Heterophylli (*Yi Mu Cao*), blackened Herba Schizonepetae Tenuifoliae (*Jing Jie Sui*), blackened Rhizoma Zingiberis (*Hei Jiang*), mix-fried Radix Glycyrrhizae (*Gan Cao*)

2. *Zhu Yu Zhi Beng Tang Jia Jian* (Dispel Stasis & Stop Flooding Decoction with Additions & Subtractions)

Ingredients: Resina Myrrhae (*Mo Yao*), Feces Trogopterori Seu Pteromi (*Wu Ling Zhi*), Radix Salviae Miltiorrhizae (*Dan Shen*), Radix Ligustici Wallichii (*Chuan Xiong*), carbonized Cortex Radicis Moutan (*Dan Pi*), Radix Angelicae Sinensis (*Dang Gui*), Pollen Typhae (*Pu Huang*), stir-fried Gelatinum Corii Asini (*E Jiao*), stir-fried Folium Artemisiae Argyii (*Ai Ye*)

3. *Ge Xia Zhu Yu Tang Jia Wei* **(Below the Diaphragm Dispel Stasis Decoction with Added Flavors)**

Ingredients: Radix Angelicae Sinensis (*Dang Gui*), Radix Ligustici Wallichii (*Chuan Xiong*), Radix Rubrus Paeoniae Lactiflorae (*Chi Shao*), Semen Pruni Persicae (*Tao Ren*), Flos Carthami Tinctorii (*Hong Hua*), Fructus Citri Aurantii (*Zhi Ke*), Rhizoma Coydalis Yanhusuo (*Yuan Hu*), Feces Trogopterori Seu Pteromi (*Wu Ling Zhi*), Cortex Radicis Moutan (*Dan Pi*), Radix Linderae Strychnifoliae (*Wu Yao*), processed Rhizoma Cyperi Rotundi (*Xiang Fu*), Radix Glycyrrhizae (*Gan Cao*), Radix Acyranthis Bidentatae (*Niu Xi*), Fructus Foeniculi Vulgaris (*Xiao Hui Xiang*)

4. Unnamed formula from *Zhong Yi Fu Ke Zhi Liao Shou Ce (A Handbook of Chinese Medical Gynecology Treatments)*

Ingredients: Radix Angelicae Sinensis (*Dang Gui*), Radix Ligustici Wallichii (*Chuan Xiong*), cooked Radix Rehmanniae (*Shu Di*), Radix Rubrus Paeoniae Lactiflorae (*Chi Shao*), Radix Linderae Strychnifoliae (*Wu Yao*), Radix Auklandiae Lappae (*Mu Xiang*), scorched Folium Artemisae Argyii (*Ai Ye*), Gelatinum Corii Asini (*E Jiao*), Herba Leonuri Heterophylli (*Yi Mu Cao*)

Key patterns to memorize	
1. Repletion patterns	**A. Replete heat (damp heat)** **B. Depressive heat** **C. Blood stasis**
2. Vacuity patterns	**A. Qi vacuity** **B. Kidney yang vacuity** **C. Kidney yin vacuity - vacuity heat**
3. Mixed repletion & vacuity pattern	**Phelgm rheum or phlegm dampness**

5

Scanty Menstruation

Scanty menstruation is defined as a noticeable reduction in the volume of the menses which otherwise continues to come at regular intervals. It also includes menstruation which only lasts one to two days. As with the foregoing TCM disease categories, most women who come to the clinic will not necessarily mention this as their major complaint. Rather it tends to turn up during the questioning concerning the menstruation. Often scanty menstruation accompanies delayed menstruation, and, when both of these occur together, they may evolve into blocked menstruation.

Typically, most women, as they approach menopause, notice a reduction in the amount of their menstrual discharge. If the woman is in her mid to late 40s, this should not be regarded as abnormal, nor does it require treatment *per se*. If, however, the patient has other perimenopausal complaints, reduction in menstrual volume can help make the pattern discrimination.

Disease causes, disease mechanisms

Scanty menstruation, similar to delayed menstruation discussed above, may be regarded as a species of not bleeding when or, in this case, as fully as a woman should. This means that its disease mechanisms are none other than insufficiency of blood and obstruction of its free and uninhibited flow.

Insufficiency of blood may be due to any of the three viscera responsible for blood engenderment and transformation. However, mostly it is due to dysfunction of the spleen and kidneys. If, due to faulty diet, excessive thinking and worry, or overwork and fatigue, spleen qi becomes too weak to disperse and transform water and grains, the latter heaven root of blood engenderment and transformation may also be too weak to engender and transform the blood. On the other hand, if, due to congenital insufficiency, too early or too frequent childbearing, prolonged exhaustion, drug use, premature aging, and too much sex, kidney yin becomes vacuous and debilitated, the former heaven root of blood engenderment and transformation will likewise be insufficient. In either case, the sea of blood will be relatively vacuous and thus menstruation itself is insufficient.

In terms of obstruction, enduring qi stagnation due to stress and frustration may give rise to blood stasis. Blood stasis may also be due to trauma and iatrogenesis. In addition, phlegm dampness may obstruct the free and uninhibited flow of blood in the lower burner. In this case, there may be a mixed repletion/vacuity condition where phlegm fills up and obstructs the channels but also spleen qi vacuity and dampness results in insufficient latter heaven production of blood. Phlegm dampness is usually due to faulty diet but may be aggravated by lack of exercise. It is also possible for cold damp evils to obstruct the flow of blood and damage the *chong* and *ren*. In this case, blood stasis is due to cold congelation.

In modern society, oral birth control pills are a common iatrogenic cause of scanty menstruation. Oral contraceptives appear to cause or aggravate blood stasis in some women and cause or aggravate kidney vacuity in others. Both these are potential mechanisms leading to scanty menstruation.

Treatment based on pattern discrimination

Blood vacuity

Main symptoms: A scanty, pale red discharge even reduced to drops or menses which only last a day or two, an empty, bearing down sensation in the lower abdomen, dry, moistureless skin, a lusterless facial complexion, dizziness, blurred vision, heart palpitations, tinnitus, lack of warmth in the hands and feet, low back and knee soreness and weakness, a pale tongue with thin, white fur, and a vacuous, fine or fine, weak pulse

This category mainly covers spleen qi vacuity resulting in blood vacuity. However, one should note that there are signs and symptoms above of heart blood vacuity and even incipient kidney vacuity as well. This is because of the interconnection and interdependence of these three viscera which engender and transform the blood.

Treatment principles: Supplement the blood and boost the qi, support the spleen

Guiding formulas:

1. *Ren Shen Zi Xue Tang Jia Wei* (Ginseng Enrich the Blood Decoction with Added Flavors)

Ingredients: Radix Panacis Ginseng (*Ren Shen*) or Radix Codonopsitis Pilosulae (*Dang Shen*), Radix Dioscoreae Oppositae (*Shan Yao*), Sclerotium Poriae Cocos (*Fu Ling*), cooked Radix Rehmanniae (*Shu Di*), Radix Angelicae Sinensis (*Dang Gui*), Radix Ligustici Wallichii (*Chuan Xiong*), Radix Albus Paeoniae Lactiflorae (*Bai Shao*)

Additions & subtractions: Zhao Rei-ling suggests adding Radix Salviae Miltiorrhizae (*Dan Shen*) and Radix Cyathulae Officinalis (*Chuan Niu Xi*) for the treatment of scanty menstruation. Zhao also says that, if there is spotting, delete Ligusticum and add Semen Cuscutae (*Tu Si Zi*) and Fructus Corni Officinalis (*Shan Zhu Yu*).

2. *Si Wu Tang Jia Wei* (Four Materials Decoction with Added Flavors)

Ingredients: Cooked Radix Rehmanniae (*Shu Di*), Radix Angelicae Sinensis (*Dang Gui*), Radix Albus Paeoniae Lactiflorae (*Bai Shao*), Radix Ligustici Wallichii (*Chuan Xiong*), Radix Pseudostellariae (*Tai Zi Shen*), Fructus Lycii Chinensis (*Gou Qi Zi*), Radix Salviae Miltiorrhizae (*Dan Shen*), Gelatinum Corii Asini (*E Jiao*), Rhizoma Atractylodis Macrocephalae (*Bai Zhu*)

In both these formulas there are ingredients which quicken as well as supplement the blood. This is because, if there is insufficiency of blood, blood stasis is then a common complication. If the blood becomes too scanty, the vessels are not filled and, therefore, they fail to promote free and uninhited flow. The Chinese word for stasis is made out of the character for silt surrounded by the disease radical. If there is not enough volume in a stream, its flow will not be vigorous and hence it will precipitate silt.

3. *Shi Quan Da Bu Tang* (Ten [Ingredients] Completely & Greatly Supplementing Decoction)

Ingredients: Radix Astragali Membranacei (*Huang Qi*), Cortex Cinnamomi Cassiae (*Rou Gui*), Radix Panacis Ginseng (*Ren Shen*), cooked Radix Rehmanniae (*Shu Di*), Rhizoma Atractylodis Macrocephalae (*Bai Zhu*), Radix Angelicae Sinensis (*Dang Gui*), Radix Albus Paeoniae Lactiflorae (*Bai Shao*), Radix Ligustici Wallichii (*Chuan Xiong*), Sclerotium Poriae Cocos (*Fu Ling*), mix-fried Radix Glycyrrhizae (*Gan Cao*)

This formula is made up of the ingredients of *Si Jun Zi Tang* (Four Gentlemen Decoction) and *Si Wu Tang* (Four Materials Decoction) plus Astragalus and Cinnamon to more forcefully promote the engenderment and transformation of qi and blood.

Additions: Radix Auklandiae Lappae (*Mu Xiang*) and Rhizoma Corydalis Yanhusuo (*Yan Hu Suo*) can be added to any of the above formulas if there is insidious pain in the lower abdomen.

4. Unnamed formula from *Concise Traditional Chinese Gynecology*

Ingredients: Radix Angelicae Sinensis (*Dang Gui*), Radix Albus Paeoniae Lactiflorae (*Bai Shao*), cooked Radix Rehmanniae (*Shu Di*), Radix Salviae Miltiorrhizae (*Dan Shen*), Herba Lycopi Lucidi (*Ze Lan*)

This formula is for blood vacuity uncomplicated by significant qi vacuity but with an element of blood stasis.

5. *Qi Wu Tang* (Seven Materials Decoction)

Ingredients: Radix Angelicae Sinensis (*Dang Gui*), Radix Ligustici Wallichii (*Chuan Xiong*), Radix Albus Paeoniae Lactiflorae (*Bai Shao*), wine-steamed cooked Radix Rehmanniae (*Shu Di*), Rhizoma Curcumae Zedoariae (*Peng Zhu*), Rhizoma Curcumae Longae (*Chuan Jiang*), Radix Auklandiae Lappae (*Mu Xiang*)

This formula is suggested by Du Jie-hui for the treatment of scanty menstruation due to blood vacuity but obviously complicated by stagnation and stasis. Du gives the therapeutic principles for the use of this formula as nourishing and quickening the blood, rectifying the qi, and freeing the flow of the channels (or menses).

6. *Li Yin Fu Yang Si Wu Tang* (Rectify Yin & Support Yang Four Materials Decoction)

Ingredients: Radix Angelicae Sinensis (*Dang Gui*), Radix Ligustici Wallichii (*Chuan Xiong*), Radix Albus Paeoniae Lactiflorae (*Bai Shao*), cooked Radix Rehmanniae (*Shu Di*), blackened Rhizoma Zingiberis (*Hei Jiang*), Cortex Cinnamomi Cassiae (*Rou Gui*), Fructus Evodiae Rutecarpae (*Zhu Yu*), Fructus Piperis Longi (*Bi Ba*)

Du Jie-hui recommends this formula for the treatment of blood vacuity scanty or late menstruation complicated by cold congelation. This formula nourishes and quickens the blood, warms the channels (or menses), and rectifies the qi.

Kidney vacuity

Main symptoms: Menstruation scanty in amount, color fresh red or pale red, low back and knee soreness and weakness, pain in the heels of the feet, possible dizziness and tinnitus, a pale tongue with scanty fluids, and a deep, fine, forceless pulse

As stated, these signs and symptoms add up to a liver blood-kidney yin vacuity. However, the pattern name is simply kidney vacuity. This is because kidney yin and yang are very closely related and interdependent. As the reader will see, several of the formulas given below supplement both kidney yin and yang.

Treatment principles: Enrich and supplement the liver and kidneys, nourish blood and regulate the menses

Guiding formulas:

1. *Bu Shen Tiao Jing Tang* (Supplement the Kidneys & Regulate the Menses Decoction)

Ingredients: Radix Angelicae Sinensis (*Dang Gui*), Fructus Corni Officinalis (*Shan Zhu Yu*), Radix Dioscoreae Oppositae (*Shan Yao*), Semen Cuscutae (*Tu Si Zi*), Placenta Hominis (*Zi He Che*), Herba Epimedii (*Xian Ling Pi*), Radix Morindae Officinalis (*Ba Ji Rou*), Radix Cyathulae Officinalis (*Chuan Niu Xi*), mix-fried Radix Glycyrrhizae (*Gan Cao*), Caulis Milletiae Seu Spatholobi (*Ji Xue Teng*)

2. *Dang Gui Di Huang Yin* (Dang Gui & Rehmannia Drink)

Ingredients: Radix Angelicae Sinensis (*Dang Gui*), cooked Radix Rehmanniae (*Shu Di*), Fructus Corni Officinalis (*Shan Zhu Yu*), Cortex Eucommiae Ulmoidis (*Du Zhong*), Radix Dioscoreae Oppositae (*Shan Yao*), Radix Cyathulae Officinalis (*Chuan Niu Xi*), mix-fried Radix Glycyrrhizae (*Gan Cao*)

Additions: For fear of cold and cold extremities, add Radix Morindae Officinalis (*Ba Ji Tian*), Fructus Rubi Chingii (*Fu Pen Zi*), Semen Cuscutae (*Tu Si Zi*)

3. Unnamed formula from *Concise Traditional Chinese Gynecology*

Ingredients: Semen Cuscutae (*Tu Si Zi*), cooked Radix Rehmanniae (*Shu Di*), Fructus Lycii Chinensis (*Gou Qi Ji*), Cortex Eucommiae Ulmoidis (*Du Zhong*), Radix Achyranthis Bidentatae (*Huai Niu Xi*)

4. *Yi Shen Yang Xin Tang* (Boost the Kidneys & Nourish the Heart Decoction)

Ingredients: Cooked Radix Rehmanniae (*Shu Di*), Fructus Lycii Chinensis (*Gou Qi Zi*), Semen Cuscutae (*Tu Si Zi*), Herba Cistanchis Deserticolae (*Rou Cong Rong*), Cortex Eucommiae Ulmoidis (*Du Zhong*), Fructus Alpiniae Oxyphyllae (*Yi Zhi Ren*), Semen Zizyphi Spinosae (*Zao Ren*), Semen Biotae Orientalis (*Bai Zi Ren*), Sclerotium Pararadicis Poriae Cocos (*Fu Shen*), Herba Lycopi Lucidi (*Ze Lan*)

This formula boosts the kidneys, nourishes the heart, and both supplements and quickens the blood.

Blood stasis

Main symptoms: Scanty menses colored purple and black with clots, lower abdominal distention and pain resisting pressure, pain relieved after the passage of blood clots, tongue purple and dark or with static spots or macules, and a fine, bowstring, deep, and/or choppy pulse. If blood stasis is due to qi stagnation, there is rib-side distention and pain and the pulse is definitely bowstring.

Treatment principles: Quicken the blood and transform stasis

Guiding formulas:

1. *Tao Hong Si Wu Tang Jia Wei* (Persica & Carthamus Four Materials Decoction with Added Flavors)

Ingredients: Radix Angelicae Sinensis (*Dang Gui*), Radix Albus Paeoniae Lactiflorae (*Bai Shao*), cooked Radix Rehmanniae (*Shu Di*), Radix Ligustici Wallichii (*Chuan Xiong*), Flos Carthami Tinctorii (*Hong Hua*), Semen Pruni Persicae (*Tao Ren*), Rhizoma Cyperi Rotundi (*Xiang Fu*), Rhizoma Curcumae Zedoariae (*E Zhu*), Cortex Cinnamomi Cassiae (*Rou Gui*), Radix Cyathulae Officinalis (*Chuan Niu Xi*)

This formula is for fairly substantial blood stasis complicated by cold and qi stagnation.

2. *Tao Hong Si Wu Tang Jia Jian* (Persica & Carthamus Four Materials Decoction with Additions & Subtractions)

Ingredients: Semen Pruni Persicae (*Tao Ren*), Flos Carthami Tinctorii (*Hong Hua*), Radix Albus Paeoniae Lactiflorae (*Bai Shao*), Radix Angelicae Sinensis (*Dang Gui*), cooked Radix Rehmanniae (*Shu Di*), Rhizoma Cyperi Rotundi (*Xiang Fu*), Radix Linderae Strychnifoliae (*Wu Yao*)

This formula is for blood stasis with obvious qi stagnation.

3. *Tong Yu Jian* (Free the Flow of Stasis Drink)

Ingredients: Rhizoma Alismatis (*Ze Xie*), Radix Auklandiae Lappae (*Mu Xiang*), Fructus Crataegi (*Shan Zha*), Pericarpium Citri Reticulatae Viride (*Qing Pi*), Radix Linderae Strychnifoliae (*Wu Yao*), Flos Carthami Tinctorii (*Hong Hua*), Extremitas Radicis Angelicae Sinensis (*Gui Wei*)

This formula is for blood stasis with more prominent qi stagnation and complicated by food stagnation and dampness.

4. *Xiao Yao San Jia Chuan Xiong Yu Jin* (Rambling Powder plus Ligusticum & Curcuma)

Ingredients: Radix Bupleuri (*Chai Hu*), Radix Angelicae Sinensis (*Dang Gui*), Radix Albus Paeoniae Lactiflorae (*Bai Shao*), Rhizoma Atractylodis Macrocephalae (*Bai Zhu*), Sclerotium Poriae Cocos (*Fu Ling*), Herba Menthae Haplocalycis (*Bo He*), mix-fried Radix Glycyrrhizae (*Gan Cao*), uncooked Rhizoma Zingiberis (*Sheng Jiang*), Radix Ligustici Wallichii (*Chuan Xiong*), Tuber Curcumae (*Yu Jin*)

This formula is for scanty menstruation with purplish clots and rib-side and abdominal pain due to stagnant qi and blood stasis.

Liver depression qi stagnation

Main symptoms: Scanty, possibly delayed menstruation, amount scanty, color dark red, premenstrual breast, rib-side, and/or abdominal distention and pain worse with emotional stress, irritability, a normal, pale, or dark tongue with thin, white fur, and a bowstring or fine and bowstring pulse

Treatment principles: Course the liver and rectify the qi, nourish the blood and regulate the menses

Guiding formula: *Hei Xiao Yao San* (Black Rambling Powder)

Ingredients: Radix Bupleuri (*Chai Hu*), Rhizoma Atractylodis Macrocephalae (*Bai Zhu*), Sclerotium Poriae Cocos (*Fu Ling*), mix-fried Radix Glycyrrhizae (*Gan Cao*), cooked Radix Rehmanniae (*Shu Di*), Radix Angelicae Sinensis (*Dang Gui*), Radix Albus Paeoniae Lactiflorae (*Bai Shao*)

Du Jie-hui suggests unmodified *Xiao Yao San* (Rambling Powder) for the treatment of qi stagnation scanty menstruation. Du is the only major Chinese authority to list this as a mechanism of scanty menstruation. In this case, the liver is depressed and the spleen is vacuous. Because the spleen is vacuous, it fails in its duty to engender and transform the blood. Personally, I do feel that this is a valid category, if a mixed one. Since the qi moves the blood, if the qi is stagnant, the blood flow will tend to be sluggish. If the spleen is vacuous, as is assumed in the use of *Xiao Yao San*, the blood will also tend to be scanty. In this case, there need not be actual blood stasis as well.

Phlegm dampness

Main symptoms: Scanty menstruation, bodily fatigue, lassitude of the spirit, feet and lower limbs sore and weak, chest and epigastric fullness and opression, excessive phlegm turbidity, white, glossy or slimy tongue fur, and a bowstring, slippery or deep, fine pulse. If there is more phlegm obstructing the channels (or menses), the pulse will be slippery and bowstring. But, if there is more dampness encumbering spleen function and the engenderment and transformation of blood, the pulse will be deep and fine.

Treatment principles: Dispel phlegm, transform dampness, and fortify the spleen

Guiding formulas:

1. *Xiong Gui Er Chen Tang* (Ligusticum & Dang Gui Two Aged [Ingredients] Decoction)

Ingredients: Rhizoma Pinelliae Ternatae (*Ban Xia*), Sclerotium Poriae Cocos (*Fu Ling*), Radix Glycyrrhizae (*Gan Cao*), Pericarpium Citri Reticulatae (*Chen Pi*), uncooked Rhizoma Zingiberis (*Sheng Jiang*), Radix Ligustici Wallichii (*Chuan Xiong*), Radix Angelicae Sinensis (*Dang Gui*)

Additions: One may add Rhizoma Atractylodis (*Cang Zhu*) and Cortex Magnoliae Officinalis (*Hou Pu*) to further transform dampness and Radix Auklandiae Lappae (*Mu Xiang*) and Fructus Amomi (*Sha Ren*) to rectify the qi and fortify the spleen.

2. Unnamed formula from *Concise Traditional Chinese Gynecology*

Ingredients: Processed Rhizoma Atractylodis (*Cang Zhu*), processed Rhizoma Cyperi Rotundi (*Zhi Xiang Fu*), stir-fried Fructus Citri Aurantii (*Zhi Ke*), Pericarpium Citri Reticulatae (*Chen Pi*), Radix Salviae Miltiorrhizae (*Dan Shen*)

3. *Kai Yu Er Chen Tang* (Open Depression Two Aged [Ingredients] Decoction)

Ingredients: Exocarpium Citri Rubri (*Ju Pi*), Sclerotium Poriae Cocos (*Fu Ling*), Rhizoma Atractylodis (*Cang Zhu*), Rhizoma Cyperi Rotundi (*Xiang Fu*), Radix Ligustici Wallichii (*Chuan Xiong*), processed Rhizoma Pinelliae Ternatae (*Ban Xia*), Pericarpium Citri Reticulatae Viride (*Qing Pi*), Rhizoma Curcumae Zedoariae (*E Zhu*), Radix Auklandiae Lappae (*Mu Xiang*), Radix Glycyrrhizae (*Gan Cao*), Semen Arecae Catechu (*Bing Lang*), uncooked Rhizoma Zingiberis (*Sheng Jiang*)

Du Jie-hui recommends this formula for the treatment of simultaneous qi stagnation and phlegm obstruction resulting in either scanty menstruation or blocked menstruation. This formula moves the qi and resolves depression, dries dampness and transforms phlegm.

4. *Si Wu Er Chen Tang* (Four Materials Two Aged [Ingredients] Decoction)

Ingredients: Rhizoma Pinelliae Ternatae (*Ban Xia*), Radix Glycyrrhizae (*Gan Cao*), Pericarpium Citri Reticulatae (*Chen Pi*), Sclerotium Poriae Cocos (*Fu Ling*), Radix Angelicae Sinensis (*Dang Gui*), Radix Ligustici Wallichii (*Chuan Xiong*), Radix Albus Paeoniae Lactiflorae (*Bai Shao*), cooked Radix Rehmanniae (*Shu Di*), uncooked Rhizoma Zingiberis (*Sheng Jiang*)

This formula is for the treatment of phlegm obstruction scanty menstruation, delayed menstruation, and blocked menstruation. It dries dampness and transforms phlegm, nourishes the blood and regulates the menses.

5. *Er Chen Jia Xiong Gui Tang* (Two Aged [Ingredients] plus Ligusticum & Dang Gui Decoction)

Ingredients: Pericarpium Citri Reticulatae (*Chen Pi*), Sclerotium Poriae Cocos (*Fu Ling*), Radix Angelicae Sinensis (*Dang Gui*), Radix Ligustici Wallichii (*Chuan Xiong*), stri-fried Rhizoma Cyperi Rotundi (*Chao Xiang Fu*), Fructus Citri Aurantii (*Zhi Ke*), Rhizoma Pinelliae Ternatae (*Ban Xia*), Radix Glycyrrhizae (*Gan Cao*), Talcum (*Hua Shi*), uncooked Rhizoma Zingiberis (*Sheng Jiang*)

Du Jie-hui says this formula eliminates phlegm and percolates dampness, quickens the blood and regulates the menses. It is recommended for phlegm obstruction scanty menstruation, delayed menstruation, and blocked menstruation.

6. *Cang Po Er Chen Tang Jia Wei* (Atractylodes & Magnolia Two Aged [Ingredients] Decoction with Added Flavors)

Ingredients: Rhizoma Atractylodis (*Cang Zhu*), Cortex Magnoliae Officinalis (*Hou Po*), Pericarpium Citri Reticulatae (*Chen Pi*), Rhizoma Pinelliae Ternatae (*Ban Xia*), Sclerotium Poriae Cocos (*Fu Ling*), Radix Glycyrrhizae (*Gan Cao*), Rhizoma Cyperi Rotundi (*Xiang Fu*), Radix Ligustici Wallichii (*Chuan Xiong*), Herba Leonuri Heterophylli (*Kun Cao*)

Within this formula, Atractylodes and Poria fortify the spleen, dry dampness, and transform phlegm. Orange Peel and Magnolia move the qi and transform phlegm. Pinellia transforms phlegm and harmonizes the middle. Cyperus, Ligusticum, and Leonurus move the qi and quicken the blood, regulate and rectify the *chong* and *ren*.

Additions: If there is simultaneous spleen & stomach vacuity weakness with a sallow yellow facial complexion, shortness of breath, spontaneous perspiration, diminished appetite, loose stools, and a bland, tasteless mouth or superficial edema, the main formula should be combined with *Si Jun Zi Tang* (Four Gentlemen Decoction): Radix Panacis

Ginseng (*Ren Shen*), Rhizoma Atractylodis Macrocephalae (*Bai Zhu*), Sclerotium Poriae Cocos (*Fu Ling*), and mix-fried Radix Glycyrrhizae (*Gan Cao*). This is in order to fortify the spleen and boost the qi. If there is simultaneous blood vacuity with dizziness, blurred vision, heart palpitations, racing heart, poor memory, scanty sleep, chapped lips which are a pale white color, and late menstruation with insidious menstrual pain, the main formula should be combined with *Si Wu Tang* (Four Materials Decoction): Radix Angelicae Sinensis (*Dang Gui*), cooked Radix Rehmanniae (*Shu Di*), Radix Albus Paeoniae Lactiflorae (*Bai Shao*), Radix Ligustici Wallichii (*Chuan Xiong*). This is in order to nourish the blood and regulate the menses. If there is simultaneous blood stasis with purple, dark menstrual blood or sticky, thick menses with clots, piercing pain in the lower abdomen which refuses pressure, premenstrual breast distention and pain, a dark, purplish tongue or one with static patches, the main formula should be combined with *Tao Hong Si Wu Tang* (Persica & Carthamus Four Materials Decoction): Radix Angelicae Sinensis (*Dang Gui*), Radix Rubrus Paeoniae Lactiflorae (*Chi Shao*), uncooked Radix Rehmanniae (*Sheng Di*), Radix Ligustici Wallichii (*Chuan Xiong*), Semen Pruni Persicae (*Tao Ren*), Flos Carthami Tinctorii (*Hong Hua*). This is in order to quicken the blood and transform stasis, thus treating phlegm and stasis at the same time.

Blood cold

Main symptoms: The blood does not move easily. The amount of the menses is scanty. There is lower abdominal cold or chilly pain. Warmth makes the menses flow more easily. The tongue is purplish and dark with thin, white fur. The pulse is deep and tight.

If yin cold is excessive and victorious, yin qi will take advantage of yang. The *chong* and *ren* suffer damage and the qi and blood are not transported. The menstrual water becomes congealed and static and the blood does not move easily.

Treatment principles: Warm the channels (or menses) and scatter cold, quicken the blood and regulate the menses

Guiding formula: *Wen Jing Tang* (Warm the Channels [or Menses] Decoction)

Ingredients: Fructus Evodiae Rutecarpae (*Wu Zhu Yu*), Cortex Cinnamomi Cassiae (*Rou Gui*), Radix Angelicae Sinensis (*Dang Gui*), Radix Ligustici Wallichii (*Chuan Xiong*), Radix Albus Paeoniae Lactiflorae (*Bai Shao*), Gelatinum Corii Asini (*E Jiao*), Tuber Ophiopogonis Japonici (*Mai Dong*), Cortex Radicis Moutan (*Dan Pi*), Radix Panacis Ginseng (*Ren Shen*), Rhizoma Pinelliae Ternatae (*Ban Xia*), uncooked Rhizoma Zingiberis (*Sheng Jiang*), Radix Glycyrrhizae (*Gan Cao*)

Discussion

Scanty menstruation is frequently encountered in clinical practice. It, too, typically responds quite well to Chinese medicinal therapy. Because blood vacuity leads to blood stasis and *vice versa*, even if all the signs and symptoms point to blood vacuity, if there are clots in the discharge, one should also include blood-quickening, stasis-transforming medicinals. Thin women or those beyond their mid to late 30s usually suffer from at least some element of yin and/or yang vacuity. Therefore, they usually need kidney supplements.

Prognosis

All varieties of scanty menstruation are usually amenable to treatment and tend to show almost immediate improvement. If a response is not forthcoming, blood stasis may be complicating either blood vacuity or kidney vacuity. In that case, add Flos Carthami Tinctorii (*Hong Hua*) and Herba Leonuri Heterophylli (*Yi Mu Cao*) or Semen Leonuri Heterophylli (*Chong Wei Zi*) to quicken the blood and transform stasis. It is said that these medicinals quicken the blood without damaging it. Other such medicinals are Herba Lycopi Lucidi (*Ze Lan*) and Radix Salviae Miltiorrhizae (*Dan Shen*).

Dietary therapy

Some women in the West have scanty menstruations at least in part because of having adopted vegetarianism. As mentioned above, blood is engendered and transformed out of the *wei* or "flavor" part of foods. This is the heavy, enriching, yin portion of foods. Vegetables and grains are not proportionally high in flavor as opposed to qi. It is animal foods which provide humankind with foods rich in flavor which are also enriching and nourishing to the blood.

If a woman grew up eating meat and then switches to vegetarianism as a young adult, if she lives in a temperate climate, and works as most contemporary women do, she may find that, after several years of vegetarianism, her menses get scanty and/or delayed. In this case, it is very difficult to get a good therapeutic result without adding some red meat to the diet. This does not mean a lot of red meat, but at least two to three ounces several times per week. This can be cooked with black soybeans, dark green leafy, and orange red root vegetables. If the woman cannot stomach the idea of actually eating flesh, then she can make a soup out of marrow bones with the above beans and vegetables or she can use canned beef or chicken stock.

Over the years, I have had this conversation with literally scores of women. Those who have tried adding a little red meat or, at the very least, some meat broths back into their diets have all noticed a definite increase in the amount of their menstrual blood and more energy and warmth in their bodies. If the woman is a vegetarian for religious or ethical reasons, she may have to make a choice between her health and her spiritual or ethical beliefs, which most certainly is each woman's perogative. But a perosn may not be able to have it all.

Key patterns to memorize	
1. Repletion patterns	A. Blood stasis B. Liver depression qi stagnation C. Cold congelation

2. Vacuity patterns	A. Blood vacuity
	B. Kidney vacuity
	    i. Liver-kidney yin vacuity
	    ii. Kidney yin & yang vacuity

3. Mixed repletion/vacuity pattern	Phlegm dampness

Addenda: Menstruation comes, starts & stops

There are two more possible disease categories having to do with irregularities in the flow and its amount. These are menstruation coming but then starting and stopping irregularly and menstruation which is sometimes profuse or excessive and sometimes scanty and has no fixed amount. Most Chinese gynecology texts do not discuss these, but the authors of *Fu Ke San Bai Zheng (Three Hundred Gynecological Conditions)* do.

Disease causes, disease mechanisms: The menses come on time but wind cold invades the blood chamber, taking advantage of vacuity. Thus the blood becomes obstructed and cannot move downward. I would caution the reader, however, that this disease mechanism is not necessarily categorically complete.

Main symptoms: Menses come on time but then they stop, sometimes continue, sometimes cease. They may come thereafter two to three times per month. There is a greenish blue, yellowish facial complexion, occasional pain in the abdomen, alternating fever and chills, a dark tongue or possible static spots or macules, and a bowstring and/or choppy pulse.

Treatment principles: Supplement and warm liver blood, course evils and scatter wind

Guiding formula: *Si Wu Tang He Xiao Chai Hu Tang Jia Jian* (Four Materials Decoction plus Minor Bupleurum Decoction with Additions & Subtractions)

Ingredients: Radix Angelicae Sinensis (*Dang Gui*), Radix Ligustici Wallichii (*Chuan Xiong*), uncooked Radix Rehmanniae (*Sheng Di*), Radix Albus Paeoniae Lactiflorae (*Bai Shao*), Radix Bupleuri (*Chai Hu*), Radix Scutellariae Baicalensis (*Huang Qin*), Rhizoma Pinelliae Ternatae (*Ban Xia*), Radix Codonopsitis Pilosulae (*Dang Shen*), Radix Glycyrrhizae (*Gan Cao*), Cortex Radicis Moutan (*Dan Pi*), Rhizoma Corydalis Yanhusuo (*Xuan Hu Suo*), Rhizoma Atractylodis Macrocephalae (*Bai Zhu*), uncooked Rhizoma Zingiberis (*Sheng Jiang*), Fructus Zizyphi Jujubae (*Da Zao*)

Menstrual water (sometimes) profuse, (sometimes) scanty, no fixed amount

Disease causes, disease mechanisms: This condition is mostly due to spleen qi vacuity weakness and liver qi depression and binding. If enduring depression transforms into fire and heat forces the blood to move frenetically outside its pathways or if the spleen becomes so weak that it cannot contain the blood within its vessels, the amount of the menses is profuse or excessive. However, when there is only qi stagnation without heat not moving the blood or spleen vacuity not engendering and transforming the blood, there is scanty menstruation.

Treatment principles: Course the liver and rectify the qi, clear heat and eliminate vexation

Guiding formula: *Qing Liang San* (Clearing & Cooling Powder)

Ingredients: Fructus Viticis (*Man Jing Zi*), Herba Schizonepetae Tenuifoliae (*Jing Jie*), Folium Bambusae (*Zhu Ye*), Fructus Gardeniae Jasminoidis (*Shan Zhi*), Radix Glycyrrhizae (*Gan Cao*), uncooked Radix Rehmanniae (*Sheng Di*), Radix Albus Paeoniae Lactiflorae (*Bai Shao*), Fructus Amomi (*Sha Ren*), Cortex Radicis Moutan (*Dan Pi*), Radix Scutellariae Baicalensis (*Huang Qin*), uncooked Rhizoma Zingiberis (*Sheng Jiang*)

This formula is a modification of *Dan Zhi Xiao Yao San* (Moutan & Gardenia Rambling Powder). I would probably suggest sticking closer to the standard formula, since the above formula does not really address spleen vacuity. Schizonepeta is a good addition as is Scutellaria if there is more prominent heat. If one uses uncooked Rehmannia, Amomum does then help protect the spleen from being damaged by Rehmannia's enriching, slimy nature.

6

Flooding & Leaking

Beng lou is a compound term. *Beng* means flooding or avalanche. *Lou* means a leak or a trickle. As a compound term, *beng lou* or flooding and leaking refers to functional uterine bleeding in modern Western medicine. The difference between flooding and leaking and profuse menstruation is that flooding and leaking does not occur at regular periodic intervals. Therefore, it can also be referred to as metrorrhagia or bleeding from the uterus at other than the time of the menses. In some cases, this bleeding begins with menstruation but then continues on after the menstruation would have normally been expected to stop. In other cases, it may occur at any time during a woman's cycle. In some instances, some Chinese authors will use the term flooding to mean excessively or greatly profuse menstruation.

Although flooding and leaking describes two distinct types of uterine bleeding, one abrupt and profuse, sometimes referred to as blood flooding, and the other, enduring and scanty, sometimes referred to as downward leaking, these two are interrelated and can transform one into the other. As species of abnormal bleeding, their mechanisms are none other than those previously discussed above under menstruation ahead of schedule and profuse menstruation. Some Chinese gynecology texts discuss either flooding and leaking or profuse menstruation, but not both, since their mechanisms, pattern discrimination, and treatments are essentially the same. As discussed above, I do think there is a logical reason for discussing both these categories in order to better present to Western practitioners the Chinese methodology of disease discrimination so that Western practitioners can better understand how to apply these categories to their patients who mostly present with modern Western disease categories. Therefore, the clinician is strongly advised to refer to the chapter on profuse menstruation for an even wider selection of possible guiding formulas.

Disease causes, disease mechanisms

As with all other species of abnormal menstrual bleeding, the disease mechanisms involved in flooding and leaking are none other than heat, blood stasis, and qi vacuity. Evil heat causing abnormal uterine bleeding may be replete or vacuous, damp or depressive. The various disease causes for these various types of evil heat have been discussed above. No matter what the cause or the type, evil heat makes the blood move frenetically outside its pathways. The numerous causes of blood stasis amongst modern women have also been discussed above. Blood stasis prevents the fresh blood from returning or gathering in its channels. Qi vacuity can be of two types. The first is spleen qi vacuity. Often this spleen vacuity is complicated by accumulation of phlegm rheum in constitutionally obese patients. It may also be due to central qi fall in turn due to loss of blood provoked by some other mechanism. Because the kidneys rule opening and closing and especially the opening and closing of the two lower yin or orifices, because the blood and essence share a common source, and because the kidneys are the former heaven root of spleen qi, enduring bleeding may exhaust and weaken the kidneys, either yin or yang depending upon the mechanisms at work, the patient's age, and their constitution. It is also possible for kidney vacuity due to age, taxation, enduring disease, or congenital insufficiency to lead directly to loss of astringency and securing and, therefore, loss of regulation of the *chong* and *ren*, remembering that the *ren* or conception vessel's qi is primarily kidney qi.

There are three common scenarios which I tend to see in clinical practice. First, liver qi may turn into depressive heat, overeating hot, spicy, oily, greasy foods, or drinking alcohol may cause full heat, or damp heat may either invade the uterus externally or be engendered internally. Any one of these species of evil heat may cause the blood to move frenetically outside its pathways. This then typically results in flooding. Eventually this flooding results in blood vacuity and, because there just is not the same volume of blood available in the sea of blood, flooding turns to leakage.

This leakage may persist for an indefinite period of time as long as the disease mechanism has not been rebalanced. However, because the blood is the mother of qi, after some time, enough blood has been lost that the qi also deserts and fails to contain the blood within its vessels. Leakage then turns to flooding once again. But this time, the flooding is due to spleen vacuity or central qi fall.

Once again, however, the woman only has so much blood and, therefore, this second round of flooding eventually gives way to leakage again. At this point, often replete or depressive heat has transformed into vacuity heat and qi vacuity has weakened the kidneys' ability to secure the essence. If this leakage is not brought under control and its mechanisms remedied, it may alternate back and forth between flooding to leaking to flooding to leaking.

The second common scenario I see involves spleen qi vacuity and phlegm rheum or dampness in obese women. Even if there is the presence of phlegm dampness, typically the initial flooding is due to spleen qi vacuity failing to contain the blood within its vessels. In this cases also, flooding may result in blood vacuity and insufficiency which then leads to the flooding transforming into leakage. This leakage may then, over time, transform back into flooding for the same reasons described above. However, in my experience, flooding due to spleen qi vacuity in obese or overweight patients often does not transform into leakage. Rather, it is either treated and stops completely or the woman is able to recuperate on her own to the point where her qi returns and the flooding stops only later to flood again if she gets exhausted or eats the wrong foods.

The third flooding and leaking scenario I tend to see in my clinical practice is in women who are in their late 30s and 40s who develop spotting and leakage due, in part, to kidney weakness. In this case, leakage tends to be recurrent each month, either at midcycle due to depressive, damp, or vacuity heat, before the actual start of the menses due to qi and yang vacuity, or after the menses have supposedly finished due to yin vacuity and/or blood stasis. It is possible for this leakage to worsen over time and transform into flooding due to central qi fall and then return to leakage again when the sea of blood becomes relatively vacuous, but mostly it continues on as leakage. This does not mean, however, that all women in their late 30s and older will start with leakage. Nonetheless, in women in their 40s, even if they commence with flooding due to flaring of liver fire or depressive liver heat, they tend to move fairly quickly to a situation in which yin vacuity-vacuity heat and kidney qi not securing play their part.

Most often, blood stasis is not the main cause of flooding and leaking. More often, blood stasis complicates other mechanisms resulting in abnormal uterine bleeding. As discussed above, when blood stasis is involved, this stasis must be eliminated before the bleeding will be brought to a complete and satisfactory cessation.

Treatment based on pattern discrimination

Replete blood heat

Main symptoms: The menses are excessive in amount and do not cease or, suddenly, a large volume discharges downward. Their color is deep red. They are thick in consistency, may smell offensively, and may have clots and lumps. There is lower abdominal pain which resists pressure, heart vexation, and profuse dreaming. The four limbs are feverish and there is constipation and reddish urine. The mouth is thirsty, desiring cold drinks. The facial complexion is dark red, the tongue fur is yellow and dry, and the pulse is surging and large or bowstring, rapid, and forceful depending upon the disease mechanism causing the heat.

Treatment principles: Clear heat, cool the blood, and stop flooding

Guiding formulas:

1. *Qing Re Gu Jing Tang* (Clear Heat & Secure the Menses Decoction)

Ingredients: Uncooked Radix Rehmanniae (*Sheng Di*), Cortex Radicis Lycii Chinensis (*Di Gu Pi*), Plastrum Testudinis (*Gui Ban*), Concha Ostreae (*Mu Li*), Gelatinum Corii Asini (*E Jiao*), Fructus Gardeniae Jasminoidis (*Zhi Zi*), stir-fried Radix Sanguisorbae (*Di Yu*), Radix Scutellariae Baicalensis (*Huang Qin*), carbonized Petiolus Et Folium Trachycarpi (*Zong Tan*), Nodus Rhizomatis Nelumbinis Nuciferae (*Ou Jie*), Radix Glycyrrhizae (*Gan Cao*)

Additions: Han Bai-ling suggests adding Cortex Radicis Moutan (*Dan Pi*) and Radix Albus Paeoniae Lactiflorae (*Bai Shao*) to cool the blood and constrain yin. Prof. Song and Yu suggest the same formula by name but instead of Nodus Rhizomatis Nelumbinis and Radix Glycyrrhizae, they include Crinis Carbonisatus (*Xue Yu Tan*) and Radix Panacis Quinque-folii (*Xi Yang Shen*). Then, to these ingredients, they suggest adding Radix Glehniae Littoralis (*Sha Shen*) and Tuber Ophiopogonis Japonici (*Mai Dong*). Zhang En-qin *et al.*, in *Zhong Yi Lin Chuang Ge Ke (Various Clinical Specialties in Chinese Medicine)*, give the following variation: Radix Scutellariae Baicalensis (*Huang Qin*), stri-fried Fructus Gardeniae Jasminoidis (*Zhi Zi*), uncooked Radix Rehmanniae (*Sheng Di*), Cortex Radicis Lycii Chinensis (*Di Gu Pi*), uncooked Radix Sanguisorbae (*Di Yu*), Herba Leonuri Heterophylli (*Yi Mu Cao*), Gelatinum Corii Asini (*E Jiao*), carbonized, aged Folium Et Petiolus Trachycarpi (*Chen Zong Tan*), calcined Concha Ostreae (*Mu Li*).

2. *Gu Jing Wan Jia Jian* (Secure the Menses Pills with Additions & Subtractions)

Ingredients: Stir-fried Cortex Phellodendri (*Huang Bai*), stri-fried Radix Scutellariae Baicalensis (*Huang Qin*), processed Rhizoma Cyperi Rotundi (*Xiang Fu*), stir-fried Radix Sanguisorbae (*Di Yu*), Crinis Carbonisatus (*Xue Yu Tan*), Radix Albus Paeoniae Lactiflorae (*Bai Shao*), Cortex Toonae (*Chun Geng Pi*), carbonized Radix Rubiae Cordifoliae (*Qian Cao*), roasted Radix Cynanchi Atrati (*Bai Wei*)

Additions: For liver channel effulgent fire, add Folium Mori Albi (*Sang Ye*) and Radix Gentianae Scabrae (*Long Dan Cao*) to clear the liver and discharge fire.

3. Unnamed formula from *Concise Traditional Chinese Gynecology*

Ingredients: Mix-fried Plastrum Testudinis (*Gui Ban*), Radix Scutellariae Baicalensis (*Huang Qin*), Cortex Phellodendri (*Huang Bai*), uncooked Radix Rehmanniae (*Sheng Di*), Cortex Toonae Sinensis (*Chun Geng Bai Pi*)

4. *Jie Du Si Wu Tang Jia Wei* (Resolve Toxins Four Materials Decoction with Added Flavors)

Ingredients: Radix Scutellariae Baicalensis (*Huang Qin*), Rhizoma Coptidis Chinensis (*Huang Lian*), Cortex Phellodendri (*Huang Bai*), Fructus Gardeniae Jasminoidis (*Zhi Zi*), Radix Angelicae Sinensis (*Dang Gui*), Radix Albus Paeoniae Lactiflorae (*Bai Shao*), cooked Radix Rehmanniae (*Shu Di*), Radix Ligustici Wallichii (*Chuan Xiong*), Radix Rubiae Cordifoliae (*Qian Cao*)

The first eight ingredients of this formula when used alone comprise *Wen Qing Yin* (Warming & Clearing Drink) which may also be used for excessive menstrual or uterine bleeding due to internal heat. Depending upon whether ones uses uncooked Rehmannia or cooked Rehmannia or white Peony or red Peony, one can make both of these formulas more nourishing and enriching or cooling and quickening.

5. *Qin Lian Si Wu Tang* (Scutellaria & Coptis Four Materials Decoction)

Ingredients: Radix Scutellariae Baicalensis (*Huang Qin*), Rhizoma Coptidis Chinensis (*Huang Lian*), Radix Angelicae Sinensis (*Dang Gui*), Radix Albus Paeoniae Lactiflorae (*Bai Shao*), uncooked Radix Rehmanniae (*Sheng Di*), Radix Ligustici Wallichii (*Chuan Xiong*)

This formula is given by Jane B. Tang in an article titled "Uterine Bleeding - 'Collapse and Dripping'" appearing in *Fu Ke Bing (Gynecological Diseases)*.[22] Dr. Tang notes that Dang Gui is often omitted since it quickens the blood. However, it can be use carbonized. Dr. Tang gives this formula simply for bleeding due to blood heat. The additions she then gives make it clear this formula can be modified to treat replete, vacuous, and depressive heats and complications due to blood stasis and loss of astringency.

Additions & subtractions: For depressive heat, add stir-fried Fructus Gardeniae Jasminoidis (*Zhi Zi*). For complicating blood stasis, add stir-fried Pollen Typhae (*Pu Huang*). For excessive bleeding due to blood heat, add carbonized Cacumen Biotae Orientalis (*Ce Bai Ye*) and carbonized Radix Sanguisorbae (*Di Yu*). For kidney essence or yin vacuity, substitute carbonized uncooked Radix Rehmanniae (*Sheng Di*) for cooked Rehmannia. For loss of astringency and constraint, add carbonized Receptaculum Nelumbinis Nuciferae (*Lian Fang*) and carbonized Nodus Rhizomatis Nelumbinis Nuciferae (*Ou Jie*). For bleeding due to heat arising from the *yang ming*, add carbonized Radix Et Rhizoma Rhei (*Da Huang*) and Rhizoma Imperatae Cylindricae (*Bai Mao Geng*).

---

[22] *Fu Ke Bing*, California Certified Acupuncturists Association, Oakland, CA, 1988, p. 160-172

6. *Hei Pu Huang San Jia Jian* (Blackened Pollen Typhae Powder with Additions & Subtractions)

Ingredients: Blackened, stir-fried Pollen Typhae (*Pu Huang*), stir-fried Gelatinum Corii Asini (*E Jiao*), Radix Ligustici Wallichii (*Chuan Xiong*), stir-fried Radix Albus Paeoniae Lactiflorae (*Bai Shao*), stir-fried uncooked Radix Rehmanniae (*Sheng Di*), Cortex Radicis Moutan (*Dan Pi*), blackened, stir-fried Herba Schizonepetae Tenuifoliae (*Jing Sui*), blackened, stir-fried Radix Sanguisorbae (*Di Yu*), carbonized Folium Et Petriolus Trachycarpi (*Zong Tan*), Crinis Carbonisatus (*Xue Yu Tan*)

Damp heat

Main symptoms: This category is subdivided depending upon whether dampness predominates or heat predominates. If dampness predominates, there will be bloody discharge with pasty fluids or watery, thick discharge. The facial complexion is sallow yellow or there is facial edema. There is heaviness and dizziness of the head, and the essence spirit is listless and fatigued. The chest is oppressed and there may be abdominal lumps. There is a sticky, slimy sensation inside the mouth and the tongue fur is thin, white, and slimy. The pulse is relaxed (retarded) and slippery.

If heat predominates, the bloody discharge is excessive in amount. The blood is colored purple, has an offensive odor, and is sticky or pasty in consistency. The facial complexion is red or the body is hot and there is spontaneous perspiration. The mouth has a bitter taste and is dry. Urination is short and red. Defecation is difficult and bound or there is diarrhea which is not smoothly flowing. The tongue is red with slimy, yellow fur and the pulse is slippery and rapid.

Treatment principles: If heat predominates, the principle is mainly to clear heat assisted by eliminating dampness. If dampness predominates, the principle is mainly to eliminate dampness assisted by clearing heat.

Guiding formulas:

1. *Jia Wei Dan Zhi Xiao Yao San* (Moutan & Gardenia Rambling Powder)

Ingredients: Cortex Radicis Moutan (*Dan Pi*), scorched Fructus Gardeniae Jasminoidis (*Zhi Zi*), Radix Bupleuri (*Chai Hu*), Herba Menthae Haplocalycis (*Bo He*), Fructus Meliae Toosendan (*Chuan Lian*), Radix Scutellariae Baicalensis (*Huang Qin*), Rhizoma Atractylodis Macrocephalae (*Bai Zhu*), Radix Albus Paeoniae Lactiflorae (*Bai Shao*), Semen Biotae Orientalis (*Bai Zi Ren*), Radix Angelicae Sinensis (*Dang Gui*), Gelatinum Corii Asini (*E Jiao*), carbonized Radix Sanguisorbae (*Di Yu Tan*), and a small amount of vinegar

This formula is given by Song and Yu for predominant heat in damp heat flooding and leaking. This formula can also be used as the guiding formula with modification if flooding and leaking are due to depressive heat.

2. *Sheng Yang Chu Shi Tang Jia Wei* (Upbear Yang & Eliminate Dampness Decoction with Added Flavors)

Ingredients: Radix Et Rhizoma Notopterygii (*Qiang Huo*), Radix Bupleuri (*Chai Hu*), Rhizoma Atractylodis (*Cang Zhu*), Radix Ledebouriellae Divaricatae (*Fang Feng*), mix-fried Radix Glycyrrhizae (*Gan Cao*), Rhizoma Cimicifugae (*Sheng Ma*), Sclerotium Polypori Umbellati (*Zhu Ling*), Rhizoma Alismatis (*Ze Xie*), Fructus Alpiniae Oxyphyllae (*Yi Zhi Ren*), Rhizoma Pinelliae Ternatae (*Ban Xia*), Massa Medica Fermentata (*Shen Qu*), Fructus Germinatus Hordei Vulgaris (*Mai Ya*), Pericarpium Citri Reticulatae (*Chen Pi*), Radix Scutellariae Baicalensis (*Huang Qin*), carbonized Radix Sanguisorbae (*Di Yu Tan*)

This formula is given by Song and Yu for predominant dampness in damp heat flooding and leaking. It is one of Li Dong-yuan's formulas. It eliminates dampness by upbearing yang and disinhibiting the qi mechanism. If clear yang is upborne, then turbid yin can be downborne. In addition, it not only uses bitter, cold to clear heat but uses exterior-resolving, yang-upbearing medicinals to out-thrust heat.

Vacuity blood heat

Main symptoms: Menstruation dribbles on but does not cease. The amount of blood is scanty and its color is pale red. The abdomen is not distended or painful. There is dizziness and heart palpitations, impaired memory, blurred vision, dry, scaly skin, and heat in the center of the hands, feet, and heart. The facial complexion is a vacuous red (meaning that the face is pale with a slight red flush). The tongue is dry, red, and without fur. The pulse is vacuous, fine, and a little rapid.

Treatment principles: Nourish yin, cool the blood, and stop bleeding

Guiding formulas:

1. *Di Gu Pi Yin* (Cortex Lycii Drink)

Ingredients: Cortex Radicis Lycii Chinensis (*Di Gu Pi*), Radix Bupleuri (*Chai Hu*), Rhizoma Anemarrhenae Aspheloidis (*Zhi Mu*), mix-fried Radix Glycyrrhizae (*Gan Cao*), Carapax Amydae Sinensis (*Bie Jia*), Radix Scutellariae Baicalensis (*Huang Qin*), Radix Panacis Ginseng (*Ren Shen*), Sclerotium Rubrum Poriae Cocos (*Chi Fu Ling*), uncooked Rhizoma Zingiberis (*Sheng Jiang*), Fructus Pruni Mume (*Wu Mei*)

Additions: To the above standard ingredients, Han Bai-ling says to add stir-fried Radix Sanguisorbae (*Di Yu*), carbonized Folium Et Petriolus Trachycarpi (*Zong Tan*), Gelatinum Corii Asini (*E Jiao*), Plastrum Testudinis (*Gui Ban*), Radix Dipsaci (*Chuan Duan*), and Ramulus Loranthi Seu Visci (*Ji Sheng*) to enrich yin and stop bleeding.

2. *Qing Re Gu Jing Tang* (Clear Heat & Secure the Menses Decoction)

Ingredients: Uncooked Radix Rehmanniae (*Sheng Di*), Radix Scutellariae Baicalensis (*Huang Qin*), Fructus Gardeniae Jasminoidis (*Zhi Zi*), Radix Cortex Lycii Chinensis (*Di Gu Pi*), Nodus Rhizomatis Nelumbinis Nuciferae (*Ou Jie*), uncooked Radix Sanguisorbae (*Di Yu*), Gelatinum Corii Asini (*E Jiao*), Plastrum Testudinis (*Gui Ban*), uncooked Conchae Ostreae (*Mu Li*), carbonized Folium Et Petriolus Trachycarpi (*Zong Tan*), Radix Glycyrrhizae (*Gan Cao*)

3. *Bao Yin Jian Jia Jian* (Protect Yin Decoction with Additions & Subtractions)

Ingredients: Uncooked Radix Rehmanniae (*Sheng Di*), Radix Scutellariae Baicalensis (*Huang Qin*), Cortex Phellodendri (*Huang Bai*), Gelatinum Corii Asini (*E Jiao*), Fructus Ligustri Lucidi (*Nu Zhen Zi*), Herba Ecliptae Prostratae (*Han Lian Cao*), Herba Leonuri Heterophylli (*Yi Mu Cao*), Radix Albus Paeoniae Lactiflorae (*Bai Shao*), Radix Dioscoreae Oppositae (*Shan Yao*)

4. *Xue Beng Xiao Fang* (Blood Flooding Effective Formula)

Ingredients: Cooked Radix Coquitus Rehmanniae (*Shu Di*), Radix Angelicae Sinensis (*Dang Gui*), Radix Albus Paeoniae Lactiflorae (*Bai Shao*), clam shell stri-fried Gelatinum Corii Asini (*E Jiao*), Herba Schizonepetae Tenuifoliae (*Jing Jie Sui*), Radix Sanguisorbae (*Di Yu*), Radix Ligustici Wallichii (*Chuan Xiong*)

Du Jie-hui recommends this formula for the treatment of yin vacuity blood heat flooding and leaking. It enriches yin and nourishes the blood, stops bleeding and regulates the menses.

5. *Jia Wei Gu Yin Jian* (Added Flavors Secure Yin Decoction)

Ingredients: Uncooked Radix Rehmanniae (*Sheng Di*), Radix Albus Paeoniae Lactiflorae (*Bai Shao*), Gelatinum Corii Asini (*E Jiao*), uncooked Os Draconis (*Long Gu*), uncooked Concha Ostreae (*Mu Li*), Sclerotium Pararadicis Poriae Cocos (*Fu Shen*), Radix Dioscoreae Oppositae (*Shan Yao*), Calcium Uratum (*Qiu Shi*), Rhizoma Anemarrhenae Aspheloidis (*Zhi Mu*), Cortex Phellodendri (*Huang Bai*)

This formula enriches yin, clears heat, and secures flooding. It is indicated for the treatment of flooding and leaking due to yin vacuity blood heat. The previous formula nourishes yin blood more, while this formula supplements the kidneys, enriches yin, and secures and constrains more.

6. Unnamed formula from *Nu Ke Jing Wei (Profundities from the Gynecological Classics)*

Ingredients: Uncooked Radix Rehmanniae (*Sheng Di*), earth stir-fried Rhizoma Atractylodis Macrocephalae (*Bai Zhu*), uncooked Radix Astragali Membranacei (*Huang Qi*), whole Radix Angelicae Sinensis (*Quan Dang Gui*), Fructus Corni Officinalis (*Shan Zhu Yu*), calcined Os Draconis (*Long Gu*), calcined Concha Ostreae (*Mu Li*), uncooked Radix Albus Paeoniae Lactiflorae (*Bai Shao*), stir-fried Radix Rubiae Cordifoliae (*Qian Cao*), Os Sepiae Seu Sepiellae (*Wu Zei Gu*), carbonized Petiolus Trachycarpi (*Zong Lu*), Herba Agrimoniae Pilosae (*He Xian Cao*), true Gelatinum Corii Asini (*E Jiao*), uncooked Radix Glycyrrhizae (*Gan Cao*)

This formula is for yin vacuity-vacuity heat combined with qi vacuity. Therefore, there is leaking alternating with blood flooding during which the blood is thin and watery.

Additions & subtractions: If, after administering the above formula, the flooding and leaking disappear, subtract the blood-cooling, heat-clearing, stop bleeding medicinals — Agrimonia, Rubia, Trachycarpus, and Sepia. Instead of calcined Dragon Bone and Oyster Shell, use uncooked Dragon Bone and Oyster Shell in order to reduce their astringing, constraining effect and to strengthen their enriching yin. Replace uncooked Rehmannia with cooked Radix Rehmanniae (*Shu Di*) to also strengthen the enrichment of yin and nourishment of blood, thus preventing the engenderment of blood heat. Add Radix Dioscoreae Oppositae (*Huai Shan Yao*), scorched Cortex Eucommiae Ulmoidis (*Du Zhong*), and Ramulus Loranthi Seu Visci (*Sang Ji Sheng*) to supplement the spleen and kidneys and secure the *chong* and *ren*. Add processed Rhizoma Cyperi Rotundi (*Xiang Fu*) to regulate and rectify the qi and blood. If there is heat, it is ok to clear heat using Cortex Radicis Lycii Chinensis (*Di Gu Pi*). Administer this formula until the qi becomes normally flowing and the blood is quickened and there will be a cure.

Qi stagnation depressive heat

Main symptoms: The menses dribble on and do not cease. Sometimes the amount is more and sometimes less. The blood is clotty and lumpy and colored purple and dark or dull. There is lower abdominal distention and pain which refuses pressure, rib-side distention, a tendency to sighing, dizziness, excessive anger, and a dark, dusky facial complexion. The tongue is dark with white or yellowish fur and the pulse is bowstring, rapid, and forceful.

Treatment principles: Course the liver and rectify the qi, clear heat and stop flooding

Guiding formulas:

1. *Xiao Yao San* (Rambling Powder)

Ingredients: Radix Bupleuri (*Chai Hu*), Radix Angelicae Sinensis (*Dang Gui*), Radix Albus Paeoniae Lactiflorae (*Bai Shao*), Rhizoma Atractylodis Macrocephalae (*Bai Zhu*), Sclerotium Poriae Cocos (*Fu Ling*), Herba Menthae Haplocalycis (*Bo He*), mix-fried Radix Glycyrrhizae (*Gan Cao*), uncooked Rhizoma Zingiberis (*Sheng Jiang*)

Although Han Bai-ling gives qi stagnation as a cause of flooding and leaking, by itself, simple qi stagnation does not cause uterine bleeding. It is only when qi stagnation transforms into heat that heat forces the blood to move frenetically outside its pathways. The above formula is for simple liver depression qi stagnation with an element of spleen and blood vacuity. Usually, one thinks of *Dan Zhi Xiao Yao Wan* (Moutan & Gardenia Rambling Powder) as the standard guiding formula for depressive heat flooding and leaking. That formula has been discussed above under damp heat flooding and leaking and is discussed again in terms of depressive heat below. Also below are Han Bai-ling's modifications for qi stagnation depressive heat flooding and leaking to be added to the above standard guiding formula. Although Han Bai-ling says to add Radix Scutellariae Baicalensis (*Huang Qin*) and uncooked Radix Rehmanniae (*Sheng Di*) to the above formula only if heat is prominent, there must be heat before simple qi stagnation results in profuse menstruation or flooding and leaking.

Additions: If the amount of blood is excessive, add stir-fried Radix Sanguisorbae (*Di Yu*) and carbonized Petiolus Et Folium Trachycarpi (*Zong Tan*). If heat is prominent, add Radix Scutellariae Baicalensis (*Huang Qin*) and uncooked Radix Rehmanniae (*Sheng Di*) to clear heat and cool the blood. If lower abdominal distention is prominent, add Fructus Meliae Toosendan (*Chuan Lian Zi*), Fructus Immaturus Citri Aurantii (*Zhi Shi*), and Radix Linderae Strychnifoliae (*Wu Yao*) to rectify the qi and disperse distention. If there is piercing pain in the lower abdomen, add Radix Ligustici Wallichii (*Chuan Xiong*) and Radix Salviae Miltiorrhizae (*Dan Shen*) to quicken the blood and transform stasis.

2. *Dan Zhi Xiao Yao San Jia Jian* (Moutan & Gardenia Rambling Powder with Additions & Subtractions)

Ingredients: Radix Bupleuri (*Chai Hu*), Radix Albus Paeoniae Lactiflorae (*Bai Shao*), Cortex Radicis Moutan (*Dan Pi*), Fructus Gardeniae Jasminoidis (*Zhi Zi*), Rhizoma Atractylodis Macrocephalae (*Bai Zhu*), Sclerotium Poriae Cocos (*Fu Ling*), mix-fried Radix Glycyrrhizae (*Gan Cao*), Herba Menthae Haplocalycis (*Bo He*), uncooked Rhizoma Zingiberis (*Sheng Jiang*)

Additions: If rib-side or abdominal distention and pain are prominent, add carbonized Rhizoma Cyperi Rotundi (*Xiang Fu*), carbonized Fructus Meliae Toosendan (*Chuan Lian Zi*), and/or Tuber Curcumae (*Yu Jin*) to move the qi and stop pain. If bleeding is excessive, add Herba Agrimoniae Pilosae (*Xian He Cao*) and carbonized Radix Sanguisorbae (*Di Yu*) to stop bleeding. If bleeding has caused blood and yin vacuity, add carbnoized uncooked Radix Rehmanniae (*Sheng Di*).

3. *Fu Pi Shu Gan Tang* (Support the Spleen & Course the Liver Decoction)

Ingredients: Radix Bupleuri (*Chai Hu*), Radix Albus Paeoniae Lactiflorae (*Bai Shao*), Radix Adenophorae Strictae (*Nan Sha Shen*), stir-fried Pollen Typhae (*Pu Huang*), Crinis Carbonsatus (*Xue Yu Tan*), carbonized Folium Artemisiae Argyii (*Ai Ye*), Rhizoma Atractylodis Macrocephalae (*Bai Zhu*), Sclerotium Poriae Cocos (*Fu Ling*), Herba Menthae Haplocalycis (*Bo He*), uncooked Rhizoma Zingiberis (*Sheng Jiang*)

This formula is for flooding and leaking due to anger damaging the liver, a purple colored discharge with clots, lower abdominal distention, chest and epigastric fullness and oppression, shortness of breath, lassitude of the spirit, decreased appetite, and indigestion. This formula is a modification of *Xiao Yao San* (Rambling Powder) and the signs and symptoms suggest liver depression qi stagnation with qi vacuity. Personally, if there were shortness of breath and fatigue, I would probably add Radix Astragali Membranacei (*Huang Qi*) and Radix Panacis Ginseng (*Ren Shen*) or Radix Codonopsitis Pilosulae (*Dang Shen*) to fortify the spleen and boost the qi more.

4. Unnamed formula from *Nu Ke Jing Wei (Profundities from the Gynecological Classics)*

Ingredients: Fine uncooked Radix Rehmanniae (*Sheng Di*), stir-fried Radix Albus Paeoniae Lactiflorae (*Bai Shao*), whole Radix Angelicae Sinensis (*Quan Dang Gui*), old Radix Ligustici Wallichii (*Chuan Xiong*), scorched Fructus Gardeniae Jasminoidis (*Shan Zhi*), Cortex Radicis Moutan (*Dan Pi*), carbonized Cacumen Biotae Orientalis (*Ce Bai*), carbonized Petiolus Et Folium Trachycarpi (*Zong Lu*), carbonized Herba Schizonepetae Tenuifoliae (*Jie Sui*), Herba Agrimoniae Pilosae (*He Xian Cao*), Rhizoma Corydalis Yanhusuo (*Yan Hu Suo*), Fructus Meliae Toosendan (*Chuan Lian Rou*), uncooked Radix Glycyrrhizae (*Gan Cao*)

This formula is given by Lu Guo-zhi and Song Shu-de for qi stagnation blood stasis flooding and leaking. However, based on its ingredients there is also depressive heat.

Additions: If the discharged blood's amount is excessive and qi follows blood's perishing with spirit clouding and heart palpitations, then, in emergency, use Radix Panacis Quinqefolii (*Xi Yang Shen*), 4g. Decoct and administer in order to rescue yin and return yang, quiet the spirit and tranquilize the orientation. If afterwards there is severe lumbar pain with dizziness and vertigo, add true Gelatinum Corii Asini (*E Jiao*) and Fructus Corni Officinalis (*Shan Zhu Yu*). If there is constipation, add Radix Et Rhizoma Rhei (*Da Yun Pian*).

Blood stasis

Main symptoms: The menses are dribbling and astringent but do not stop or, after they stop, they suddenly discharge profusely with bloody clumps and lumps. The color of the blood is purple and dull or dark. There is piercing pain in the lower abdomen which refuses pressure, dizziness, heart vexation, profuse dreaming, a distended feeling in the four extremities, a deep red facial complexion, a red tongue and static macules on the sides of the tongue, and a bowstring, choppy, forceful pulse.

Treatment principles: Quicken the blood, move stasis, and stop flooding

Guiding formulas:

1. *Tao Hong Si Wu Tang* (Persica & Carthamus Four Materials Decoction)

Ingredients: Radix Angelicae Sinensis (*Dang Gui*), Radix Ligustici Wallichii (*Chuan Xiong*), uncooked Radix Rehmanniae (*Sheng Di*), Radix Rubrus Paeoniae Lactiflorae (*Chi Shao*), Semen Pruni Persicae (*Tao Ren*), Flos Carthami Tinctorii (*Hong Hua*)

Additions: To the above, Han Bai-ling says to add Radix Achyranthis Bidentatae (*Niu Xi*) and Radix Salviae Miltiorrhizae (*Dan Shen*). If the bleeding is profuse, add carbonized Pollen Typhae (*Pu Huang*), stir-fried Radix Sanguisorbae (*Di Yu*), and Radix Pseudoginseng (*San Qi*). If there is also heat, add Radix Scutellariae Baicalensis (*Huang Qin*). If there is constipation, add a small amount of Radix Et Rhizoma Rhei (*Da Huang*). Zhang En-qin *et al.* suggest adding stir-fried Pollen Typhae (*Pu Huang*), stir-fried Feces Trogopterori Seu Pteromi (*Ling Zhi*), Radix Rubiae Cordifoliae (*Qian Cao*), carbonized Herba Cephalano-ploris Segeti (*Xiao Ji*), and Radix Pseudoginseng (*San Qi*). Then, to these, if there is more prominent abdominal distention, add Fructus Meliae Toosendan (*Chuan Lian Zi*) and Rhizoma Cyperi Rotundi (*Xiang Fu*). If there is a dry, bitter mouth and excessive, red blood, add Herba Agrimoniae Pilosae (*Xian He Cao*), Radix Sanguisorbae (*Di Yu*), and Radix Rubiae Cordifoliae (*Qian Cao Geng*).

2. *Si Wu Tang He Shi Xiao San Jia Wei* **from** *Bai Ling Fu Ke (Bai-ling's Gynecology)* **(Four Materials Decoction plus Loose a Smile Powder with Added Flavors)**

Ingredients: Radix Angelicae Sinensis (*Dang Gui*), uncooked Radix Rehmanniae (*Sheng Di*), Radix Rubrus Paeoniae Lactiflorae (*Chi Shao*), Radix Ligustici Wallichii (*Chuan Xiong*), Pollen Typhae (*Pu Huang*), Feces Trogopterori Seu Pteromi (*Wu Ling Zhi*), Radix Pseudoginseng (*San Qi*), carbonized Radix Rubiae Cordifoliae (*Qian Cao Tan*), Gelatinum Corii Asini (*E Jiao*)

3. *Si Wu Tang He Shi Xiao San Jia Wei* **from** *Zhong Yi Fu Ke (Chinese Medical Gynecology)* **(Four Materials Decoction plus Loose a Smile Powder with Added Flavors)**

Ingredients: Pollen Typhae (*Pu Huang*), Feces Trogopterori Seu Pteromi (*Wu Ling Zhi*), processed Rhizoma Cyperi Rotundi (*Xiang Fu*), processed Resina Olibani (*Ru Xiang*), stir-fried Radix Albus & Rubrus Paeoniae Lactiflorae (*Chi Bai Shao*), large uncooked Radix Rehmanniae (*Sheng Di*), Radix Ligustici Wallichii (*Chuan Xiong*), Radix Pseudoginseng (*San Qi*), Cortex Radicis Moutan (*Dan Pi*), stir-fried Radix Scutellariae Baicalensis (*Dan Qin*), carbonized Radix Angelicae Sinensis (*Dang Gui*)

Additions: If blood stasis flooding and leaking is due to endometrial inflammation or tumor, Zhu Cheng-han says it is ok to add heat-clearing, toxin-resolving medicinals to the above guiding formula.

4. *Si Wu Tang He Shi Xiao San Jia Wei* **according to Jane B. Tang**

Ingredients: Radix Angelicae Sinensis (*Dang Gui*), uncooked Radix Rehmanniae (*Sheng Di*), Radix Rubrus Paeoniae Lactiflorae (*Chi Shao*), Radix Ligustici Wallichii (*Chuan Xiong*), Pollen Typhae (*Pu Huang*), Feces Trogopterori Seu Pteromi (*Wu Ling Zhi*), carbonized Radix Rubiae Cordifoliae (*Qian Cao Geng*), Semen Pruni Persicae (*Tao Ren*), Flos Carthami Tinctorii (*Hong Hua*)

Additions: If there is heavy bleeding, add Radix Pseudoginseng (*San Qi*).

5. Unnamed formula from *Concise Traditional Chinese Gynecology*

Ingredients: Stir-fried, blackened Radix Angelicae Sinensis (*Dang Gui*), Radix Rubrus Paeoniae Lactiflorae (*Chi Shao*), Feces Trogopterori Seu Pteromi (*Wu Ling Zhi*), Pollen Typhae (*Pu Huang*), Herba Leonuri Heterophylli (*Yi Mu Cao*)

6. *Chu Yu Zhi Xue Fang* (Eliminate Stasis & Stop Bleeding Formula)

Ingredients: Radix Angelicae Sinensis (*Dang Gui*), Radix Rubrus Paeoniae Lactiflorae (*Chi Shao*), Herba Artemisiae Anomalae (*Liu Ji Nu*), Rhizoma Cyperi Rotundi (*Xiang Fu*), Sanguis Draconis (*Xue Jie*), uncooked Pollen Typhae (*Pu Huang*), Feces Trogopterori Seu Pteromi (*Wu Ling Zhi*), Radix Rubiae Cordifoliae (*Qian Cao*), Herba Leonuri Heterophylli (*Yi Mu Cao*), Radix Pseudoginseng (*San Qi*)

Additions: If excessive blood loss has led to qi and blood vacuity, add Radix Codonopsitis Pilosulae (*Dang Shen*), Radix Astragali Membranacei (*Huang Qi*), and Rhizoma Cimicifugae (*Sheng Ma*) to supplement the qi, upbear, and lift in order to prevent qi fall and blood desertion.

7. *Zhu Yu Zhi Xue Tang* (Dispel Stasis & Stop Bleeding Decoction)

Ingredients: Wine stir-fried uncooked Radix Rehmanniae (*Sheng Di*), Radix Et Rhizoma Rhei (*Da Huang*), Radix Rubrus Paeoniae Lactiflorae (*Chi Shao*), stir-fried Fructus Citri Aurantii (*Zhi Ke*), vinegar mix-fried Plastrum Testudinis (*Gui Ban*), Cortex Radicis Moutan (*Dan Pi*), Extremitas Radicis Angelicae Sinensis (*Dang Gui Wei*), stir-fried Semen Pruni Persicae (*Tao Ren*)

Fu Qing-zhu gives this formula in *Nu Ke Xian Fang (Immortal Formulas in Gynecology)* for the treatment of blood flooding due to injury and fall or, in other words, due to traumatic injury affecting the pelvis and uterus. In this case, blood stasis is created which results in blood flooding. Fu Qing-zhu says that after one *ji* or prescription, *i.e.*, one *bao* or packet, the aching should be less. After two packets, the aching should have stopped. And after three packets, the bleeding should also have completely stopped.

8. *Ping Gan Kai Yu Zhi Beng Tang* (Level the Liver, Open Depression & Stop Bleeding Decoction)

Ingredients: Vinegar stir-fried Radix Albus Paeoniae Lactiflorae (*Bai Shao*), earth stir-fried Rhizoma Atractylodis Macrocephalae (*Bai Zhu*), Cortex Radicis Moutan (*Dan Pi*), Radix Angelicae Sinensis (*Dang Gui*), Guangdong Radix Pseudoginseng (*Guang San Qi*), Radix Glycyrrhizae (*Gan Cao*), wine stir-fried uncooked Radix Rehmanniae (*Sheng Di*), blackened Herba Schizonepetae Tenuifoliae (*Jie Sui*), Radix Bupleuri (*Chai Hu*)

This formula is from Fu Qing-zhu's *Nu Ke Xian Fang (Immortal Formulas in Gynecology)* under the heading depression and binding blood flooding. Fu Qing-zhu's editor says that if carbonized Rhizoma Dryopteridis (*Guan Chong*) is added, the effect will be even better. Du Jie-hui says this formula is for the treatment of liver depression and blood stasis flooding and leaking. It courses the liver and resolves depression, quickens the blood and stops bleeding.

9. *Jiao Hong Yin* ([Donkey Skin] Glue & Carthamus Drink)

Ingredients: Gelatinum Corii Asini (*E Jiao*), whole Radix Angelicae Sinensis (*Quan Dang Gui*), Flos Carthami Tinctorii (*Hong Hua*), Semen Benincasae Hispidae (*Dong Gua Zi*)

Du Jie-hui recommends this formula for the treatment of blood stasis flooding and leaking. It nourishes the blood and frees the flow of the vessels, dispels stasis and stops bleeding. In this case, blood stasis gathering and stagnating make it so the blood cannot return or gather in the channels. Thus there is flooding and leaking which will not recover or leakage which changes into flooding. This formula is especially useful for the treatment of uterine bleeding in older women. In perimenopausal women, the menses may not come for some time. But then, when it does, it may only dribble and drip without stopping, or sometimes it may be profuse and sometimes scanty. If one has used securing and constraining but without cure, use this formula, increasing the amount of Carthamus up to 24 grams.

10. *Zhu Yu Zhi Beng Tang* (Dispel Stasis & Stop Flooding Decoction)

Ingredients: Radix Angelicae Sinensis (*Dang Gui*), Feces Trogopterori Seu Pteromi (*Wu Ling Zhi*), stir-fried Cortex Radicis Moutan (*Dan Pi*), stir-fried Radix Salviae Miltiorrhizae (*Dan Shen*), Pollen Typhae (*Pu Huang*), stir-fried Gelatinum Corii Asini (*E Jiao*), Radix Ligustici Wallichii (*Chuan Xiong*), carbonized Folium Artemisiae Argyii (*Ai Ye*), Resina Myrrhae (*Mo Yao*), Radix Pseudoginseng (*San Qi*), Os Sepiae Seu Sepiellae (*Wu Zhi Gu*), Os Draconis (*Long Gu*), Concha Ostreae (*Mu Li*)

Zhang Xue-wen, author of *Yu Xue Zheng Zhi (Static Blood Patterns & Treatments)*, recommends this formula for stasis and stagnation flooding and leaking. Zhang says this formula dispels stasis and stops flooding at the same time as it heavily settles pain.

Qi vacuity

Main symptoms: If the menses continue to dribble and drip without cessation, eventually this continuous loss of blood will lead to a sudden, large down-pouring. The color of the blood is pale red and is clear and thin in consistency. There is slight abdominal pain which does not resist pressure, shortness of breath, fatigue and sluggishness, sweating with movement, dizziness, heart palpitations, lack of warmth in the four extremities, lassitude and fatigue of the essence spirit, a pale, white, bloodless facial complexion, lack of strength in the low back and knees, a pale, wet tongue or a white, fat tongue with teeth marks on its edges, and a vacuous, large or soggy, scallion stalk, or fine, weak pulse.

Treatment principles: Fortify the spleen and boost the qi, secure the *chong* and stop bleeding

Guiding formulas:

1. *Bu Zhong Yi Qi Tang* **(Supplement the Center & Boost the Qi Decoction)**

Ingredients: Radix Astragali Membranacei (*Huang Qi*), Rhizoma Atractylodis Macrocephalae (*Bai Zhu*), Radix Codonopsitis Pilosulae (*Dang Shen*), Rhizoma Cimicifugae (*Sheng Ma*), Radix Angelicae Sinensis (*Dang Gui*), Radix Bupleuri (*Chai Hu*), Pericarpium Citri Reticulatae (*Chen Pi*), Radix Glycyrrhizae (*Gan Cao*)

Additions: If the amount of blood loss is excessive, add stir-fried Radix Sanguisorbae (*Di Yu*), carbonized Pollen Typhae (*Pu Huang*), and carbonized Folium Et Petriolus Trachycarpi (*Zong Tan*). If there is slippery desertion, add Os Draconis (*Long Gu*), Conchae Ostreae (*Mu Li*), and Os Sepiae Seu Sepiellae (*Hai Piao Xiao*). If there are heart palpitations and loss of sleep, add Semen Zizyphi Spinosae (*Zao Ren*) and Radix Polygalae Tenuifoliae (*Yuan Zhi*). If flooding transforms into leakage and continues on for years without stopping, Wan Mi-zhai says this is due to central qi fall and the source qi not securing. For this, Master Wan recommends administering *Bu Zhong Yi Qi Tang* simultaneously with *Lu Jiao Shuang Wan* (Degelatinized Deer Antler Pills). Master Wan gives the ingredients of this second formula as: Radix Ligustici Wallichii (*Chuan Xiong*), vinegar-processed Rhizoma Cyperi Rotundi (*Xiang Fu*), mix-fried Radix Glycyrrhizae (*Gan Cao*), Radix Dipsaci (*Chuan Xu Duan*), Cornu Degelatinum Cervi (*Lu Jiao Shuang*), Semen Biotae Orientalis (*Bai Zi Ren*), Radix Angelicae Sinensis (*Dang Gui*), Sclerotium Pararadicis Poriae Cocos (*Fu Shen*), calcined Os Draconis (*Long Gu*), and clam shell stir-fried Gelatinum Corii Asini (*E Jiao*).

2. *Gui Pi Tang* **(Restore the Spleen Decoction)**

Ingredients: Radix Panacis Ginseng (*Ren Shen*), Radix Astragali Membranacei (*Huang Qi*), Radix Angelicae Sinensis (*Dang Gui*), Arillus Euphoriae Longanae (*Long Yan Rou*), Rhizoma Atractylodis Macrocephalae (*Bai Zhu*), Radix Auklandiae Lappae (*Mu Xiang*), Sclerotium Poriae Cocos (*Fu Ling*), Radix Polygalae Tenuifoliae (*Yuan Zhi*), Semen Zizyphi Spinosae (*Suan Zao Ren*), mix-fried Radix Glycyrrhizae (*Gan Cao*), uncooked Rhizoma Zingiberis (*Sheng Jiang*), Fructus Zizyphi Jujubae (*Da Zao*)

Additions & subtractions: Han Bai-ling says to add stir-fried Radix Sanguisorbae (*Di Yu*) and carbonized Pollen Typhae (*Pu Huang*) and delete Auklandia which is acrid and dispersing and consumes and wastes the qi. Han Bai-ling also gives as a category blood vacuity flooding and leaking. However, this is nothing other than spleen qi and heart blood vacuity. Blood loss affects the heart and keeps the qi from being engendered, since blood is the mother of the qi. But it is still spleen qi insufficiency which fails to contain the blood within its vessels. For this pattern, Han Bai-ling uses *Gui Pi Tang* plus the addition of Concha Ostreae (*Mu Li*), Semen Biotae Orientalis (*Bai Ren*), Gelatinum Corii Asini (*E Jiao*), and stir-fried Radix Sanguisorbae (*Di Yu*) to secure the *chong* and stop bleeding.

3. *Gu Ben Zhi Xue Tang* (Secure the Root & Stop Bleeding Decoction)

Ingredients: Cooked Radix Rehmanniae (*Shu Di*), earth stir-fried Rhizoma Atractylodis Macrocephalae (*Bai Zhu*), Radix Codonopsitis Pilosulae (*Dang Shen*), uncooked Radix Astragali Membranacei (*Huang Qi*), wine-washed Radix Angelicae Sinensis (*Dang Gui*), blackened Rhizoma Zingiberis (*Hei Jiang*)

Fu Qing-zhu gives this formula for the treatment of blood flooding dimness and darkness. This dimness and darkness refer to dimming of vision on the verge of blacking out due to insufficient blood filling the sea of marrow. Fu Qing-zhu explains this type of flooding and leaking as being due to vacuity fire. Based on the ingredients of this formula, this is a combination of kidney yin vacuity and qi and blood vacuity resulting in vacuity fire.

Additions & subtractions: Fu Qing-zhu's editor says to substitute Radix Panacis Ginseng (*Ren Shen*) for Codonopsis for stronger supplementation in case of desertion and that one can add carbonized Rhizoma Dryopteridis (*Guan Chong*) to more effectively stop bleeding if necessary. Carbonized Dryopteridis was a favorite hemostatic of this editor. Prof. Song and Yu suggest deleting Dang Gui and adding processed Radix Polygoni Mutliflori (*Shou Wu*) and Os Sepiae Seu Sepiellae (*Hai Piao Xiao*). Zhang En-qin *et al.* suggest deleting Dang Gui, substituting Radix Panacis Ginseng (*Ren Shen*) for Codonopsis, and adding Rhizoma Cimicifugae (*Sheng Ma*), Radix Dioscoreae Oppositae (*Shan Yao*), Os Sepiae Seu Sepiellae (*Wu Zei Gu*), and Herba Leonuri Heterophylli (*Yi Mu Cao*). The addition of Herba Leonuri Heterophylli is based on the presence of blood stasis complicating vacuity. If there is fear of cold, chilled extremities, and soreness and weakness of the low back and knees, delete cooked Rehmannia, Dioscorea, and Os Sepiae and add Colla Cornu Cervi (*Lu Jiao Jiao*), Semen Cuscutae (*Tu Si Zi*), and Cortex Eucommiae Ulmoidis (*Du Zhong*). If the blood is pale red and there is dizziness, tinnitus, and soreness and weakness of the low back and knees, delete blackened Ginger, Cimicifuga, Os Sepiae, and Dioscorea and add Fructus Ligustri Lucidi (*Nu Zhen Zi*), Herba Ecliptae Prostratae (*Han Lian Cao*), and Colla Cornu Cervi (*Lu Jiao Jiao*).

4. *Jia Jian Dang Gui Bu Xue Tang* (Additions & Subtractions Dang Gui Supplement the Blood Decoction)

Ingredients: Wine-washed Radix Angelicae Sinensis (*Dang Gui*), uncooked Radix Astragali Membranacei (*Huang Qi*), Folium Mori Albi (*Sang Ye*), Radix Pseudoginseng (*Guang San Qi*)

This is another of Fu Qing-zhu's formulas for the treatment of blood flooding. Fu Qing-zhu gives this formula under the heading old (woman's) blood flooding. Fu Qing-zhu says that, after 50 years of age, the *tian gui* is exhausted. This means that yin fluids are exhausted. Normally the menses cease because of this. However, if kidney fire becomes greatly stirred, vacuity fire may cause the blood to move frenetically outside its pathways. But, because the blood and essence share a common source as do the blood and fluids, this bleeding tends to be more leakage than flooding. Fu Qing-zhu says that two *ji* of the above formula will slow or stop the bleeding and that four *ji* should keep it from recurring again.

Additions: However, if leakage continues to occur, it is because the older woman's yin essence is vacuous. After giving four *ji* of the above formula, one can add Rhizoma Atractylodis Macrocephalae (*Bai Zhu*), cooked Radix Rehmanniae (*Shu Di*), Fructus Corni Officinalis (*Shan Zhu Rou*), Tuber Ophiopogonis Japonici (*Mai Dong*), and Fructus Schisandrae Chinensis (*Bei Wu Wei*). As Fu Qing-zhu says, if one gives 100 *ji* of this formula, the root of blood leakage will be exhausted and eliminated. Fu Qing-zhu's editor also says that if a white-haired or hoary, *i.e.*, a really old woman, has blood flooding, one must certainly tie the qi vigorously in the blood chamber. In that case, one should add carbonized Rhizoma Dryopteridis (*Guan Chong*) and carbonized Hangzhou Radix Albus Paeoniae Lactiflorae (*Hang Shao*) to the above original formula. Although Fu Qing-zhu says that the mechanism behind this type of flooding and leaking is vacuity heat, this formula relies on the principles of nourishing the blood and enriching yin in order to spontaneously cool the blood. At the same time, it supplements the qi in order to constrain, secure, and contain the blood. Therefore, I have chosen to place this formula under the qi vacuity category.

5. *Gu Ben Zhi Beng Tang Jia Jian* (Secure the Root & Stop Bleeding Decoction with Additions & Subtractions)

Ingredients: Stir-fried Radix Codonopsitis Pilosulae (*Dang Shen*), stir-fried Rhizoma Atractylodis Macrocephalae (*Bai Zhu*), mix-fried Radix Glycyrrhizae (*Gan Cao*), processed Rhizoma Polygonati (*Huang Jing*), Radix Albus Paeoniae Lactiflorae (*Bai Shao*), mix-fried Radix Astragali Membranacei (*Huang Qi*), Hallyositum Rubrum (*Chi Shi Zhi*), Fructus Psoraleae Corylifoliae (*Bu Gu Zhi*), Os Sepiae Seu Sepiellae (*Wu Zei Gu*)

Zhu Cheng-han, in *Zhong Yi Fu Ke (Chinese Medical Gynecology)*, gives the above modified version of Fu Qing-zhu's formula.

Additions: If the amount of blood loss is excessive, the facial complexion is sallow and white, and there is sweating, lack of warmth in the hands and feet, and the pulse becomes minute and weak, this is characteristic of yang vacuity desertion and expiry. In this case, it is ok to add scalded Radix Lateralis Praeparatus Aconiti Carmichaeli (*Fu Pian*), calcined Os Draconis (*Long Gu*), and calcined Concha Ostreae (*Mu Li*). If the heart and spleen are both vacuous, add mix-fried Radix Polygalae Tenuifoliae (*Yuan Zhi*) and Semen Biotae Orientalis (*Bai Zi Ren*). If there is sometimes flooding and sometimes leaking which will not stop but absence of lower abdominal distention or pain, add Fructus Pruni Mume (*Wu Mei*), calcined Os Draconis (*Long Gu*), and calcined Concha Ostreae (*Mu Li*) to secure and astringe the *chong* and *ren*.

6. *Yin Jing Zhi Xue Tang* (Lead the Essence & Stop Bleeding Decoction)

Ingredients: Earth stir-fried Rhizoma Atractylodis Macrocephalae (*Bai Zhu*), Sclerotium Poriae Cocos (*Fu Ling*), Radix Codonopsitis Pilosulae (*Dang Shen*), cooked Radix Rehmanniae (*Shu Di*), Fructus Corni Officinalis (*Shan Zhu Rou*), blackened Rhizoma Zingiberis (*Hei Jiang*), Cortex Phellodendri (*Huang Bai*), wine stir-fried Semen Plantaginis (*Che Qian Zi*), Herba Schizonepetae Tenuifoliae (*Jing Sui*)

Fu Qing-zhu gives this formula under the heading of bleeding due to sexual intercourse. If, every time after sexual intercourse there is flowing of blood which will not stop, even if this bleeding is not extreme, over time the qi and blood will both be damaged. This may then lead to blocked menstraution and the formation of concretions and conglomerations, accumulations and gathering or abdominal masses. Fu Qing-zhu attributes this flooding and leaking to excessive sexual desire leading to male essence penetrating the blood vessels. If the blood vessels are delicate and fragile, due to qi and blood vacuity, this penetration may result in their breaking and leaking.

7. Unnamed formula from *Concise Traditional Chinese Gynecology*

Ingredients: Radix Codonopsitis Pilosulae (*Dang Shen*), stir-fried Rhizoma Atractylodis Macrocephalae (*Bai Zhu*), mix-fried Radix Glycyrrhizae (*Gan Cao*), Radix Astragali Membranacei (*Huang Qi*), carbonized Herba Schizonepetae Tenuifoliae (*Jing Jie*)

8. *Gu Chong Tang* (Secure the *Chong* Decoction)

Ingredients: Radix Astragali Membranacei (*Huang Qi*), Rhizoma Atractylodis Macro-cephalae (*Bai Zhu*), Fructus Corni Officinalis (*Shan Zhu Rou*), Radix Albus Paeoniae Lactiflorae (*Bai Shao*), calcined Concha Ostreae (*Mu Li*), calcined Os Draconis (*Long Gu*), Os Sepiae Seu Sepiellae (*Hai Piao Xiao*), Fructus Schisandrae Chinensis (*Wu Wei Zi*), carbonized Folium Et Petriolus Trachycarpi (*Zong Tan*), Radix Rubiae Cordifoliae (*Qian Cao*)

This is a formula taught to me by Dr. Chen Wei in a formula and prescription class at the

Shanghai College of Traditional Chinese Medicine. According to Dr. Chen, it is indicated for uterine bleeding and abnormal vaginal discharge due to spleen-stomach vacuity.

Additions: If complicated by yang vacuity, add Radix Panacis Ginseng (*Ren Shen*) and Radix Lateralis Praeparatus Aconiti Carmichaeli (*Fu Zi*).

9. *Liu Yuan San* (Lodge the Source Powder)

Ingredients: Clam shell stir-fried Gelatinum Corii Asini (*E Jiao*), earth stir-fried Rhizoma Atractylodis Macrocephalae (*Bai Zhu*), Sclerotium Poriae Cocos (*Fu Ling*), Radix Albus Paeoniae Lactiflorae (*Bai Shao*), Radix Ligustici Wallichii (*Chuan Xiong*), Radix Angelicae Sinensis (*Dang Gui*), cooked Radix Rehmanniae (*Shu Di*), Radix Angelicae Dahuricae (*Bai Zhi*), Rhizoma Cimicifugae (*Sheng Ma*), Rhizoma Cyperi Rotundi (*Xiang Fu*), Radix Sanguisorbae (*Di Yu*), Radix Dipsaci (*Chuan Duan*), Pollen Typhae (*Pu Huang*), Radix Glycyrrhizae (*Gan Cao*)

This formula boosts the qi and nourishes the blood, dispels stasis and stops flooding. It is indicated by Du Jie-hui for the treatment of spleen-kidney vacuity flooding and leaking possibly complicated by blood stasis.

10. *Xue Beng Ji Yu Fang* (Blood Flooding Immediately Curing Formula)

Ingredients: Rhizoma Cimicifugae (*Sheng Ma*), Radix Bupleuri (*Chai Hu*), Radix Ligustici Wallichii (*Chuan Xiong*), Radix Angelicae (*Bai Zhi*), Herba Schizonepetae Tenuifoliae (*Jing Jie Sui*), Radix Angelicae Sinensis (*Dang Gui*)

Du Jie-hui suggests this formula for spleen vacuity flooding which will not recuperate or heal. It upbears yang and stops flooding.

Kidney vacuity patterns

A. Yin vacuity

Main symptoms: The amount of bleeding is scanty or continuously dripping and dribbling. Its color is bright or fresh red. There is dizziness, tinnitus, vexatious heat in the five hearts, heart palpitations, loss of sleep, tidal fever, night sweats, low back and knee soreness and weakness or lumbar pain, pain in the heels or feet, no abdominal distention or pain, a dry red tongue with scant or no fur, a dry mouth but no particular thirst, a red face and red cheeks, and a bowstring, fine, rapid pulse.

Treatment principles: Enrich yin and supplement the kidneys, secure the *chong* and stop bleeding

Guiding formulas:

1. *Liu Wei Di Huang Tang Jia Jian* (Six Flavors Rehmannia Pills with Additions & Subtractions) according to Sun Jiu-ling

Ingredients: Cooked Radix Rehmanniae (*Shu Di*), stri-fried Radix Dioscoreae Oppositae (*Shan Yao*), Herba Ecliptae Prostratae (*Han Lian Cao*), Fructus Ligustri Lucidi (*Nu Zhen Zi*), Fructus Lycii Chinensis (*Gou Qi Zi*), Sclerotium Poriae Cocos (*Fu Ling*), Rhizoma Alismatis (*Ze Xie*), Cortex Radicis Moutan (*Dan Pi*), mix-fried Plastrum Testudinis (*Gui Ban*), Gelatinum Corii Asini (*E Jiao*), Herba Agrimoniae Pilosae (*Xian He Cao*)

2. *Liu Wei Di Huang Tang Jia Wei* (Six Flavors Rehmannia Pills with Added Flavors) according to Jane B. Tang

Ingredients: Cooked Radix Rehmanniae (*Shu Di*), Radix Dioscoreae Oppositae (*Shan Yao*), Fructus Corni Officinalis (*Shan Zhu Rou*), Cortex Radicis Moutan (*Dan Pi*), Rhizoma Alismatis (*Ze Xie*), Sclerotium Poriae Cocos (*Fu Ling*), Concha Ostreae (*Mu Li*), Os Draconis (*Long Gu*), Os Sepiae Seu Sepiellae (*Wu Zei Gu*), carbonized Folium Et Petriolus Trachycarpi (*Zong Lu Tan*), Radix Polygoni Multiflori (*He Shou Wu*), Herba Ecliptae Prostratae (*Han Lian Cao*), Gelatinum Plastri Testudinis (*Gui Ban Jiao*), Gelatinum Corii Asini (*E Jiao*)

3. *Zuo Gui Wan Jia Jian* (Restore the Left [Kidney] Pills with Additions & Subtractions)

Ingredients: Cooked Radix Rehmanniae (*Shu Di*), Radix Dioscoreae Oppositae (*Shan Yao*), Fructus Lycii Chinensis (*Gou Qi Zi*), Fructus Corni Officinalis (*Shan Zhu Rou*), Semen Cuscutae (*Tu Si Zi*), Gelatinum Plastri Testudinis (*Gui Jiao*), Fructus Ligustri Lucidi (*Nu Zhen Zi*), Herba Ecliptae Prostratae (*Han Lian Cao*), carbonized Cacumen Biotae Orientalis (*Ce Bai Ye*)

4. *Yu Yin Tang* (Heal Yin Decoction)

Ingredients: Cooked Radix Rehmanniae (*Shu Di*), Radix Dioscoreae Oppositae (*Shan Yao*), Radix Dipsaci (*Chuan Duan*), Ramulus Loranthi Seu Visci (*Sang Ji Sheng*), Fructus Corni Officinalis (*Shan Zhu Rou*), Os Sepiae Seu Sepiellae (*Hai Piao Xiao*), Plastrum Testudinis (*Gui Ban*), Conchae Ostreae (*Mu Li*), Radix Albus Paeoniae Lactiflorae (*Bai Shao*), Gelatinum Corii Asini (*E Jiao*), stir-fried Radix Sanguisorbae (*Di Yu*)

Additions: If bleeding is excessive in amount, increase the amount of Sanguisorba and add carbonized Folium Et Petriolus Trachycarpi (*Zong Tan*) and carbonized Pollen Typhae (*Pu Huang*). If heat is prominent, add salt-processed Cortex Phellodendri (*Huang Bai*), Cortex Radicis Lycii Chinensis (*Di Gu Pi*), and Rhizoma Anemarrhenae Aspheloidis (*Zhi Mu*). If there is qi fall, add Rhizoma Cimicifugae (*Sheng Ma*).

5. Unnamed formula from *Concise Traditional Chinese Gynecology*

Ingredients: Fructus Ligustri Lucidi (*Nu Zhen Zi*), Herba Ecliptae Prostratae (*Han Lian Cao*), mix-fried Plastrum Testudinis (*Gui Ban*), Fructus Corni Officinalis (*Shan Zhu Rou*)

6. *Xue Beng Fang* (Blood Flooding Formula)

Ingredients: Stir-fried Radix Angelicae Sinensis (*Dang Gui*), uncooked Pollen Typhae (*Pu Huang*), Radix Achyranthis Bidentatae (*Niu Xi*), Radix Salviae Miltiorrhizae (*Dan Shen*), Radix Rubrus Paeoniae Lactiflorae (*Chi Shao*), Radix Albus Paeoniae Lactiflorae (*Bai Shao*), processed Rhizoma Cyperi Rotundi (*Xiang Fu*), Dolomitum (*Hua Rui Shi*), carbonized cooked Radix Et Rhizoma Rhei (*Shu Jun*), Sanguis Draconis (*Xue Jie*)

This formula is for blood flooding due to liver-kidney vacuity complicated by blood stasis.

7. *Bu Shen Tiao Jing Tang* (Supplement the Kidneys & Regulate the Menses)

Ingredients: Cooked Radix Rehmanniae (*Shu Di*), processed Radix Polygoni Multiflori (*Shou Wu*), Fructus Lycii Chinensis (*Gou Qi*), Rhizoma Polygonati (*Huang Jing*), Ramulus Loranthi Seu Visci (*Sang Ji Sheng*), Cornu Degelatinum Cervi (*Lu Jiao Shuang*), Fructus Rosae Laevigatae (*Jin Ying Zi*), Semen Cuscutae (*Tu Si Zi*), Radix Dipsaci (*Xu Duan*), Radix Codonopsitis Pilosulae (*Dang Shen*), Rhizoma Atractylodis Macrocephalae (*Bai Zhu*), Radix Glycyrrhizae (*Gan Cao*)

This formula enriches the kidneys and boosts yin, stops bleeding and regulates the menses. It is indicated for the treatment of kidney yin vacuity flooding and leaking.

8. *Zhi Bai Di Huang Wan* (Anemarrhena & Phellodendron Rehmannia Pills)

Ingredients: Rhizoma Anemarrhenae Aspheloidis (*Zhi Mu*), Cortex Phellodendri (*Huang Bai*), cooked Radix Rehmanniae (*Shu Di*), Fructus Corni Officinalis (*Shan Zhu Yu*), Radix Dioscoreae Oppositae (*Shan Yao*), Sclerotium Poriae Cocos (*Fu Ling*), Cortex Radicis Moutan (*Dan Pi*), Rhizoma Alismatis (*Ze Xie*)

Additions: For massive bleeding, add Radix Sanguisorbae (*Di Yu*) and Radix Rubiae Cordifoliae (*Qian Cao Geng*). For systemic yin vacuity, add Plastrum Testudinis (*Gui Ban*) and Gelatinum Corii Asini (*E Jiao*). If there is dizziness, add Fructus Ligustri Lucidi (*Nu Zhen Zi*) and Herba Ecliptae Prostratae (*Han Lian Cao*). If there is dry mouth and sore throat, add Radix Scrophulariae Ningpoensis (*Yuan Shen*) and Tuber Ophiopogonis Japonici (*Mai Dong*).

B. Yang vacuity

Main symptoms: The amount of bleeding is scanty or dribbles and drips continuously. Its color is pale red or watery and thin. There is chilly pain in the abdomen desiring warmth and pressure. The facial complexion is dark and dusky. There is dizziness and vertigo, fear of cold and chilled extremities. Both the lower and upper back are sore and painful. Urination is frequent, clear, and long or incontinent. There is terminal dribbling after urination. The face and limbs may be swollen and edematous. There may also be white vaginal discharge pouring down. The stools may be loose and flimsy. The tongue is pale and moist with thin, white fur. The mouth is not dry and there is no thirst. The pulse is fine and weak or deep and weak.

Treatment principles: Warm the kidneys and invigorate yang, secure the *chong* and stop bleeding

Guiding formulas:

1. *Lu Rong Wan* (Cornu Parvum Cervi Pills)

Ingredients: Cornu Parvum Cervi (*Lu Rong*), Hallyositum Rubrum (*Chi Shi Zhi*), Limonitum (*Yu Yu Liang*), Radix Lateralis Praeparatus Aconiti Carmichaeli (*Fu Zi*), carbonized Folium Artemisiae Argyii (*Ai Ye*), carbonized Cacumen Biotae Orientalis (*Ce Bai Ye*), Radix Angelicae Sinensis (*Dang Gui*), cooked Radix Rehmanniae (*Shu Di*), Radix Dipsaci (*Chuan Duan*)

Additions: Han Bai-ling, who gives this formula for the treatment of kidney yang vacuity flooding and leaking, says to add Cortex Eucommiae Ulmoidis (*Du Zhong*), Radix Morindae Officinalis (*Ba Ji Tian*), Radix Dioscoreae Oppositae (*Shan Yao*), and Os Draconis (*Long Gu*). If the amount of bleeding is excessive, add stir-fried Radix Sanguisorbae (*Di Yu*). If there is qi fall, add Rhizoma Cimicifugae (*Sheng Ma*). If there is loose stools or diarrhea, add Rhizoma Atractylodis Macrocephalae (*Bai Zhu*).

2. *You Gui Wan* (Restore the Right [Kidney] Pills)

Ingredients: Cooked Radix Rehmanniae (*Shu Di*), stir-fried Radix Dioscoreae Oppositae (*Shan Yao*), Fructus Lycii Chinensis (*Gou Qi Zi*), Radix Lateralis Praeparatus Aconiti Carmichaeli (*Fu Zi*), mix-fried Radix Glycyrrhizae (*Gan Cao*), Cortex Eucommiae Ulmoidis (*Du Zhong*), Cortex Cinnamomi Cassiae (*Rou Gui*)

Additions & subtractions: Sun Jiu-ling says to delete mix-fried Licorice, Eucommia, and Cinnamon and to add Gelatinum Cornu Cervi (*Lu Jiao Jiao*), Fructus Ligustri Lucidi (*Nu Zhen Zi*), Semen Cuscutae (*Tu Si Zi*), blast-fried carbonized Rhizoma Zingiberis (*Pao*

Jiang), Os Sepiae Seu Sepiellae (*Wu Zei Gu*), and Radix Dipsaci (*Chuan Xu Duan*). Song and Yu suggest deleting Cinnamon from the standard formula and adding Radix Astragali Membranacei (*Huang Qi*), Radix Dipsaci (*Xu Duan*), Radix Polygoni Multiflori (*He Shou Wu*), carbonized Rhizoma Zingiberis (*Jiang Tan*), and carbonized Radix Angelicae Sinensis (*Dang Gui*).

3. Unnamed formula from *Concise Traditional Chinese Gynecology*

Ingredients: Colla Cornu Cervi (*Lu Jiao Jiao*), Fructus Psoraleae Corylifoliae (*Bu Gu Zhi*), carbonized Folium Artemisiae Argyii (*Ai Ye*), Radix Codonopsitis Pilosulae (*Dang Shen*), stir-fried Rhizoma Atractylodis Macrocephalae (*Bai Zhu*)

4. *Jin Gui Shen Qi Wan Jia Jian* (*Golden Cabinet* Kidney Qi Pills with Additions & Subtractions)

Ingredients: Cortex Cinnamomi Cassiae (*Rou Gui*), cooked Radix Rehmanniae (*Shu Di*), Fructus Corni Officinalis (*Shan Zhu Rou*), Radix Dioscoreae Oppositae (*Shan Yao*), Cortex Radicis Moutan (*Dan Pi*), Sclerotium Poriae Cocos (*Fu Ling*), Rhizoma Alismatis (*Ze Xie*), Gelatinum Cornu Cervi (*Lu Jiao Jiao*), blast-fried carbonized Rhizoma Zingiberis (*Pao Jiang*), carbonized Folium Artemisiae Argyii (*Ai Ye*), Os Sepiae Seu Sepiellae (*Wu Zei Gu*), Hallyositum Rubrum (*Chi Shi Zhi*), Fructus Psoraleae Corylifoliae (*Bu Gu Zhi*), carbonized Petiolus Et Folium Trachycarpi (*Zong Lu Tan*), carbonized Receptaculum Nelumbinis Nuciferae (*Lian Fang*), carbonized Cortex Eucommiae Ulmoidis (*Du Zhong*), carbonized Radix Rubiae Cordifoliae (*Qian Cao Gen*), carbonized Fructus Pruni Mume (*Wu Mei*), stir-fried Pollen Typhae (*Pu Huang*)

5. *Jiao Ai Tang* ([Donkey Skin] Glue & Mugwort Decoction)

Ingredients: Gelatinum Corii Asini (*E Jiao*), Folium Artemisiae Argyii (*Ai Ye*), mix-fried Radix Glycyrrhizae (*Gan Cao*), cooked Radix Rehmanniae (*Shu Di*), Radix Albus Paeoniae Lactiflorae (*Bai Shao*), Radix Angelicae Sinensis (*Dang Gui*), Radix Ligustici Wallichii (*Chuan Xiong*)

Du Jie-hui recommends this formula for the treatment of kidney yang vacuity flooding and leaking. It is, perhaps, more commonly thought of for the treatment of stirring fetus disquietude (*tai dong bu an*). Du says that it warms the kidneys and secures the *chong*, stops bleeding and regulates the menses. Personally, this would not be my choice for kidney yang vacuity flooding and leaking.

6. Unnamed formula from *Nu Ke Jing Wei (Profundities from the Gynecological Classics)*

Ingredients: Whole Radix Angelicae Sinensis (*Quan Dang Gui*), Os Sepiae Seu Sepiellae (*Wu Zei Gu*), Gelatinum Cornu Cervi (*Lu Jiao Jiao*), true Gelatinum Corii Asini (*E Jiao*), baked dry Rhizoma Zingiberis (*Gan Jiang*), vinegar-processed Folium Artemisiae Argyii (*Ai Ye*), large Radix Codonopsitis Pilosulae (*Dang Shen*), uncooked Radix Astragali Membranacei (*Huang Qi*), carbonized Herba Schizonepetae Tenuifoliae (*Jie Sui*), large cooked Radix Rehmanniae (*Shu Di*), old Radix Ligustici Wallichii (*Chuan Xiong*), mix-fried Radix Glycyrrhizae (*Gan Cao*), earth stir-fried Rhizoma Atractylodis Macrocephalae (*Bai Zhu*), Rhizoma Cimicifugae (*Sheng Ma*)

Additions: If there is lumbar soreness and pain and the hands and feet lack warmth, add Semen Cuscutae (*Tu Si Zi*) and Ramulus Cinnamomi Cassiae (*Gui Zhi*). If there are loose stools and diarrhea, add Fructus Terminaliae Chebulae (*He Zi Rou*). If the amount of blood lost is excessive and there is heart fluster, add scorched Semen Zizyphi Spinosae (*Zao Ren*) and cinnabar-processed Sclerotium Pararadicis Poriae Cocos (*Fu Shen*).

Phlegm rheum

Main symptoms: There is blood exiting from the vaginal tract. It may be excessive like a flood or dribbling and dripping like a leak. It may contain blood clots like a sticky substance. Discharging is slightly soothing, while stopping leads to oppression. Mostly this occurs to fat women. Simultaneously, there may be abdominal fullness, abdominal oppression, distention, and pain, or palpitations above the navel. There is also scanty appetite and profuse phlegm, a pale tongue with white, slimy fur, and a deep, slippery or soggy, fine, and slippery pulse.

Treatment principles: Eliminate phlegm and downbear counterflow, regulate and rectify the *chong* and *ren*

Guiding formulas:

1. *Cang Bai Er Chen Tang Jia Wei* (Atractylodes & Atractylodes Macrocephala Two Aged [Ingredients] Decoction with Added Flavors)

Ingredients: Rhizoma Atractylodis (*Cang Zhu*), Rhizoma Atractylodis Macrocephalae (*Bai Zhu*), Pericarpium Citri Reticulatae (*Chen Pi*), Rhizoma Pinelliae Ternatae (*Ban Xia*), Sclerotium Poriae Cocos (*Fu Ling*), Radix Glycyrrhizae (*Gan Cao*), Galla Rhi Chinensis (*Wu Bei Zi*), Concha Ostreae (*Mu Li*), Rhizoma Arisaematis (*Nan Xing*), Crinis Carbonisatus (*Xue Yu Tan*), blast-fried, carbonized Rhizoma Zingiberis (*Pao Jiang*)

Within this formula, *Er Chen Tang* dries dampness and transforms phlegm. Atractylodes, Atractylodes Macrocephala, and Arisaema are added to strengthen the fortification of the spleen, drying of dampness, and eliminating of phlegm. Chinese Nutgall and Oyster Shell are able to disperse phlegm and scatter nodulation. They are also able to astringe flow and stop bleeding. Carbonized Hair and blast-fried, carbonized Ginger stop bleeding but without retaining stasis.

271

2. *Er Chen Tang Jia Wei* (Two Aged [Ingredients] Decoction with Added Flavors)

Ingredients: Rhizoma Pinelliae Ternatae (*Ban Xia*), Pericarpium Citri Reticulatae (*Chen Pi*), Sclerotium Poriae Cocos (*Fu Ling*), Radix Glycyrrhizae (*Gan Cao*), Radix Angelicae Sinensis (*Dang Gui*), Radix Albus Paeoniae Lactiflorae (*Bai Shao*), Fructus Citri Aurantii (*Zhi Ke*)

Additions: For cold phlegm, add the juice of uncooked Rhizoma Zingiberis (*Jiang Zhi*). For phlegm fire, add Rhizoma Belamcandae (*She Gan*) and Pulvis Indigonis (*Qing Dai*). For phlegm dampness, add Rhizoma Atractylodis (*Cang Zhu*) and Rhizoma Atractylodis Macrocephalae (*Bai Zhu*). For dry phlegm, add Semen Trichosanthis Kirlowii (*Gua Lou Ren*), Radix Trichosanthis Kirlowii (*Tian Hua Fen*), and/or Semen Pruni Armeniacae (*Xing Ren*). For food stagnation complicating phlegm, select from Fructus Immaturus Citri Aurantii (*Zhi Shi*), Semen Raphani Sativi (*Lai Fu Zi*), Fructus Crataegi (*Shan Zha*), Massa Medica Fermentata (*Shen Qu*), and Fructus Chaenomelis Lagenariae (*Mu Gua*). For recalcitrant phlegm, add Rhizoma Alismatis (*Ze Xie*), Pumice (*Hai Fu Shi*), Mirabilitum (*Mang Xiao*), and Rhizoma Acori Graminei (*Shi Chang Pu*). If there is more significant blood stasis with clotty blood, add Feces Trogopterori Seu Pteromi (*Wu Ling Zhi*) and Pollen Typhae (*Pu Huang*). If spleen qi vacuity is prominent, add Radix Panacis Ginseng (*Ren Shen*) and Radix Astragali Membranacei (*Huang Qi*).

Securing the root

In TCM, there are three stages to treating flooding and leaking. The first stage is to stop the bleeding using emergency measures and employing stop-bleeding medicinals. Once any heavy bleeding is brought under control, the second stage is to correct the disease mechanism responsible for the bleeding. Often this second stage involves clearing heat, dispelling stasis, resolving depression, or transforming phlegm. The third stage is to treat the root. Treating the root means to supplement the underlying vacuity which typically caused or occurred due to the bleeding. This is referred to as securing the root in TCM gynecology. To aid in identifying the root, the following pattern discrimination is given:

Central qi vacuity

Main symptoms: Shortness of breath, sweating on movement, fatigue and exhaustion, a pale facial complexion, possible feverish feelings, dizziness on standing up, reduced appetite, loose stools, lack of strength in the four limbs, a pale, moist tongue with thin, white fur, and a deep, short, weak pulse

Treatment principles: Fortify the spleen and boost the qi, nourish the blood and clear lingering vacuity heat

Guiding formula: *Jia Wei Bu Zhong Yi Qi Tang* **(Added Flavors Supplement the Center & Boost the Qi Decoction)**

Ingredients: Mix-fried Radix Astragali Membranacei (*Huang Qi*), Radix Panacis Ginseng (*Ren Shen*), Rhizoma Atractylodis Macrocephalae (*Bai Zhu*), Pericarpium Citri Reticulatae (*Chen Pi*), Radix Angelicae Sinensis (*Dang Gui*), wine stir-fried Radix Albus Paeoniae Lactiflorae (*Bai Shao*), cooked Radix Rehmanniae (*Shu Di*), mix-fried Radix Glycyrrhizae (*Gan Cao*), white Sclerotium Poriae Cocos (*Bai Ling*), Rhizoma Cimicifugae (*Sheng Ma*), Radix Bupleuri (*Chai Hu*), Rhizoma Anemarrhenae Aspheloidis (*Zhi Mu*), Cortex Phellodendri (*Huang Bai*), uncooked Rhizoma Zingiberis (*Sheng Jiang*), Fructus Zizyphi Jujubae (*Da Zao*)

This formula is given by Wan Mi-zhai for the treatment of spleen-stomach vacuity after bleeding has stopped and internal heat has mostly been cleared.

Kidney yang vacuity

Main symptoms: Mental depression, fear of cold, chilled extremities, soreness and weakness of the low back and knees, clear, long urine, loose stools, a pale, moist tongue with white fur, and a deep, weak pulse

Treatment principles: Greatly invigorate the kidneys and support yang

Guiding formula: *You Gui Yin Jia Jian* **(Restore the Right [Kidney] Drink with Additions & Subtractions)**

Ingredients: Cooked Radix Rehmanniae (*Shu Di*), Radix Dioscoreae Oppositae (*Shan Yao*), Fructus Corni Officinalis (*Shan Zhu Rou*), Fructus Lycii Chinensis (*Gou Qi Zi*), Cortex Eucommiae Ulmoidis (*Du Zhong*), Radix Polygoni Multiflori (*He Shou Wu*), Semen Cuscutae (*Tu Si Zi*), Herba Cistanchis Deserticolae (*Rou Cong Rong*), Rhizoma Curculiginis Orchioidis (*Xian Mao*), Herba Epimedii (*Xian Ling Pi*), Fructus Ligustri Lucidi (*Nu Zhen Zi*), Herba Ecliptae Prostratae (*Han Lian Cao*), Radix Dipsaci (*Xu Duan*), Radix Angelicae Sinensis (*Dang Gui*), Gelatinum Corii Asini (*E Jiao*)

Jane B. Tang suggests taking the above medicinals each day for seven to ten days following the cessation of bleeding and then, under observation, for another two to three weeks. She says that these medicinals may be taken repeatedly even if there are signs of recuperation. However, I would caution neophytes that this formula does contain some very powerfully supplementing and potentially slimy ingredients which may adversely affect the qi mechanism.

Kidney vacuity, blood stasis

Main symptoms: Fatigue, low back and knee soreness and weakness, a pale facial complexion, abdominal pain and distention, a pale, purplish tongue or a pale, dry tongue with static spots or macules, and a deep, fine, bowstring pulse. These signs and symptoms add up to vacuity cold congelation and stagnation.

Treatment principles: Supplement the kidneys and quicken the blood

Guiding formula: Unnamed formula given by Jane B. Tang

Ingredients: Radix Bupleuri (*Chai Hu*), Radix Rubrus Paeoniae Lactiflorae (*Chi Shao*), Radix Albus Paeoniae Lactiflorae (*Bai Shao*), Herba Lycopi Lucidi (*Ze Lan*), Herba Leonuri Heterophylli (*Yi Mu Cao*), Herba Artemisiae Anomalae (*Liu Ji Nu*), Pollen Typhae (*Pu Huang*), Radix Achyranthis Bidentatae (*Niu Xi*), Caulis Milletiae Seu Spatholobi (*Ji Xue Teng*), Fructus Ligustri Lucidi (*Nu Zhen Zi*), Fructus Rubi Chingii (*Fu Pen Zi*), Semen Cuscutae (*Tu Si Zi*), Fructus Lycii Chinensis (*Gou Qi Zi*), Herba Cistanchis Deserticolae (*Rou Cong Rong*), Rhizoma Curculiginis Orchioidis (*Xian Mao*), Herba Epimedii (*Xian Ling Pi*)

Patients with no menstruation should take one *ji* of the above medicinals per day for three days and then discontinue for seven days.[23] Take nine packets per month. Patients with menstruation should take one *ji* three times during the menses. At the 12-13th day of the cycle, *i.e.*, just before or at ovulation, again take one packet per day for three days for a total of six packets per complete menstrual cycle.

Phlegm rheum

If phlegm rheum or dampness have already been eliminated and the condition of flooding and leaking has been relaxed, one should then treat the root. If there is spleen vacuity, there will be a somber white facial complexion, lassitude of the spirit, scanty intake, lower abdominal distention and dragging, non-replete stools, a pale tongue, and a vacuous, weak pulse. In that case, treatment should be based on a spleen-supplementing formula such as *Bu Zhong Yi Qi Tang* (Supplement the Center & Boost the Qi Decoction). If there is kidney yin vacuity, the symptoms are lumbar soreness and weak limbs, dizziness, tinnitus, possible vexatious heat in the five hearts, a dry mouth but no desire to drink, and a fine, rapid pulse. If there is kidney yang vacuity, there may be a cold body with chilled limbs, dark patches on the face, a relatively fat body, a pale tongue, and a deep, weak pulse. If there is yin vacuity, use *Zuo Gui*

---

[23] Some women develop amenorrhea after *beng lou*. This is what is meant here by women with no menstrual period.

Wan (Restore the Left [Kidney] Pills). If there is yang vacuity, use *You Gui Wan* (Restore the Right [Kidney] Pills). If there is chest and rib-side distention and pain, heart vexation and easy anger, occasional sighing, and a bowstring, rapid pulse, this is due to liver depression transforming into heat. Therefore it is appropriate to use *Dan Zhi Xiao Yao San* (Moutan & Gardenia Rambling Powder) in order to level or calm the liver and clear heat, quicken the blood and regulate the menses.

Discussion

Flooding and leaking is a commonly encountered problem in modern clinical practice. Most women who have hysterectomies do so because their Chinese disease category was flooding and leaking. TCM treats flooding and leaking relatively effectively. If more women resorted first to TCM for the treatment of uterine bleeding, there would be far less D & Cs and hysterectomies performed. Neither of these two surgical procedures is a radical cure for the underlying disease mechanisms causing flooding and leaking. Therefore, D & Cs must often be repeated two or three times before the Western MD decides that they are not working and then suggests a hysterectomy. Similar to profuse menstruation discussed above, Chinese medicine is most effective for treating functional uterine bleeding and is less effective for treating uterine bleeding due to uterine myomas. However, this does depend on the size and location of the myomas.

Because flooding and leaking involves the unwanted loss of blood and because blood is a pure substance in Chinese medicine, such blood loss is given priority treatment as a branch symptom. Ye Tian-shi in the Qing Dynasty formulated the three basic steps in treating flooding and leaking according to TCM. These are to block, clear, and consolidate. Blocking refers to stopping bleeding using styptics and hemostatics. Especially when there is blood flooding with voluminous blood loss, the use of symptomatic or empirical hemostatic medicinals is warranted.

Clearing refers to clearing the source. Ye Tian-shi chose the word *qing*, to clear, since most flooding and leaking involves evil heat which must be cleared according to TCM methodology. However, this term when used in the context of flooding and leaking also means to treat the root imbalance according to a discrimination of patterns no matter what the disease mechanism. If the bleeding is due to heat, that heat must be cleared. If the bleeding is due to stasis, that stasis must be eliminated. If the bleeding is due to vacuity, that vacuity must be supplemented, etc. Such clearing of the source of the bleeding is most important when treating downward leaking. Unless one accurately identifies the patterns or disease mechanisms at work in the patient causing her bleeding, even though one may reduce the bleeding symptomatically using styptics, one will not be able to bring the leakage under complete control. As discussed above under profuse menstruation, it is important not to randomly or overuse stop-bleeding medicinals since these can engender blood stasis.

Securing refers to the administration of supplementing medicinals after the flooding and leaking has been eradicated in order to help the woman engender and transform the qi and blood that she lost. The Chinese phrase is *gu ben.* In this case, the *ben* or root implied here is the righteous qi. This righteous qi actually has two roots, the kidneys which are the former heaven root and the spleen-stomach which are the latter heaven root. Such post-bleeding supplementation is especially important in cases involving qi and blood vacuity, kidney vacuity, vacuity heat, and loss of constraining or securing. If such vacuities are not redressed, they will set the stage for repeat episodes of bleeding in the future or may lead to blocked menstruation. This is why Song and Yu suggest that, after clearing heat in vacuity heat flooding and leaking, one should administer *Liu Wei Di Huang Wan* (Six flavors Rehmannia Pills) to enrich yin and secure the root. On the other hand, one must take care not to use too many rich, slimy medicinals, *i.e.*, blood and yin supplements, which can gum up the qi mechanism, thus impairing digestion and the latter heaven root.

In terms of stopping bleeding, often carbonized or stir-fried medicinals are used. Carbonizing means to reduce the medicinal to an ash. Traditionally it is believed that carbonizing potentizes a medicinal's hemostatic function. This is because carbonizing turns the medicinal black and black is the color of water-cold. However, the medicinal still retains its other TCM functions. Therefore, when carbonized medicinals are used, they should still be employed according to a discrimination of patterns correlated with the medicinal's other functions. The following list provides a basis for such discrimination.

Carbonized Folium Artemisiae Argyii (*Ai Ye*) and blast-fried carbonized Rhizoma Zingiberis (*Pao Jiang*) warms the channels and stops bleeding.

Carbonized Receptaculum Nelumbinis Nuciferae (*Lian Fang*) and carbonized Nodus Rhizomatis Nelumbinis Nuciferae (*Ou Jie*) constrain, secure, and stop bleeding.

Carbonized Cortex Eucommiae Ulmoidis (*Du Zhong*) and carbonized uncooked Radix Rehmanniae (*Sheng Di*) nourish kidney essence and stop bleeding.

Carbonized Rhizoma Cyperi Rotundi (*Xiang Fu*) moves and rectifies the qi.

Carbonized Cacumen Biotae Orientalis (*Ce Bai Ye*), carbonized Radix Scutellariae Baicalensis (*Huang Qin*), and carbonized Radix Sanguisorbae Officinalis (*Di Yu*) clear heat from the blood and stop bleeding.

Stir-fried Pollen Typhae (*Pu Huang*) quickens the blood and stops bleeding.

Carbonized Petiolus Et Folium Trachycarpi (*Zong Lu Tan*) astringes and stops bleeding when excessive blood has already been lost.

Carbonized Radix Rubiae Cordifoliae (*Qian Cao Gen*) quickens the blood, rectifies the qi, and stops bleeding.

Carbonized Rhizoma Cimicifugae (*Sheng Ma*) and blackened Herba Schizonepetae Tenuifoliae (*Jing Sui*) upbear the qi and stop bleeding.

Carbonized Fructus Pruni Mume (*Wu Mei*) secures the qi and stops bleeding.

The excessive use of carbonized medicinals may, however, cause hindrance to the discharge of blood stasis. Therefore, they should be used cautiously in cases where there is complicating lower abdominal pain. Recent research in China, reported by Philippe Sionneau in *Pao Zhi: An Introduction to the Use of Processed Chinese Medicinals* also published by Blue Poppy Press, suggests that carbonizing certain stop-bleeding medicinals may not be necessary and that their blood-stopping ability is actually reduced by carbonizing.

As mentioned above, it is also important to note that uterine bleeding may be due to uterine neoplasia, either benign or malignant. Western gynecological examination and diagnosis is, therefore, recommended to rule out the possibility of cancer. Uterine fibroids are classified as concretions and conglomerations, accumulations and gatherings in TCM gynecology. These are discussed in traditional Chinese gynecology texts in the *za bing* or miscellaneous disease section.

Acupuncture & moxibustion

One can use the same acupuncture & moxibustion treatments to stop bleeding during acute episodes of flooding as in the treatment of profuse menstruation.

Nursing

Sexual intercourse should be avoided during the course of treatment for flooding and leaking so as not to damage the fragile and delicate blood vessels. Patients should also avoid greasy, spicy, hot, acrid foods so as to avoid the creation of evil heat. On the other hand, neither should one eat uncooked or chilled foods for fear of damaging the central qi and its containment of the blood. Cold and sour foods should be avoided so as not to cause stagnation and astringency. Women experiencing excessive blood loss should rest in bed and be sure to replace body fluids by drinking plenty of fluids.

Prognosis

In general, all patterns of flooding and leaking are amenable to treatment with TCM internal medicine. The key to successful treatment is accurate discrimination of each patient's patterns and, therefore, the accurate rebalancing of each patient's disease mechanism. It is relatively easy to bring blood flooding under control. It is often more difficult to completely put a stop to leakage and dribbling. As mentioned above under profuse menstruation, when a satisfactory result is not obtained, it is often due to either not quickening the blood and tranforming stasis appropriately or not astringing and securing the kidneys.

Western women who suffer from flooding and leaking in their late 30s and 40s almost always have a combination of heat (depressive, damp, and/or vacuity), liver depression, spleen qi vacuity, and kidney yang vacuity. Therefore, even when these women have been diagnosed as having a uterine myoma, they typically do require forceful supplementation along with any other appropriate clear, moving, or attacking therapies. Therefore, the formula I most commonly use in the treatment of flooding and leaking in patients in this age range is *Bu Zhong Yi Qi Tang* (Supplement the Center & Boost the Qi Decoction) with additions and subtractions. Sometimes, the dosage of Radix Astragali Membranacei (*Huang Qi*) will be as high as 60g and the dosage of Radix Panacis Ginseng (*Ren Shen*) may reach 30g.

As explained above, in Western women this age, the symptoms of kidney yang vacuity may only be concomitant lumbar pain, frequent, especially nighttime, urination, cold feet, and decreased libido. When these occur, it is important to include ingredients, such as Cortex Eucommiae Ulmoidis (*Du Zhong*), Radix Dipsaci (*Xu Duan*), etc.

When there is a uterine myoma causing the flooding and leaking, my advice is to attempt to bring the flooding and leaking under control with Chinese medicinals and acupuncture-moxibustion. If it cannot be brought under control after three menstrual cycles, then the woman should seriously consider a myomectomy if she is a candidate for that procedure. If the woman is nearing menopause and Chinese medicinals are sufficient to stop the bleeding, the woman should remain on the Chinese medicinals until she has passed through menopause, after which time the myoma(s) will probably recede on thier own due to their estrogen dependency. For younger women or for those who Chinese medicine is ineffective, myomectomy can provide significant relief from the discomfort and fatigue associated with large myomas and their attendant bleeding. In that case, Chinese medicine can be used to prepare the woman for surgery and to speed her recovery afterwards.

Key patterns to memorize	
1. Blood heat	A. Replete heat B. Vacuity heat C. Depressive heat D. Damp heat
2. Blood stasis	
3. Vacuity patterns	A. Spleen vacuity B. Kidney qi not securing
4. Mixed repletion/vacuity pattern	Phlegm rheum

Addenda: Killed blood heart pain

If a woman has blood flooding and this is accompanied by heart pain, this is called killed blood heart pain.

Disease causes, disease mechanisms: This is associated with heart blood-spleen qi vacuity. In this case, there is a lack of free flow in the vessels of the heart due to insufficiency of qi and blood.

Main symptoms: Profuse uterine bleeding, thin, watery blood, heart pain, a sallow yellow facial complexion, fatigue, lassitude of the spirit, dizziness when standing up, lack of strength, shortness of breath, disinclination to speak, possible spontaneous perspiration on movement

Treatment principles: Use sweet, warm formulas to nourish and construct the qi and blood.

Guiding formula: Unnamed formula from *Zhong Yi Zhi Liao Fu Nu Bing (The Chinese Medical Treatment of Gynecological Diseases)*

Ingredients: Radix Codonopsitis Pilosulae (*Dang Shen*), earth stir-fried Rhizoma Atractylodis Macrocephalae (*Bai Zhu*), cooked Radix Rehmanniae (*Shu Di*), Radix Angelicae Sinensis (*Dang Gui*), Radix Ligustici Wallichii (*Chuan Xiong*), Radix Albus Paeoniae Lactiflorae (*Bai Shao*), Sclerotium Poriae Cocos (*Fu Ling*), mix-fried Radix Astragali Membranacei (*Huang Qi*), Cortex Cinnamomi Cassiae (*Rou Gui*), mix-fried Radix Glycyrrhizae (*Gan Cao*), uncooked Rhizoma Zingiberis (*Sheng Jiang*), Fructus Zizyphi Jujubae (*Hong Zao*)

Uterine myomas

Because uterine myomas are frequently the Western medical cause of flooding and leaking, especially in women in their late 30s and throughout their 40s, I have added three functional translations taken from the contemporary Chinese gynecological literature. The first is a textbook discussion of the treatment of uterine myomas based on pattern discrimination. This is then followed by two Chinese TCM journal articles with case histories, exemplifying their actual clinical treatment in the People's Republic of China today. In general, uterine myomas are considered a species of difficult to treat, knotty disease within TCM. If the myoma is larger than a robin's egg, its disappearance in less than six months of consistent TCM treatment is not likely. However, even though Chinese medicinals are not all that effective for shrinking and making fibroids disappear completely, they can often stop the flooding and leaking that commonly accompany fibroids.

(From *Zhong Yi Fu Ke Lin Chuang Jing Hua [The Clinical Effloresence of Chinese Medical Gynecology]*) by Wang Bo-jiu & Wang Qi-ming, Sichuan Science & Technology Press, Chengdu, 1989)

Treatment based on pattern discrimination

1. Qi stagnation blood stasis

Main symptoms: Uterine concretions and lumps, menstrual irregularity, menses amount profuse, premenstrual tension, painful menstruation, lumbar distention, soreness, and pain, a dark, purplish tongue, and a deep, choppy pulse

Treatment principles: Soften the hard and scatter nodulation, move the qi and quicken the blood

Guiding formulas:

1. *Jia Wei Gui Zhi Fu Ling Wan* (Added Flavors Cinnamon Twig & Poria Pills)

Ingredients: Ramulus Cinnamomi Cassiae (*Gui Zhi*), Semen Pruni Persicae (*Tao Ren*), Radix Rubrus Paeoniae Lactiflorae (*Chi Shao*), Cortex Radicis Moutan (*Dan Pi*), Semen Vaccariae Segetalis (*Wang Bu Liu Xing*), Herba Sargassii (*Hai Zao*), 40g @, Sclerotium Poriae Cocos (*Fu Ling*), Radix Angelicae Sinensis (*Dang Gui*), Spica Prunellae Vulgaris (*Xia Ku Cao*), Radix Bupleuri (*Chai Hu*), Radix Salviae Miltiorrhizae (*Dan Shen*), 60g @, Rhizoma Curcumae Zedoariae (*E Zhu*), Rhizoma Sparganii (*San Leng*), 30g @, vinegar stir-fried Carapax Amydae Sinensis (*Bie Jia*), Concha Ostreae (*Mu Li*), 50g @. Grind the above flavors into powder and make into pills with honey. Take 10 pills each time, three times each day.

2. *Ruan Jian Hua Yu Xiao Liu Fang* (Soften the Hard, Transform Stasis & Disperse Tumors Formula)

Ingredients: Radix Salviae Miltiorrhizae (*Dan Shen*), 15g, Herba Sargassii (*Hai Zao*), 15g, Spica Prunellae Vulgaris (*Xia Ku Cao*), 30g, Rhizoma Curcumae Zedoariae (*E Zhu*), 9g, Rhizoma Sparganii (*San Leng*), 9g, Thallus Algae (*Kun Bu*), 15g, Concha Cyclinae (*Hai Ge Ke*), 15g, Bulbus Fritillariae Thunbergii (*Zhe Bei Mu*), 9g, Radix Angelicae Sinensis (*Dang Gui*), 9g, *Ji Xue Teng Gao* (Milletia Paste), 15g, Cortex Radicis Moutan (*Dan Pi*), 9g, Resina Olibani (*Ru Xiang*), 6g, Resina Myrrhae (*Mo Yao*), 6g, Semen Citri Reticulatae (*Ju He*), 15g, Radix Cynanchi Atrati (*Bai Wei*), 15g. Make into fine powder and form into pills with honey. Each pill should weigh 10g. Take one pill each time, three times each day.

2. Cold congelation blood stasis

Main symptoms: Besides the qi stagnation and blood stasis manifestations discussed above, there is simultaneously a bluish green, grey or ashen facial complexion, dread of bodily chill, chilly abdominal pain, a bluish green tongue with thin, white fur, and a slow, choppy pulse.

Treatment principles: Warm the channels and scatter cold, quicken the blood and transform stasis

Guiding formulas:

1. *Jia Jian Jian Dan Dan* (Additions & Subtractions Glaring Elixir)

Ingredients: Radix Lateralis Praeparatus Aconiti Carmichaeli (*Fu Zi*), 40g, Flouritum (*Zi Shi Ying*), 30g, Radix Salviae Miltiorrhizae (*Dan Shen*), 40g, Cortex Cinnamomi Cassiae (*Rou Gui*), 20g, Rhizoma Corydalis Yanhusuo (*Yan Hu Suo*), 20g, Radix Auklandiae Lappae (*Guang Mu Xiang*), 20g, Sanguis Draconis (*Xue Jie*), 15g, Hirudo (*Shui Zhi*), 25g, Semen Arecae Catechu (*Bing Lang*), 25g, Semen Pruni Persicae (*Tao Ren*), 30g, Rhizoma Sparganii (*San Leng*), 30g, Squama Manitis Pentadactylis (*Jia Zhu*), 30g, Radix Codonopsitis Pilosulae (*Dang Shen*), 30g, Radix Angelicae Sinensis (*Dang Gui*), 30g, *Ji Xue Teng Gao* (Milletia Paste), 30g. Grind into fine powder. Dissolve the Milletia Paste in water and use this to make into pills. Take six to nine grams each time, three times each day.

2. *Jia Wei Xiang Leng Wan* (Added Flavors Fragrant Sparganium Pills)

Ingredients: Rhizoma Sparganii (*San Leng*), 6g, Pericarpium Citri Reticulatae Viride (*Qing Pi*), 9g, Fructus Meliae Toosendan (*Chuan Lian Zi*), 9g, Fructus Foeniculi Vulgaris (*Xiao Hui Xiang*), 9g, Rhizoma Curcumae Zedoariae (*E Zhu*), 6g, Cortex Cinnamomi Cassiae (*Rou Gui*), 6g, Radix Lateralis Praeparatus Aconiti Carmichaeli (*Fu Zi*), 6g, Radix Ligustici

Wallichii (*Chuan Xiong*), 9g, Radix Angelicae Sinensis (*Dang Gui*), 9g, Fructus Aurantii (*Zhi Ke*), 9g, Radix Bupleuri (*Chai Hu*), 10g, Semen Citri Reticulatae (*Ju He*), 15g, Spica Prunellae Vulgaris (*Xia Ku Cao*), 15g, Herba Sargassii (*Hai Zao*), 15g

3. Liver depression qi stagnation

Main symptoms: Headache, head distention, emotional depression, vexation and agitation, easy anger, chest, rib-side, and lower abdominal pain, vision problems, profuse dreams, diminished eating, indigestion, menstrual cycle abnormalities, dribbling and dripping without cease or flooding, a dark, red tongue with yellow fur, and a bowstring or bowstring, rapid pulse. The tongue may be red with no fur and the pulse may be bowstring, fine, and rapid.

Treatment methods: Soothe the liver and rectify the qi, quicken the blood and transform stasis

Guiding formulas:

1. *Jia Wei Chai Hu Shu Gan Tang* (Added Flavors Bupleurum Soothe the Liver Decoction)

Ingredients: Radix Bupleuri (*Chai Hu*), 9g, Radix Albus Paeoniae Lactiflorae (*Bai Shao*), 15g, Fructus Immaturus Aurantii (*Zhi Shi*), 9g, Radix Glycyrrhizae (*Gan Cao*), 3g, Radix Ligustici Wallichii (*Chuan Xiong*), 6g, Rhizoma Cyperi Rotundi (*Xiang Fu*), 9g, Cortex Radicis Moutan (*Dan Pi*), 9g, Fructus Gardeniae Jasminoidis (*Shan Zhi Zi*), 9g, Semen Citri Reticulatae (*Ju He*), 12g, green Folium Citri Reticulatae (*Ju Ye*), 9g, Radix Salviae Miltiorrhizae (*Dan Shen*), 30g, Semen Vaccariae Segetalis (*Wang Bu Liu Xing*), 12g, Pericarpium Citri Reticulatae Viride (*Qing Pi*), 9g

2. *Jia Wei Yi Guan Jian* (Added Flavors One Link Decoction)

Ingredients: Uncooked Radix Rehmanniae (*Sheng Di*), 30g, Tuber Ophiopogonis Japonici (*Mai Dong*), 12g, Fructus Meliae Toosendan (*Chuan Lian Zi*), 9g, Radix Angelicae Sinensis (*Dang Gui*), 9g, Radix Glehniae Littoralis (*Bai Sha Shen*), 9g, Fructus Lycii Chinensis (*Gou Qi*), 9g, Semen Citri Reticulatae (*Ju He*), 12g, Semen Litchi Sinensis (*Li Zhi He*), 12g, Semen Pruni Persicae (*Tao Ren*), 9g, Rhizoma Sparganii (*San Leng*), 6g, Rhizoma Curcumae Zedoariae (*E Zhu*), 6g

4. Damp heat pouring downward

Main symptoms: Vaginal discharge profuse in amount, sticky and slimy in consistency with a fishy, foul odor, lower abdominal sagging, distention, and pain, possible fever, lumbosacral soreness and distention, yellow or yellow, slimy tongue fur, and a slippery, rapid pulse

Treatment principles: Clear heat and resolve toxins, quicken the blood and transform stasis

Guiding formula: *Jin Lian Hong Jiang Jie Du Tang* **(Lonicera, Forsythia, Sargentodoxa & Patrinia Resolve Toxins Decoction)**

Ingredients: Flos Lonicerae Japonicae (*Jin Yin Hua*), 24g, Fructus Forsythiae Suspensae (*Lian Qiao*), 15g, Caulis Sargentodoxae (*Hong Teng*) 24g, Herba Patriniae Heterophyllae Cum Radice (*Bai Jiang Cao*), 24g, Semen Coicis Lachryma-jobi (*Yi Yi Ren*), 24g, Cortex Radicis Moutan (*Dan Pi*), 12g, Fructus Gardeniae Jasminoidis (*Shan Zhi Zi*), 9g, Radix Rubrus Paeoniae Lactiflorae (*Chi Shao*), 12g, Semen Pruni Persicae (*Tao Ren*), 9g, Rhizoma Corydalis Yanhusuo (*Yan Hu Suo*), 9g, processed Resina Myrrhae (*Ru Xiang*), 6g, processed Resina Myrrhae (*Mo Yao*), 6g, Fructus Meliae Toosendan (*Chuan Lian Zi*), 3 pieces

Additions: If qi and blood are insufficient, add Radix Codonopsitis Pilosulae (*Dang Shen*), Radix Angelicae Sinensis (*Dang Gui*), and Gelatinum Corii Asini (*E Jiao*). If the menses are profuse and the menstrual period is long, add Radix Rubiae Cordifoliae (*Qian Cao*), powdered Radix Pseudoginseng (*San Qi*, swallowed down with the decoction), and Herba Leonuri Heterophylli (*Yi Mu Cao*). If there is painful menstruation, add Feces Trogopterori Seu Pteromi (*Wu Ling Zhi*) and Pollen Typhae (*Pu Huang*). If there is loss of sleep, add Radix Polygoni Multiflori (*He Shou Wu*) or Caulis Polygoni Multiflori (*Ye Jiao Teng*) and Semen Zizyphi Spinosae (*Suan Zao Ren*).

Acupuncture treatment method:

Main points: *Guan Yuan* (CV 4), *Zi Hu* (right Ki 13), *Qi Hai* (CV 6), *Zhong Ji* (CV 3), *Bao Men* (left Ki 13)

Auxiliary points: *San Yin Jiao* (Sp 6), *Xue Hai* (Sp 10), *Zhong Wan* (CV 12), *Zu San Li* (St 36), *Nei Guan* (Per 6), *Guan Yuan Shu* (Bl 26), *Ge Shu* (Bl 17), *Shen Shu* (Bl 23)

Needling method: Each time, choose all the main points and two auxiliary points. Use medium strong stimulation and retain the needles from 20-30 minutes. Do one time each day, with 10-15 times equalling one course of treatment.

Although the above article does accurately identify the most commonly occurring species of repletion at work in this disease, it does not adequately deal with the spleen and/or kidney vacuities that usually also complicate these repletions or which, in fact, are the root mechanisms of these repletions.

(From "Chen Hui-lin's Experiences in Treating Uterine Myomas — Including an Analysis of the Clinical Data of 239 Cases" by Zeng Zhen & Shen Xiao-heng, *Shang Hai Zhong Yi Yao Za Zhi [Shanghai Journal of Chinese Medicine & Medicinals]*, #12, 1995, p. 3-5)

Chen Hui-lin is an old Chinese doctor with more than 50 years clinical experience who is especially good at gynecology. Dr. Chen treats uterine myomas on the basis of a Western medical diagnosis combined with Chinese medical pattern discrimination. Dr. Chen also bases his treatment on a combination of treatment based on pattern discrimination and treatment based on the menstrual cycle. Likewise, his treatment combines transforming stasis and dispersing and scattering myomas with supporting the righteous and banking the root, regulating and rectifying the *chong* and *ren*.

Integrated Western medicine diagnosis & Chinese medicine pattern discrimination

Prior to treatment, all Dr. Chen's gynecology patients receive a gynecological examination and ultrasonography in order to make a Western medical diagnosis. This is then combined with the pattern discrimination which is made on the basis of the clinical symptoms, tongue examination, and pulse examination. Dr. Chen divides uterine myoma patients into four basic patterns.

1. Qi stagnation blood stasis: Emotional depression, chest oppression, sighing, susceptibility to sorrow, excessive worry, bilateral premenstrual breast distention and pain, lower abdominal soreness and distention, a bowstring pulse, and thin tongue fur

2. Heat burning blood stasis: Vexation and agitation, easy anger, a dry mouth, a bitter taste in the mouth, difficult defecation, yellow urine, a rapid pulse

3. Cold congelation blood stasis: A bluish-greenish white facial complexion, fear of cold, chilled limbs, loose stools, clear urination, especially severe menstrual movement abdominal pain, liking for warmth, a pale tongue, and a tight pulse

4. Bodily vacuity blood stasis: Dizziness, lack of strength, lassitude of the spirit, low back and knee soreness and weakness, heart fluster, shortness of breath, a fine, forceless pulse, and a fat tongue with the marks of the teeth on its edges or a red tongue with scanty fur

Treatment method

Dr. Chen's main method of treating uterine myomas is to use *Zi Gong Ji Liu Fang* (Uterine Myoma Formula) with additions and subtractions depending on the symptoms. This formula is composed of: Rhizoma Sparganii (*San Leng*), Rhizom Curcumae Zedoariae (*E Zhu*), Radix Angelicae Sinensis (*Dang Gui*), Radix Salviae Miltiorrhizae (*Dan Shen*), Pericarpium Citri Reticulatae Viride (*Qing Pi*), Pericarpium Citri Reticulatae (*Chen Pi*), Fructus Aurantii (*Zhi Ke*), Radix Linderae Strychnifoliae (*Wu Yao*), Rhizoma Corydalis Yanhusuo (*Yuan Hu*), Rhizoma Pinelliae Ternatae (*Ban Xia*), Herba Sargassii (*Hai Zao*), Thallus Algae (*Kun Bu*), Concha Ostreae (*Mu Li*), Bulbus Fritillariae (*Bei Mu*), Fructus Germinatus Oryzae Sativae (*Gu Ya*), Fructus Germinatus Hordei Vulgaris (*Mai Ya*).

Additions: If there is cold congelation blood stasis, Dr. Chen adds Ramulus Cinnamomi Cassiae (*Gui Zhi*) and Herba Asari Cum Radice (*Xi Xin*). If there is burning heat blood stasis, Dr. Chen adds Radix Scutellariae Baicalensis (*Huang Qin*) and Radix Et Rhizoma Rhei (*Da Huang*). If there is bodily vacuity blood stasis, Dr. Chen adds Radix Astragali Membranacei (*Huang Qi*), Rhizoma Atractylodis Macrocephalae (*Bai Zhu*), Herba Epimedii (*Xian Ling Pi*), etc. If there is qi stagnation blood stasis, Dr. Chen adds double amounts of Sparganium and Zedoaria. From the cessation of menstruation, depending upon whether the body is strong or weak and depending on the accompanying clinical symptoms, Dr. Chen administers 10-20 packets [each month].

In order to increase the effect of dispersing and scattering the myoma, these are combined with *Hai Zao Jing* (Sargassium Crystals), *Xiao Jin Dan* (Small Golden Elixir), *Xia Ku Cao Gao* (Prunella Paste), or other such prepared [*i.e.*, patent] Chinese medicines. Mirabilitum (*Pi Xiao*) is applied externally to the affected area.

Modifying the treatment based on an integration of the clinical symptoms & the menstrual cycle

1. Heavy menstruation: One week prior to the onset of menstruation, *Zi Gong Ji Liu Fang* is halted and is replaced by *Gu Jing She Xue Fang* (Secure the Menses & Contain the Blood Formula). This consists of: Radix Codonopsitis Pilosulae (*Dang Shen*), Radix Astragali Membranacei (*Huang Qi*), Os Sepiae Seu Sepiellae (*Wu Zei Gu*), Semen Cuscutae (*Tu Si Zi*), Herba Agrimoniae Pilosae (*Xian He Cao*), Os Draconis (*Long Gu*), Concha Ostreae (*Mu Li*), Radix Sanguisorbae (*Di Yu*), *Shi Hui Wan* (Ten Ashes Pills), Herba Ecliptae Prostratae (*Han Lian Cao*), Fructus Rosae Laevigatae (*Jin Ying Zi*), Gelatinum Corii Asini (*E Jiao Zhu*), Rhizoma Bletillae Striatae (*Bai Ji*). If, after administering these medicinals, the bleeding is still excessive and will not stop, then the patient is also administered *Gong Xue*

Yi Hao Jiao Nang (Uterine Bleeding No. 1 Gelatin Capsules). These consist of: Carbonized Nodus Nelumbinis Nuciferae (*Ou Jie*), Fructus Terminaliae Chebulae (*He Zi*), Radix Pseudoginseng (*Shen San Qi*), and Rhizoma Bletillae Striatae (*Bai Ji*) ground up into powder and placed in gelatin capsules. These are given two to three pills each time, three times each day. Or dicyone, vitamin C, vitamin B₆, etc. are given by intravenous injection, one time each day continuously for three days.

2. Painful menstruation: Three to five days prior to the onset of menstruation, *Zi Gong Ji Liu Fang* is halted and is replaced by *Tong Jing Fang* (Painful Menstruation Formula). This is comprised of: Radix Angelicae Sinensis (*Dang Gui*), Semen Pruni Persicae (*Tao Ren*), Flos Carthami Tinctorii (*Hong Hua*), Radix Ligustici Wallichii (*Chuan Xiong*), Fructus Crataegi (*Shan Zha*), Radix Achryanthis Bidentatae (*Niu Xi*), Rhizoma Corydalis Yanhusuo (*Yuan Hu*), Fructus Aurantii (*Zhi Ke*), Rhizoma Cyperi Rotundi (*Xiang Fu*), Herba Lycopi Lucidi (*Ze Lan*), Radix Glycyrrhizae (*Gan Cao*), *Shi Xiao San* (Loose a Smile Powder). If aching and pain is especially severe, *Xiang Gui Huo Xue Gao* (Cyperus & Cinnamon Quicken the Blood Paste) plus *Qi Li San* (Seven *Li* Powder) are applied to *Guan Yuan* (CV 4), *Shen Que* (CV 8), and other painful spots. Or one can use Rhizoma Cyperi Rotundi (*Xiang Fu*), Cortex Cinnamomi Cassiae (*Rou Gui*), and Lignum Aquilariae Agallochae (*Chen Xiang*) stir-fried with salt and applied hot externally over the abdominal region.

3. Infertility: After the menses have ceased, *Zi Gong Ji Liu Fang* is administered with modifications based on pattern discrimination. However, in addition, suitable amounts of Herba Epimedii (*Xian Ling Pi*), Rhizoma Curculiginis Orchioidis (*Xian Mao*), Herba Cynomorii Songarici (*Suo Yang*), Radix Morindae Officinalis (*Ba Ji Tian*), etc. are added in order to supplement the kidneys and fill the essence. After the basal body temperature rises, *Zi Gong Ji Liu Fang* is halted and is replaced by *Fu Ke Tiao Li Fang* (Gynecological Regulating & Rectifying Formula). This formula consists of: Radix Codonopsitis Pilosulae (*Dang Shen*), Radix Astragali Membranacei (*Huang Qi*), Sclerotium Poriae Cocos (*Fu Ling*), Rhizoma Atractylodis Macrocephalae (*Bai Zhu*), Radix Angelicae Sinensis (*Dang Gui*), Radix Albus Paeoniae Lactiflorae (*Bai Shao*), Ramulus Loranthi Seu Visci (*Sang Ji Sheng*), Radix Dipsaci (*Chuan Duan*), Rhizoma Cobotii Barometsis (*Gou Ji*), Radix Glycyrrhizae (*Gan Cao*). During the menses, this is replaced by *Tong Guan Fang* (Free the Flow of the Tubes Formula). This formula is comprised of: Radix Angelicae Sinensis (*Dang Gui*), Radix Ligustici Wallichii (*Chuan Xiong*), Radix Salviae Miltiorrhizae (*Dan Shen*), Herba Leonuri Heterophylli (*Yi Mu Cao*), Flos Carthami Tinctorii (*Hong Hua*), Rhizoma Corydalis Yanhusuo (*Yuan Hu*), Tuber Curcumae (*Yu Jin*), Radix Achryanthis Bidentatae (*Niu Xi*), Folium Artemisiae Argyii (*Ai Ye*), Fructus Liquidambaris Taiwaniae (*Lu Lu Tong*), unidentified (*Hong Yue Li Hua*).

4. Anemia: After the cessation of menstruation, depending on whether the amount of blood discharged is excessive or scanty, five to seven packets of *Fu Ke Tiao Li Fang* are administered. If anemia is severe, Radix Codonopsitis Pilosulae (*Dang Shen*) and Radix Astragali Membranacei (*Huang Qi*) are used in amounts of up to 15-30 grams. In addition, Fructus Lycii Chinensis (*Qi Zi*), Gelatinum Corii Asini (*E Jiao*), and other such supplementing the blood medicinals are added. If lumbar soreness and pain are severe, *Yao Tong Fang* (Lumbar Pain Formula) is used. This consists of: Radix Angelicae Sinensis (*Dang Gui*), Radix Dipsaci (*Chuan Duan*), Ramulus Loranthi Seu Visci (*Sang Ji Sheng*), Radix Angelicae Pubescentis (*Du Huo*), Fructus Psoraleae Corylifoliae (*Bu Gu Zhi*), Radix Drynariae (*Gu Sui Bu*), Semen Cuscutae (*Tu Si Zi*), Cortex Eucommiae Ulmoidis (*Du Zhong*), *Qing E Wan* (Young Girl Pills). If vaginal discharge is excessive, *Zhi Dai Fang* (Treat Vaginal Discharge Formula) is used. This consists of: Uncooked Radix Rehmanniae (*Sheng Di*), Flos Celosiae Cristatae (*Ji Guan Hua*), Rhizoma Atractylodis Macrocephalae (*Bai Zhu*), Semen Nelumbinis Nuciferae (*Lian Rou*), Radix Ligustici Wallichii (*Chuan Xiong*), Rhizoma Atractylodis (*Cang Zhu*), Flos Dolichoris Lablab (*Bian Dou Hua*), Os Sepieae Seu Sepiellae (*Hai Piao Xiao*), black Fructuficatio Tremellae (*Hei Mu Er*), Concha Ostreae (*Mu Li*), *Zhen Ling Dan* (Shockingly Clever Elixir). If abdominal pain is severe even at ordinary times, *Fu Tong Fang* (Abdominal Pain Formula) is used. This is comprised of: Rhizoma Corydalis Yanhusuo (*Yuan Hu*), Rhizoma Atractylodis (*Cang Zhu*), Semen Arecae Catechu (*Bing Lang*), Rhizoma Alpiniae Officinari (*Gao Liang Jiang*), Sclerotium Poriae Cocos (*Fu Ling*), Cortex Cinnamomi Cassiae (*Rou Gui*), Flos Caryophylli (*Ding Xiang*), Rhizoma Sparganii (*San Leng*), Rhizoma Zedoariae (*E Zhu*), Pericarpium Citri Reticulatae Viride (*Qing Pi*), Fructus Amomi (*Sha Ren*), Rhizoma Cyperi Rotundi (*Xiang Fu*).

To any of the above formulas, Spica Prunellae Vulgaris (*Xia Ku Cao*), Concha Ostreae (*Mu Li*), Bulbus Frtillariae (*Bei Mu*), Rhizoma Dioscoreae Bulbiferae (*Huang Yao Zi*), Herba Sargassii (*Hai Zao*), Endothelium Corneum Gigeriae Galli (*Ji Nei Jin*), etc. can be added in order to soften the hard and scatter nodulation. In those over 50 years of age, if their menses still are shifting, *Ling Zhi Wan* (Campsis & Anemarrhena Pills) are also administered in order to look forward to an early cessation of menstruation. This formula is comprised of: Flos Campsitis (*Ling Xiao Hua*), Rhizoma Anemarrhenae Aspheloidis (*Zhi Mu*), Rhizoma Alismatis (*Ze Xie*), Cortex Phellodendri (*Huang Bai*), Radix Sophorae Flavescentis (*Ku Shen*), Cortex Radicis Moutan (*Dan Pi*), Glauberitum (*Han Shi Shi*), etc. If menstruation is profuse, then radiation of the ovaries may also be used to cease menstruation.

Clinical survey

Between Feb. 1990 and December 1993, Dr. Chen treated 154 cases of uterine myoma based on pattern discrimination as described above. These were referred to as Dr. Chen's group. These were compared to 85 women with uterine myomas who received treatment with *Gui Zhi Fu Ling Chong Ji* (Cinnamon Twig & Poria Soluble Granules). These were referred to as the *Gui Ling* group. In Dr. Chen's group, the youngest woman was 23 and the oldest was 55, with a median age of 37.65 plus or minus 10.47 years. In the *Gui Ling* group, the youngest woman was 22 and the oldest was 56, with a median age of 38.21 plus or minus 9.97 years. In Dr. Chen's group, the shortest course of disease was two months and the longest was 10 years, with a median duration of 18.42 plus or minus 27.38 months. In the *Gui Ling* group, the shortest course of disease was three months and the longest was nine years, with a median duration of 19.21 plus or minus 30.21 months. In Dr. Chen's group, 39 women were not married and 154 were married. Of the married women, 35 had not given birth, while 80 had already given birth. In the *Gui Ling* group, 27 women were not married and 58 women were married. Of these married women, 18 had not given birth and 40 had already given birth.

In Dr. Chen's group, 69 women's uteri were enlarged similar to 50-60 days of pregnancy, 62 to more than two months of pregnancy, and 23 to more than three months of pregnancy. Fifty-one had painful menstruation, 85 had profuse menstruation, 37 had lengthened menstruation, 77 had lumbar soreness and pain, 43 had increased vaginal discharge, and 37 had anemia. In the *Gui Ling* group, in 35 cases, their uteri were enlarged similar to 50-60 days of pregnancy, 33 to more than two months of pregnancy, and 17 to more than three months of pregnancy. Twenty-nine had painful menstruation, 45 had profuse menstruation, 22 had lengthened menstruation, 41 had lumbar soreness and pain, 24 had increased vaginal discharge, and 21 had anemia.

The women in the *Gui Ling* group received *Gui Zhi Fu Ling Chong Ji* manufactured by the No. 2 Shanghai Chinese Medicinal Co. These consist of: Ramulus Cinnamomi Cassaie (*Gui Zhi*), Sclerotium Poriae Cocos (*Fu Ling*), Radix Paeoniae Lactilforae (*Shao Yao*), Cortex Radicis Moutan (*Dan Pi*), Semen Pruni Persicae (*Tao Ren*). A half packet was taken each time, two times each day. Treatment for one whole month equalled one course of treatment and everyone in this study was treated for three whole months or more. After treatment, all these women underwent gynecological examinations and ultrasonography in order to determine the size of their uteri and changes in their clinical symptoms were assessed. Treatment efficacy was ascertained using the Ridit analysis method.

Criteria of treatment outcomes

Markedly effective: The uterus became smaller or the main accompanying conditions took a turn for the better or disappeared.

Effective: There was no change in the size of the uterus. However, the main accompanying conditions either were improved or disappeared.

Ineffective: There was no change in the size of the uterus or it got larger and there was no marked change in the accompanying conditions.

Treatment outcomes

Dr. Chen's protocol was judged markedly effective in 48 cases, effective in 89 cases, and ineffective in 17 cases. Thus the total effectiveness rate in Dr. Chen's group was 88.96%. In the *Gui Ling* group, that protocol was judged markedly effective in 19 cases, effective in 44 cases, and ineffective in 22 cases. Thus the total effectiveness rate in the *Gui Ling* group was 74.12%. This means that there was a marked statistical difference in effect between these two groups (P <0.01). Further, in Dr. Chen's group, 83.76% of the cases experienced some reduction in size of their uteri, while in the comparison group, only 65.88% experienced a reduction in the size of their uteri. Among those women with uteri similar to 50-60 days of pregnancy, Dr. Chen's protocol was very markedly more effective than the *Gui Ling* protocol. However, in those women whose uteri were two to three months of pregnancy or more in size, there was no marked difference in effect between these two protocols. In terms of profuse menstruation and anemia, Dr. Chen's protocol was markedly more effective (P<0.05). In terms of the painful menstruation, lengthened menstruation, lumbar soreness and pain, and increased vaginal discharge, Dr. Chen's protocol was somewhat more effective than the comparison protocol, but this difference was not statistically significant.

Dr. Chen's protocol was 90.7% effective in women with the qi stagnation blood stasis pattern. It was 89.84% effective in women with the cold congelation blood stasis pattern. It was 80.77% effective in women with the heat burning blood stasis pattern. And it was 91.49% effective in women with the bodily vacuity blood stasis pattern. Based on Ridit analysis method, the differences in effect between these four groups was not marked (P>0.05). In the *Gui Ling* group, that protocol was 65.22% effective in those with qi stagnation blood stasis pattern, was 95% effective for those with cold congelation blood stasis pattern, was 52.63% effective for those with heat burning blood stasis pattern, and was 82.61% in those with bodily vacuity blood stasis pattern. These differences were marked statistically significant (P<0.05). Those with the cold congelation pattern got the best effect, those with the bodily vacuity pattern got the second best effect, those with the qi stagnation pattern got the third best effect, and those with the heat burning pattern got the least effect from the *Gui Zhi Fu Ling Chong Ji* protocol. In comparison, Dr. Chen's patients with the burning heat blood stasis pattern and the qi stagnation blood stasis pattern got a markedly better treatment effect than the women in the *Gui Ling* group with those same patterns experienced. The difference in effect between the members of the two groups with the other two patterns was not statistically significant (P > 0.05).

(From "The Treatment of 45 Cases of Uterine Myoma with *Bu Zhong Yi Qi Tang Jia Jian* [Supplement the Center & Boost the Qi Decoction with Additions & Subtractions]" by Wang Dao-qing *et al.*, *Zhe Jiang Zhong Yi Za Zhi [Zhejiang Journal of Traditional Chinese Medicine]*, #1, 1994, p. 15)

Uterine myoma is a commonly seen benign tumor in gynecology departments. It is categorized in our national medicine (*i.e.*, TCM) as concretions and conglomerations. The authors have used *Bu Zhong Yi Qi Tang* with additions and subtractions to treat this disease with good results.

Of the 45 women treated with this protocol, 17 were between 25-39 years of age, 25 between 40-49, and three were 50 years old or older. The disease course had lasted from two to 12 months in 25 cases, one to two years in 18 cases, and three to five years in two cases. Diagnosis was based on ultrasonography and all these women's uteri were approximately the size of a three month pregnant woman's. Most of these women also had profuse menstruation, prolonged menstruation, a shortened cycle, abdominal distention and hardness, and other such symptoms.

The formula consisted of: Radix Astragali Membranacei (*Huang Qi*), Thallus Algae (*Kun Bu*), Os Draconis (*Long Gu*), and Concha Ostreae (*Mu Li*), 30g @, Radix Codonopsitis Pilosulae (*Dang Shen*), Rhizoma Atractylodis Macrocephalae (*Bai Zhu*), Pericarpium Citri Reticulatae (*Chen Pi*), Herba Cistanchis Deserticolae (*Rou Cong Rong*), Spica Prunellae Vulgaris (*Xia Ku Cao*), and Herba Sargassii (*Hai Zao*), 15g @, and Rhizoma Cimicifugae (*Sheng Ma*) and Radix Bupleuri (*Chai Hu*), 10g @. These were decocted in water and administered, one *ji* per day divided in morning and evening doses.

If there was excessive precipitation of blood, carbonized Radix Sanguisorbae (*Di Yu*) and Herba Agrimoniae Pilosae (*Xian He Cao*), 15g @, were added. In addition, *Yun Nan Bai Yao* (Yunnan White Medicine), was given two times per day, 0.5g per dose. If there was abdominal pain, Feces Trogopterori Seu Pteromi (*Wu Ling Zhi*) and stir-fried Pollen Typhae (*Chao Pu Huang*), 9g @, were added. If there was blood heat, uncooked Radix Rehmanniae (*Sheng Di*) and Radix Scutellariae Baicalensis (*Huang Qin*), 15g @, were added. If there was blood vacuity, Radix Angelicae Sinensis (*Dang Gui Shen*), 6g, and Gelatinum Corii Asini (*E Jiao*), 9g, were added. If there was downward leaking which would not stop or a continuous yellow abnormal vaginal discharge, Flos Immaturus Sophorae Japonicae (*Huai Hua*), 6g, and Hallyositum Rubrum (*Chi Shi Zhi*), 10g, were added. If the precipitated blood was not excessive or after treatment the precipitated blood became less, Rhizoma Sparganii (*San Leng*) and Rhizoma Curcumae Zedoariae (*E Zhu*), 10g @, were added. In addition, *Bu Zhong Yi Qi Wan* (Supplement the Center & Boost the Qi Pills) were administered two times per day, nine grams per dose.

After administering from 20-60 *ji* of these medicinals, 20 cases were cured. This meant that their symptoms disappeared, that their myomas were dispersed and scattered, and that their uteri were normal. Eighteen cases were obviously improved. This meant that their symptoms disappeared and that their myoma was 1/3 the size or smaller than when treatment began. Five cases got some improvement. This meant that their symptoms obviously diminished but their myomas did not obviously get smaller. And two cases experienced no improvement. Thus, the total amelioration rate was 95.5%.

Case history: Liu X X, 35 years old, Yi nationality. This woman's menses had been excessive for the last five years. She also experienced prolonged menstruation which lasted from six to fifteen days. The amount of the menstruate was excessive, dark purplish, and contained clots. She also had heart palpitations, lack of strength, a distended, hard abdomen, a bowstring pulse, and a dark red tongue with thin, yellow fur. Ultrasonography revealed a uterine myoma 6.6 x 5.1 x 4.5cm in size. The patient was given the basic formula with uncooked Radix Rehmanniae (*Sheng Di*), Radix Scutellariae Baicalensis (*Huang Qin*), carbonized Radix Sanguisorbae (*Di Yu*), and Herba Agrimoniae Pilosae (*Xian He Cao*), 15g @. In addition, she was given *Yun Nan Bai Yao*, 0.5g per dose, two times per day.

After nine *ji*, her bleeding had diminished and her abdominal hardness and distention had also lessened. Therefore, she was given the basic formula with Rhizoma Sparganii (*San Leng*) and Rhizoma Curcumae Zedoariae (*E Zhu*), 10g @. *Yun Nan Bai Yao* was suspended and *Bu Zhong Yi Qi Wan* were given, nine grams each time, two times per day. After another 24 *ji*, her menstrual cycle was normal, ultrasonography showed that the uterine myoma had disappeared, her uterus was normal, and the disease was cured.

According to the authors' discussion, qi is the commander of the blood. Therefore, blood follows the movement of the qi. If the channels and network vessels are open and free flowing, the entire body is constructed and nourished. Conversely, qi vacuity may lead to stasis. If the qi stagnates, the blood will become static. In addition, if the qi is vacuous, it may not be able to contain the blood and thus the blood will be lost. If there is qi vacuity, the blood will not throb (*i.e.*, pulse or move) smoothly and there will be blood stasis. If there is qi vacuity, there may also be downward fall. Blood will stagnate in the uterus and become gatherings and accumulations over many days. This then can become a tumor.

Based on the ancient saying, "In order to treat the blood, treat the qi", *Bu Zhong Yi Qi Tang Jia Jian* may be used to treat this condition. Within that formula, Codonopsis and Astragalus supplement the center and boost the qi. Orange Peel and Atractylodes fortify the spleen and rectify the qi. Bupleurum and Cimicifuga upbear the fallen and guard the qi. Dragon Bone, Oyster Shell, and Cistanches soften the hard and scatter nodulation while boosting the essence qi. Prunella scatters stasis binding and disperses tumors. Sargassium and Algae disperse and transform concretions and conglomerations. Uncooked Rehmannia, Scutellaria, carbonized Sanguisorba, and Agrimonia cool the blood and stop bleeding. Sparganium and Zedoaria quicken the blood and transform stasis. Feces Trogopeterori and stir-fried Pollen Typhae move stasis and stop pain. Dang Gui and Donkey Skin Glue supplement and nourish the blood. Flos Immaturus Sophorae and Hallyositum Rubrum clear damp heat and secure desertion. Thus taken as a whole, this formula is able to transform stasis without stirring the blood and to stop bleeding without retaining stasis. Thus stasis is dispelled without damaging the righteous, the tumor is dispersed, and the disease is cured.

7

Blocked Menstruation

Amenorrhea is called *jing bi* or *bi jing* in Chinese Medicine. *Bi* means blockage or something that is closed or shut. *Jing* refers to the menses. As a compound term, *bi jing* gives just the opposite impression of flooding and leaking. In blocked menstruation, the door or dam is shut closed or obstructed, while in flooding and leaking, the door or dam is open or leaking. Blocked menstruation is also sometimes referred to as *bu yue* or no moon or monthly flow. The term blocked menstruation in Chinese clearly identifies this as a pathological absence of menstruation as distinct from normal menopause which is not pathological. In other words, it is not merely the absence of menstruation but a pathological absence of menstruation. Therefore, I have chosen to stick to the literal Chinese name for this disease category rather than using the Western medical term amenorrhea which does simply translate from Greek as no monthly flow.

If a woman has not menstruated by the time she is 18 years old, this is defined as primary amenorrhea. Whereas, if a woman's menstrual cycle has become established but then ceases for three months or more, this is called secondary amenorrhea. Primary and secondary amenorrhea are Western medical categories which have been adopted by modern TCM.

Blocked menstruation often evolves from delayed menstruation and/or scanty menstruation. It is essentially a problem of not bleeding or discharging blood when and as one should.

Disease causes, disease mechanisms

Because blocked menstruation is a species of not discharging blood when the woman should, its mechanisms are only two. Either there is not enough blood to fill to overflowing the uterus on a regular basis or something is inhibiting the free flow of blood, thus preventing its discharge.

If there is not enough blood to fill the chalice of the uterus or sea of blood, this can be due to either failure in its engenderment and transformation or consumption and wasting of the blood. If faulty or insufficient blood engenderment and transformation is the cause, one must once again go back to the three viscera which engender and transform the blood — the heart, spleen, and kidneys.

Emotional disturbances can cause the heart to fail to perform its function of turning the blood red. Overthinking, worry, lack of exercise, excessive fatigue, insufficient nutrition, and faulty diet, *i.e.*, eating too many sweets, too much chilled, uncooked, or fluid engendering foods, may damage the spleen and hinder the latter heaven root of blood production. Or, due to congenital insufficiency, excessive sex, prolonged and unremitting fatigue, enduring disease, drug abuse, oral contraceptive use, and age, the kidneys may become vacuous and debilitated. Since the kidneys are the former heaven root of blood production and since the essence and blood share a common source, kidney vacuity may also result in insufficient blood production.

It is also possible that, though blood production is unimpaired, the blood that is made is being consumed and wasted. This may be due to excessive fluid loss, since it is said that blood and fluids share a common source. For instance, profuse sweating during a febrile disease may result in consumption of the blood. Not only that, but heat may also damage and consume the blood. If there is chronic fever, even a low-grade one, this may damage the blood as well. Therefore, blocked menstruation may be encountered as the sequela of a *wen bing* or warm disease. In addition, excessive blood loss during birth or following a bout of flooding or leaking or excessive consumption of blood and yin due to numerous pregnancies and prolonged breast-feeding may all also consume the blood and lead to blocked menstruation.

In terms of evil qi blocking or obstructing the free flow of menstrual blood, there are three main types of blockage. The first is damp cold congelation and stagnation resulting in blood stasis. This may be due to exposure to dampness and cold, such as encountered in China where there is no central heating and women may have to work outside, for instance in rice paddies, exposed for long hours to dampness and cold. Cold congeals and constricts the blood and causes stasis. While dampness is a yin evil which obstructs and hinders the free flow of yang qi which is responsible for moving the blood. Evil dampness and cold may also be engendered by overeating fluid-engendering, uncooked, or chilled foods and especially eating cold, frozen, chilled foods and drinks just before the expected onset of the menses such as ice cream, frozen yogurt, and chilled, refrigerated juices.

The second cause of blockage and obstruction is due to qi stagnation and blood stasis. Due to emotional upset, stress, and frustration, liver qi may become depressed and bound. The qi moves the blood and the liver rules coursing and discharge. If liver depression qi stagnation arises, it may, over time, result in blood stasis. However, blood stasis may also be caused directly by trauma, iatrogenesis, and chronic disease. If blood stasis arises before liver qi, because blood is the mother of the qi, eventually the qi will tend to become stagnant as well. Since the emotions are the subjective experience of the flow of qi, this is one reason why blood stasis often also causes emotional disturbances.

The third cause of blockage of the menses is phlegm dampness. As mentioned above, phlegm can obstruct the *jing* and this *jing* can mean both the channels and the menses. Whereas, dampness can obstruct the free flow of qi. Phlegm dampness is mostly due to faulty diet and lack of exercise, although some people are constitutionally predisposed to this condition. Typically, over time, phlegm dampness becomes complicated by stagnant qi and blood stasis.

Therefore, it is said in the *Nei Jing Su Wen (Inner Classic Simple Questions)*: "If the menstrual matter does not come, the *bao mai* is blocked." Zhang Zhong-jing, in the *Jin Gui Yao Lue (Essentials from the Golden Cabinet)*, amplified this when he said: "Women's diseases caused by vacuity, accumulation chill, or bound qi may result in the menstrual water being cut off." And Zhu Dan-xi reiterated these same facts when he said:

> If the menses are not free-flowing, this may be due to induced abortions and excessive births. Suffering from tidal fever may use up the blood. Emission of night sweats may consume the blood. Or disharmony of the spleen and stomach and diminished intake of food and drink may not engender the blood ... Or the seven affects may damage the heart and heart qi may become stuck and bound. Thus diseased blood cannot move.

Treatment based on pattern discrimination

Han Bai-ling says that treatment of blocked menstruation should be predicated on the four examinations and eight principles, a discrimination of the causes of the disease and also on the place or part that is diseased. In other words, blocked menstruation should be categorized as to viscera or bowels, channel or network vessels, vacuity or repletion, cold or heat. Following this methodology, vacuity should be supplemented, repletion should be drained, cold should be warmed, and heat should be cleared. This is a basic recapitulation of TCM's treatment based on pattern discrimination methodology.

Vacuity patterns

1. Qi & blood vacuity weakness

Main symptoms: The menses become progressively later and scantier. The color of the blood is pale. This eventually evolves into blocked menstruation. The facial complexion is sallow yellow. There is dizziness and vertigo, heart palpitations, shortness of breath, lassitude of the spirit, weak limbs, lusterless hair, reduced food intake, loose stools, a pale tongue, and a fine, relaxed (retarded), weak; deep, and retarded; or fine, small, forceless pulse.

Treatment principles: Boost the qi and fortify the spleen, nourish the blood and free the flow of the menses

Guiding formulas:

1. *Ren Shen Yang Rong Tang Jia Jian* (Ginseng Nourish the Constructive Decoction) according to Han Bai-ling

Ingredients: Radix Codonopsitis Pilosulae (*Dang Shen*), Radix Albus Paeoniae Lactiflorae (*Bai Shao*), Rhizoma Atractylodis Macrocephalae (*Bai Zhu*), Sclerotium Poriae Cocos (*Fu Ling*), Radix Glycyrrhizae (*Gan Cao*), Radix Angelicae Sinensis (*Dang Gui*), cooked Radix Rehmanniae (*Shu Di*), Radix Salviae Miltiorrhizae (*Dan Shen*), Fructus Craetagi (*Shan Zha*), Radix Astragali Membranacei (*Huang Qi*), Radix Cyathulae Officinalis (*Chuan Niu Xi*)

2. *Ren Shen Yang Rong Tang Jia Jian* (Ginseng Nourish the Constructive Decoction) according to Zhang En-qin *et al.*

Ingredients: Radix Panacis Ginseng (*Ren Shen*), Radix Astragali Membranacei (*Huang Qi*), Rhizoma Atractylodis Macrocephalae (*Bai Zhu*), Sclerotium Poriae Cocos (*Fu Ling*), Fructus Schisandrae Chinensis (*Wu Wei Zi*), Radix Angelicae Sinensis (*Dang Gui*), cooked Radix Rehmanniae (*Shu Di*), Radix Albus Paeoniae Lactiflorae (*Bai Shao*), Cortex Cinnamomi Cassiae (*Rou Gui*), Placenta Hominis (*Zi He Che*)

Additions: For blocked menstruation due to profuse postpartum bleeding, add Cornu Parvum Cervi (*Lu Rong*).

3. *Nu Ke Ba Zhen Wan Jia Jian* (Women's Eight Pearls Pills with Additions & Subtractions)

Ingredients: Stir-fried Radix Codonopsitis Pilosulae (*Dang Shen*), stir-fried Rhizoma Atractylodis Macrocephalae (*Bai Zhu*), uncooked Radix Astragali Membranacei (*Huang Qi*), mix-fried Radix Glycyrrhizae (*Gan Cao*), whole Radix Angelicae Sinensis (*Quan Dang Gui*), stir-fried Radix Ligustici Wallichii (*Chuan Xiong*), Radix Albus Paeoniae Lactiflorae (*Bai Shao*), Semen Leonuri Heterophylli (*Chong Wei Zi*), processed Rhizoma Cyperi Rotundi (*Xiang Fu*), Flos Carthami Tinctorii (*Hong Hua*)

This formula's ingredients presuppose a degree of qi stagnation and blood stasis complicating what otherwise is a predominantly vacuity condition.

4. Unnamed formula from *Concise Traditional Chinese Gynecology*

Ingredients: Radix Angelicae Sinensis (*Dang Gui*), Radix Albus Paeoniae Lactiflorae (*Bai Shao*), Radix Astragali Membranacei (*Huang Qi*), Radix Codonopsitis Pilosulae (*Dang Shen*), Pericarpium Citri Reticulatae (*Chen Pi*), Radix Salviae Miltiorrhizae (*Dan Shen*)

As quoted above, the *Nei Jing (Inner Classic)* says that, if there is blocked menstruation, the *bao mai* is blocked. The *bao mai* is the vessel which connects the heart to the uterus. Therefore, to say that the *bao mai* is blocked implies some involvement with the heart. The inclusion of Salvia in this formula takes this viscus's involvement into account.

5. *Shi Quan Da Bu Tang* (Ten [Ingredients] Completely & Greatly Supplementing Decoction)

Ingredients: Radix Astragali Membranacei (*Huang Qi*), Cortex Cinnamomi Cassiae (*Rou Gui*), Radix Panacis Ginseng (*Ren Shen*), cooked Radix Rehmanniae (*Shu Di*), Rhizoma Atractylodis Macrocephalae (*Bai Zhu*), Radix Angelicae Sinensis (*Dang Gui*), Radix Albus Paeoniae Lactiflorae (*Bai Shao*), Radix Ligustici Wallichii (*Chuan Xiong*), Sclerotium Poriae Cocos (*Fu Ling*), mix-fried Radix Glycyrrhizae (*Gan Cao*)

Song and Yu recommend this formula for women whose blood has become vacuous postpartum by excessive breast-feeding.

Additions: Guo Yuan recommends this formula for blocked menstruation due to qi and blood, yin and yang vacuity. In this case, Guo recommends adding Radix Morindae Officinalis (*Ba Ji Tian*) and Pericarpium Citri Reticulatae (*Chen Pi*).

6. *Bu Zhong Yi Qi Tang* (Supplement the Center & Boost the Qi Decoction)

Ingredients: Radix Astragali Membranacei (*Huang Qi*), Radix Panacis Ginseng (*Ren Shen*), Rhizoma Atractylodis Macrocephalae (*Bai Zhu*), mix-fried Radix Glycyrrhizae (*Gan Cao*), Radix Angelicae Sinensis (*Dang Gui*), Pericarpium Citri Reticulatae (*Chen Pi*), Rhizoma Cimicifugae (*Sheng Ma*), Radix Bupleuri (*Chai Hu*)

Song and Yu give this as a guiding formula for blocked menstruation due primarily to spleen and stomach vacuity weakness.

7. *Gui Pi Tang* (Restore the Spleen Decoction)

Ingredients: Radix Panacis Ginseng (*Ren Shen*), Radix Astragali Membranacei (*Huang Qi*), Rhizoma Atractylodis Macrocephalae (*Bai Zhu*), Sclerotium Poriae Cocos (*Fu Ling*), Semen Zizyphi Spinosae (*Suan Zao Ren*), Arillus Euphoriae Longanae (*Long Yan Rou*), Radix

Auklandiae Lappae (*Mu Xiang*), mix-fried Radix Glycyrrhizae (*Gan Cao*), Radix Angelicae Sinensis (*Dang Gui*), mix-fried Radix Polygalae Tenuifoliae (*Yuan Zhi*)

Han Bai-ling gives this as a guiding formula for the treatment of blocked menstruation primarily due to spleen qi-heart blood vacuity. In this case, there is no abdominal distention or pain. The facial complexion is pale white. The tongue is pale and moist. There is dizziness and impaired memory, heart palpitations and sweating, continuous white vaginal discharge, lack of warmth of the four extremities, reduced appetite for food and drink, wasting and emaciation of the muscles and flesh, loose stools, facial edema and swollen extremities, and a vacuous, relaxed (retarded) pulse.

Additions & subtractions: The authors of *Zhong Yi Fu Ke Xue (A Study of Chinese Medical Gynecology)* suggest that if worry has caused vacuity detriment to the spleen, one should remove Auklandia and Dang Gui and add Radix Astragali Membranacei (*Huang Qi*), Fructus Psoraleae Corylifoliae (*Bu Gu Zhi*), Rhizoma Cyperi Rotundi (*Xiang Fu*), and Pericarpium Citri Reticulatae (*Chen Pi*). Yu Yo-yuan has a very interesting discussion of this formula under women without moon (flow). Based on a quote from the *Nei Jing (Inner Classic)*, Yu says that the heart and spleen may be damaged by unjustifiable desires for the unobtainable. Such desires cause depression in the heart. The heart is not able to engender the blood and the blood is not able to nourish the spleen. The stomach then loses its ability to absorb and receive. Water and grains decline and become scanty, and the finest essence qi is not transformed. The blood vessels, therefore, wither and the menstrual matter is not able to periodically descend. For this, Yu Yo-yuan recommends using *Gui Pi Tang* with Cornu Cervi Parvum (*Lu Rong*) and Tuber Ophiopogonis Japonici (*Mai Men Dong*). Yu then quotes Wu Shu-qing that if a person has hidden feelings and unjustifiable desires, it is difficult for them to relax. This leads to depression and lack of ease. Lack of ease leads to the heart qi not being open and the spleen qi not transforming. Water and grains become scanty and are not able to be transformed into qi and blood. The sea of blood is not filled and thus there is no menstruation. Wu Shu-qing advises that, for this condition, *Gui Pi Tang* should be used plus Radix Albus Paeoniae Lactiflorae (*Bai Shao*) and Radix Bupleuri (*Chai Hu*). If there is fever and emaciation, the wasting is due to the stomach's governing the flesh and muscles. In this case, use *Gui Pi Tang* with Cortex Radicis Moutan (*Dan Pi*), Fructus Gardeniae Jasminoidis (*Zhi Zi*), Cortex Radicis Lycii Chinensis (*Di Gu Pi*), and Radix Albus Paeoniae Lactiflorae (*Bai Shao*).

8. *Fu Zi Li Zhong Wan Jia Jian* (Aconite Rectify the Center Pills with Additions & Subtractions)

Ingredients: Radix Lateralis Praeparatus Aconiti Carmichaeli (*Fu Zi*), Radix Panacis Ginseng (*Ren Shen*), Rhizoma Atractylodis Macrocephalae (*Bai Zhu*), dry Rhizoma Zingiberis

(*Gan Jiang*), mix-fried Radix Glycyrrhizae (*Gan Cao*), Radix Morindae Officinalis (*Ba Ji Tian*), Fructus Psoraleae Corylifoliae (*Bu Gu Zhi*), Radix Angelicae Sinensis (*Dang Gui*), Radix Astragali Membranacei (*Huang Qi*)

Guo Yuan suggests this formula for the treatment of blocked menstruation due to spleen-kidney yang vacuity. Guo gives the signs and symptoms of this pattern as menstruation behind schedule or blocked menstruation, a yellowish white or sallow white facial complexion, facial edema, swollen lower limbs, wheezing and heart palpitations due to movement, sweating, lack of warmth in the hands and feet, fear of cold, desire for warmth, soreness and weakness of the low back and knees, diminished appetite, loose stools, a pale tongue with thin, white fur, and a deep, fine, or vacuous pulse. This formula is then prescribed based on the principles of warming yang and fortifying the spleen, nourishing the blood and freeing the flow of the menses.

9. *Shen Ling Bai Zhu San Jia Gui Xiong* (Ginseng, Poria & Atractylodes Powder plus Dang Gui & Ligusticum)

Ingredients: Radix Panacis Ginseng (*Ren Shen*), Semen Nelumbinis Nuciferae (*Lian Zi Rou*), Radix Dioscoreae Oppositae (*Shan Yao*), Rhizoma Atractylodis Macrocephalae (*Bai Zhu*), Sclerotium Poriae Cocos (*Fu Ling*), Semen Dolichoris Lablab (*Bai Bian Dou*), Semen Coicis Lachryma-jobi (*Yi Yi Ren*), Fructus Amomi (*Sha Ren*), Radix Platycodi Grandiflori (*Jie Geng*), mix-fried Radix Glycyrrhizae (*Gan Cao*), Radix Angelicae Sinensis (*Dang Gui*), Radix Ligustici Wallichii (*Chuan Xiong*)

This formula is for the treatment of qi and blood vacuity blocked menstruation with an emphasis on spleen qi vacuity.

2. Liver-kidney insufficiency

Main symptoms: If a young woman has reached 18 years of age and her menses have not come, if at the beginning of the tide it is comparatively slow or tardy, or if the menses come but they eventually become later and scantier and evolve into blocked menstruation, this is suggestive of liver-kidney vacuity. Other signs and symptoms include a dark, gloomy facial complexion, dizziness and tinnitus, soreness and weakness of the low back and knees, possibly a dry mouth and throat, tidal fever, night sweats, both cheeks tidally red, heat in the center of the hands, feet, and heart, dry skin, dry, astringent eyelids, constipation, scanty, reddish urination, heart palpitations, either a red or a pale tongue with scant fur, and a deep, bowstring or deep, fine pulse. However, it is also possible to find a floating pulse at the inch and/or cubit positions if yin fails to control yang.

This pattern is a combination of liver blood and kidney yin vacuities. If kidney yin is more vacuous, the tongue will be red and the pulse will be fine. If liver blood is more vacuous, the tongue will be pale with a possible red tip and the pulse will be bowstring. The exact presenting signs and symptoms also depend on how much vacuity heat is present. If there is vacuity heat, the pulse will also be rapid.

Treatment principles: Supplement the kidneys, nourish the liver, and regulate the menses. If there is vacuity heat, the principles are to nourish yin and clear heat.

Guiding formulas:

1. *Liu Wei Di Huang Wan Jia Jian* (Six Flavors Rehmannia Pills with Additions & Subtractions)

Ingredients: Cooked Radix Rehmanniae (*Shu Di*), Fructus Corni Officinalis (*Shan Zhu Rou*), Cortex Radicis Moutan (*Dan Pi*), Sclerotium Poriae Cocos (*Fu Ling*), Radix Dioscoreae Oppositae (*Shan Yao*), Radix Angelicae Sinensis (*Dang Gui*), Radix Albus Paeoniae Lactiflorae (*Bai Shao*), Gelatinum Corii Asini (*E Jiao*), Caulis Milletiae Seu Spatholobi (*Ji Xue Teng*), Radix Cyathulae Officinalis (*Chuan Niu Xi*), Herba Epimedii (*Xian Ling Pi*)

This formula presupposes a slight element of yang vacuity as well as some blood stasis.

2. *Liu Wei Di Huang Tang* (Six Flavors Rehmannia Decoction)

Ingredients: Cooked Radix Rehmanniae (*Shu Di*), Fructus Corni Officinalis (*Zhu Rou*), Radix Dioscoreae Oppositae (*Shan Yao*), Rhizoma Alismatis (*Ze Xie*), Cortex Radicis Moutan (*Dan Pi*), Sclerotium Poriae Cocos (*Fu Ling*)

Song and Yu give the standard ingredients for *Liu Wei Di Huang Wan* but call it *Liu Wei Di Huang Tang*. My supposition is that this minor name change is meant to merely indicate that this formula should be given in decoction. Song and Yu specifically indicate this formula for kidney vacuity blocked menstruation due to bedroom, *i.e.*, sexual, taxation.

3. *Gui Shen Wan Jia Jian* (Restore the Kidneys Pills with Additions & Subtractions)

Ingredients: Semen Cuscutae (*Tu Si Zi*), Cortex Eucommiae Ulmoidis (*Du Zhong*), Fructus Lycii Chinensis (*Gou Qi Zi*), Fructus Ligustri Lucidi (*Nu Zhen Zi*), Herba Ecliptae Prostratae (*Han Lian Cao*), Fructus Corni Officinalis (*Shan Zhu Rou*), Radix Angelicae Sinensis (*Dang Gui*), cooked Radix Rehmanniae (*Shu Di*), Radix Dioscoreae Oppositae (*Shan Yao*), Sclerotium Poriae Cocos (*Fu Ling*)

4. *Zi Lu Xian Zong Tang Jia Wei* (Placenta & Deer [Antler] Immortals Gathering Decoction with Added Flavors)

Ingredients: Placenta Hominis (*Zi He Che*), Gelatinum Cornu Cervi (*Lu Jiao Jiao*), Radix Angelicae Sinensis (*Dang Gui*), Radix Ligustici Wallichii (*Chuan Xiong*), cooked Radix Rehmanniae (*Shu Di*), Radix Albus Paeoniae Lactiflorae (*Bai Shao*), Fructus Rubi Chingii (*Fu Pen Zi*), Semen Cuscutae (*Tu Si Zi*), Fructus Lycii Chinensis (*Gou Qi Zi*), Fructus Schisandrae Chinensis (*Wu Wei Zi*), Semen Plantaginis (*Che Qian Zi*), Rhizoma Curculiginis Orchioidis (*Xian Mao*), Herba Epimedii (*Xian Ling Pi*), Radix Cyathulae Officinalis (*Chuan Niu Xi*)

This formula is given by Sun Jiu-ling for the treatment of kidney yin vacuity so severe that there is kidney essence vacuity as well. Sun gives the cause of this as extreme blood loss during labor. Sun quotes the *Nu Ke She Yao (The Essentials for Absorbing Gynecology)* to substantiate the connection between the blood and essence:

> Blood is the essence qi of water and grains. It is united with and regulated by the five viscera and shed and displayed by the six bowels. In men, it is transformed into essence. In women, it becomes milk above and menstrual water below.

5. Unnamed formula from *Concise Traditional Chinese Gynecology*

Ingredients: Cooked Radix Rehmanniae (*Shu Di*), Fructus Lycii Chinensis (*Gou Qi Zi*), Semen Cuscutae (*Tu Si Zi*), Radix Salviae Miltiorrhizae (*Dan Shen*), Radix Achyranthis Bidentatae (*Huai Niu Xi*)

Additions: If yin vacuity is affecting yang, add Radix Codonopsitis Pilosulae (*Dang Shen*), Rhizoma Atractylodis Macrocephalae (*Bai Zhu*), and Herba Epimedii (*Xian Ling Pi*). If yin vacuity affecting yang is even more severe, also add Placenta Hominis (*Zi He Che*) and Cornu Parvum Cervi (*Lu Rong*).

6. *Bai Zi Ren Wan* (Biota Seed Pills)

Ingredients: Semen Biotae Orientalis (*Bai Zi Ren*), Radix Achyranthis Bidentatis (*Niu Xi*), Herba Lycopi Lucidi (*Ze Lan*), Radix Dipsaci (*Chuan Xu Duan*), cooked Radix Rehmanniae (*Shu Di*), Herba Selaginellae Tamariscinae (*Juan Bo*)

Song and Yu recommend this formula if there is blood vacuity with fire.

7. *Yi Guan Jian Jia Wei* (One Link Decoction with Added Flavors)

Ingredients: Radix Glehniae Littoralis (*Bei Sha Shen*), stir-fried Tuber Ophiopogonis Japonici (*Mai Dong*), Fructus Meliae Toosendan (*Chuan Lian Zi*), whole Radix Angelicae

Sinensis (*Quan Dang Gui*), large uncooked Radix Rehmanniae (*Sheng Di*), Fructus Lycii Chinensis (*Gan Qi Zi*), scalded Carapax Amydae (*Bie Jia*), stir-fried Rhizoma Anemarrhenae Aspheloidis (*Chao Zhi Mu*), stir-fried Cortex Phellodendri (*Huang Bai*), stir-fried Radix Rubrus Paeoniae Lactiflorae (*Chi Shao*), Cortex Radicis Moutan (*Dan Pi*), Semen Leonuri Heterophylli (*Chong Wei Zi*)

This formula is for yin vacuity with internal heat. Zhu Cheng-han lists the signs and symptoms appropriate for the use of this formula as an emaciated, weak bodily constitution, afternoon tidal fever, a dry mouth and throat, enduring blocked menstruation, lumbar soreness, heart vexation, night sweats, cough, withered, dry skin and flesh, insidious lower abdominal pain, a red tongue with scant fur in the center, and a fine, rapid pulse.

8. *Bu Shen Di Huang Wan* (Supplement the Kidneys Rehmannia Pills)

Ingredients: Cooked Radix Rehmanniae (*Shu Di*), Rhizoma Anemarrhenae Aspheloidis (*Zhi Mu*), salt-processed Cortex Phellodendri (*Huang Bai*), Rhizoma Alismatis (*Ze Xie*), Radix Dioscoreae Oppositae (*Shan Yao*), Radix Polygalae Tenuifoliae (*Yuan Zhi*), Sclerotium Poriae Cocos (*Fu Ling*), Cortex Radicis Moutan (*Dan Pi*), Semen Zizyphi Spinosae (*Zao Ren*), Radix Scrophulariae Ningpoensis (*Yuan Shen*), Tuber Ophiopogonis Japonici (*Mai Dong*), Folium Bambusae (*Zhu Ye*), Plastrum Testudinis (*Gui Ban*), Ootheca Mantidis (*Sang Piao Xiao*), Fructus Corni Officinalis (*Shan Zhu Rou*)

Additions: Han Bai-ling says that, if there is cough with bleeding, add Gelatinum Corii Asini (*E Jiao*) and Rhizoma Imperatae Cylindricae (*Mao Gen*). This formula could be seen as a modification of either *Tian Wang Bu Xin Dan* (Heavenly Emperor Supplement the Heart Elixir) or *Liu Wei Di Huang Wan* (Six Flavors Rehmannia Pills). Han Bai-ling gives it under the heading blood vacuity blocked menstruation. The signs and symptoms he lists under this heading include yin vacuity and vacuity heat. He does not give a heading for liver-kidney yin vacuity.

9. *Zuo Gui Wan* (Restore the Left [Kidney] Pills)

Ingredients: Cooked Radix Rehmanniae (*Shu Di*), Radix Dioscoreae Oppositae (*Shan Yao*), Fructus Lycii Chinensis (*Gou Qi Zi*), Fructus Corni Officinalis (*Shan Zhu Yu*), Semen Cuscutae (*Tu Si Zi*), Radix Cyathulae Officinalis (*Chuan Niu Xi*), Gelatinum Cornu Cervi (*Lu Jiao Jiao*), Gelatinum Plastri Testudinis (*Gui Ban Jiao*)

This formula is suggested by Guo Yuan for blocked menstruation due to liver-kidney yin vacuity.

10. *Dang Gui Yu Zhu San* (Dang Gui Dispel Stasis Powder)

Ingredients: Radix Angelicae Sinensis (*Dang Gui*), Radix Albus Paeoniae Lactiflorae (*Bai Shao*), Radix Rubrus Paeoniae Lactiflorae (*Chi Shao*), Radix Ligustici Wallichii (*Chuan Xiong*), uncooked Radix Rehmanniae (*Sheng Di*), Radix Et Rhizoma Rhei (*Da Huang*), Mirabilitum (*Mang Xiao*), Radix Glycyrrhizae (*Gan Cao*)

This formula enriches yin, nourishes the blood, and discharges heat. It treats yin vacuity, blood dryness blocked menstruation. In this case, there is accumulated heat in the stomach and intestines. The stools are dry and bound. Heat damages yin, resulting in scanty and/or delayed menstruation and eventually blocked menstruation. This formula can also be used for blood stasis blocked menstruation accompanied by constipation.

Additions & subtractions: If one does not have dry, bound stools, delete Rhubarb and Mirabilitum and add Rhizoma Anemarrhenae Aspheloidis (*Zhi Mu*) and Semen Trichosanthis Kirlowii (*Gua Lou Ren*) to clear and moisten.

3. Lung yin & blood vacuity

Main symptoms: The menses are not free-flowing. There is a dry cough with blood in the spittle, chest pain, shortness of breath, red lips, red cheeks, heat in the center of the hands, feet, and heart, a pale face which is flushed red, a dry, red tongue with no fur, and a fine, rapid pulse.

This pattern specifically describes blocked menstruation due to pulmonary tuberculosis.

Treatment principles: Nourish yin and moisten the lungs, engender fluids and stop cough

Guiding formulas:

1. *Bai He Gu Jin Tang* (Lily Secure Metal Decoction)

Ingredients: Bulbus Lilii (*Bai He*), cooked Radix Rehmanniae (*Shu Di*), uncooked Radix Rehmanniae (*Sheng Di*), Tuber Ophiopogonis Japonici (*Mai Dong*), Radix Albus Paeoniae Lactiflorae (*Bai Shao*), Radix Scrophulariae Ningpoensis (*Yuan Shen*), Bulbus Fritillariae Cirrhosae (*Chuan Bei Mu*), Radix Angelicae Sinensis (*Dang Gui*), Radix Platycodi Grandiflori (*Jie Geng*), Radix Glycyrrhizae (*Gan Cao*)

Additions: If there is bloody cough, add Cortex Radicis Moutan (*Dan Pi*) and Rhizoma Imperatae Cylindricae (*Mao Gen*) to cool the blood and stop bleeding.

2. *Yi Guan Jian* (One Link Decoction)

Ingredients: Uncooked Radix Rehmanniae (*Sheng Di*), Radix Glehniae Littoralis (*Bei Sha Shen*), Tuber Ophiopogonis Japonici (*Mai Dong*), Radix Angelicae Sinensis (*Dang Gui*), Fructus Lycii Chinensis (*Gou Qi Zi*), Fructus Meliae Toosendan (*Chuan Lian Zi*)

Additions: For a bitter taste in and dry mouth, add Rhizoma Coptidis Chinensis (*Huang Lian*). For constipation, add Fructus Trichosanthis Kirlowii (*Gua Lou*). For profuse night sweats, add Cortex Radicis Lycii Chinensis (*Di Gu Pi*). For relatively more phlegm, add Bulbus Fritillariae Thunbergii (*Zhe Bei Mu*). For vexatious heat and thirst, add Rhizoma Anemarrhenae Aspheloidis (*Zhi Mu*) and Gypsum Fibrosum (*Shi Gao*).

4. Heart yin & blood vacuity

Main symptoms: Blocked menstruation after the menses having stopped suddenly in the middle of menstruation, no pain and no distention in the lower abdomen, heart palpitations and timidity or nervousness, heart palpitations when scared or nervous, sweating on movement, loss of sleep, the power to remember diminished, facial complexion pale but flushed red, tongue fur dry and light, and a vacuous, fine pulse

Treatment principles: Enrich yin, engender blood, and nourish the heart

Guiding formula: *Tian Wang Bu Xin Dan* (Heavenly Emperor Supplement the Heart Elixir)

Ingredients: Uncooked Radix Rehmanniae (*Sheng Di*), Radix Scrophulariae Ningpoensis (*Yuan Shen*), Radix Panacis Ginseng (*Ren Shen*), Radix Salviae Miltiorrhizae (*Dan Shen*), Sclerotium Pararadicis Poriae Cocos (*Fu Shen*), Radix Platycodi Grandiflori (*Jie Geng*), Radix Polygalae Tenuifoliae (*Yuan Zhi*), Semen Zizyphi Spinosae (*Zao Ren*), Semen Biotae Orientalis (*Bai Ren*), Tuber Asparagi Cochinensis (*Tian Dong*), Tuber Ophiopogonis Japonici (*Mai Dong*), Radix Angelicae Sinensis (*Dang Gui*), Fructus Schisandrae Chinensis (*Wu Wei Zi*)

5. Kidney qi insufficiency

Main symptoms: Blocked menstruation, facial complexion dull and dark, lower and upper back soreness and pain, weary limbs, dizziness and tinnitus, a feeling of chilly pain in the lower abdomen which desires warmth and pressure, clear, thin vaginal discharge, a pale, moist tongue with thin fur, and a deep, fine, forceless or deep, weak pulse

Although this pattern is called kidney qi insufficiency by Zhu Cheng-han, the signs and symptoms clearly evidence that this is a yang vacuity. This is confirmed by Han Bai-ling's calling this pattern kidney yang vacuity. Zhu Cheng-han says that, if the kidney qi becomes insufficient, essence and blood will become vacuous and scanty, leading to the *chong mai* not being filled and the *ren mai* not being free-flowing. If the *chong* and *ren* both are vacuous and empty, the menses become stuck and cannot move. Therefore, this pattern describes both an essence blood vacuity and an insufficiency of kidney qi or yang to warm and motivate the menses.

Treatment principles: Warm and supplement kidney yang, regulate and rectify the *chong* and *ren*

Guiding formulas:

1. Unnamed formula from *Zhong Yi Fu Ke (Chinese Medical Gynecology)*

Ingredients: Herba Epimedii (*Xian Ling Pi*), Semen Cuscutae (*Tu Si Zi*), Cortex Cinnamomi Cassiae (*Shang Rou Gui*), Folium Eucommiae Ulmoidis (*Du Zhong Ye*), Caulis Milletiae Seu Spatholobi (*Ji Xue Teng*), stir-fried Radix Ligustici Wallichii (*Chao Chuan Xiong*), Radix Albus Paeoniae Lactiflorae (*Bai Shao*), processed Rhizoma Cyperi Rotundi (*Zhi Xiang Fu*), Semen Leonuri Heterophylli (*Chong Wei Zi*), Flos Carthami Tinctorii (*Hong Hua*), Flos Rosae Rugosae (*Yue Ji Hua*)

As Zhu Cheng-han mentions, due to lack of motivation from kidney yang, cold and damp obstruct the *bao mai,* giving rise to chilly pain in the lower abdomen. This means that if there is such chilly pain, there is complicating blood stasis and this accounts for the inclusion of blood-quickening ingredients, such as Semen Leonuri and Carthamus.

2. *Gu Yin Jian* (Secure Yin Decoction)

Ingredients: Radix Panacis Ginseng (*Ren Shen*), Radix Dioscoreae Oppositae (*Shan Yao*), cooked Radix Rehmanniae (*Shu Di*), Fructus Corni Officinalis (*Shan Zhu Rou*), Semen Cuscutae (*Tu Si Zi*), Radix Polygalae Tenuifoliae (*Yuan Zhi*), Fructus Schisandrae Chinensis (*Wu Wei Zi*), mix-fried Radix Glycyrrhizae (*Gan Cao*)

Additions: Han Ba-ling says to add Radix Lateralis Praeparatus Aconiti Carmichaeli (*Fu Zi*), Cortex Cinnamomi Cassiae (*Rou Gui*), and Fructus Psoraleae Corylifoliae (*Bu Gu Zhi*) to the above formula in order to warm the kidneys and invigorate yang.

3. *Zuo Gui Yin Jia Jian* (Restore the Left [Kidney] Drink with Additions & Subtractions)

Ingredients: Cooked Radix Rehmanniae (*Shu Di*), Gelatinum Cornu Cervi (*Lu Jiao Jiao*), Semen Cuscutae (*Tu Si Zi*), Fructus Rubi Chingii (*Fu Pen Zi*), Rhizoma Cibotti Barometsis (*Gou Ji*), Semen Trigonellae Foeni-greaci (*Hu Lu Ba*), Herba Epimedii (*Xian Ling Pi*), Rhizoma Polygonati (*Huang Jing*), Spica Prunellae Vulgaris (*Xia Gu Cao*)

This formula is given by Zhang En-qin *et al.* for the treatment of polycystic ovarian syndrome with amenorrhea or infrequent periods due to kidney vacuity with symptoms of emaciation, hirsutism or pilosity, lumbar soreness, dizziness, fear of cold, loose stools, a pale tongue with thin, white coating, and a deep, fine pulse. This is a mixed yin and yang vacuity pattern as evidenced by the therapeutic principles given: warm the kidneys, boost the essence, and scatter nodulation. Therefore, although it uses as its guiding formula a classic yin-supplementing formula, I have chosen to list it under this kidney yang vacuity section.

Prunella is added to this formula based on its ability to scatter nodulation. In modern TCM gynecology, ovarian cysts are typically, at least in part, a type of phlegm nodulation.

Pilosity or excessive hair growth is an interesting symptom in women. According to the *Nei Jing (Inner Classic)*, men have hair on their face because they do not discharge their blood downward each month. This leaves them with relatively more blood and especially more blood in their upper bodies as compared to women. One should remember that hair is the surplus of the blood. Women's blood, on the other hand, at least until menopause, goes downward to nourish their uterus. This leaves their upper body with relatively less blood and so less facial hair. If yang counterflows upward, even if this upward counterflow is due to yang vacuity, this can carry blood upward as well, resulting in increased facial hair. Typically in such cases, yang must be led back downward to its lower source.

Repletion patterns

1. Qi stagnation blood stasis

Main symptoms: The number of menses becomes less and eventually the menses do not move. There is dizziness, heart vexation, easy anger, breast distention and pain, chest and rib-side distention and fullness, hiccups, twitching and spasm of the sinew vessels, and a sore feeling in the extremities and body. The facial complexion is dusky and stagnant. There may also be a bitter mouth and dry throat, constipation, and reddish urine. The tongue is slightly yellowish and may have macules or spots of static blood on its borders. The tongue may also be purplish. The tongue fur is thin and white. The pulse may be small and bowstring; bowstring and forceful; deep and bowstring; fine and choppy; or deep and choppy.

The exact signs and symptoms of this pattern depend upon the relative amounts of stagnant qi and blood stasis as well as on whether or not there is transformative heat.

Treatment principles: Course the liver and rectify the qi, quicken the blood and transform stasis

Guiding formulas:

1. *Wu Yao San* (Lindera Powder)

Ingredients: Radix Linderae Strychnifoliae (*Wu Yao*), Rhizoma Curcumae Zedoariae (*E Zhu*), Cortex Cinnamomi Cassiae (*Rou Gui Xin*), Radix Angelicae Sinensis (*Dang Gui*), Semen Pruni Persicae (*Tao Ren*), Pericarpium Citri Reticulatae Viride (*Qing Pi*), Radix Auklandiae Lappae (*Mu Xiang*)

This formula is for predominant qi stagnation complicated by blood stasis.

Additions & subtractions: Han Bai-ling says to add Radix Ligustici Wallichii (*Chuan Xiong*) and Radix Rubrus Paeoniae Lactiflorae (*Chi Shao*). If there is heat, delete Cinnamon and add a small amount of Radix Et Rhizoma Rhei (*Da Huang*).

2. *Xiao Yao San Jia Wei* (Rambling Powder with Added Flavors)

Ingredients: Radix Bupleuri (*Chai Hu*), Radix Angelicae Sinensis (*Dang Gui*), Radix Albus Paeoniae Lactiflorae (*Bai Shao*), Rhizoma Atractylodis Macrocephalae (*Bai Zhu*), Sclerotium Poriae Cocos (*Fu Ling*), mix-fried Radix Glycyrrhizae (*Gan Cao*), Herba Menthae Haplocalycis (*Bo He*), uncooked Rhizoma Zingiberis (*Sheng Jiang*), Semen Pruni Persicae (*Tao Ren*), Flos Carthami Tinctorii (*Hong Hua*), Cortex Radicis Moutan (*Dan Pi*), Radix Achyranthis Bidentatae (*Niu Xi*)

Song and Yu suggest this formula for blocked menstruation due to qi depression resulting in stagnation.

3. *Xiao Yao San Jia Jian* (Rambling Powder with Additions & Subtractions)

Ingredients: Radix Angelicae Sinensis (*Dang Gui*), Radix Albus Paeoniae Lactiflorae (*Bai Shao*), Radix Rubrus Paeoniae Lactiflorae (*Chi Shao*), Radix Bupleuri (*Chai Hu*),

Sclerotium Poriae Cocos (*Fu Ling*), stir-fried Rhizoma Atractylodis Macrocephalae (*Bai Zhu*), Pericarpium Citri Reticulatae (*Chen Pi*), Semen Pruni Persicae (*Tao Ren*), Flos Carthami Tinctorii (*Hong Hua*), blast-fried Rhizoma Zingiberis (*Pao Jiang*), Radix Glycyrrhizae (*Gan Cao*)

4. *Si Ni San He Gui Zhi Fu Ling Wan Jia Wei* (Four Counterflows Powder plus Cinnamon Twig & Poria Pills with Added Flavors)

Ingredients: Stir-fried Radix Bupleuri (*Chai Hu*), Radix Rubrus Paeoniae Lactiflorae (*Chi Shao*), Radix Albus Paeoniae Lactiflorae (*Bai Shao*), uncooked Radix Glycyrrhizae (*Gan Cao*), stir-fried Fructus Citri Aurantii (*Zhi Ke*), processed Rhizoma Cyperi Rotundi (*Xiang Fu*), Semen Pruni Persicae (*Tao Ren*), Flos Carthami Tinctorii (*Hong Hua*), Ramulus Cinnamomi Cassiae (*Gui Zhi*), Cortex Radicis Moutan (*Dan Pi*), Cortex Sclerotii Poriae Cocos (*Fu Ling Pi*), Tian Tai Radix Linderae Strychnifoliae (*Tai Wu Yao*), Semen Leonuri Heterophylli (*Chong Wei Zi*)

5. *Xue Fu Zhu Yu Tang* (Blood Mansion Dispel Stasis Decoction)

Ingredients: Semen Pruni Persicae (*Tao Ren*), Flos Carthami Tinctorii (*Hong Hua*), Radix Angelicae Sinensis (*Dang Gui*), Radix Rubrus Paeoniae Lactiflorae (*Chi Shao*), Radix Achyranthis Bidentatae (*Niu Xi*), Radix Bupleuri (*Chai Hu*), Radix Platycodi Grandiflori (*Jie Geng*), Fructus Citri Aurantii (*Zhi Ke*), uncooked Radix Rehmanniae (*Sheng Di*), Radix Glycyrrhizae (*Gan Cao*)

If there is more abdominal pain than distention, this is categorized as predominately blood stasis. In this case, the above formula is more appropriate.

Additions: Han Bai-ling suggests adding Radix Scutellariae Baicalensis (*Huang Qin*) and Fructus Gardeniae Jasminoidis (*Zhi Zi*) if there is heat. If there is constipation, add a small amount of Radix Et Rhizoma Rhei (*Da Huang*).

6. *Xue Fu Zhu Yu Tang Jia Jian* (Blood Mansion Dispel Stasis Decoction with Additions & Subtractions) according to Zhang En-qin *et al.*

Ingredients: Semen Pruni Persicae (*Tao Ren*), Flos Carthami Tinctorii (*Hong Hua*), Radix Angelicae Sinensis (*Dang Gui*), Radix Salviae Miltiorrhizae (*Dan Shen*), Radix Ligustici Wallichii (*Chuan Xiong*), Radix Rubrus Paeoniae Lactiflorae (*Chi Shao*), Cortex Cinnamomi Cassiae (*Gui Xin*), Radix Cyathulae Officinalis (*Chuan Niu Xi*), Fructus Citri Aurantii (*Zhi Ke*), Radix Linderae Strychnifoliae (*Wu Yao*), Rhizoma Cyperi Rotundi (*Xiang Fu*)

7. Unnamed formula from *Concise Traditional Chinese Gynecology*

Ingredients: Radix Bupleuri (*Chai Hu*), processed Rhizoma Cyperi Rotundi (*Xiang Fu*), Radix Angelicae Sinensis (*Dang Gui*), Flos Carthami Tinctorii (*Hong Hua*), Semen Pruni Persicae (*Tao Ren*)

8. *Tong Zhi Jian Jia Wei* (Free the Flow of Stagnation Decoction with Added Flavors)

Ingredients: Semen Pruni Persicae (*Tao Ren*), Radix Salviae Miltiorrhizae (*Dan Shen*), Herba Lycopi Lucidi (*Ze Lan*), Radix Achyranthis Bidentatae (*Niu Xi*), Extremitas Radicis Angelicae Sinensis (*Gui Wei*), Flos Carthami Tinctorii (*Hong Hua*), Fructus Crataegi (*Shan Zha*), Rhizoma Cyperi Rotundi (*Xiang Fu*), Radix Linderae Strychnifoliae (*Wu Yao*), Pericarpium Citri Reticulatae Viride (*Qing Pi*), Radix Auklandiae Lappae (*Mu Xiang*), Rhizoma Alismatis (*Ze Xie*)

This formula is from the *Jing Yue Quan Shu ([Zhang] Jing-yue's Complete Book)*. It is for more prominent blood stasis blocked menstruation.

9. *Tu Niu Xi San* (Achyranthese Powder)

Ingredients: Radix Achyranthis Bidentatae (*Tu Niu Xi*), Extremitas Radicis Angelicae Sinensis (*Gui Wei*), Semen Pruni Persicae (*Tao Ren*), Flos Carthami Tinctorii (*Hong Hua*)

Du Jie-hui recommends this formula for the treatment of qi stagnation blood stasis blocked menstruation. It supplements and quickens the blood, dispels stasis and frees the flow of the channels or menses.

10. *Tong Jing Huo Xue Tang* (Free the Flow of the Menses & Quicken the Blood Decoction)

Ingredients: Cortex Radicis Moutan (*Dan Pi*), Herba Schizonepetae Tenuifoliae (*Jing Jie Sui*), Radix Rubrus Paeoniae Lactiflorae (*Chi Shao*), Radix Angelicae Sinensis (*Dang Gui*), Radix Ligustici Wallichii (*Chuan Xiong*), uncooked Radix Rehmanniae (*Sheng Di*), cooked Radix Rehmanniae (*Shu Di*), Semen Pruni Persicae (*Tao Ren*), Flos Carthami Tinctorii (*Hong Hua*), Herba Lycopi Lucidi (*Ze Lan*), Rhizoma Corydalis Yanhusuo (*Yan Hu Suo*), Rhizoma Cyperi Rotundi (*Xiang Fu*), Radix Salviae Miltiorrhizae (*Dan Shen*), Radix Cyathulae Officinalis (*Chuan Niu Xi*)

Du Jie-hui also recommends this formula for the treatment of qi stagnation blood stasis blocked menstruation. It nourishes and quickens the blood, transforms stasis and frees the channels or menses.

11. *Da Huang Zhe Chong Wan* (Rhubarb & Eupolyphaga Pills)

Ingredients: Radix Et Rhizoma Rhei (*Da Huang*), Radix Scutellariae Baicalensis (*Huang Qin*), Radix Glycyrrhizae (*Gan Cao*), Semen Pruni Persicae (*Tao Ren*), Semen Pruni Armeniacae (*Xing Ren*), Radix Albus Paeoniae Lactiflorae (*Bai Shao*), dry Radix Rehmanniae (*Di Huang*), Resina Rhi Vernicifluae (*Gan Qi*), Tabanus (*Meng Chong*), Hirudo (*Shui Zhi*), Holotrichia Vermiculus (*Qi Cao*), Eupolyphaga Seu Ophistoplastia (*Zhe Chong*)

This formula is for blood stasis with concretions and conglomerations, heat, and constipation. It breaks the blood and disperses concretions. Therefore, it should be used with care and only if there is both blood stasis and concretions and conglomerations.

2. Cold damp congelation & stagnation

Main symptoms: Blocked menstruation, chilly pain in the lower abdomen, a heavy, dragging, or bearing down, distended feeling, desire for warmth but resistance to pressure, continuous white vaginal discharge, lack of warmth in the four extremities, chest oppression, hiccups, a greenish-bluish white facial complexion, and a greenish blue, dark tongue with white, glossy fur, and a deep, relaxed (retarded), and forceful or deep and slow pulse

Sun Jiu-ling says that this pattern may be due either to being caught in a downpour of rain or wading in the water during the menses, affection by wind cold, overeating chilled, uncooked foods, or taking too many cold and cooling medicinals. Cold congeals the blood, the qi mechanism is inhibited, and stasis obstructs the *chong* and *ren*, thus giving rise to blocked menstruation. If this condition is due to external contraction of wind cold, there will also be fear of cold and headache with soreness and distention of the lower and upper back.

Treatment principles: Warm the channels (or menses) and scatter cold, dry dampness and transform stasis

Guiding formulas:

1. *Wen Jing Tang Jia Jian* (Warm the Channels [or Menses] Decoction with Additions & Subtractions)

Ingredients: Stir-fried Ramulus Cinnamomi Cassiae (*Gui Zhi*), Folium Artemisiae Argyii (*Ai Ye*), stir-fried Radix Angelicae Sinensis (*Dang Gui*), stir-fried Radix Ligustici Wallichii (*Chuan Xiong*), stir-fried Radix Rubrus Paeoniae Lactiflorae (*Chi Shao*), stir-fried Radix Albus Paeoniae Lactiflorae (*Bai Shao*), scalded Fructus Evodiae Rutecarpae (*Zhu Yu*), stir-fried Radix Salviae Miltiorrhizae (*Dan Shen*), processed Rhizoma Cyperi Rotundi (*Xiang Fu*), Folium Perillae Frutescentis (*Su Ye*)

Zhu Cheng-han says that if there is menstrual pain after the menses come, use *Dang Gui Wan* (Dang Gui Pills) to regulate and rectify the menstrual blood.

2. *Shao Fu Zhu Yu Tang* (Lower Abdomen Dispel Stasis Decoction)

Ingredients: Stir-fried Fructus Foeniculi Vulgaris (*Xiao Hui Xiang*), stir-fried dry Rhizoma Zingiberis (*Gan Jiang*), Rhizoma Corydalis Yanhusuo (*Yan Hu Suo*), Radix Angelicae Sinensis (*Dang Gui*), Radix Ligustici Wallichii (*Chuan Xiong*), Resina Myrrhae (*Mo Yao*), Cortex Tubiformis Cinnamomi Cassaie (*Guan Gui*), Radix Rubrus Paeoniae Lactiflorae (*Chi Shao*), Pollen Typhae (*Pu Huang*), stir-fried Feces Trogopterori Seu Pteromi (*Wu Ling Zhi*)

3. *He Xue Tong Jing Tang* (Harmonize the Blood & Free the Flow of the Channels [or Menses] Decoction)

Ingredients: Radix Angelicae Sinensis (*Dang Gui*), cooked Radix Rehmanniae (*Shu Di*), Rhizoma Sparganii (*San Leng*), Rhizoma Curcumae Zedoariae (*E Zhu*), Radix Auklandiae Lappae (*Mu Xiang*), Cortex Cinnamomi Cassiae (*Rou Gui*), Flos Carthami Tinctorii (*Hong Hua*), Lignum Sappanis (*Su Mu*), Sanguis Draconis (*Xue Jie*)

This formula contains ingredients which break the blood, but also medicinals which enter and free the flow of the network vessels. Therefore, it ma be used when there is enduring disease entering the network vessels combined with cold congelation.

4. *Wu Zhu Yu Tang* (Evodia Decoction)

Ingredients: Fructus Evodiae Rutecarpae (*Wu Zhu Yu*), Radix Angelicae Sinensis (*Dang Gui*), ginger-processed Rhizoma Pinelliae Ternatae (*Ban Xia*), Radix Ledebouriellae Divaricatae (*Fang Feng*), Radix Ligustici Wallichii (*Chuan Xiong*), Sclerotium Poriae Cocos (*Fu Ling*), Cortex Cinnamomi Cassiae (*Rou Gui*), Cortex Radicis Moutan (*Dan Pi*), Tuber Ophiopogonis Japonici (*Mai Dong*), Herba Asari Cum Radice (*Xi Xin*), dry Rhizoma Zingiberis (*Gan Jiang*), Radix Auklandiae Lappae (*Mu Xiang*), mix-fried Radix Glycyrrhizae (*Gan Cao*)

Song and Yu suggest this formula if it is mostly an exterior pattern.

5. *Hu Po San* (Amber Powder)

Ingredients: Rhizoma Sparganii (*San Leng*), Rhizoma Curcumae Zedoariae (*E Zhu*), Succinum (*Hu Po*), Radix Albus Paeoniae Lactiflorae (*Bai Shao*), Herba Artemisiae Anomalae (*Liu Ji Nu*), Cortex Radicis Moutan (*Dan Pi*), Cortex Cinnamomi Cassiae (*Rou Gui*), Radix Linderae Strychnifoliae (*Wu Yao*), Rhizoma Corydalis Yanhusuo (*Yan Hu Suo*)

Song and Yu suggest this formula if it is mostly an interior pattern accompanied by concretions and conglomerations. Sparganium and Zedoaria break the blood and Amber enters and frees the flow of the network vessels.

3. Phlegm dampness obstruction & stagnation

Main symptoms: Blocked menstruation, a fat, plump body, chest and rib-side fullness and oppression, vomiting and nausea with profuse phlegm, lack of strength, lassitude and fatigue, lumbar soreness, edema and swelling, profuse white colored vaginal discharge, a fat tongue with slimy, white fur, and a slippery, bowstring, deep, and/or small pulse

This is usually a mixed vacuity/repletion pattern. Spleen qi vacuity is usually the root of phlegm engenderment. Once phlegm is produced, it may obstruct the *jing*, meaning both the channels and the menses. Because of spleen vacuity, there may also be concomitant blood vacuity, and, because of phlegm dampness, there may also be concomitant qi stagnation and blood stasis. It is also possible for there to be kidney yang vacuity or spleen-kidney dual vacuity.

Treatment principles: Dry dampness and transform phlegm, quicken the blood and free the flow of the channels or menses. Zhu Cheng-han says to move the qi rather than to quicken the blood. This reflects that this pattern is typically complicated by liver depression qi stagnation.

Guiding formulas:

1. *Cang Fu Dao Tan Wan* (Atractylodes & Cyperus Abduct Phlegm Pills)

Ingredients: Rhizoma Atractylodis (*Cang Zhu*), processed Rhizoma Cyperi Rotundi (*Xiang Fu*), Pericarpium Citri Reticulatae (*Chen Pi*), Sclerotium Poriae Cocos (*Fu Ling*), Fructus Citri Aurantii (*Zhi Ke*), processed Rhizoma Pinelliae Ternatae (*Ban Xia*), Rhizoma Arisaematis (*Nan Xing*), mix-fried Radix Glycyrrhizae (*Gan Cao*), uncooked Rhizoma Zingiberis (*Sheng Jiang*)

2. *Cang Fu Dao Tan Wan Jia Wei* (Atractylodes & Cyperus Abduct Phlegm Pills with Added Flavors)

Ingredients: Ginger-processed Rhizoma Pinelliae Ternatae (*Ban Xia*), Pericarpium Citri Reticulatae (*Chen Pi*), Sclerotium Poriae Cocos (*Fu Ling*), uncooked Radix Glycyrrhizae (*Gan Cao*), aged Rhizoma Arisaematis (*Nan Xing*), aged Rhizoma Atractylodis (*Cang Zhu*), stir-fried Fructus Citri Aurantii (*Zhi Ke*), uncooked Rhizoma Zingiberis (*Sheng Jiang*), stir-fried Radix Ligustici Wallichii (*Chuan Xiong*), scorched Massa Medica Fermentata (*Liu Qu*), processed Rhizoma Cyperi Rotundi (*Xiang Fu*)

3. *Cang Fu Dao Tan Wan Jia Jian* (Atractylodes & Cyperus Abduct Phlegm Pills with Additions & Subtractions)

Ingredients: Rhizoma Atractylodis (*Cang Zhu*), Rhizoma Cyperi Rotundi (*Xiang Fu*), Pericarpium Citri Reticulatae (*Chen Pi*), processed Rhizoma Pinelliae Ternatae (*Zhi Ban Xia*), Thallus Algae (*Kun Bu*), Spica Prunellae Vulgaris (*Xia Gu Cao*), Bulbus Fritillariae (*Bei Mu*), Squama Manitis Pentadactylis (*Shan Jia*), Rhizoma Shancigu (*Shan Ci Gu*), Spina Gleditschiae Sinensis (*Zao Ci*), Fructus Citri Aurantii (*Zhi Ke*), Sclerotium Poriae Cocos (*Fu Ling*)

Zhang En-qin *et al.* give this formula under polycystic ovarian syndrome due to phlegm dampness manifested by amenorrhea or infrequent menstruation, obesity, pilosity or hirsutism, a pale, fat tongue with white, slimy fur, and a deep, relaxed (retarded) pulse. Gleditschia is now being used in the People's Republic of China in order to "ripen" ovarian cysts based on a combination of modern Western and TCM diagnoses. Traditionally, Gleditschia is used to ripen pus so that welling abscesses would rupture and suppurate.

4. *Hou Pu Er Chen Tang* (Magnolia Two Aged [Ingredients] Decoction)

Ingredients: Cortex Magnoliae Officinalis (*Chuan Bu*), Pericarpium Citri Reticulatae (*Chen Pi*), ginger-processed Rhizoma Pinelliae Ternatae (*Ban Xia*), Sclerotium Poriae Cocos (*Fu Ling*)

This formula primarily transforms phlegm and eliminates dampness. It does not directly quicken the blood or transform stasis.

5. *Jia Wei Si Wu Er Chen Tang* (Added Flavors Four Materials Two Aged [Ingredients] Decoction)

Ingredients: Extremitas Radicis Angelicae Sinensis (*Gui Wei*), Radix Rubrus Paeoniae Lactiflorae (*Chi Shao*), Radix Ligustici Wallichii (*Chuan Xiong*), uncooked Radix Rehmanniae (*Sheng Di*), Pericarpium Citri Reticulatae (*Chen Pi*), Rhizoma Pinelliae Ternatae (*Ban*

Xia), Cortex Radicis Moutan (*Dan Pi*), Sclerotium Poriae Cocos (*Fu Ling*), Herba Sargassii (*Hai Zao*), Flos Carthami Tinctorii (*Hong Hua*), Rhizoma Cyperi Rotundi (*Xiang Fu*)

This formula is for the treatment of damp turbidity with blood stasis resulting in blocked menstruation.

6. *Bu Zhong Yi Qi Tang* (Supplement the Center & Boost the Qi Decoction)

Ingredients: Radix Astragali Membranacei (*Huang Qi*), Radix Codonopsitis Pilosulae (*Dang Shen*), scorched Rhizoma Actractylodis Macrocephalae (*Bai Zhu*), Sclerotium Poriae Cocos (*Fu Ling*), Radix Angelicae Sinensis (*Dang Gui*), Rhizoma Cimicifugae (*Sheng Ma*), Radix Bupleuri (*Chai Hu*), Pericarpium Citri Reticulatae (*Chen Pi*), Radix Glycyrrhizae (*Gan Cao*), uncooked Rhizoma Zingiberis (*Sheng Jiang*), Fructus Zizyphi Jujubae (*Da Zao*)

Guo Yuan suggests this formula for the treatment of phlegm dampness obstruction and stagnation resulting in blocked menstruation. This formula is most often thought of as a central qi supplement and lifter of the fallen. However, it does include qi-rectifying medicinals and at least one phlegm-transformer. Its use is based on the statement that the spleen is the root of phlegm engenderment. By fortifying the spleen and boosting the qi, the qi mechanism is disinhibited. Thus the clear is upborne and the turbid is downborne, and qi can move and transform liquids. The use of this formula is predicated on this condition being most defintely a mixed vacuity/repletion one.

7. *Jia Jian Xiang Sha Liu Jun Zi Tang* (Additions & Subtractions Auklandia & Amomum Six Gentlemen Decoction)

Ingredients: Radix Panacis Ginseng (*Ren Shen*), Sclerotium Poriae Cocos (*Fu Ling*), Rhizoma Atractylodis Macrocephalae (*Bai Zhu*), processed Rhizoma Pinelliae Ternatae (*Ban Xia*), Pericarpium Citri Reticulatae (*Chen Pi*), Radix Auklandiae Lappae (*Mu Xiang*), Fructus Amomi (*Sha Ren*), Radix Angelicae Sinensis (*Dang Gui*), Radix Ligustici Wallichii (*Chuan Xiong*)

Du Jie-hui recommends this formula for the treatment of phlegm dampness obstruction and stagnation blocked menstruation. It fortifies the spleen, dries dampness, and transforms phlegm, quickens the blood and frees the channels or menses. Personally, I recommend using *Bu Zhong Yi Qi Tang* as the guiding formula if fatigue and dizziness on standing up are the most prominent spleen vacuity symptoms and using this formula if diarrhea or loose stools are the most prominent spleen vacuity symptoms.

8. *Miao Ying Wan* (Wonderously Responding Pills)

Ingredients: Radix Panacis Ginseng (*Ren Shen*), honey mix-fried Radix Astragali Membranacei (*Huang Qi*), earth stir-fried Rhizoma Atractylodis Macrocephalae (*Bai Zhu*), wine-washed Radix Rehmanniae (*Di Huang*), Pericarpium Citri Reticulatae (*Chen Pi*), processed Rhizoma Pinelliae Ternatae (*Ban Xia*), wine-washed Radix Angelicae Sinensis (*Dang Gui*), Sclerotium Poriae Cocos (*Fu Ling*), wine stir-fried Rhizoma Atractylodis (*Cang Zhu*), Talcum (*Hua Shi*), mix-fried Radix Glycyrrhizae (*Gan Cao*)

This formula boosts the qi and fortifies the spleen, transforms phlegm and eliminates dampness, and it regulates the menses. It is indicated for the treatment of simultaneous phlegm dampness obstruction and stagnation and qi vacuity blocked or scanty menstruation.

4. Fire effulgence

Shen Zhong-li, in *Zhong Yi Fu Ke Lin Chuang Shou Ce (A Clinical Handbook of Chinese Medical Gynecology)*, gives this pattern of blocked menstruation which I have not encountered anywhere else in the Chinese gynecological literature. In my clinical experience, I do believe I have seen this pattern and, therefore, I am including it even though other Chinese gynecological authorities do not. Dr. Shen says that liver depression may transform into fire. Because of the upward counterflow this engenders, the heart qi is thus not able to flow freely downward. The *chong* and *ren* are not free-flowing and hence there is blocked menstruation. This is different from heart yin and blood vacuity. In this case, the heat affecting the heart is depressive heat, a form of replete heat due to liver depression qi stagnation.

Main symptoms: Blocked menstruation does not descend, heart vexation, easy anger, constipated stools, hot, red urination, insomnia, restlessness, a red or crimson tongue with scanty fur, and a fine, bowstring, rapid pulse

Treatment principles: Level or calm the liver and drain fire, clear the heart and free the flow of the channels or menses

Guiding formulas:

1. *San Huang Si Wu Tang Jia Jian* (Three Yellows Four Materials Decoction with Additions & Subtractions)

Ingredients: Radix Scutellariae Baicalensis (*Huang Qin*), Rhizoma Coptidis Chinensis (*Huang Lian*), Cortex Phellodendri (*Huang Bai*), uncooked Radix Rehmanniae (*Sheng Di*), uncooked Radix Et Rhizoma Rhei (*Da Huang*), Radix Angelicae Sinensis (*Dang Gui*),

Radix Albus Paeoniae Lactiflorae (*Bai Shao*), Radix Ligustici Wallichii (*Chuan Xiong*), Radix Rubiae Cordifoliae (*Qian Cao*), Radix Auklandiae Lappae (*Mu Xiang*), Radix Polygalae Tenuifoliae (*Yuan Zhi*), Caulis Polygoni Multiflori (*Ye Jiao Teng*), Radix Glehniae Littoralis (*Sha Shen*)

2. Empirical formula

Ingredients: Uncooked Radix Rehmanniae (*Sheng Di*), Radix Polygalae Tenuifoliae (*Yuan Zhi*), Tuber Ophiopogonis Japonici (*Mai Dong*), Herba Artemisiae Capillaris (*Yin Chen*), Radix Gentianae Scabrae (*Long Dan Cao*), Fructus Gardeniae Jasminoidis (*Shan Zhi*), Radix Rubrus Paeoniae Lactiflorae (*Chi Shao*), Semen Pruni Persicae (*Tao Ren*), Fructus Meliae Toosendan (*Jin Ling Zi*), Radix Cynanchi Atrati (*Bai Wei*)

3. Empirical formula

Ingredients: Radix Salviae Miltiorrhizae (*Dan Shen*), Radix Scrophulariae Ningpoensis (*Yuan Shen*), Tuber Ophiopogonis Japonici (*Mai Dong*), Tuber Asparagi Cochinensis (*Tian Dong*), Semen Biotae Orientalis (*Bai Zi Ren*), uncooked Radix Rehmanniae (*Sheng Di*), Radix Angelicae Sinensis (*Dang Gui*), Radix Codonopsitis Pilosulae (*Dang Shen*), Fructus Schisandrae Chinensis (*Wu Wei Zi*), Semen Pruni Persicae (*Tao Ren*), Radix Polygoni Multiflori (*Shou Wu*), Fructus Ligustri Lucidi (*Nu Zhen Zi*)

Discussion

Before administering precipitating and attacking, blood-quickening and stasis-transforming ingredients for the treatment of supposed blocked menstruation, one must be sure to rule out pregnancy. With the advent of cheap, accurate, home pregnancy tests, this is easily done. One should also not treat a woman for blocked menstruation if, right from menarche, she has regularly only had one or two menses per year. Some women menstruate on a regular cycle of 60, 90, 180, or 360 days. The key here to discriminating such idiosyncratic but nonetheless normal physiological cycles is the fact that the woman's menses have always been like this and that they come at a regular cycle without other complicating signs and symptoms.

If blocked menstruation is accompanied by the presence of concretions and conglomerations, *i.e.*, abdominal mass, the patient should be referred to a Western MD for a gynecological exam, including ultrasound and bimanual palpation. It is important to rule out possible malignancy. If blocked menstruation is accompanied by galactorrhea or weeping from the nipples, the woman should also be referred to a Western MD. In this case, blood work and possible x-ray of the sella turcica may be necessary to rule out a pituitary tumor, such as a chromophobe adenoma. Galactorrhea-amenorrhea syndrome is dealt with in the addenda below.

If the woman's blocked menstruation is due to vacuous and insufficient blood, it is important that she be treated with supplementing and nourishing medicinals. If attacking medicinals are used inappropriately, the patient will be iatrogenically injured and will tend to manifest more severe kidney and yin vacuity signs and symptoms.

Prognosis

As with so many of the menstrual diseases, blocked menstruation due to blood stasis in turn due to an historical cause or event is usually relatively easy to treat and there is little recidivism. If due to qi depression leading to blood stasis, it is usually relatively easy to promote menses, but then it may be more difficult to completely and lastingly eliminate all menstrual irregularities.

Both vacuity and replete cold species of blocked menstruation typically respond well to TCM treatment with vacuity cold sometimes taking longer but often responding surprisingly fast.

Blood and yin vacuity, on the other hand, often do not respond as well. This is especially so if the yin insufficiency is constitutional. In this case, persistence is what is required. If there is vacuity heat as well as blood and yin vacuity, this typically makes the case even more difficult. Most women with yin vacuity and vacuity fire are quite nervous and tend not to stick with any one treatment long enough to get lasting results. Their minds jump around and so they tend to jump around from doctor to doctor, therapy to therapy, when, in fact, the best thing for them would be to do a hundred day rest cure. Many female athletes suffer from yin vacuity with vacuity fire blocked menstruation.

Phlegm dampness obstruction and stasis can also be recalcitrant to treatment. This is often a complicated scenario where there may be simultaneous kidney yin and/or yang vacuity, blood stasis, qi stagnation, and/or qi and blood vacuity. Such cases require very careful pattern discrimination where each element is parsed out and attended to appropriately. If one is not getting any result with women with very stubborn blocked menstruation where there is definite qi stagnation and blood stasis, it is sometimes useful to try adding some phlegm-transforming, nodulation-scattering medicinals to wash away any phlegm. This is based on the idea that phlegm often plays a part in curious or strange diseases and also that, since qi moves and transforms fluids, if there is enduring qi stagnation, phlegm will tend to accumulate. In cases of phlegm dampness obstruction and stagnation, it is usually important for the patient to avoid dairy products, eggs, heavy, greasy meats, or any other foods which would tend to aggravate phlegm dampness. In obviously obese patients, increased exercise is also quite important.

Most women with amenorrhea are anovulatory and typically have a monophasic or flat line BBT graph. Having women suffering from blocked menstruation chart their BBT may, therefore, at first sight seem superfluous. However, charting the BBT in women with blocked menstruation does give both the patient and practitioner some idea of how the treatment is going and may help staging of treatment methods and formulas. If the woman's BBT goes up, then the practitioner can tell the woman that she will be menstruating typically 14 days after this rise in temperature. If this same woman also suffers from some premenstrual complaints or painful menstruation, the practitioner can then know to change their treatment methods and formula in order to deal with such premenstrual symptoms or menstrual pain. In addition, after the menses come, continuing to chart the BBT can tell whether the woman has ovulated on time and can help stage the use of articifical regulation of the menstrual cycle methods. These consist of promoting follicular development in the postmenstruum by primarily nourishing the blood and supplementing the kidneys, promoting ovulation during the intermenstruum by warming and invigorating yang, quickening the blood and freeing the flow of the network vessels. Since growth of yin reaching its apogee during the intermenstruum also means possible engenderment of dampness, dampness-eliminating, phlegm-transforming medicinals may also be added during this phase if there is a tendency to phlegm damp obstruction and stagnation.

Key patterns to memorize	
1. Repletion patterns	**A. Qi stagnation blood stasis** **B. Phlegm damp obstruction & stagnation** **C. Cold damp congelation & stagnation** **D. Liver fire effulgence**

2. Vacuity patterns	**A. Spleen vacuity**
	B. Lung yin vacuity
	C. Heart yin vacuity
	D. Kidney vacuity
	     i. Kidney yin vacuity
	     ii. Kidney yang vacuity

Addenda: Special types of blocked menstruation dealt with separately in the Chinese gynecological literature

1. Galactorrhea-amenorrhea

Disease causes, disease mechanisms

If the spleen and kidneys are both vacuous, they are not able to contain and secure. Thus breast milk spills over spontaneously. If qi and blood are both vacuous, the sea of blood will be empty and vacuous. Thus the *chong* qi counterflows upward. On the one hand there is blocked menstruation below. On the other, there is hirsutism above. If emotional depression damages the liver, the liver may lose its orderly reaching. In that case, the *chong* qi may also counterflow upward, causing or contributing to both blocked menstruation and hirsutism. If this depression transforms into heat, heat will force the blood to move frenetically outside its pathways. The reader should remember the saying, "The menses move down and become the menstrual water; they move upward and become the breast milk." Therefore, galactorrhea can be seen as a species of heat forcing the blood to move frenetically outside its pathways. If there are concretions and conglomerations in the brain, *i.e.*, a pituitary tumor, stasis and phlegm mixed with dampness obstruct and stagnate in the breast and uterine network vessels. Because of static or old blood, fresh or new blood is not engendered. On the one hand, this causes blocked menstruation due to a combination of blood stasis and blood vacuity. On the other, it prevents the blood (in this case the milk) from returning to its channels. Thus the breast milk spills over outside.

Treatment based on pattern discrimination

1. Spleen-kidney insufficiency

Main symptoms: The menses have been blocked for some time and do not descend. However the breast milk spontaneously spills over. It is watery in consistency and pale in color. The breasts are slack and soft and there is dizziness, vertigo, low back and knee soreness and weakness, scanty appetite, loose stools, lack of warmth in the four limbs, a pale tongue with thin fur, and a fine pulse.

Treatment principles: Fortify the spleen and supplement the kidneys, fill the essence and contain the milk

Guiding formulas:

1. Unnamed empirical formula from *Zhong Yi Fu Ke Lin Chuang Shou Ce (A Clinical Handbook of Chinese Medical Gynecology)*

Ingredients: Radix Codonopsitis Pilosulae (*Dang Shen*), Radix Astragali Membranacei (*Huang Qi*), Radix Angelicae Sinensis (*Dang Gui*), cooked Radix Rehmanniae (*Shu Di*), Radix Ligustici Wallichii (*Chuan Xiong*), Radix Albus Paeoniae Lactiflorae (*Bai Shao*), Gelatinum Corii Asini (*E Jiao*), Cornu Degelatinum Cervi (*Lu Jiao Shuang*), Radix Dipsaci (*Chuan Duan*), Folium Photiniae Serrulatae (*Shi Nan Ye*)

2. Unnamed formula from *Zhong Yi Fu Ke Lin Chuang Shou Ce (A Clinical Handbook of Chinese Medical Gynecology)*

Ingredients: Radix Astragali Membranacei (*Huang Qi*), stir-fried Rhizoma Atractylodis Macrocephalae (*Bai Zhu*), Sclerotium Poriae Cocos (*Fu Ling*), Herba Epimedii (*Xian Ling Pi*), Radix Morindae Officinalis (*Ba Ji Rou*), Herba Cynomorii Songarici (*Suo Yang*), Radix Angelicae Sinensis (*Dang Gui*), Radix Polygoni Multiflori (*Shou Wu*), Pericarpium Citri Reticulatae (*Chen Pi*), Galla Rhois Chinensis (*Wu Bei Zi*), Semen Cuscutae (*Tu Si Zi*)

Additions: If there are loose stools, add blast-fried Rhizoma Zingiberis (*Pao Jiang*), Fructus Psoraleae Corylifoliae (*Bu Gu Zhi*), and carbonized Fructus Crataegi (*Shan Zha*). If there is lumbar pain, add Cortex Eucommiae Ulmoidis (*Du Zhong*) and Ramulus Loranthi Seu Visci (*Sang Ji Sheng*). If there is blocked menstruation, add Flos Carthami Tinctorii (*Hong Hua*), Rhizoma Curcumae Zedoariae (*E Zhu*), and Herba Leonuri Heterophylli (*Yi Mu Cao*). For scanty appetite, add Radix Auklandiae Lappae (*Mu Xiang*), Fructus Amomi (*Sha Ren*), and Massa Medica Fermentata (*Liu Qu*).

2. Qi & blood dual vacuity

Main symptoms: Due to excessive postpartum blood loss or failure of the spleen to transform and engender the qi and blood, there may be blocked menstruation which does not descend, spillage over outside of breast milk which is clear in color and watery in consistency, dizziness, lack of strength, a somber white facial complexion, heart palpitations, heart fluster, shortness of breath, faint voice, a pale tongue with thin fur, and a fine, weak pulse.

Treatment principles: Supplement the qi and nourish the blood, fortify the spleen and contain the milk

Guiding formula: *Shi Quan Da Bu Tang Jia Jian* (Ten [Ingredients] Completely & Greatly Supplementing Decoction with Additions & Subtractions)

Ingredients: Radix Codonopsitis Pilosulae (*Dang Shen*), mix-fried Radix Astragali Membranacei (*Huang Qi*), Rhizoma Atractylodis Macrocephalae (*Bai Zhu*), Radix Albus Paeoniae Lactiflorae (*Bai Shao*), Radix Angelicae Sinensis (*Dang Gui*), Radix Dioscoreae Oppositae (*Shan Yao*), Fructus Psoraleae Corylifoliae (*Bu Gu Zhi*), Caulis Milletiae Seu Spatholobi (*Ji Xue Teng*), Fructus Germinatus Hordei Vulgaris (*Mai Ya*), Fructus Schisandrae Chinensis (*Wu Wei Zi*), Cortex Cinnamomi Cassiae (*Rou Gui*), Radix Angelicae Dahuricae (*Bai Zhi*)

Additions: If there are heart palpitations and heart fluster, add Radix Polygalae Tenuifoliae (*Yuan Zhi*) and stir-fried Semen Zizyphi Spinosae (*Zao Ren*). If there is shortness of breath and faint voice, add Rhizoma Cimicifugae (*Sheng Ma*) and Radix Bupleuri (*Chai Hu*). If there is dizziness, add Fructus Lycii Chinensis (*Gou Qi Zi*) and Fructus Tribuli Terrestris (*Bai Ji Li*). If there is a sallow yellow facial complexion, add Gelatinum Corii Asini (*E Jiao*). If the spill-over of milk is moderately excessive, add Actinolitum (*Chi Shi Zhi*), Ootheca Mantidis (*Sang Piao Xiao*), and Galla Rhois Chinensis (*Wu Bei Zi*).

3. Liver depression qi stagnation

Main symptoms: Emotional depression, belching, blocked menstruation which does not descend, spontaneous spilling over of breast milk or spilling over of breast milk on the outside when squeezed, breast distention and pain, palpable lumps, chest and rib-side distention and pain, a thin tongue coating, and a bowstring pulse

Treatment principles: Course the liver and resolve depression, rectify the qi and free the flow of the channels or menses

Guiding formulas:

1. *Xiao Yao San Jia Jian* (Rambling Powder with Additions & Subtractions)

Ingredients: Radix Bupleuri (*Chai Hu*), Radix Angelicae Sinensis (*Dang Gui*), Radix Rubrus & Albus Paeoniae Lactiflorae (*Chi Bai Shao*), Rhizoma Atractylodis Macrocephalae (*Bai Zhu*), Sclerotium Poriae Cocos (*Fu Ling*), Herba Menthae Haplocalycis (*Bo He*), Radix Glycyrrhizae (*Gan Cao*), Flos Carthami Tinctorii (*Hong Hua*), whole Fructus Trichosanthis Kirlowii (*Quan Gua Lou*), Semen Vaccariae Segetalis (*Wang Bu Liu Xing*), Fructus Akebiae Trifoliatae (*Ba Yue Zha*), Cortex Albizziae Julibrissinis (*He Huan Pi*), Fructus Germinatus Hordei Vulgaris (*Mai Ya*)

2. Unnamed formula from *Zhong Yi Fu Ke Lin Chuan Shou Ce (A Clinical Handbook of Chinese Medical Gynecology)*

Ingredients: Radix Bupleuri (*Chai Hu*), stir-fried Rhizoma Atractylodis Macrocephalae (*Bai Zhu*), stir-fried Radix Albus Paeoniae Lactiflorae (*Bai Shao*), Radix Angelicae Sinensis (*Dang Gui*), Radix Ligustici Wallichii (*Chuan Xiong*), Fructus Germinatus Oryzae Sativae & Hordei Vulgaris (*Gu Mai Ya*), Tuber Curcumae (*Yu Jin*), Radix Linderae Strychnifoliae (*Wu Yao*), Radix Auklandiae Lappae (*Mu Xiang*), Fructus Citri Sacrodactylis (*Fo Shou Pian*), Lignum Aquilaria Agallochae Massa Medica Fermentata (*Chen Xiang Qu*), scorched Fructus Crataegi (*Shan Zha*), Semen Leonuri Heterophylli (*Chong Wei Zi*)

4. Blood stasis obstructing the network vessels

Main symptoms: Blocked menstruation which does not descend, lower abdominal distention and pain which refuses pressure, spontaneous spilling over of breast milk, breast distention and pain, blurred vision or possible concretions and conglomerations in the brain, a dark tongue with a thin coating, and a bowstring pulse

Treatment principles: Quicken the blood and transform concretions, regulate the menses and contain the milk

Guiding formulas:

1. Unnamed formula from *Zhong Yi Fu Ke Lin Chuang Shou Ce (A Clinical Handbook of Chinese Medical Gynecology)*

Ingredients: Radix Salviae Miltiorrhizae (*Dan Shen*), Radix Rubrus Paeoniae Lactiflorae (*Chi Shao*), Spica Prunellae Vulgaris (*Xia Ku Cao*), Geotrupes Laevistriatus (*Qiang Liang*), Bombyx Batryticatus (*Jiang Can*), Lumbricus (*Di Long*), Rhizoma Curcumae Zedoariae (*E Zhu*), Radix Angelicae Dahuricae (*Bai Zhi*), Fructus Germinatus Hordei Vulgaris (*Mai Ya*), Feces Trogopeterori Seu Pteromi (*Wu Ling Zhi*), Pollen Typhae (*Pu Huang*), Herba Leonuri Heterophylli (*Yi Mu Cao*)

2. *Tao Hong Si Wu Tang Jia Jian* (Persica & Carthamus Four Materials Decoction with Additions & Subtractions)

Ingredients: Semen Pruni Persicae (*Tao Ren*), Flos Carthami Tinctorii (*Hong Hua*), Radix Angelicae Sinensis (*Dang Gui*), Radix Ligustici Wallichii (*Chuan Xiong*), Radix Rubrus Paeoniae Lactiflorae (*Chi Shao*), cooked Radix Rehmanniae (*Shu Di*), Rhizoma Corydalis Yanhusuo (*Yan Hu Suo*), Fructus Meliae Toosendan (*Jin Ling Zi*), Rhizoma Cyperi Rotundi (*Xiang Fu*), Thallus Algae (*Kun Bu*), Concha Ostreae (*Mu Li*), Lumbricus (*Di Long*), Radix Angelicae Dahuricae (*Bai Zhi*), powdered Buthus Martensi (*Quan Xie*)

3. Unnamed formula from *Zhong Yi Fu Ke Lin Chuang Shou Ce (A Clinical Handbook of Chinese Medical Gynecology)*

Ingredients: Radix Codonopsitis Pilosulae (*Dang Shen*), Radix Astragali Membranacei (*Huang Qi*), mix-fried Squama Manitis Pentadactylis (*Shan Jia*), Lumbricus (*Di Long*), Semen Benicasae Hispidae (*Dong Kui Zi*), Herba Cistanchis Deserticolae (*Rou Cong Rong*), Fructus Lycii Chinensis (*Qi Zi*), Nidus Vespae (*Lu Feng Fang*), Rhizoma Acori Graminei (*Chang Pu*), Herba Cynomorii Songarici (*Suo Yang*), Spica Prunellae Vulgaris (*Xia Ku Cao*), calcined Concha Ostreae (*Mu Li*), fragrant Radix Angelicae Dahuricae (*Bai Zhi*)

2. Contraceptive medicinals leading to amenorrhea

Disease causes, disease mechanisms

Most of these patients have constitutional visceral vacuity. After taking contraceptive medicinals, the *chong* and *ren* qi and blood function suffers restraint and the essence blood is insufficient. Thus the sea of blood is empty and vacuous. Or, after taking such medicinals, spleen movement and transportation suffers obstruction. Phlegm and dampness are thus engendered internally.

Treatment based on pattern discrimination

1. Spleen-Kidney insufficiency

Main symptoms: After taking contraceptive medicinals, the menstrual blood becomes progressively more watery and scanty until it becomes blocked. There is dizziness, tinnitus, low back and knee soreness and weakness, long-term indifference to sexual desire, a pale tongue, and a fine, deep pulse.

Treatment principles: Fortify the spleen, warm the kidneys, and free the flow of the channels or menses

Guiding formulas:

1. *Wen Shen Tong Jing Fang Jia Wei* (Warm the Kidneys & Free the Flow of the Menses Formula with Added Flavors)

Ingredients: Wine-processed Radix Angelicae Sinensis (*Dang Gui*), Radix Albus Paeoniae Lactiflorae (*Bai Shao*), cooked Radix Rehmanniae (*Shu Di*), Rhizoma Atractylodis Macrocephalae (*Bai Zhu*), Radix Morindae Officinalis (*Ba Ji*), Semen Cuscutae (*Tu Si Zi*), Herba Cistanchis Deserticolae (*Rou Cong Rong*), Radix Ligustici Wallichii (*Chuan Xiong*), powdered Placenta Hominis (*Zi He Che*), Radix Codonopsitis Pilosulae (*Dang Shen*),

Fructus Cnidii Monnieri (*She Chuang Zi*), Semen Pruni Persicae (*Tao Ren*), Rhizoma Acori Graminei (*Chang Pu*)

Additions & subtractions: If there are loose stools, remove Persica and Cistanches and add blast-fried Rhizoma Zingiberis (*Pao Jiang*) and Folium Artemisiae Argyii (*Ai Ye*).

2. Empirical formula

Ingredients: Radix Angelicae Sinensis (*Dang Gui*), Radix Codonopsitis Pilosulae (*Dang Shen*), Radix Albus Paeoniae Lactiflorae (*Bai Shao*), Rhizoma Polygonati (*Huang Jing*), Radix Dipsaci (*Chuan Duan*), Semen Cuscutae (*Tu Si Zi*), Rhizoma Curculiginis Orchioidis (*Xian Mao*), Herba Epimedii (*Xian Ling Pi*), Radix Morindae Officinalis (*Ba Ji Tian*), Flouritum (*Zi Shi Ying*), Rhizoma Cyperi Rotundi (*Xiang Fu*)

2. Liver-kidney yin vacuity

Main Symptoms: After taking contraceptive medicinals, the menstrual water becomes blocked and stops. There is spontaneous spill-over of breast milk which is scanty in amount and clear and watery in consistency, dizziness, tinnitus, low fever in the afternoon, heart vexation, sleeplessness, dry mouth and parched throat, a red tongue with scanty fluids, and a fine, rapid pulse.

Treatment principles: Supplement the kidneys and fill the essence, clear heat and enrich yin

Guiding formulas:

1. *Tiao Gan Tang Jia Jian* (Regulate the Liver Decoction with Additions & Subtractions)

Ingredients: Radix Angelicae Sinensis (*Dang Gui*), stir-fried Radix Albus Paeoniae Lactiflorae (*Bai Shao*), Radix Dioscoreae Oppositae (*Shan Yao*), Fructus Corni Officinalis (*Shan Zhu Yu*), Cortex Eucommiae Ulmoidis (*Du Zhong*), Gelatinum Corii Asini (*E Jiao*), Radix Morindae Officinalis (*Ba Ji*), Tuber Ophiopogonis Japinici (*Mai Dong*), Fructus Ligustri Lucidi (*Nu Zhen Zi*), Cortex Radicis Lycii Chinensis (*Di Gu Pi*), uncooked Radix Rehmanniae (*Sheng Di*), Fructus Germinatus Hordei Vulgaris (*Mai Ya*)

2. *Liu Zi Tang* (Six Seeds Decoction)

Ingredients: Radix Angelicae Sinensis (*Dang Gui*), stir-fried Radix Albus Paeoniae Lactiflorae (*Bai Shao*), Radix Angelicae Dahuricae (*Bai Zhi*), whole Fructus Trichosanthis Kirlowii (*Quan Gua Lou*), Fructus Corni Officinalis (*Shan Zhu Yu*), Fructus Ligustri Lucidi

(*Nu Zhen Zi*), Fructus Schisandrae Chinensis (*Wu Wei Zi*), Galla Rhois Chinensis (*Wu Bei Zi*), Semen Cuscutae (*Tu Si Zi*), Fructus Lycii Chinensis (*Qi Zi*), Fructus Rosae Laevigatae (*Jin Ying Zi*), Radix Codonopsitis Pilosulae (*Dang Shen*)

3. Liver depression qi stagnation

Main symptoms: After taking contraceptive medicinals, the menstrual water becomes blocked and stops. There is breast distention, scanty appetite, possible nausea, thin tongue fur, and a bowstring pulse.

Treatment principles: Course the liver and resolve depression, rectify the qi and free the flow of the channels or menses

Guiding formulas:

1. *Chai Hu Shu Gan San Jia Jian* (Bupleurum Course the Liver Powder with Additions & Subtractions)

Ingredients: Radix Bupleuri (*Chai Hu*), Tuber Curcumae (*Yu Jin*), Fructus Citri Aurantii (*Zhi Ke*), stir-fried Radix Albus Paeoniae Lactiflorae (*Bai Shao*), Rhizoma Cyperi Rotundi (*Xiang Fu*), Radix Ligustici Wallichii (*Chuan Xiong*), Rhizoma Curcumae Zedoariae (*E Zhu*), Radix Glycyrrhizae (*Gan Cao*), Fructus Meliae Toosendan (*Chuan Lian Zi*), Rhizoma Corydalis Yanhusuo (*Yan Hu Suo*), Fructus Foeniculi Vulgaris (*Xiao Hui Xiang*), Fructus Crataegi (*Shan Zha*), Herba Angelicae Anomalae (*Liu Ji Nu*)

2. Unnamed formula from *Zhong Yi Fu Ke Lin Chuang Shou Ce (A Clinical Handbook of Chinese Medical Gynecology)*

Ingredients: Radix Angelicae Sinensis (*Dang Gui*), Radix Rubrus & Albus Paeoniae Lactiflorae (*Chi Bai Shao*), Radix Bupleuri (*Chai Hu*), Sclerotium Poriae Cocos (*Fu Ling*), Fructus Ligustri Lucidi (*Nu Zhen Zi*), Tuber Curcumae (*Yu Jin*), Radix Echinopsis Seu Rhaponitici (*Lou Lu*), Rhizoma Acori Gaminei (*Chang Pu*), Radix Angelicae Dahuricae (*Bai Zhi*), Caulis Lonicerae Japonicae (*Ren Dong Teng*), Herba Epimedii (*Xian Ling Pi*), Retinervus Fascicularis Luffae Cylindricae (*Si Gua Lou*)

This formula is for liver depression qi stagnation, however, there is still an ingredient that supplements the kidneys and invigorates yang—Epimedium. This shows how this condition typically does include some element of kidney vacuity. In addition, Luffa enters and frees the flow of the network vessels.

3. Obesity condition amenorrhea

Disease causes, disease mechanisms

This is mostly due to unfulfilled feelings and emotional depression. The spleen's movement and transformation thus lose their duty. Dampness gathers and fat congeals. Hence the *bao luo* suffers obstruction.

Treatment based on pattern discrimination

1. Spleen-kidney yang vacuity

Main symptoms: An obese body and blocked menstruation, dizziness, lassitude of the spirit, lack of strength, somnolence, scanty appetite, loose stools, chest oppression, profuse phlegm, a somber white facial complexion, low back and lower leg pain and suffering, scanty urination, skin distention, a pale tongue with slimy, white fur, and a soggy, fine, slippery pulse

Treatment principles: Fortify the spleen and warm the kidneys, transform dampness, abduct phlegm, and free the flow of the channels or menses

Guiding formula: *Di Tan Tang Jia Jian* (Wash Away Phlegm Decoction with Additions & Subtractions)

Ingredients: Pericarpium Citri Reticulatae (*Chen Pi*), ginger-processed Rhizoma Pinelliae Ternatae (*Ban Xia*), Sclerotium Poriae Cocos (*Fu Ling*), Hawthornberry Massa Medica Fermentata (*Shan Zha Qu*), Six (Ingredients) Massa Medica Fermentata (*Liu Qu*), Rhizoma Curcumae Zedoariae (*E Zhu*), Rhizoma Atractylodis Macrocephalae (*Bai Zhu*), Rhizoma Arisaemais (*Nan Xing*), Rhizoma Acori Graminei (*Chang Pu*), Ramulus Cinnamomi Cassiae (*Gui Zhi*), Caulis Milletiae Seu Spatholobi (*Ji Xue Teng*), processed Rhizoma Cyperi Rotundi (*Xiang Fu*), Herba Epimedii (*Xian Ling Pi*)

Once the power of the appetite has increased, one can take *Ba Zhen Tang* (Eight Pearls Decoction) with Radix Dipsaci (*Chuan Duan*), Radix Astragali Membranacei (*Huang Qi*), Ramulus Cinnamomi Cassiae (*Gui Zhi*), and Caulis Milletiae Seu Spatholobi (*Ji Xue Teng*). If the menstrual water moves downward, one can use *Gui Shen Wan* (Restore the Kidneys Pills) to regulate and supplement the *chong* and *ren*.

2. Liver depression qi binding

Main symptoms: Obese body and blocked menstruation, headache, easy anger, a red face with upbearing fire, a dry mouth, bound stools, effulgent appetite, chest oppression, swelling and distention of the body and limbs, a red tongue with thin fur, and a fine, bowstring pulse

Treatment principles: Clear the liver and drain fire, quicken the blood, rectify the qi, and regulate the menses

Guiding formula: Empirical formula

Ingredients: Uncooked Radix Rehmanniae (*Sheng Di*), Cortex Radicis Moutan (*Dan Pi*), Radix Rubrus Paeoniae Lactiflorae (*Chi Shao*), Radix Bupleuri (*Chai Hu*), Fructus Gardeniae Jasminoidis (*Shan Zhi*), Radix Et Rhizoma Rhei (*Da Huang*), Cortex Phello-dendri (*Huang Bai*), Radix Cyathulae Officinalis (*Chuan Niu Xi*), Herba Lycopi Lucidi (*Ze Lan Ye*), Tuber Curcumae (*Yu Jin*)

Once liver qi has been regulated and the above conditions are ameliorated, then administer the following formula: Radix Angelicae Sinensis (*Dang Gui*), Radix Rubrus Paeoniae Lactiflorae (*Chi Shao*), uncooked Radix Rehmanniae (*Sheng Di*), Herba Lycopi Lucidi (*Ze Lan Ye*), Radix Salviae Miltiorrhizae (*Dan Shen*), Herba Leonuri Heterophylli (*Yi Mu Cao*), Herba Patriniae Heterophyllae Cum Radice (*Bai Jiang Cao*), Herba Brucnerae Cruciatae (*Gui Jian Yu*), Herba Angelicae Anomale (*Liu Ji Nu*)

After the menses move, one can then administer *Gui Shen Wan* (Restore the Kidneys Pills) or *Liu Wei Di Huang Wan* (Six Flavors Rehmannia Pills) to regulate and boost the liver and kidneys.

4. Stein-Leventhal syndrome amenorrhea

Disease causes, disease mechanisms

If postpartum a great deal of blood has been lost, the liver and kidney essence and blood may become insufficient. In that case, the sea of blood is empty, the brain loses the blood which nourishes it, and there may be blocked menstruation. It is also possible that the spleen and kidneys are constitutionally insufficient or, after loss of blood, spleen and kidney yang qi may follow the discharged blood. Thus the fire of the gate of life becomes debilitated and is not able to warm and steam. The sea of blood is empty and vacuous and blocked menses do not descend. If postpartum there has been a great loss of blood, the heart qi may also become vacuous and weak and the brain may lose its nourishing blood. The heart and brain thus do not interact and the menstrual blood does not move. In addition, it is possible for liver depression-depressive heat to manifest simultaneously with kidney vacuity. In fact, this is a clinically common presentation among my patients. And lastly, qi stagnation and blood stasis may also manifest in sufferers of Stein-Leventhal syndrome blocked menstruation.

Treatment based on pattern discrimination

1. Liver-kidney yin vacuity

Main symptoms: Blocked menstruation, dizziness, tinnitus, lassitude of the spirit, lack of strength, low back and knee pain and weakness, heart vexation, no sleep, dry mouth, parched throat, constipated stools, reddish urine, a red tongue with scanty fluids and fur, and a fine, weak pulse

Treatment principles: Enrich yin and fill the essence, boost the kidneys and regulate the menses

Guiding formulas:

1. *Bu Shen Di Huang Tang Jia Jian* (Supplement the Kidneys Rehmannia Decoction with Additions & Subtractions)

Ingredients: Cooked Radix Rehmanniae (*Shu Di*), Tuber Ophiopogonis Japonici (*Mai Dong*), Rhizoma Anemarrhenae Aspheloidis (*Zhi Mu*), Cortex Phellodendri (*Huang Bai*), Rhizoma Alsimatis (*Ze Xie*), Radix Dioscoreae Oppositae (*Shan Yao*), Radix Polygalae Tenuifoliae (*Yuan Zhi*), Cortex Radicis Moutan (*Dan Pi*), Radix Scrophulariae Ningpoensis (*Xuan Shen*), Fructus Corni Officinalis (*Shan Zhu Yu*), Plastrum Testudinis (*Gui Ban*), Ootheca Mantidis (*Sang Piao Xiao*)

2. Unnamed formula from *Zhong Yi Fu Ke Lin Chuang Shou Ce (A Clinical Handbook of Chinese Medical Gynecology)*

Ingredients: Uncooked & cooked Radix Rehmanniae (*Sheng Shu Di*), Tuber Ophiopogonis Japonici (*Mai Dong*), Radix Polygalae Tenuifoliae (*Yuan Zhi*), Semen Biotae Orientalis (*Bai Zi Ren*), Radix Dioscoreae Oppositae (*Shan Yao*), Radix Polygoni Multiflori (*Shou Wu*), Fructus Corni Officinalis (*Shan Zhu Yu*), Gelatinum Corii Asini (*E Jiao*), Gelatinum Plastri Testudinis (*Gui Ban Jiao*), Caulis Milletiae Seu Spatholobi (*Ji Xue Teng*), Fructus Ligustri Lucidi (*Nu Zhen Zi*), Fructus Lycii Chinensis (*Qi Zi*), mix-fried Radix Glycyrrhizae (*Gan Cao*)

2. Spleen-kidney yang vacuity

Main symptoms: Sudden onset blocked menstruation, fear of cold, chilled limbs, essence spirit withering, lassitude of the spirit, falling hair, scarce and faded, practically no vaginal discharge, vaginal meatus dry and astringent, no interest in sexual desire, loose stools, clear urination, a pale tongue with a thin coating, and a deep, fine, weak pulse

Treatment principles: Warm the kidneys and fortify the spleen, boost the essence and free the flow of the channels or menses

Guiding formula: *Jia Jian Cong Rong Tu Si Zi Wan* (Additions & Subtractions Cistanches & Cuscuta Pills)

Ingredients: Semen Cuscutae (*Tu Si Zi*), Fructus Rubi Chingii (*Fu Pen Zi*), Herba Cistanchis Deserticolae (*Cong Rong*), Fructus Lycii Chinensis (*Qi Zi*), Ramulus Loranthi Seu Visci (*Sang Ji Sheng*), large cooked Radix Rehmanniae (*Shu Di*), Radix Angelicae Sinensis (*Dang Gui*), Folium Artemisiae Argyii (*Ai Ye*), powdered Placenta Hominis (*Zi He Che*), Radix Astragali Membranacei (*Huang Qi*)

Additions & subtractions: If there are loose stools, add blast-fried Rhizoma Zingiberis (*Pao Jiang*) and Radix Morindae Officinalis (*Ba Ji Rou*) and remove Cistanches.

3. Heart & brain not interacting

Main symptoms: Blocked menstruation, dizziness, vertigo, lumbar pain, tinnitus, heart palpitations, racing heart, shortness of breath, lack of strength, insomnia, impaired memory, listless essence spirit, a pale tongue with thin fur, and a fine, weak pulse

These signs and symptoms are essentially a heart blood-spleen qi vacuity pattern with the addition of kidney vacuity as well, *i.e.*, lumbar pain.

Treatment principles: Nourish the heart and supplement the blood, boost the kidneys and supplement the brain

Guiding formula: Unnamed formula from *Zhong Yi Fu Ke Lin Chuang Shou Ce (A Clinical Handbook of Chinese Medical Gynecology)*

Ingredients: Radix Codonopsitis Pilosulae (*Dang Shen*), Radix Astragali Membranacei (*Huang Qi*), Radix Angelicae Sinensis (*Dang Gui*), stir-fried Radix Albus Paeoniae Lactiflorae (*Bai Shao*), stir-fried Rhizoma Atractylodis Macrocephalae (*Bai Zhu*), Gelatinum Corii Asini (*E Jiao*), Fructus Schisandrae Chinensis (*Wu Wei Zi*), Radix Polygalae Tenuifoliae (*Yuan Zhi*), Herba Cynomorii Songarici (*Suo Yang*), Herba Epimedii (*Xian Ling Pi*), Fructus Ligustri Lucidi (*Nu Zhen Zi*), Gelatinum Cornu Cervi (*Lu Jiao Jiao*), Rhizoma Polygonati (*Huang Jing*), processed Radix Polygoni Multiflori (*Shou Wu*), *He Che Da Zao Wan* (Placenta Great Creation Pills, patent medicine), Radix Ligustici Wallichii (*Chuan Xiong*)

4. Liver depressive heat & kidney vacuity

Main symptoms: Blocked menstruation, irritability, red eyes and face, a bitter taste in the mouth, low back pain, cold feet, absent or decreased sexual desire, chest and rib-side fullness and oppression, a dark red tongue with thin, possibly yellow fur, and a bowstring, fine, rapid pulse

Treatment principles: Course the liver and rectify the qi, clear heat and resolve depression, supplement the kidneys and invigorate yang

Guiding formula: *Qing Gan Bu Shen Tang* (Clear the Liver & Supplement the Kidneys Decoction)

Ingredients: Cortex Radicis Moutan (*Dan Pi*), stir-fried Fructus Gardeniae Jasminoidis (*Shan Zhi*), Radix Bupleuri (*Chai Hu*), Radix Angelicae Sinensis (*Dang Gui*), Pericarpium Citri Reticulatae Viride (*Qing Pi*), uncooked Radix Rehmanniae (*Sheng Di*), Rhizoma Polygonati (*Huang Jing*), Herba Epimedii (*Xian Ling Pi*), Fructus Psoraleae Corylifoliae (*Bu Gu Zhi*), Squama Manitis Pentadactylis (*Shan Jia*)

5. Qi stagnation blood stasis

Main symptoms: Emotional depression, vexation and agitation, easy anger, lower abdominal distention and fullness refusing pressure, possible chest fullness and rib-side pain, delayed menstruation, amount diminished, containing small clots, if severe, blocked menstruation, anovulation, infertility, excessive hair, fat body, bilateral ovarian enlargement, a dark or purplish tongue with possible static spots or macules, and a fine, bowstring or deep, choppy pulse

Treatment principles: Move the qi and quicken the blood, dispel stasis and free the flow of the channels or menses

Guiding formula: *Ge Xia Zhu Yu Tang* (Below the Diaphragm Dispel Stasis Decoction)

Ingredients: Radix Linderae Strychnifoliae (*Wu Yao*), Fructus Aurantii (*Zhi Ke*), Radix Angelicae Sinensis (*Dang Gui*), Flos Carthami Tinctorii (*Hong Hua*), Radix Ligustici Wallichii (*Chuan Xiong*), Rhizoma Cyperi Rotundi (*Xiang Fu*), Radix Rubrus Paeoniae Lactiflorae (*Chi Shao*), Semen Pruni Persicae (*Tao Ren*), Cortex Radicis Moutan (*Dan Pi*), Rhizoma Corydalis Yanhusuo (*Yan Hu Suo*), Feces Trogopterori Seu Pteromi (*Wu Ling Zhi*), Radix Glycyrrhizae (*Gan Cao*)

5. Tubercular amenorrhea

Due to the tuberculosis bacillus invading the reproductive organs, this may give rise to tubercular pelvic inflammatory disease. If this is not treated in a timely manner, it may eventually destroy the endometrium, resulting in blocked menstruation.

Disease causes, disease mechanisms

If the natural endowment is vacuous and weak, tuberculosis germs may enter, taking advantage of vacuity, invading the *bao luo* and *bao gong*. This may then lead to the *chong* and *ren* suffering detriment. The sea of blood thus becomes empty and vacuous and this results in blocked menstruation.

Key points in diagnosis

1. This disease is basically a form of tuberculosis.

2. The onset of this disease is marked by a menstruation which gets progressively more watery and scant until it becomes blocked menstruation. This is accompanied in most cases by afternoon tidal fever, red cheeks, night sweats, and other such signs of yin vacuity.

Treatment based on pattern discrimination

1. Lung-kidney yin vacuity

Main symptoms: Blocked menstruation, dizziness, tinnitus, low back and knee soreness and weakness, yellow colored vaginal discharge, dry cough, scanty phlegm, afternoon tidal fever, both cheeks red, a dry mouth, parched throat, a red tongue with thin fur and scanty fluids, and a fine, rapid pulse

Treatment principles: Boost the kidneys and nourish the lungs, clear heat and regulate the menses

Guiding formulas:

1. *Bai He Gu Jin Tang Jia Jian* (Lily Secure Metal Decoction with Additions & Subtractions)

Ingredients: Uncooked Radix Rehmanniae (*Sheng Di*), cooked Radix Rehmanniae (*Shu Di*), Tuber Ophiopogonis Japonici (*Mai Dong*), Bulbus Lilii (*Bai He*), Radix Paeoniae Lactiflorae (*Shao Yao*), Radix Angelicae Sinensis (*Dang Gui*), Radix Scutellariae Baicalensis (*Huang Qin*), Radix Stemonae (*Bai Bu*), Bulbus Fritillariae Cirrhosae (*Chuan Bei*), Herba Lycopi Lucidi (*Ze Lan*)

2. *Kang Lao Tong Jing Fang* (Combat Consumption & Free the Flow of the Channels [or Menses] Formula)

Ingredients: Radix Salviae Miltiorrhizae (*Dan Shen*), Radix Stemonae (*Bai Bu*), Radix Scutellariae Baicalensis (*Huang Qin*), Tuber Ophiopogonis Japonici (*Mai Dong*), Radix Scrophulariae Ningpoensis (*Xuan Shen*), Radix Gentianae Macrophyllae (*Qin Jiao*), mix-fried Carapax Amydae Sinensis (*Bie Jia*), Cortex Radicis Lycii Chinensis (*Di Gu Pi*), Flos Lonicerae Japonicae (*Yin Hua*), Herba Angelicae Anomalae (*Liu Ji Nu*), Fructus Cinidii Monnieri (*She Chuang Zi*), Radix Glycyrrhizae (*Gan Cao*)

Additions: If the skin is scaly and rough, add Gelatinum Corii Asini (*E Jiao*), Flos Carthami Tinctorii (*Hong Hua*), and *Da Huang Zhe Chong Wan* (Rhubarb & Eupolyphaga Pills, a patent medicine). If there are night sweats, add Fructus Schisandrae Chinensis (*Wu Wei Zi*) and Radix Et Rhizoma Oryzae Glutinosae (*Nuo Dao Geng*). For lack of strength, add Radix Pseudostellariae (*Tai Zi Shen*). For scanty appetite, add Fructus Germinatus Hordei Vulgaris (*Mai Ya*) and Fructus Amomi (*Sha Ren*).

2. Qi & blood vacuity weakness

Main symptoms: Blocked menstruation, dizziness, lack of strength, lassitude of the spirit, low fever in the afternoon, no thought for taking grains, a pale tongue with thin fur, and a fine, weak pulse

Treatment principles: Supplement the qi and nourish the blood, boost the kidneys and regulate the menses

Guiding formula: Unnamed formula from *Zhong Yi Zhi Liao Fu Nu Bing (The Chinese Medical Treatment of Gynecological Diseases)*

Ingredients: Radix Astragali Membranacei (*Huang Qi*), Radix Codonopsitis Pilosulae (*Dang Shen*), Radix Angelicae Sinensis (*Dang Gui*), cooked Radix Rehmanniae (*Shu Di*), Tuber Ophiopogonis Japonici (*Mai Dong*), Radix Dioscoreae Oppositae (*Shan Yao*), Sclerotium Poriae Cocos (*Fu Ling*), Pericarpium Citri Reticulatae (*Chen Pi*), mix-fried Carapax Amydae Sinensis (*Bie Jia*), mix-fried Radix Stemonae (*Bai Bu*), Concha Cyclinae (*Hai Ge Ke*), Radix Scutellariae Baicalensis (*Huang Qin*), Radix Pseudoginseng (*San Qi*), Semen Cuscutae (*Tu Si Zi*)

6. Ceased menstruation in a young girl

A young girl's menses have already come but then again do not come for several months. This is called young girl's ceased menstruation.

Disease causes: Lack of movement in a young girl's menstruation is mostly caused by yang vacuity and blood weakness. Fire is exuberant and water is deficient.

Main symptoms: The menses stop and cease and there is generalized fever, tidal fever, and progressive emaciation with each passing day

Treatment principles: Nourish yin and boost the blood. However, do not use cooling medicinals.

Guiding formulas:

1. Unnamed formula from *Zhong Yi Zhi Liao Fu Nu Bing (Chinese Medical Treatments for Women's Diseases)*

Ingredients: Semen Biotae Orientalis (*Bai Zi Ren*), wine stir-fried Radix Achyranthis Bidentatae (*Niu Xi*), Herba Menthae Haplocalycis (*Bo He*), Herba Lycopi Lucidi (*Ze Lan Ye*), Sichuan Radix Dipsaci (*Chuan Xu Duan*), cooked Radix Rehmanniae (*Shu Di*)

2. Unnamed formula from *Zhong Yi Zhi Liao Fu Nu Bing (Chinese Medical Treatments for Women's Diseases)*

Ingredients: Herba Lycopi Lucidi (*Ze Lan Ye*), Radix Angelicae Sinensis (*Dang Gui*), Radix Glycyrrhizae (*Gan Cao*)

Although Lycopus is a blood-quickening medicinal, it does not damage the blood when there is concomitant blood vacuity.

7. Enduring, enduring blocked menstruation

A woman, due to disease or constitutional deficiency weakness, may have enduring, enduring blocked menstruation.

Disease causes: This is mostly caused by internal damage by the seven affects.

Main symptoms: Progressive bodily emaciation, lack of strength in the four limbs, no thought for food or drink, essence exhausted, lassitude of the spirit

Treatment principles: Nourish yin and rectify the blood

Guiding formula: Unnamed formula from *Zhong Yi Zhi Liao Fu Nu Bing (Chinese Medical Treatments for Women's Diseases)*

Ingredients: Fructus Zizyphi Jujubae (*Hong Zao*), red sugar (*Hong Tang*), uncooked Rhizoma Zingiberis (*Sheng Jiang*), Radix Indigoferae Tinctoriae (*Ma Lan Dou Gen*), 60g @. Decoct together and divide in two. Take two times per day. Take continuously without stopping until the menstrual water comes.

8. Widow's ceased menstruation

If a widow's menstruation does not move, this is called widow's ceased menstruation.

Disease causes: A widow's solitary yin lacks yang. Desire causes stirring but does not obtain satisfaction. Regret accumulates and does not obtain release. Thus depression results in blocked menstruation.

Main symptoms: Aversion to wind, bodily fatigue, a red facial complexion, heart vexation, spontaneous sweating which does not stop

Treatment principles: Rectify the qi and quicken the blood, clear heat and cool the blood

Guiding formula: Unnamed formula from *Zhong Yi Zhi Liao Fu Nu Bing (Chinese Medical Treatments for Women's Diseases)*

Ingredients: Radix Bupleuri (*Chai Hu*), Pericarpium Viridis Citri Reticulatae (*Qing Pi*), Radix Rubrus Paeoniae Lactiflorae (*Chi Shao*), Cortex Radicis Moutan (*Dan Pi*), Cortex Radicis Lycii Chinensis (*Di Gu Pi*), processed Rhizoma Cyperi Rotundi (*Xiang Fu*), stir-fried Fructus Gardeniae Jasminoidis (*Zhi Zi*), stir-fried Rhizoma Atractylodis (*Cang Zhu*), Radix Ligustici Wallichii (*Chuan Xiong*), bran stir-fried Massa Medica Fermentata (*Shen Qu*), 9g @, wine stir-fried uncooked Radix Rehmanniae (*Sheng Di*), 12g, Fructus Forsythiae Suspensae (*Lian Qiao*), Radix Glycyrrhizae (*Gan Cao*), 6g @. Decoct in water and take after meals.

(From Zhong Yi Zi Xue Cong Shu [The Chinese Medical Self-study Series], Vol II, "Gynecology", Hebei Science & Technology Press, Shijiazhuang, 1987)

BLOCKED MENSTRUATION:
VACUITY & REPLETION

	REPLETION PATTERNS	VACUITY PATTERNS
CHEST & ABDOMEN	Chest oppression, lower abdominal pain or distention, pressure makes worse	No sensation of distention or oppression within the chest or abdomen, or abdominal distention and pain which likes pressure and rubbing
FORMAL BODY	Formal body not debilitated or obesity	Formal body vacuous and debilitated, or as if withered firewood
PULSE & TONGUE	Pulse wiry with force or deep & choppy. Tongue coating yellow or white and slimy; substance purplish	Pulse fine & weak or fine & choppy. Tongue coating thin or scanty; tongue substance pale or bright red

(From *Zhong Yi Fu Ke Xue [A Study of Chinese Medical Gynecology]* by Liu Min-ru, Sichuan Science & Technology Press, Chengdu, 1992)

THE DIFFERENTIATION OF BLOCKED MENSTRUATION FROM EARLY PREGNANCY

Clinical Signs & Symptoms	Blocked Menstruation	Early Pregnancy
	Before developing blocked menstruation, mostly have menstrual irregularity. It is does suddenly stop & cease, usually there will be lower abdominal distention and pain or other such pathological symptoms.	Menses mostly normal and then suddenly stops & ceases. Typically have pregnant reactions.
Pulse Image	mostly deep & choppy or vacuous & fine	slippery & uninhibited
Gynecological Examination	no sign of pregnancy	has signs of pregnancy
Pregnancy test	negative	positive

8

Painful Menstruation

Dysmenorrhea is called *tong jing* in Chinese. *Tong* means pain and *jing* refers to menstruation. Therefore, *tong jing* means pain, principally of the lower abdomen but also including the low back, sacrum, hips, and thighs, occurring just before, during, or just after the menses. In Chinese, this is sometimes also referred to as menstrual movement abdominal pain. The pain may be either crampy, sharp and stabbing, dragging and heavy, or pulling and tight. It may feel either hot or cold. It can be either mild or so intense as to be incapacitating and unbearable. In some cases, painful menstruation may be accompanied by nausea, vomiting, chilling of the extremities, cold sweats, headache, dizziness, or diarrhea.

Painful menstruation is often a patient's major complaint. This may be lifelong or of recent onset. Painful menstruation is often associated with the modern Western medical disease categories endometriosis, endometritis (adnexitis, salpingitis, ovarian cystitis, etc.), uterine myomas (a.k.a. fibroids), retroverted uterus, etc. Because painful menstruation is so common and also associated with a number of Western diseases, it is of utmost importance that the practitioner of TCM gynecology be competent in the diagnosis and treatment of this disease category.

Disease causes, disease mechanisms

Painful menstruation, as its name states, is a species of pain or *tong*. The basic dictum in Chinese medicine regarding pain is:

Tong zhi bu tong
Bu tong zhi tong

If there is pain, there is no free flow;
If there is no free flow, there is pain.

337

Based on this dictum which every TCM practitioner is expected to know by heart, it is clear that painful menstruation has to do with lack of free flow. Lack of free flow may be due to either repletion or vacuity. Evil qi may lodge, block, and obstruct the flow of qi and blood, thus resulting in lack of free flow and, therefore, pain. Insufficiency of righteous qi (including blood, yin, and/or yang) may result in lack of qi to move the blood, lack of yin and blood to nourish the sinews and vessels, or lack of yang to warm the channels and uterus. Repletions obstructing the uninhibited free flow of the menstrual water include stagnant qi, blood stasis, replete cold and dampness, damp heat, depressive heat, and worm accumulation. Vacuities include qi vacuity, blood vacuity, liver-kidney yin vacuity, vacuity heat, and vacuity cold.

Stagnant qi is usually associated with liver depression in turn due to stress and frustration. If qi stagnation endures, it may give rise to blood stasis. Blood stasis, however, may also be caused by trauma, including lower abdominal surgery, IUDs, OCs, abortions and miscarriages, and sex during menstruation. Accumulation of cold and dampness blocking the free flow of qi and blood is usually caused by exposure to external cold and dampness and overeating uncooked, chilled foods, sour foods, and fluid-engendering foods, such as sugar. Damp heat which wrestles and binds with stagnant qi and blood stasis may be due either to external invasion, including sexual transmission, overeating fluid-engendering, hot foods, such as greasy, spicy foods and alcohol, or enduring internal heat and spleen dampness. Depressive heat is the same as liver depression qi stagnation which has transformed into heat. Depressive heat is usually due to more extreme emotional stress and frustration. Worm accumulation may also obstruct the free flow of the menses. It is usually associated with damp heat in turn due to spleen vacuity and dampness and faulty diet.

If spleen qi becomes weak and fails to upbear clear yang, the abdominal contents may fall. The qi and blood thus cannot flow freely through the channels and network vessels in the lower burner and, therefore, there is pain and discomfort. Spleen qi vacuity weakness may be due to faulty diet, overtaxation, under-exercise, or excessive worry and thinking. If blood and yin are vacuous, they will fail to nourish the sinews and vessels, which then tend to contract, thus inhibiting the free flow of qi and blood. Blood vacuity may be due to faulty diet, worry and overthinking, or any other factor which damages the spleen and/or heart. If blood vacuity endures or is accompanied by yin vacuity, this becomes liver blood-kidney yin vacuity. Liver-kidney yin vacuity may be due to insufficient natural endowment, enduring disease, bedroom, *i.e.*, sexual, taxation, drug use, or simply aging.

When yin becomes vacuous and insufficient, yang may come out of control, giving rise to signs and symptoms of vacuity heat. Because the pain is due to liver blood-kidney yin vacuity, many TCM gynecology texts do not list this as a separate pattern. However, because many Western women present with this species of painful menstruation and because its signs and symptoms do not exactly fit any of the above scenarios, I am listing it here as a separate category. Likewise, most Chinese gynecology texts do not list vacuity cold of the uterus as a disease mechanism or pattern. Han Bai-ling, however, does. In this case, age, congenital insufficiency, drug use, excessive sex, enduring disease, or extreme exhaustion may exhaust the yang, thus leading to its inability to warm the channels and uterus and motivate the qi and blood. Since cold by its very nature leads to constriction and congelation, vacuity cold due to yang vacuity also leads to blood stasis.

Treatment based on pattern discrimination

Repletion patterns

1. Qi stagnation, blood stasis

Main symptoms: Lower abdominal distention and pain one or two days before menstruation or during the first part of menstruation which is aggravated by pressure. If qi stagnation is more prominent, there is more distention and cramping and the condition is aggravated by stress and emotional upset. If blood stasis is more prominent, there is more pain than distention and the pain tends to be fixed and lancinating. In addition, severe pain is usually categorized as blood stasis. The flow tends to be scanty or does not flow easily. The blood is typically purplish and dark. The more blood stasis, the more and larger the clots (except in the case of endometriosis). There is usually a relief of pain after blood clots are discharged (again, except in the case of endometriosis). If qi stagnation is pronounced, there is also chest, breast, and rib-side distention and pain. The tongue is purplish and dark or has static spots or macules and the pulse is deep and bowstring or deep and choppy. Poking pain with deep intercourse or dyspareunia is also a symptom of blood stasis (commonly indicating the likelihood of endometriosis).

Treatment principles: Rectify the qi and quicken the blood, move stasis and stop pain

Guiding formulas:

1. *Ge Xia Zhu Yu Tang* (Below the Diaphragm Dispel Stasis Decoction)

Ingredients: Radix Angelicae Sinensis (*Dang Gui*), Radix Ligustici Wallichii (*Chuan Xiong*), Radix Rubrus Paeoniae Lactiflorae (*Chi Shao*), Semen Pruni Persicae (*Tao Ren*), Flos Carthami Tinctorii (*Hong Hua*), Fructus Citri Aurantii (*Zhi Ke*), Rhizoma Corydalis Yanhusuo (*Yan Hu Suo*), Feces Trogopterori Seu Pteromi (*Wu Ling Zhi*), Cortex Radicis Moutan (*Dan Pi*), Radix Linderae Strychnifoliae (*Wu Yao*), Rhizoma Cyperi Rotundi (*Xiang Fu*), Radix Glycyrrhizae (*Gan Cao*)

2. *Xue Fu Zhu Yu Tang* (Blood Mansion Dispel Stasis Decoction)

Ingredients: Semen Pruni Persicae (*Tao Ren*), Flos Carthami Tinctorii (*Hong Hua*), Radix Angelicae Sinensis (*Dang Gui*), Radix Ligustici Wallichii (*Chuan Xiong*), Radix Rubrus Paeoniae Lactiflorae (*Chai Hu*), Radix Cyathulae Officinalis (*Chuan Niu Xi*), Radix Bupleuri (*Chai Hu*), Radix Platycodi Grandiflori (*Jie Geng*), Fructus Citri Aurantii (*Zhi Ke*), uncooked Radix Rehmanniae (*Sheng Di*), Radix Glycyrrhizae (*Gan Cao*)

Additions: If distention is worse than pain, add Rhizoma Cyperi Rotundi (*Xiang Fu*) and Tuber Curcumae (*Yu Jin*). If there is breast pain and distention, add Spica Prunella Vulgaris (*Xia Gu Cao*) and Fructus Aesculi (*Suo Luo Zi*). If the discharge of clots is difficult, add Rhizoma Sparganii (*San Leng*) and Rhizoma Curcumae Zedoariae (*E Zhu*). If pain is severe, add Feces Trogopterori Seu Pteromi (*Wu Ling Zhi*) and Pollen Typhae (*Pu Huang*).

3. Sun Jiu-ling's *Xue Fu Zhu Yu Tang Jia Jian* (Blood Mansion Dispel Stasis Decoction with Additions & Subtractions)

Ingredients: Radix Angelicae Sinensis (*Dang Gui*), stir-fried Semen Pruni Persicae (*Tao Ren*), Flos Carthami Tinctorii (*Hong Hua*), Radix Ligustici Wallichii (*Chuan Xiong*), Radix Rubrus Paeoniae Lactiflorae (*Chi Shao*), Feces Trogopterori Seu Pteromi (*Wu Ling Zhi*), Rhizoma Corydalis Yanhusuo (*Yan Hu Suo*), Rhizoma Cyperi Rotundi (*Xiang Fu*), Fructus Citri Aurantii (*Zhi Ke*), Radix Auklandiae Lappae (*Mu Xiang*), Radix Achyranthis Bidentatae (*Chuan Niu Xi*), Radix Glycyrrhizae (*Gan Cao*)

4. Han Bai-ling's *Xue Fu Zhu Yu Tang Jia Jian* (Blood Mansion Dispel Stasis Decoction with Additions & Subtractions)

Ingredients: Radix Angelicae Sinensis (*Dang Gui*), uncooked Radix Rehmanniae (*Sheng Di*), Semen Pruni Persicae (*Tao Ren*), Flos Carthami Tinctorii (*Hong Hua*), Fructus Citri Aurantii (*Zhi Ke*), Radix Rubrus Paeoniae Lactiflorae (*Chi Shao*), Radix Bupleuri (*Chai Hu*), Radix Ligustici Wallichii (*Chuan Xiong*), Radix Platycodi Grandiflori (*Jie Geng*), Radix Achyranthis Bidentatae (*Niu Xi*), uncooked Radix Glycyrrhizae (*Gan Cao*)

Additions: If there is heat, add Radix Scutellariae Baicalensis (*Huang Qin*). If there is constipation, add a little Radix Et Rhizoma Rhei (*Da Huang*).

5. Zhu Cheng-han's *Xue Fu Zhu Yu Tang Jia Jian* (Blood Mansion Dispel Stasis Decoction with Additions & Subtractions)

Ingredients: Radix Angelicae Sinensis (*Dang Gui*), Radix Ligustici Wallichii (*Chuan Xiong*), Radix Rubrus Paeoniae Lactiflorae (*Chi Shao*), Semen Pruni Persicae (*Tao Ren*),

Flos Carthami Tinctorii (*Hong Hua*), Radix Achyranthis Bidentatae (*Niu Xi*), Rhizoma Cyperi Rotundi (*Xiang Fu*), Pericarpium Citri Reticulatae Viride (*Qing Pi*), Fructus Citri Aurantii (*Zhi Ke*), Radix Auklandiae Lappae (*Mu Xiang*), Rhizoma Corydalis Yanhusuo (*Yan Hu Suo*)

6. *Qing Re Tiao Xue Tang* (Clear Heat & Regulate the Blood Decoction)

Ingredients: Radix Albus Paeoniae Lactiflorae (*Bai Shao*), uncooked Radix Rehmanniae (*Sheng Di*), Rhizoma Coptidis Chinensis (*Huang Lian*), Rhizoma Curcumae Zedoariae (*E Zhu*), Radix Angelicae Sinensis (*Dang Gui*), Radix Ligustici Wallichii (*Chuan Xiong*), Flos Carthami Tinctorii (*Hong Hua*), Rhizoma Corydalis Yanhusuo (*Yan Hu Suo*), Semen Pruni Persicae (*Tao Ren*), Rhizoma Cyperi Rotundi (*Xiang Fu*), Cortex Radicis Moutan (*Dan Pi*)

This formula is for stagnant qi and blood stasis which have given rise to transformative heat. The blood is fresh red in color but contains clots. The tongue fur is yellow and the pulse is rapid along with the other signs which denote qi stagnation and blood stasis. In this case, the treatment principles are to clear heat and cool the blood, quicken the blood and transform stasis.

7. *Jia Wei Wu Yao Tang* (Added Flavors Lindera Decoction)

Ingredients: Radix Linderae Strychnifoliae (*Wu Yao*), Fructus Amomi (*Sha Ren*), Radix Auklandiae Lappae (*Mu Xiang*), Rhizoma Corydalis Yanhusuo (*Yan Hu Suo*), processed Rhizoma Cyperi Rotundi (*Xiang Fu*), mix-fried Radix Glycyrrhizae (*Gan Cao*), uncooked Rhizoma Zingiberis (*Sheng Jiang*), Radix Angelicae Sinensis (*Dang Gui*), Radix Salviae Miltiorrhizae (*Dan Shen*)

This formula is for more pronounced qi stagnation as opposed to blood stasis. Although the majority of the ingredients are qi-rectifiers, blood-quickening medicinals are added due to the reciprocal relationship between the qi and blood. Readers should note that Lindera is particularly indicated if menstrual or lower abdominal pain follows the course of the liver channel on the sides of the lower abdomen.

8. *Ba Wu Tang* (Eight Materials Decoction)

Ingredients: Radix Angelicae Sinensis (*Dang Gui*), Radix Ligustici Wallichii (*Chuan Xiong*), Radix Albus Paeoniae Lactiflorae (*Bai Shao*), Rhizoma Corydalis Yanhusuo (*Yan Hu Suo*), Fructus Meliae Toosendan (*Chuan Lian Zi*), Radix Auklandiae Lappae (*Mu Xiang*), Semen Arecae Catechu (*Bing Lang*), cooked Radix Rehmanniae (*Shu Di*)

9. *Tao Hong Si Wu Tang Jia Wei* (Persica & Carthamus Four Materials Decoction with Added Flavors)

Ingredients: Flos Carthami Tinctorii (*Hong Hua*), Semen Pruni Persicae (*Tao Ren*), Radix Angelicae Sinensis (*Dang Gui*), Radix Albus Paeoniae Lactiflorae (*Bai Shao*), Radix Ligustici Wallichii (*Chuan Xiong*), cooked Radix Rehmanniae (*Shu Di*), Rhizoma Corydalis Yanhusuo (*Yan Hu Suo*), Rhizoma Cyperi Rotundi (*Xiang Fu*), Herba Leonuri Heterophylli (*Yi Mu Cao*), Radix Auklandiae Lappae (*Mu Xiang*)

This formula is for blood stasis complicated by qi stagnation and an element of blood vacuity. The readers should remember that *Tao Hong Si Wu Tang* is the standard guiding formula for blood vacuity- blood stasis.

10. *Tong Jing Fang* (Painful Menstruation Formula)

Ingredients: Stir-fried Radix Angelicae Sinensis (*Dang Gui*), Radix Ligustici Wallichii (*Chuan Xiong*), Radix Salviae Miltiorrhizae (*Dan Shen*), Radix Cyathulae Officinalis (*Chuan Niu Xi*), Radix Rubrus Paeoniae Lactiflorae (*Chi Shao*), Ramulus Cinnamomi Cassiae (*Gui Zhi*), processed Rhizoma Cyperi Rotundi (*Xiang Fu*), Rhizoma Corydalis Yanhusuo (*Yan Hu Suo*), Sanguis Draconis (*Xue Jie*), Resina Myrrhae (*Mo Yao*)

Zhang En-qin *et al.* give this formula for endometriosis due to qi stagnation, blood stasis. The signs and symptoms Zhang *et al.* list as the indications for this formula are headed by severe pain in the lower abdomen before, during, or after menstruation accompanied by a dragging pain in the lumbosacral region and anus. These are accompanied by a purplish red tongue with thin, white fur and a bowstring, fine pulse.

11. *Sheng Hua Tang Jia Wei* (Engendering & Transforming Decoction with Added Flavors)

Ingredients: Radix Angelicae Sinensis (*Dang Gui*), Radix Ligustici Wallichii (*Chuan Xiong*), Semen Pruni Persicae (*Tao Ren*), Radix Rubrus Paeoniae Lactiflorae (*Chi Shao*), Flos Carthami Tinctorii (*Hong Hua*), Radix Achyranthis Bidentatae (*Niu Xi*), Rhizoma Cyperi Rotundi (*Xiang Fu*), Radix Linderae Strychnifoliae (*Wu Yao*), Rhizoma Corydalis Yanhusuo (*Yan Hu Suo*), Radix Glycyrrhizae (*Gan Cao*), blast-fried Rhizoma Zingiberis (*Pao Jiang*)

This formula is a modification of Fu Qing-zhu's famous postpartum formula, *Sheng Hua Tang*. It is indicated, due to the inclusion of blast-fried Ginger, when blood stasis is complicated by an element of vacuity cold. However, given the above modifications, here blood stasis and qi stagnation are much more important than any cold.

12. *Tiao Jing Yin* (Regulate the Menses Drink)

Ingredients: Radix Angelicae Sinensis (*Dang Gui*), Radix Achyranthis Bidentatae (*Niu Xi*), Fructus Crataegi (*Shan Zha*), Rhizoma Cyperi Rotundi (*Xiang Fu*), Pericarpium Citri Reticulatae Viride (*Qing Pi*), Sclerotium Poriae Cocos (*Fu Ling*)

Du Jie-hui suggests this formula for the treatment of qi stagnation, blood stasis painful menstruation. It moves the qi and quickens the blood, regulates the menses and stops pain. It is particularly useful, due to the inclusion of Crataegus, if there are clots in the menstruate which look like pieces of meat.

13. *Jia Jian Chai Hu Shu Gan Tang* (Additions & Subtractions Bupleurum Soothe the Liver Decoction)

Ingredients: Radix Bupleuri (*Chai Hu*), Radix Albus Paeoniae Lactiflorae (*Bai Shao*), Rhizoma Cyperi Rotundi (*Xiang Fu*), Radix Ligustici Wallichii (*Chuan Xiong*), Radix Angelicae Sinensis (*Dang Gui*), Rhizoma Corydalis Yanhusuo (*Yan Hu Suo*), Fructus Immaturus Citri Seu Ponciri (*Zhi Shi*), Folium Artemisiae Argyii (*Ai Ye*), Cortex Cinnamomi Cassaie (*Rou Gui*), Radix Glycyrrhizae (*Gan Cao*)

This formula is primarily for qi stagnation painful menstruation.

14. *Jia Jian Xiao Yao San* (Additions & Subtractions Rambling Powder)

Ingredients: Radix Bupleuri (*Chai Hu*), Rhizoma Atractylodis Macrocephalae (*Bai Zhu*), Radix Albus Paeoniae Lactiflorae (*Bai Shao*), Radix Angelicae Sinensis (*Dang Gui*), Rhizoma Cyperi Rotundi (*Xiang Fu*), Feces Trogopterori Seu Pteromi (*Wu Ling Zhi*), Pollen Typhae (*Pu Huang*), Sclerotium Poriae Cocos (*Fu Ling*), Rhizoma Corydalis Yanhusuo (*Yan Hu Suo*), Cortex Albizziae Julibrissin (*He Huan Pi*)

This formula is also for liver depression qi stagnation but complicated by definite blood stasis.

Additions: If blood binding, stasis, and obstruction are severe with abdominal distention and pain and the menses are tardy and do not descend, add Semen Pruni Persicae (*Tao Ren*), Flos Carthami Tinctorii (*Hong Hua*), and Radix Cyathulae Officinalis (*Chuan Niu Xi*). If liver depression transforms into fire, add Radix Gentianae Scabrae (*Long Dan Cao*), Cortex Radicis Moutan (*Dan Pi*), and Fructus Gardeniae Jasminoidis (*Shan Zhi*). If liver yin is insufficient and liver yang is hyperactive, reduce the amount of Bupleurum and add Spica Prunellae Vulgaris (*Xia Gu Cao*), Fructus Ligustri Lucidi (*Nu Zhen Zi*), and Herba Ecliptae Prostratae (*Han Lian Cao*). If qi and blood are both vacuous and deficient, add Radix

Codonopsitis Pilosulae (*Dang Shen*) and Radix Astragali Membranacei (*Huang Qi*). If there is lower origin yang vacuity and the *chong* and *ren* are insufficient, add Radix Morindae Officinalis (*Ba Ji Tian*), Semen Cuscutae (*Tu Si Zi*), and Placenta Hominis (*Zi He Che*). If the menses are late and there is lower abdominal rigidity and tension, add Folium Artemisiae Argyii (*Ai Ye*) and Cortex Cinnamomi Cassiae (*Rou Gui*).

These additions exemplify that painful menstruation due to qi stagnation and blood stasis may be complicated by a number of other patterns. In my experience, it is common to use two or even three of these different additions when using a guiding formula such as *Xiao Yao San* for painful menstruation.

2. Cold damp congelation & stagnation

Main symptoms: Menstrual pain in the abdomen as if a knife were being twisted, desires warmth but resists pressure, obtainment of warmth followed by relaxation, amount of the menstruate astringent and scanty, does not flow freely, color purple, dark, and lusterless or the color of black bean juice, clots, counterflow inversion of the four extremities, a greenish-bluish white facial complexion, a cyanotic, purple tongue with glossy moisture inside the mouth, and a deep, slow, forceful or deep and tight pulse

Treatment principles: Warm the channels (or menses), scatter cold, and quicken the blood

Guiding formulas:

1. *Shao Fu Zhu Yu Tang* (Lower Abdomen Dispel Stasis Decoction)

Ingredients: Fructus Foeniculi Vulgaris (*Xiao Hui Xiang*), blast-fried or dry Rhizoma Zingiberis (*Pao Jiang* or *Gan Jiang*), Rhizoma Corydalis Yanhusuo (*Yan Hu Suo*), Feces Trogopterori Seu Pteromi (*Wu Ling Zhi*), Resina Myrrhae (*Mo Yao*), Radix Ligustici Wallichii (*Chuan Xiong*), Radix Angelicae Sinensis (*Dang Gui*), uncooked Pollen Typhae (*Pu Huang*), Cortex Cinnamomi Cassiae (*Rou Gui*), Radix Rubrus Paeoniae Lactiflorae (*Chi Shao*)

Additions: If there is pronounced accompanying dampness, Zhang Rei-ling suggests adding Rhizoma Atractylodis (*Cang Zhu*) and Sclerotium Poriae Cocos (*Fu Ling*) to disinhibit dampness and transform turbidity. To these, Sun Jiu-ling adds Rhizoma Cyperi Rotundi (*Xiang Fu*) to more effectively rectify the qi. If there is copious, clear urine and soreness and weakness of the low back and knees, add Radix Lateralis Praeparatus Aconiti Carmichaeli (*Fu Zi*) and Folium Artemisiae Argyii (*Ai Ye*).

2. *Wu Zhu Yu Tang* (Evodia Decoction)

Ingredients: Fructus Evodiae Rutecarpae (*Wu Zhu Yu*), Radix Angelicae Sinensis (*Dang Gui*), Radix Platycodi Grandiflori (*Jie Geng*), Herba Asari Cum Radice (*Xi Xin*), Radix Ledebouriellae Divaricatae (*Fang Feng*), dry Rhizoma Zingiberis (*Gan Jiang*), cooked Radix Rehmanniae (*Shu Di*), mix-fried Radix Glycyrrhizae (*Gan Cao*)

This formula is effective for first aid relief of vomiting, nausea, headache, and chilling accompanying painful menstruation.

3. *Wen Jing Tang* (Warm the Channels [or Menses] Decoction) from *Fu Ren Da Quan Liang Fang (A Compendium of Fine Formulas for Women)*

Ingredients: Radix Angelicae Sinensis (*Dang Gui*), Radix Ligustici Wallichii (*Chuan Xiong*), Radix Albus Paeoniae Lactiflorae (*Bai Shao*), Rhizoma Curcumae Zedoariae (*E Zhu*), Radix Panacis Ginseng (*Ren Shen*), Radix Achyranthis Bidentatae (*Niu Xi*), Cortex Cinnamomi Cassiae (*Gui Xin*), Cortex Radicis Moutan (*Dan Pi*), mix-fried Radix Glycyrrhizae (*Zhi Gan Cao*)

Additions: Professors Song and Yu suggest adding Radix Linderae Strychnifoliae (*Wu Yao*), blast-fried Rhizoma Zingiberis (*Pao Jiang*), and Semen Coicis Lachryma-jobi (*Yi Yi Ren*) when this formula is used for the treatment of painful menstruation due to cold and dampness causing blood stasis.

4. Unnamed formula from *Concise Traditional Chinese Gynecology*

Ingredients: Ramulus Cinnamomi Cassiae (*Gui Zhi*), Fructus Evodiae Rutecarpae (*Wu Zhu Yu*), Feces Trogopterori Seu Pteromi (*Wu Ling Zhi*), Rhizoma Corydalis Yanhusuo (*Yan Hu Suo*), Rhizoma Atractylodis (*Cang Zhu*)

5. *Gui Zhi Fu Ling Wan* (Cinnamon Twig & Poria Pills)

Ingredients: Cortex Radicis Moutan (*Dan Pi*), Radix Rubrus Paeoniae Lactiflorae (*Chi Shao*), Semen Pruni Persicae (*Tao Ren*), Sclerotium Poriae Cocos (*Fu Ling*), Ramulus Cinnamomi Cassiae (*Gui Zhi*)

This formula is for blood stasis tinged with an element of cold and dampness.

6. *San Jie Fang* (Scatter Nodulation Formula)

Ingredients: Stir-fried Radix Angelicae Sinensis (*Dang Gui*), Radix Salviae Miltiorrhizae (*Dan Shen*), Radix Rubrus Paeoniae Lactiflorae (*Chi Shao*), Radix Cyathulae Officinalis

(*Chuan Niu Xi*), processed Rhizoma Cyperi Rotundi (*Xiang Fu*), Ramulus Cinnamomi Cassaie (*Gui Zhi*), Herba Sargassii (*Hai Zao*), mix-fried Squama Manitis Pentadactylis (*Chuan Shan Jia Pian*), Spina Gleditschiae Sinensis (*Zao Jiao Ci*), Sanguis Draconis (*Xue Jie*), Rhizoma Curcumae Zedoariae (*E Zhu*)

This formula is given by Zhang En-qin *et al.* under the heading endometriosis due to cold congelation and blood stasis. The signs and symptoms given are chilly pain in the lower abdomen before, during, or after menstruation, fear of cold, chilled extremities, sore lower back lacking strength, a dark tongue with thin, white fur and a deep, slow pulse.

The use of Sargassium, Squama Manitis, Spina Gleditschiae, and Zedoaria to disperse nodulation is based on the finding of nodules on the posterior fornix and isthmus of the uterus during internal gynecological exam. This is an example of integrated Chinese-Western gynecology.

7. *Dang Gui Si Ni Tang Jia Wei* (Dang Gui Four Counterflows Decoction with Added Flavors)

Ingredients: Radix Angelicae Sinensis (*Dang Gui*), Ramulus Cinnamomi Cassiae (*Gui Zhi*), Radix Rubrus Paeoniae Lactiflorae (*Chi Shao*), Herba Asari Cum Radice (*Xi Xin*), Caulis Akebiae Mutong (*Mu Tong*), mix-fried Radix Glycyrrhizae (*Gan Cao*), Fructus Zizyphi Jujubae (*Da Zao*), Fructus Evodiae Rutecarpae (*Wu Zhu Yu*)

8. *Chu Tong San* (Eliminate Pain Powder)

Ingredients: Blast-fried Rhizoma Curcumae Zedoariae (*Peng Zhu*), Radix Angelicae Sinensis (*Dang Gui*), Rhizoma Corydalis Yanhusuo (*Yan Hu Suo*), Feces Trogopterori Seu Pteromi (*Wu Ling Zhi*), Cortex Cinnamomi Cassiae (*Rou Gui*), stir-fried Rhizoma Alpiniae Officinari (*Liang Jiang*), roasted, stir-fried Pollen Typhae (*Pu Huang*), Resina Myrrhae (*Mo Yao*)

Du Jie-hui gives this formula for the treatment of cold congelation, blood stasis painful menstruation. This formula scatters cold, transforms stasis, and stops pain.

9. *Wen Jing Tang* (Warm the Channels [or Menses] Decoction) from the *Jin Gui Yao Lue (Essentials from the Golden Cabinet)*

Ingredients: Fructus Evodiae Rutecarpae (*Wu Zhu Yu*), Radix Panacis Ginseng (*Ren Shen*), Radix Angelicae Sinensis (*Dang Gui*), Radix Ligustici Wallichi (*Chuan Xiong*), Ramulus Cinnamomi Cassiae (*Gui Zhi*), Gelatinum Corii Asini (*E Jiao*), Cortex Radicis Moutan (*Dan Pi*), Radix Albus Paeoniae Lactiflorae (*Bai Shao*), Rhizoma Pinelliae Ternatae (*Ban Xia*), Tuber Ophiopogonis Japonici (*Mai Dong*), uncooked Rhizoma Zingiberis (*Sheng Jiang*), Radix Glycyrrhizae (*Gan Cao*)

Additions: If there is abdominal pain and vomiting, add Rhizoma Alpiniae Officinari (*Gao Liang Jiang*), and more Evodia. If there is diarrhea and chilled extremities, add Fructus Psoraleae Corylifoliae (*Bu Gu Zhi*) and Fructus Zanthoxyli Bungeani (*Chuan Jiao*). If there is lower abdominal pain, add Fructus Foeniculi Vulgaris (*Xiao Hui Xiang*) and Folium Artemisiae Argyii (*Ai Ye*). If blood stasis is substantial, add Rhizoma Sparganii (*San Leng*) and Herba Lycopi Lucidi (*Ze Lan*).

10. Unnamed formula from *Nu Ke Jing Wei (Profundities from the Gynecological Classics)*

Ingredients: Whole Radix Angelicae Sinensis (*Quan Dang Gui*), Radix Rubrus Paeoniae Lactiflorae (*Chi Shao Yao*), old Radix Ligustici Wallichii (*Chuan Xiong*), large Radix Codonopsitis Pilosulae (*Dang Shen*), scalded Fructus Evodiae Rutecarpae (*Dan Wu Zhu*), carbonized blast-fried Rhizoma Zingiberis (*Pao Jiang*), superior Cortex Cinnamomi Cassiae (*Rou Gui*), Rhizoma Corydalis Yanhusuo (*Yan Hu Suo*), Resina Myrrhae (*Mo Yao*), uncooked Radix Glycyrrhizae (*Gan Cao*), Radix Cyathulae Officinalis (*Chuan Niu Xi*)

Additions & subtractions: If there are acid eructations and vomiting of clear water, add Fructus Amomi (*Suo Sha Ren*) and Rhizoma Pinelliae Ternatae (*Fa Ban Xia*). If there is stomach and epigastric pain, add Rhizoma Alpiniae Officinari (*Gao Liang Jiang*) and Concha Arcae Inflatae (*Wa Leng Zi*). If the hands and feet are not warm and there is lower abdominal pain, add Sichuan Radix Lateralis Praeparatus Aconiti Carmichaeli (*Chuan Fu Pian*). After taking these medicinals, if abdominal pain has diminished and the menstruation is free-flowing and smooth, remove the Myrrh and Cyathula and add uncooked Radix Astragali Membranacei (*Huang Qi*) and Herba Lycopi Lucidi (*Ze Lan Ye*).

3. Damp heat stasis & binding

Main symptoms: Lower abdominal tightness, distention, and pain which resists pressure occurring usually before the period and getting worse as the period approaches, amount of menses excessive, color purplish, thickish in consistency, profuse vaginal discharge which is foul-smelling and may be either yellow or white and red, acutely painful lumbar soreness, vexation and agitation, disquietude, generalized fever, a dry mouth with a bitter taste, a desire to drink, stools held back and bound, short, reddish urination, yellow, slimy tongue fur, and a bowstring, rapid pulse

Patients with this pattern usually have a history of pelvic inflammatory disease (PID), chronic vaginitis, or even a past history of appendicitis. The pain may be either one-sided, frequently in the right lower quadrant, or may be bilateral. The pain may be mostly sacral and travel down the sides or back of the leg. In more acute instances, there may even be fever and/or localized redness, pain, and heat in one or both of the knees. In this case, dampness and heat have wrestled and knotted with the blood causing stasis.

Treatment principles: Clear heat and disinhibit dampness, transform stasis and stop pain

Guiding formulas:

1. *Xiao Yao San He Ju He Wan Jia Jian* (Rambling Powder plus Orange Seed Pills with Additions & Subtractions)

Ingredients: Radix Bupleuri (*Chai Hu*), Rhizoma Atractylodis Macrocephalae (*Bai Zhu*), Sclerotium Poriae Cocos (*Fu Ling*), Radix Angelicae Sinensis (*Dang Gui*), Radix Albus Paeoniae Lactiflorae (*Bai Shao*), Semen Citri Reticulatae (*Ju He*), Fructus Meliae Toosendan (*Chuan Lian Zi*), Radix Auklandiae Lappae (*Mu Xiang*), Semen Pruni Persicae (*Tao Ren*), Rhizoma Corydalis Yanhusuo (*Yan Hu Suo*), Caulis Akebiae Mutong (*Mu Tong*), Cortex Magnoliae Officinalis (*Hou Po*), Fructus Immaturus Citri Aurantii (*Zhi Shi*), Herba Sargassii (*Hai Zao*), Thallus Algae (*Kun Bu*), Herba Laminariae Japonicae (*Hai Dai*), Caulis Sargentodoxae (*Da Xue Teng*), Herba Patriniae Heterophyllae Cum Radice (*Bai Jiang Cao*), Caulis Lonicerae Japonicae (*Ren Dong Teng*), Fructus Gardeniae Jasminoidis (*Zhi Zi*)

This formula given by Song and Yu is for damp heat due to depressive liver heat and spleen vacuity and dampness with nodulation. Orange Seeds are a qi-rectifying medicinal which enters the liver channel and also scatters nodulation. They are especially indicated for lower abdominal pain on one or both sides of the lower abdomen.

2. *Xiao Yao San Jia Er Miao San* (Rambling Powder plus Two Wonders Powder)

Ingredients: Radix Bupleuri (*Chai Hu*), Radix Angelicae Sinensis (*Dang Gui*), Radix Rubrus Paeoniae Lactiflorae (*Chi Shao*), Cortex Phellodendri (*Huang Bai*), Rhizoma Atractylodis (*Cang Zhu*), Rhizoma Atractylodis Macrocephalae (*Bai Zhu*), Sclerotium Poriae Cocos (*Fu Ling*), mix-fried Radix Glycyrrhizae (*Zhi Cao*), uncooked Rhizoma Zingiberis (*Sheng Jiang*), Herba Menthae Haplocalycis (*Bo He*)

This formula is for the treatment of unilateral or bilateral lower abdominal distention and pain, soreness and pain of the low back, and profuse vaginal discharge due to damp heat blocking the qi and blood stasis of the uterus affecting the *chong* and *ren*.

Additions: For more pronounced lower abdominal distention and pain, add processed Rhizoma Cyperi Rotundi (*Xiang Fu*) and Rhizoma Corydalis Yanhusuo (*Yan Hu Suo*). For profuse vaginal discharge, add Rhizoma Dioscoreae Hypoglaucae (*Bi Xie*), Semen Plantaginis (*Che Qian Zi*), and Cortex Toonae (*Chun Pi*). For fullness in the epigastrium and decreased food intake, add Rhizoma Pinelliae Ternatae (*Ban Xia*), Fructus Cardamomi (*Dou Kou*), and Fructus Germinatus Hordei Vulgaris (*Mai Ya*).

3. *Xue Fu Zhu Yu Tang Jia Wei* (Blood Mansion Dispel Stasis Decoction with Added Flavors)

Ingredients: Semen Pruni Persicae (*Tao Ren*), Flos Carthami Tinctorii (*Hong Hua*), Radix Angelicae Sinensis (*Dang Gui*), Radix Ligustici Wallichii (*Chuan Xiong*), Radix Rubrus Paeoniae Lactiflorae (*Chi Shao*), Radix Cyathulae Officinalis (*Chuan Niu Xi*), Radix Bupleuri (*Chai Hu*), Radix Platycodi Grandiflori (*Jie Geng*), Fructus Citri Aurantii (*Zhi Ke*), uncooked Radix Rehmanniae (*Sheng Di*), Radix Glycyrrhizae (*Gan Cao*), Semen Coicis Lachryma-jobi (*Yi Yi Ren*), Caulis Sargentodoxae (*Da Xue Teng*), Herba Patriniae Heterophyllae Cum Radice (*Bai Jiang Cao*), Fructus Meliae Toosendan (*Chuan Lian Zi*)

This formula is for more serious blood stasis but complicated by dampness and heat. In this case there is no obvious nodulation.

4. *Xuan Yu Tong Jing Tang Jia Jian* (Diffuse Stasis & Free the Flow of the Channels [or Menses] Decoction with Additions & Subtractions)

Ingredients: Radix Angelicae Sinensis (*Dang Gui*), Radix Albus Paeoniae Lactiflorae (*Bai Shao*), Radix Bupleuri (*Chai Hu*), blackened Fructus Gardeniae Jasminoidis (*Shan Zhi*), Cortex Radicis Moutan (*Dan Pi*), Rhizoma Cyperi Rotundi (*Xiang Fu*), Radix Glycyrrhizae (*Gan Cao*), Herba Patriniae Heterophyllae Cum Radice (*Bai Jiang Cao*), Rhizoma Corydalis Yanhusuo (*Yan Hu Suo*), Semen Coicis Lachryma-jobi (*Yi Yi Ren*)

This formula is also for depressive liver heat plus damp heat and blood stasis where there is not so much spleen vacuity and dampness nor such prominent blood stasis.

5. Unnamed formula from *Concise Traditional Chinese Gynecology*

Ingredients: Cortex Radicis Moutan (*Dan Pi*), Radix Angelicae Sinensis (*Dang Gui*), Radix Rubrus Paeoniae Lactiflorae (*Chi Shao*), processed Resina Olibani (*Ru Xiang*), processed Resina Myrrhae (*Mo Yao*), Semen Coicis Lachryma-jobi (*Yi Yi Ren*)

6. *San Huang San Bai Tang* (Three Yellows & Three Whites Decoction)

Ingredients: Rhizoma Coptidis Chinensis (*Huang Lian*), Cortex Phellodendri (*Huang Bai*), Radix Scutellariae Baicalensis (*Huang Qin*), Rhizoma Atractylodis Macrocephalae (*Bai Zhu*), Radix Albus Paeoniae Lactiflorae (*Bai Shao*), Hallyositum Album (*Bai Shi Zhi*), Cortex Toonae Sinensis (*Chun Bai Pi*), Rhizoma Cyperi Rotundi (*Xiang Fu*), Cacumen Biotae Orientalis (*Ce Bai Ye*)

Du Jie-hui gives this formula for the treatment of painful menstruation due to damp heat pouring down. It clears heat, transforms dampness, and stops pain.

7. *Yi Shen Tang* (Smooth Stretching Decoction)

Ingredients: Radix Angelicae Sinensis (*Dang Gui*), Radix Rubrus Paeoniae Lactiflorae (*Chi Shao*), Radix Ligustici Wallichii (*Chuan Xiong*), Flos Carthami Tinctorii (*Hong Hua*), Radix Salviae Miltiorrhizae (*Dan Shen*), Herba Leonuri Heterophylli (*Yi Mu Cao*), Rhizoma Imperatae Cylindricae (*Bai Mao Gen*), Flos Lonicerae Japonicae (*Yin Hua*), Radix Isatidis Seu Baphicacanthi (*Ban Lan Geng*), Herba Violae Yedoensitis Cum Radice (*Zi Hua Di Ding*)

Zhang Xue-wen, author of *Yu Xue Zheng Zhi (Static Blood Patterns & Treatment)*, recommends this formula for the treatment of swelling, edema, fever, low back pain, headache, sore throat, susceptibility to invasion by external evils, cynaotic lips, a dark, dusky facial color, static spots or macules on the tongue, and slimy tongue fur accompanied by either a postpartum lochia which will not flow or blocked menstruation. I find this formula useful for treating low back and lower abdominal pain associated with the onset of the period where there is swelling and fever due to a combination of blood stasis, heat, and dampness. It quickens the blood, transforms stasis, and resolves toxins, clears heat, disinhibits dampness, and disperses swelling. It can also be used for the pain of acute pelvic inflammatory disease (PID) and herpes genitalia if these diseases are associated with this pattern.

4. Liver depression, effulgent fire

Main symptoms: Aching and pain in the abdomen are commonly preceded by distention and pain in the flanks. The amount of the menstruate is excessive and colored purple. This may be accompanied by lumbar soreness, dizziness, a flushed, red face, mental-emotional irascibility, fright palpitations, red lips, a bitter taste in the mouth, a crimson red tongue with scanty fur, and a bowstring, fine, rapid pulse.

In the preceding pattern, dampness and heat may be due to liver depression and transformative heat. However, in this case, there is no particular dampness nor is blood stasis prominent. The obstruction is more qi stagnation aggravated by heat.

Treatment principles: Course the liver and regulate the qi, clear heat and resolve depression

Guiding formula: *Xuan Yu Tong Jing Tang* (Diffuse Stasis & Free the Flow of the Channels [or Menses] Decoction)

Ingredients: Radix Bupleuri (*Chai Hu*), Radix Angelicae Sinensis (*Dang Gui*), stir-fried Radix Albus Paeoniae Lactiflorae (*Bai Shao*), Cortex Radicis Moutan (*Dan Pi*), Fructus Gardeniae Jasminoidis (*Zhi Zi*), stir-fried Semen Sinapis Albae (*Bai Jie Zi*), processed Rhizoma Cyperi Rotundi (*Xiang Fu*), Tuber Curcumae (*Chuan Yu Jin*), stir-fried Radix Scutellariae Baicalensis (*Huang Qin*), uncooked Radix Glycyrrhizae (*Gan Cao*)

This formula is from Fu Qing-zhu's *Fu Qing Zhu Nu Ke (Fu Qing-zhu's Gynecology)*. Besides the fact that it contains extra ingredients to clear heat and rectify the qi, it is similar to *Dan Zhi Xiao Yao San* (Moutan & Gardenia Rambling Powder) except that it does not contain Sclerotium Poriae Cocos (*Fu Ling*) and Rhizoma Atractylodis Macrocephalae (*Bai Zhu*). If the case is complicated by spleen vacuity, as evidenced by loose stools when the period comes, these two ingredients may be added and then *Dan Zhi Xiao Yao San* becomes the guiding formula.

Vacuity patterns

1. Qi & blood vacuity weakness

Main symptoms: Slight lower abdominal aching and pain with the menses or lingering on after the flow has ceased, including a heavy, dragging feeling at the base of the perineum, alleviated by pressure and warmth, scant menstrual volume which is pale in color and thin and watery in consistency, or prolonged menstruation with copious flow but pale red, thin and watery, absence of clots, an ashen white facial complexion, possible facial edema, shortness of breath and sweating on movement, dizziness, heart palpitations, exhaustion and fatigue, lassitude of the spirit, lack of strength, soreness and weakness in the low back and knees, a pale tongue with thin, white fur, teeth marks on the sides of the tongue, and a vacuous, fine pulse

These signs and symptoms are a mixture of general signs and symptoms of qi and blood vacuity plus signs and symptoms of vacuity of the three viscera which engender and transform the blood. This is because, although this pattern mostly hinges upon the spleen's engenderment and transformation of the blood, prolonged or extreme blood vacuity may eventually affect either the heart or the kidneys.

Treatment principles: Boost the qi and nourish the blood

Guiding formulas:

1. *Shen Qi Si Wu Tang Jia Wei* (Ginseng & Astragalus Four Materials Decoction with Added Flavors)

Ingredients: Radix Panacis Ginseng (*Ren Shen*) or Radix Codonopsitis Pilosulae (*Dang Shen*), Radix Astragali Membranacei (*Huang Qi*), Radix Angelicae Sinensis (*Dang Gui*), cooked Radix Rehmanniae (*Shu Di*), Radix Albus Paeoniae Lactiflorae (*Bai Shao*), Radix Ligustici Wallichii (*Chuan Xiong*), Rhizoma Cyperi Rotundi (*Xiang Fu*), Rhizoma Corydalis Yanhusuo (*Yan Hu Suo*), Radix Glycyrrhizae (*Gan Cao*), Radix Salviae Miltiorrhizae (*Dan Shen*)

2. *Ba Zhen Yi Mu Tang* (Eight Pearls Leonurus Decoction)

Ingredients: Radix Angelicae Sinensis (*Dang Gui*), Radix Albus Paeoniae Lactiflorae (*Bai Shao*), Radix Ligustici Wallichii (*Chuan Xiong*), cooked Radix Rehmanniae (*Shu Di*), Herba Leonuri Heterophylli (*Yi Mu Cao*), Radix Codonopsitis Pilosulae (*Dang Shen*), Rhizoma Atractylodis Macrocephalae (*Bai Zhu*), Sclerotium Poriae Cocos (*Fu Ling*), mix-fried Radix Glycyrrhizae (*Gan Cao*)

This formula supplements the qi and nourishes the blood. It contains Leonurus in order to quicken the blood and transform stasis as a minor motif, remembering that blood stasis is often due to blood vacuity and static blood prevents the engenderment of fresh or new blood.

3. *Shen Yu Tang* (Sage-like Curing Decoction)

Ingredients: Radix Codonopsitis Pilosulae (*Dang Shen*), Radix Astragali Membranacei (*Huang Qi*), Radix Angelicae Sinensis (*Dang Gui*), cooked Radix Rehmanniae (*Shu Di*), Radix Albus Paeoniae Lactiflorae (*Bai Shao*), Radix Ligustici Wallichii (*Chuan Xiong*)

Additions: Professors Song and Yu suggest adding Rhizoma Cyperi Rotundi (*Xiang Fu*) and Radix Glycyrrhizae (*Gan Cao*) to the above. Zhao Rei-ling agrees with this. Whereas, Zhang En-qin *et al.* suggest adding Rhizoma Cyperi Rotundi (*Xiang Fu*) and Rhizoma Corydalis Yanhusuo (*Yan Hu Suo*).

4. Unnamed formula from *Concise Traditional Chinese Gynecology*

Ingredients: Radix Angelicae Sinensis (*Dang Gui*), Radix Albus Paeoniae Lactiflorae (*Bai Shao*), Radix Astragali Membranacei (*Huang Qi*), Radix Codonopsitis Pilosulae (*Dang Shen*), vinegar-processed Radix Bupleuri (*Chai Hu*)

5. *Bu Zhong Yi Qi Tang Jia Wei* (Supplement the Center & Boost the Qi Decoction)

Ingredients: Radix Astragali Membranacei (*Huang Qi*), Radix Codonopsitis Pilosulae (*Dang Shen*), Rhizoma Atractylodis Macrocephalae (*Bai Zhu*), mix-fried Radix Glycyrrhizae (*Gan Cao*), Radix Angelicae Sinensis (*Dang Gui*), Radix Albus Paeoniae Lactiflorae

(*Bai Shao*), Rhizoma Cimicifugae (*Sheng Ma*), Radix Bupleuri (*Chai Hu*), Pericarpium Citri Reticulatae (*Chen Pi*)

This formula is for dragging pain in the uterus due to central qi fall towards the end of or immediately after menstruation.

6. *San Cai Da Bu Wan* (The Three [Heaven, Humanity & Earth] Greatly Supplementing Pills)

Ingredients: Radix Panacis Ginseng (*Ren Shen*), Radix Astragali Membranacei (*Huang Qi*), Cortex Eucommiae Ulmoidis (*Du Zhong*), Fructus Psoraleae Corylifoliae (*Bu Gu Zhi*), Rhizoma Atractylodis Macrocephalae (*Bai Zhu*), cooked Radix Rehmanniae (*Shu Di*), Radix Angelicae Sinensis (*Dang Gui*), Radix Albus Paeoniae Lactiflorae (*Bai Shao*), Gelatinum Corii Asini (*E Jiao*), Folium Artemisiae Argyii (*Ai Ye*), Radix Dioscoreae Oppositae (*Shan Yao*), Rhizoma Cyperi Rotundi (*Xiang Fu*), Radix Ligustici Wallichii (*Chuan Xiong*)

This formula treats spleen and kidney qi and blood vacuity.

7. *Jing Hou Fu Tong Fang* (Post Menstruation Abdominal Pain Formula)

Ingredients: Wine stir-fried Radix Angelicae Sinensis (*Dang Gui*), Radix Albus Paeoniae Lactiflorae (*Bai Shao*), mix-fried Radix Glycyrrhizae (*Gan Cao*), Ramulus Cinnamomi Cassiae (*Gui Zhi*)

Du Jie-hui suggests this formula for qi and blood vacuity weakness menstrual pain. The formula's name indicates that this abdominal pain occurs after or towards the latter part of the period. This formula nourishes the blood, regulates the menses, and stops pain.

8. *Shi Quan Da Bu Wan* (Ten [Ingredients] Completely & Greatly Supplementing Pills)

Ingredients: Radix Astragali Membranacei (*Huang Qi*), Cortex Cinnamomi Cassiae (*Rou Gui*), Radix Panacis Ginseng (*Ren Shen*), cooked Radix Rehmanniae (*Shu Di*), Rhizoma Atractylodis Macrocephalae (*Bai Zhu*), Radix Angelicae Sinensis (*Dang Gui*), Radix Albus Paeoniae Lactiflorae (*Bai Shao*), Radix Ligustici Wallichii (*Chuan Xiong*), Sclerotium Poriae Cocos (*Fu Ling*), mix-fried Radix Glycyrrhizae (*Gan Gao*), uncooked Rhizoma Zingiberis (*Sheng Jiang*), Fructus Zizyphi Jujubae (*Da Zao*)

Additions: If the menstrual blood is thin and light colored, add Gelatinum Corii Asini (*E Jiao*) and Folium Artemisiae Argyii (*Ai Ye*). If the pain is severe, add Feces Trogopterori Seu Pteromi (*Wu Ling Zhi*) and Pollen Typhae (*Pu Huang*). This suggests that severe pain associated with a qi and blood vacuity pattern means that there is concomitant blood stasis. If there is diarrhea during menstruation, add Fructus Psoraleae Corylifoliae (*Bu Gu Zhi*) and

Massa Medica Fermentata (*Shen Qu*). If there is lumbar pain, add Radix Dipsaci (*Xu Duan*) and Cortex Eucommiae Ulmoidis (*Du Zhong*). If there is a bearing down sensation in the perineum, add Rhizoma Cimicifugae (*Sheng Ma*), Radix Bupleuri (*Chai Hu*), and Fructus Citri Aurantii (*Zhi Ke*)

9. *Jia Jian Wen Jing Tang* (Additions & Subtractions Warm the Channels [or Menses] Decoction)

Ingredients: Fructus Evodiae Rutecarpae (*Wu Zhu Yu*), Ramulus Cinnamomi Cassaie (*Gui Zhi*), Radix Angelicae Sinensis (*Dang Gui*), Radix Albus Paeoniae Lactiflorae (*Bai Shao*), Radix Ligustici Wallichii (*Chuan Xiong*), Gelatinum Corii Asini (*E Jiao*), Radix Codonopsitis Pilosulae (*Dang Shen*), Radix Salviae Miltiorrhizae (*Dan Shen*), Tuber Ophiopogonis Japonici (*Mai Men Dong*), Radix Dipsaci (*Xu Duan*), Ramulus Loranthi Seu Visci (*Sang Ji Sheng*), Folium Artemisiae Argyii (*Ai Ye*), Caulis Milltetiae Seu Spatholobi (*Ji Xue Teng*), Fructus Lycii Chinensis (*Gou Qi*)

The authors of *Zhong Yi Fu Ke Lin Chuang Jing Hua (The Clinical Efflorescence of Chinese Medical Gynecology)* give this as a guiding formula for qi and blood vacuity weakness painful menstruation. *Wen Jing Tang* is commonly thought of as a guiding formula for cold damp congelation and stagnation or uterine vacuity cold. In this formula, there are medicinals which supplement kidney yang (Dipsacus) and others which supplement kidney yin (Lycium). Therefore, this formula is for more than just qi and blood vacuity. It should not be used for qi and blood vacuity painful menstruation unless there are definite symptoms of cold, whether replete or vacuity cold.

10. Unnamed formula from *Nu Ke Jing Wei (Profundities from the Gynecological Classics)*

Ingredients: Body of Radix Angelicae Sinensis (*Dang Gui Shen*), large cooked Radix Rehmanniae (*Shu Di*), uncooked Radix Albus Paeoniae Lactiflorae (*Bai Shao*), old Radix Ligustici Wallichii (*Chuan Xiong*), large Radix Codonopsitis Pilosulae (*Dang Shen*), earth stir-fried Rhizoma Atractylodis Macrocephalae (*Bai Zhu*), Yunnan Sclerotium Poriae Cocos (*Yun Fu Ling*), uncooked Radix Astragali Membranacei (*Huang Qi*), vinegar-processed Radix Bupleuri (*Chai Hu*), stir-fried Fructus Citri Aurantii (*Zhi Ke*), processed Rhizoma Cyperi Rotundi (*Xiang Fu*), uncooked Radix Glycyrrhizae (*Gan Cao*)

This formula is indicated for liver depression with blood vacuity by the authors of its source text. However, looking at the ingredients and their order of listing, I would say that it is indicated for qi and blood vacuity complicated by qi stagnation. However, the important thing is looking for, being able to recognize, and being able to treat complicated, multifaceted patterns.

Additions & subtractions: If afterwards there is low back soreness and pain, add scorched Cortex Eucommiae Ulmoidis (*Du Zhong*) and golden-haried Rhizoma Cibotii Barometis (*Jin Mao Gou Ji*). If, after taking these medicinals, the chest, rib-side, and abdominal pain is greatly dispersed, remove the Bupleurum and Citrus and add Radix Dioscoreae Oppositae (*Huai Shan Yao*), Semen Biotae Orientalis (*Bai Zi Ren*), scorched Semen Zizyphi Spinosae (*Zao Ren*), and processed Rhizoma Polygonati (*Huang Jing*) to supplement and boost the heart spirit in order to engender blood.

2. Vacuity cold within the uterus

Main symptoms: Insidious lower abdominal pain with menstruation, menses typically late, desiring warmth, desiring pressure, menses color clear and watery, low back and knee soreness and weakness, lack of warmth in the four extremities, frequent urination, a pale white facial complexion, a pale, moist tongue and a deep, relaxed (retarded), and forceless pulse

Treatment principles: Warm the center, support yang, and boost the qi

Guiding formulas:

1. *Wen Shen Fu Yang Tang* (Warm the Kidneys & Support Yang Decoction)

Ingredients: Radix Panacis Ginseng (*Ren Shen*), Radix Dioscoreae Oppositae (*Shan Yao*), cooked Radix Rehmanniae (*Shu Di*), Fructus Corni Officinalis (*Shan Zhu Yu*), Fructus Evodiae Rutecarpae (*Wu Zhu Yu*), Semen Cuscutae (*Tu Si Zi*), Cortex Cinnamomi Cassiae (*Rou Gui*), Radix Lateralis Praeparatus Aconiti Carmichaeli (*Fu Zi*), Fructus Psoraleae Corylifoliae (*Bu Gu Zhi*), Rhizoma Atractylodis Macrocephalae (*Bai Zhu*)

2. *Tong Jing San Hao Fang* (Painful Menstruation No. 3 Formula) from *Zhong Yi Hu Li Xue (A Study of Chinese Medical Nursing)*

Ingredients: Radix Angelicae Sinensis (*Dang Gui*), Radix Ligustici Wallichii (*Chuan Xiong*), Radix Codonopsitis Pilosulae (*Dang Shen*), blast-fried Rhizoma Zingiberis (*Pao Jiang*), Radix Albus Paeoniae Lactiflorae (*Bai Shao*), Lignum Santali Albi (*Tan Xiang*), Rhizoma Cyperi Rotundi (*Xiang Fu*), Cortex Cinnamomi Cassaie (*Rou Gui*), Fructus Evodiae Rutecarpae (*Wu Zhu Yu*)

3. *Tong Jing Shen Fang* (Painful Menstruation Spirit-like [*i.e.*, Magic] Formula)

Ingredients: Radix Panacis Ginseng (*Ren Shen*), Radix Astragali Membranacei (*Huang Qi*), Radix Angelicae Sinensis (*Dang Gui*), Rhizoma Atractylodis Macrocephalae (*Bai Zhu*), Cortex Cinnamomi Cassiae (*Rou Gui*), Radix Lateralis Praeparatus Aconiti Carmichaeli (*Fu Zi*)

This formula boosts the qi and nourishes the blood, warms yang and stops pain. It is indicated for the treatment of yang vacuity, internal cold painful menstruation.

3. Liver-kidney vacuity detriment

Main symptoms: Insidious lower abdominal pain at the onset of the menses, pale red in color and scanty in amount, dizziness, tinnitus, lumbar pain, pain in the heels or tightness in the hands and feet, dry, scratchy throat but no particular desire to drink, a pale red tongue with thin fur, and a deep, fine pulse. The menses may also be delayed.

The pain in this case is due to liver blood and kidney yin not being sufficient to both fill the uterus and nourish the sinews. It often extends to the top of the thighs along the course of the liver channel sinews.

Treatment principles: Moisten and supplement the liver and kidneys

Guiding formulas:

1. *Tiao Gan Tang* (Regulate the Liver Decoction)

Ingredients: Radix Angelicae Sinensis (*Dang Gui*), Radix Albus Paeoniae Lactiflorae (*Bai Shao*), Radix Dioscoreae Oppositae (*Shan Yao*), Gelatinum Corii Asini (*E Jiao*), Fructus Corni Officinalis (*Shan Zhu Yu*), Radix Morindae Officinalis (*Ba Ji Tian*), Radix Glycyrrhizae (*Gan Cao*)

Additions: For lumbar pain, add Cortex Eucommiae Ulmoidis (*Du Zhong*) and Radix Dipsaci (*Xu Duan*). For bilateral abdominal pain, add Semen Citri Reticulatae (*Ju He*) and Fructus Foeniculi Vulgaris (*Xiao Hui Xiang*). For rib-side pain, add Fructus Meliae Toosendan (*Chuan Lian Zi*) and Tuber Curcumae (*Yu Jin*). For frequent urination, add Fructus Alpiniae Oxyphyllae (*Yi Zhi Ren*) and Os Sepiae Seu Sepiellae (*Hai Piao Xiao*).

2. *Xue Beng Fang* (Blood Flooding Formula)

Ingredients: Stir-fried Radix Angelicae Sinensis (*Dang Gui*), uncooked Pollen Typhae (*Pu Huang*), Radix Achyranthis Bidentatae (*Niu Xi*), Radix Salviae Miltiorrhizae (*Dan Shen*), Radix Rubrus Paeoniae Lactiflorae (*Chi Shao*), Radix Albus Paeoniae Lactiflorae (*Bai Shao*), processed Rhizoma Cyperi Rotundi (*Xiang Fu*), Dolomitum (*Hua Rui Shi*), carbonized cooked Radix Et Rhizoma Rhei (*Shu Jun*), Sanguis Draconis (*Xue Jie*)

Zhang En-qin *et al.* give this formula under endometriosis due to kidney vacuity and blood stasis. Its leading indication is pain in the lower abdomen before, during, or after menstruation. There is also profuse menstruation, a dark but pale tongue with thin, white fur, and a bowstring, fine or deep, choppy pulse. Although Zhang *et al.* categorize this formula under kidney vacuity, blood stasis, they use primarily blood-nourishing ingredients and not specifically kidney-supplementing medicinals in order to enrich the kidneys. This is based on the statements that, "The liver and kidneys share a common source", "The essence and blood share a common source", and "The blood is the manifestation of essence in a woman."

4. Vacuity heat

Main symptoms: All the vacuity yin signs and symptoms above plus heat in the center of the hands, feet, and heart, malar flushing, tidal fever, night sweats, a red facial complexion, a dry, red tongue without fur, and a bowstring, fine, rapid pulse. In this case, the menstruation tends to come earlier than it should.

This pattern is similar to the above liver blood-kidney yin vacuity but with signs and symptoms of flaring of vacuity heat. The menses tend to come early. Many Chinese sources say that if the menstruation is early due to vacuity heat, there is no pain. However, this is not always the case.

Treatment principles: Nourish yin, subdue yang, and lead fire back to its lower source

Guiding formulas:

1. *Tiao Gan Tang Jia Wei* (Regulate the Liver Decoction with Added Flavors)

Ingredients: Fructus Corni Officinalis (*Shan Zhu Yu*), Gelatinum Corii Asini (*E Jiao*), Radix Angelicae Sinensis (*Dang Gui*), Radix Albus Paeoniae Lactiflorae (*Bai Shao*), Radix Dioscoreae Oppositae (*Shan Yao*), Radix Morindae Officinalis (*Ba Ji Tian*), Radix Glycyrrhizae (*Gan Cao*), Radix Achyranthis Bidentatae (*Niu Xi*), Concha Ostreae (*Mu Li*), Cortex Eucommiae Ulmoidis (*Du Zhong*)

Although, in this case, there is flaring of vacuity fire and one might think to use bitter, cold medicinals which clear heat, Ma Long-bai says that one should not use such ingredients during the menses itself.[24] Rather, Dr. Ma suggests moistening dryness, enriching yin, and nourishing the blood to spontaneously control vacuity heat. *Tiao Gan Tang* from *Fu Qing Zhu Nu Ke (Fu qing-zhu's Gynecology)* does just that. The added ingredients to heavily subdue and guide upwardly counterflowing yang back downward are Han Bai-ling's. Because vacuity heat painful menstruation often occurs along with menstruation ahead of schedule, prior to the menses, one should treat primarily for that, using such formulas as *Liang Di Tang* (Two Di's Decoction).

---

[24] *Intractable Dysmenorrhea: Experiences of Master Physicians Shen Zhong Li and Ma Long Bai*, Self-consultation Series, trans. by C.S. Cheung, Harmonious Sunshine Cultural Center, Sunnyvale, CA, 1988, p. 9

2. *Tong Jing Er Hao Fang* **(Painful Menstruation No. 2 Formula) from** *Zhong Yi Hu Li Xue (A Study of Chinese Medical Nursing)*

Ingredients: Uncooked Radix Rehmanniae (*Sheng Di*), cooked Radix Rehmanniae (*Shu Di*), Rhizoma Stellariae Dichotomae (*Yin Chai Hu*), Rhizoma Corydalis Yanhusuo (*Yan Hu Suo*), Cortex Radicis Moutan (*Dan Pi*), Fructus Meliae Toosendan (*Chuan Lian Zi*), Radix Angelicae Sinensis (*Dang Gui*), Radix Albus Paeoniae Lactiflorae (*Bai Shao*), Sclerotium Poriae Cocos (*Fu Ling*), Radix Glycyrrhizae (*Gan Cao*)

Mixed vacuity & repletion pattern, a.k.a. heat & cold, vacuity & repletion

Main symptoms: Abdominal pain, possibly violent, associated with the menses, diminished flow, sallow, yellowish complexion, diminished appetite or peculiar cravings, bodily emaciation, alternating constipation and diarrhea, gas, possible nausea, fatigue, cold hands and feet, worsening of the condition in response to yeasted, fermented foods, sweet, damp foods which mold easily, exposure to mold, persistent or recurrent abnormal vaginal discharge, slimy, yellow fur to the rear of the tongue or flowery, peeling fur, a possibly red, cracked tongue, and a fine, bowstring or bowstring, slippery pulse. Further, women suffering from candidiasis usually have a history of OC or antibiotic use.

Treatment principles: Fortify the spleen and warm yang, clear heat and kill "worms", and quicken the blood and transform stasis

Guiding formula: *Wu Mei Wan* (Mume Pills)

Ingredients: Fructus Pruni Mume (*Wu Mei*), Fructus Zanthoxyli Bungeani (*Chuan Jiao*), Herba Asari Cum Radice (*Xi Xin*), Rhizoma Coptidis Chinensis (*Huang Lian*), Cortex Phellodendri (*Huang Bai*), dry Rhizoma Zingiberis (*Gan Jiang*), Radix Lateralis Praeparatus Aconiti Carmichaeli (*Fu Zi*), Ramulus Cinnamomi Cassiae (*Gui Zhi*), Radix Panacis Ginseng (*Ren Shen*), Radix Angelicae Sinensis (*Dang Gui*)

This formula is for the treatment of worm or parasites where there is a mixture of heat and cold, vacuity and repletion. There is both dampness and heat but also spleen vacuity and vacuity cold. This formula is most classically indicated for the treatment of biliary ascariasis with obstruction of the bile duct, intermittent abdominal pain, nausea and vomiting, and cold hands and feet. However, Prof. Tang Ji-fu of the Gynecology Hospital of Shanghai, in an article in the *Journal of the American College of Traditional Chinese Medicine*, has suggested this formula for the treatment of chronic, long-standing endometriosis where there is stagnant heat and blood stasis complicated by vacuity of righteous qi.[25]

When a patient whom I had not been able to treat successfully for either sciatic pain or sinusitis returned after several years to tell me that both of these problems plus her recurrent vaginitis responded to taking extracts of umeboshi and garlic, I immediately thought of candidiasis and then secondarily of this formula with Fructus Pruni Mume as its main or ruling ingredient. This then clarified this formula's use in the treatment of long-standing, recalcitrant, and complicated endometriosis, since endometriosis is often, at least in Western women, complicated by candidiasis. Using this formula, I have had some remarkable successes in treating long-standing and severe dysmenorrhea with nausea, vomiting, diarrhea, and chills in patients with red tongues and flowery, peeled, slimy, possibly yellow fur.

Yeung Him-che, in *Handbook of Chinese Herbs and Formulas*, includes chronic diarrhea, flowery, peeled tongue fur, and a hidden or bowstring, tight pulse as indications of this formula.[26] Bensky and Barolet, in *Chinese Herbal Medicine: Formulas & Strategies*, say it treats chronic diarrhea and dysenteric disorders with a mixture of heat and cold, weakened righteous qi, borborygmus, and a red tongue with white coating.[27] Personally, I find this formula extremely important in the treatment of painful menstruation with "parasites" when such parasites are *Candida albicans*. In modern Chinese gynecology, *Candida albicans* and other similar yeasts and fungi are considered a species of *chong* or parasites which live in the stomach and intestines.

Additions & subtractions: For severe abdominal pain, add Fructus Meliae Toosendan (*Chuan Lian Zi*) and Radix Auklandiae Lappae (*Mu Xiang*). For constipation, add Semen Arecae Catechu (*Bing Lang*) and Fructus Immaturus Citri Aurantii (*Zhi Shi*). For nausea and vomiting, add Fructus Evodiae Rutecarpae (*Wu Zhu Yu*) and Rhizoma Pinelliae Ternatae (*Ban Xia*). For chronic diarrhea, add Radix Auklandiae Lappae (*Mu Xiang*) and Radix Albus Paeoniae Lactiflorae (*Bai Shao*). If there is no coldness of the hands and feet, delete Cinnamon and Aconite. If there is more pronounced coldness and chilling, substitute Cortex Cinnamomi Cassiae (*Rou Gui*) for Ramulus Cinnamomi Cassiae (*Gui Zhi*).

---

[25] Cao Ling-xian, "Endometriosis as Treated by Traditional Chinese Medicine", trans. by C.S. Cheung & Carolyn Atkinson, *Journal of the American College of Traditional Chinese Medicine*, San Francisco, No. 1, 1983, p. 56

[26] Yeung Him-che, *Handbook of Chinese Herbs and Formulas*, Vol. 1, self-published, LA, 1985, p. 245

[27] Bensky, Dan & Barolet, Randall, *Chinese Herbal Medicine: Formulas & Strategies*, Eastland Press, Seattle, 1990, p. 466-7

Discussion

Painful menstruation may accompany a number of Western medical disease categories and is a common gynecological complaint. Chinese medicine treats painful menstruation quite well. One of the most common Western disease categories associated with painful menstruation is endometriosis. Certainly, women with either confirmed or strongly suspected endometriosis make up the largest percentage of painful menstruation in my practice. Therefore, I have added some Chinese discussions on endometriosis at the end of this chapter.

Because most of the women currently comprising my patient population are in their mid 30s and 40s, most of my painful menstruation patients present a combination of vacuity and repletion patterns. The majority of these women suffer from spleen qi and kidney yang vacuity complicated by liver depression and blood stasis. This may then be further complicated by blood and/or yin vacuity, depressive, damp, or vacuity heat, and/or phlegm nodulation. Therefore, I most commonly select guiding formulas from either the categories of depressive heat, damp heat stasis and stagnation, or qi and blood vacuity and modify these accordingly.

When women have endometriosis, they may not pass conspicuous clots in their menstruate. Endometriosis means that there is endometrial tissue growing outside the endometrium. These endometrial *foci* grow and then necrose and bleed with the menstrual cycle just as the endometrium does. In this case, the pain is due to bleeding into the abdominal cavity. In modern TCM gynecology, there is the assumption that endometriosis is associated with blood stasis, and not just blood stasis but concretions and conglomerations. In addition, because this disease is an enduring, chronic one, typically stasis has entered the network vessels.

In terms of treatment, this means that one should primarily use qi-rectifying and blood-quickening medicinals during the premenstruum but then add blood-breaking medicinals during the time in menses when the woman normally experiences menstrual pain. This may result in temporarily profuse menstruation. As long as the woman's main endometrial complaint is not profuse menstruation in the first place, this is not a problem. In addition, it is important to add medicinals which do enter and free the flow of the network vessels. As discussed above, these include tree resins, "insects", and network vessel-like ingredients. Personally, I favor using processed Resina Myrrhae (*Mo Yao*) and processed Resina Olibani (*Ru Xiang*). When used in their unprocessed form, they may cause nausea. Therefore, they should be used in their stir-fried form. If a woman cannot stomach these, one can substitute Eupolyphaga Seu Ophistoplatia (*Tu Bie Chong, Di Bie Chong, Zhe Chong*).

If the menstrual pain is located over the sides of the lower abdomen, this suggests the need for medicinals which specifically enter the liver channel. These include Radix Linderae Strychnifoliae (*Wu Yao*), Semen Citri Reticulatae (*Ju He*), and Fructus Foeniculi Vulgaris (*Xiao Hui Xiang*). Since Orange Seeds also scatter nodulation, one might consider combining them with Spica Prunellae Vulgaris (*Xia Ku Cao*) which also scatters nodulation. If there are breast lumps due to fibrocystic breasts, this suggests definite phlegm nodulation. In that case, one may also add medicinals which transform phlegm and soften the hard, such as Concha Ostreae (*Mu Li*), Rhizoma Pinelliae Ternatae (*Ban Xia*), Bulbus Fritillariae (*Bei Mu*), Radix Scrophulariae Ningpoensis (*Xuan Shen*), Squama Manitis Pentadactylis (*Chuan Shan Jia*), Semen Vaccariae Segetalis (*Wang Bu Liu Xing*), Herba Sargassii (*Hai Zao*), and Thallus Algae (*Kun Bu*).

One-sided lower abdominal pain often goes along with damp heat stasis and stagnation. If such damp heat stasis and stagnation pain is located on the right lower abdomen, one should definitely use Herba Patriniae Heterophyllae Cum Radice (*Bai Jiang Cao*). This medicinal has a special tropism for right-sided damp heat stasis and stagnation. However, whether this pain is right-sided or not, one can use Caulis Sargentodoxae (*Hong Teng* or *Da Xue Teng*). Commonly, these two medicinals are used together. Other medicinals to consider using with these are Semen Citri Reticulatae (*Ju He*), Semen Coicis Lachryma-jobi (*Yi Yi Ren*), and Fructus Meliae Toosendan (*Chuan Lian Zi*). Because damp heat stasis and stagnation often presents with liver depression and spleen vacuity, these medicinals are often incorporated into *Dan Zhi Xiao Yao San* (Moutan & Gardenia Rambling Powder) along with other appropriate ingredients.

When vomiting, nausea, chills and shivering, spontaneous perspiration, and diarrhea complicate severe painful menstruation, these are due to the severity of the pain causing chaos of the qi mechanism. Therefore, I see these as branch symptoms and tend not to pay them too much attention. Rather, I focus more attention on stopping the pain, with the assumption that if the pain is prevented or alleviated, these branch symptoms will either not arise or go away automatically. What I mean by this is that one should not let their guiding formula become too large and unfocused because of trying to treat too many symptoms at the same time. I focus on the pain and its disease mechanisms.

Acupuncture & moxibustion

Pain, like bleeding, is a branch symptom which is given priority in treatment in TCM. Therefore, during the occurrence of pain, everything possible should be done to stop that pain. Acupuncture and moxibustion are two of Chinese medicine's most effective adjunctive therapies for the relief of pain, and this is another instance where its use should be combined with internal medicinals in TCM gynecology.

For women who have either a) stagnant qi, blood stasis, b) cold damp accumulation and stasis, c) damp heat stasis and binding, or d) liver depression, effulgent fire types of dysmenorrhea, I typically recommend three acupuncture treatments in the week immediately preceding the expected due date of the menses, with the last treatment scheduled the day before its expected onset. Then, if menstruation is painful and the woman can get to my clinic, I also treat during the pain itself. Prior to the menses, I choose points to course the liver and rectify the qi, relieve depression and clear heat, quicken the blood and transform stasis, and clear heat and disinhibit dampness as appropriate.

If there is constipation associated with stagnation and stasis, needle *Tian Shu* (St 25) and *Da Chang Shu* (Bl 25). If the pain is on the sides of the abdomen, choose the meeting point of the *dai mai*, *Zu Lin Qi* (GB 41) plus *Dai Mai* (GB 26), *Wu Shu* (GB 27), *Ti Tuo Xue* (N-CA-4), *Wei Bao* (M-CA-16), or *Tong Jing* (2 *cun* below *Da Heng* [Sp 15]). If there is pain in the hips, use *Huan Tiao* (GB 30). If there is pain in the sacrum, use the *Ba Liao* (M-B-31-34). In other words, select points on channels traversing the affected areas.

If the patient has acute pain and comes to the clinic for acupuncture-moxibustion for first aid relief, *do not* needle directly into the site of pain. First select either *San Yin Jiao* (Sp 6) or *Di Ji* (Sp 8) and needle these if the pain is in the middle of the abdomen. If the pain is on the sides of the abdomen, first needle *Zu Lin Qi* (GB 41). Then wait several minutes. The pain should begin to subside. If, after 10 minutes the pain has plateaued and persists, then one can use points directly over the locus of pain. If there is cold, one can use moxa immediately on the lower abdomen and sacrum.

If the patient complains of a heavy, dragging pain towards the end of her period or in the week after, one can moxa indirectly *Bai Hui* (GV 20) to raise the yang and lift the fallen. This plus the appropriate qi supplements and boosters is usually sufficient to stop this pain. Usually one only has to administer acupuncture and moxibustion intensively in the week preceding the menses for the first three cycles. After that, the pain that is left should be so mild as to only require internal medication. In cases where the pain is acute and the patient cannot come to the clinic for first aid acupuncture-moxibustion treatment, they should be given some ready-made, pain-stopping medicine, such as *Yue Yue Hong Pian* (Moon Moon Red Tablets) or *Yan Hu Suo Zhi Tong Pian* (Corydales Stop Pain Tablets).

Compresses, plasters & enemas

When painful menstruation is due to blood stasis and cold, herbal compresses and plasters are also useful in the first couple of cycles of treatment. If blood stasis is prominent, one can use a warm castor oil compress. If cold is prominent, one can use a hot ginger compress.

For either blood stasis or cold, one can use ABC Plasters, *Sheng Shi Zhi Tong Gao* (Overcome Dampness & Stop Pain Plasters), etc. directly over the lower abdomen for first aid relief on the day of pain as long as the pain is not accompanied by excessive bleeding. Another possibility is to dissolve a substantial amount of Mirabilitum (*Mang Xiao*) in warm water and use that as a compress for blood stasis painful menstruation.

In modern China, there has been renewed interest in the use of Chinese medicinal retention enemas for the treatment of endometriosis and intra-abdominal nodulation and adhesions. The benefit of such medicinal enemas is that the medicinals are directly introduced to the lower burner without having to go through the stomach. This means that 1) more medicine gets to where it is needed and 2) one does not have to worry about attacking medicinals damaging the stomach. When such medicinal enemas are used in modern TCM gynecology, their ingredients tend to focus directly on draining the repletion. This means they contain ingredients such as Resina Myrrhae (*Mo Yao*), Resina Olibani (*Ru Xiang*), Rhizoma Curcumae Zedoariae (*E Zhu*), Rhizoma Sparganii (*San Leng*), etc. which enter the network vessels and break stasis. In particular, Lignum Sappan (*Su Mu*) is an effective ingredient in such medicinal enemas. Typically, I also include Acacia Catechu (*Er Cha*) to harmonize these ingredients within the intestines.

Such retention enemas are done one time per day beginning a couple of days after the menses have ended and continuing up to their onset again. The patient makes up a medicinal decoction with the enema ingredients just the same as if they were making a decoction to take orally. Then the dregs are removed and the liquid is allowed to cool to body temperature. The medicinal liquid is then loaded into an enema bag and the tip of the enema nozzle is inserted into the rectum with the patient laying on her back. The liquid should be retained for 20 minutes to one hour if possible. Although this method of Chinese medicinal therapy can be very effective, it is time consuming. Sadly, in my experience, many harried Western women just cannot find the time to do it.

Nursing

The authors of *Zhong Yi Hu Li Xue (A Study of Chinese Medical Nursing)* divide nursing care for painful menstruation into three subdivisions.

1. Lifestyle

A. During menstruation, women should avoid intense, violent movement, overwork and taxation, (sexual) intercourse, and (exposure to) dampness.

B. If a woman has serious menstrual pain, she should be asked to stay in bed and also to try to control or stop her longing (*i.e.,* unhealthy emotional response to frustration).

C. One should explain menstrual period hygiene. One should keep the outer yin (*i.e.,* external genitalia) clean. Avoid lack of cleanliness during the menses, sexual intercourse, and swimming.

2. Diet

A. During the menstrual period, do not eat chilled, uncooked foods, such as melons and fruits or popsicles, or hot, peppery, pungent foods.

B. For painful menstruation accompanied by vomiting and categorized as a cold pattern, one can give red sugar (*i.e.,* brown sugar) and fresh ginger taken in hot water.

3. Essence spirit (*i.e.,* mind & emotions)

A. Painful menstruation in young girls is mostly caused by a combination of misunderstanding menstrual physiology which subsequently produces psychological fear or dread. It is important for nurses to do a good job of health education. They should explain a general knowledge of menstrual physiology and hygiene to resolve and eliminate worry, longing, and apprehension.

B. For those patients with internal damage by the seven affects, liver qi depression and binding are responsible for the onset of this disease. It is important for nurses to do a good job teaching about patience and being careful of worry and longing. They should teach how to relax psychologically. Then liver qi will extend itself and thus painful menstruation is automatically relaxed.

These Chinese pieces of advice may seem a bit superficial to Western readers. However, although they may not satisfy Westerners' level of psychological sophistication, they do contain kernels of worthwhile advice.

Prognosis

Replete cold and dampness associated with blood stasis are relatively easy to treat. These can often be eliminated in only one or two cycles of treatment. Blood stasis may or may not respond to treatment quickly and easily. Whether one can eliminate it successfully or not often depends on 1) correctly identifying the full pattern, 2) correctly choosing medicinals to remedy that pattern, and 3) using a high enough dosage of medicinals. If one misses qi and blood vacuity complicated blood stasis or *vice versa*, treatment will not be effective. If one does not get medicinals into the network vessels when necessary or does not use blood-breaking medicinals when necessary, treatment will not be effective. If one uses too small a dosage of medicinals during the menses themselves, treatment will not be effective.

When blood stasis is eliminated, qi stagnation may remain, and this may prove more difficult to resolve completely. Because qi stagnation is mostly a mental-emotional problem, the patient needs to have explained how to circulate their qi through exercise and promote its free flow through relaxation. Depressive heat painful menstruation usually responds favorably to treatment with the caveat that it too often leaves a residuum of qi stagnation. Damp heat can be more difficult to treat, especially if it has been festering for a prolonged period of time. On the other hand, sometimes it responds to Chinese medical treatment very quickly. True worm accumulation is not commonly seen in the West. However, if the worms can be expelled, the case can make a startlingly quick turn-around. In the West, candidiasis associated with painful menstruation is commonly seen. It too can make a startling recovery if the patient can avoid all the foods which aggravate this condition. In some cases, candidiasis can be very recalcitrant to treatment or the patient cannot stay on the correct diet long enough to really see lasting results. In some cases, women on strict anti-candidal diets may loose too much weight and this may cause them to go off this diet. In other cases, it is the blandness of such a diet that simply is not appetizing unless the woman has the time to cook creatively.

Vacuity cold of the uterus is usually easy to treat. So is central qi fall causing heavy, dragging pain towards the end of or after menstruation . This usually only requires a single course of therapy to remedy, as long as the root cause of the spleen qi vacuity is found and remedied as well.

Blood and yin vacuity causing cramping pain in the tops and insides of the thighs is also usually easy to treat with Chinese medicinals. It typically responds in the first cycle of treatment. However, if there is vacuity heat as well, the patient will tend to be nervous and restless. This means that they typically have a short attention span and little long-term perseverance. Such patients tend to look for quick fixes and to jump from therapy to therapy. Therefore, they often do not stay with a single practitioner long enough to get a satisfactory result.

Case history: The patient was a 50 year-old woman whose major complaint was chronic fatigue immune deficiency syndrome (CFIDS). Her generalized symptoms were fatigue, lack of strength, shortness of breath, poor memory, orthostatic hypotension, easy bruising, delayed wound healing, loose stools, profuse phlegm, feeling cold at night, decreased libido, lumbar pain, urinary incontinence when she coughed or sneezed, recurent sore throats, swollen glands, neck and shoulder tension, headaches four to five times per week which were both tight and pounding and affected her occiput and vertex, dry skin, and dry eyes. Her gynecological signs and symptoms included premenstrual breast swelling and pain as well as nipple hypersensitivity, fibrocystic lumps in her breasts, premenstrual abdominal distention, lower abdominal cramps beginning one to two days before the arrival of her menses, severe menstrual cramps all over her lower abdomen and lower back, and clots in her menstruate. She also said that when her menses really began, she bled excessively heavily for at least the first day. In addition, all the symptoms she associated with chronic fatigue syndrome were much worse during her premenstruum. Although this woman was 50 years old, she still menstruated regularly on a 26-27 day cycle preceded by two days of premenstrual spotting. Her tongue was slightly swollen and dark in hue with a redder tip. The center of the top of the tongue was covered with small cracks. The tongue fur was thin and white. Her pulse was fine and a little rapid overall. In particular, both inch positions were floating, her right bar position was floating, her left bar position was fine and a little bowstring, and her left cubit position was fine and floating.

My initial pattern discrimination of this patient was spleen qi-kidney yin and yang vacuity complicated by liver depression, blood stasis, and phlegm nodulation. Therefore, my treatment principles were to fortify the spleen and boost the qi, nourish the liver and supplement the kidneys, enrich yin and clear heat, rectify the qi and quicken the blood, transform stasis and scatter nodulation. The prescription I wrote was comprised of: Radix Astragali Membranacei (*Huang Qi*), 18g, Radix Panacis Ginseng (*Ren Shen*), 6g, Radix Angelicae Sinensis (*Dang Gui*), 9g, Rhizoma Anemarrhenae Aspheloidis (*Zhi Mu*), 9g, Cortex Phellodendri (*Huang Bai*), 9g, Rhizoma Curculiginis Orchioidis (*Xian Mao*), 9g, Herba Epimedii (*Xian Ling Pi*), 9g, Radix Bupleuri (*Chai Hu*), 3g, Rhizoma Cimicifugae (*Sheng Ma*), 6g, Rhizoma Atractylodis Macrocephalae (*Bai Zhu*), 9g, Pericarpium Citri Reticulatae (*Chen Pi*), 9g, mix-fried Radix Glcycyrrhizae (*Gan Cao*), 6g, Tuber Ophiopogonis Japonici (*Mai Dong*), 12g, Spica Prunellae Vulgaris (*Xia Ku Cao*), 15g, Radix Scrophulariae Ningpoensis (*Xuan Shen*), 15g, Semen Citri Reticulatae (*Ju He*), 15g, Bulbus Fritillariae (*Bei Mu*), 9g, Semen Vaccariae Segetalis (*Wang Bu Liu Xing*), 9g, Squama Manitis Pentadactylis (*Chuan Shan Jia*), 9g. Because the patient was already on day 25 of her current cycle, and her menses began after only two days on this formula, there was no improvement in any of her menstrual symptoms that month.

After her menses were over, I removed the blood-quickening medicinals Vaccaria and Squama Manitis and added Rhizoma Pinelliae Ternatae (*Ban Xia*), 9g, and Sclerotium Poriae Cocos (*Fu Ling*), 9g, in order to further fortify the spleen and transform dampness and phlegm. Just before her menses came the next month, I put the blood-quickening medicinals back in while keeping the Pinellia and Poria. When she called me after that menstruation, she said that her PMS was much better, that the amount of menstrual bleeding was much less, and that she had not had as painful a menstruation.

Unfortunately, the next cycle, the patient was out of town. Before she left, she asked if I could have her basic prescription made up in desiccated extract form, which I did. However, on that powdered extract formula, even though theoretically the dosages were the same as when she was taking decoctions, her symptoms all came back — the heavy bleeding, the breast swelling and pain, and the painful menstruation. The third cycle she was again able to take the decocted Chinese medicinals throughout her entire cycle. Because the patient's tongue tip was no longer red and her pulse was no longer rapid, I removed the Anemarrhena and Phellodendron. Instead, during her premenstruum, I added Radix Linderae Strychnifoliae (*Wu Yao*), 9g, and Fructus Foeniculi Vulgaris (*Xiao Hui Xiang*), 9g, in order to further rectify her qi. During this premenstruum, the patient reported that she no longer had chronically swollen glands and that her fibrocystic breast lumps had markedly diminished. In addition, she had little PMS and no breast tenderness and pain. Therefore, the day before we expected her menses to start, I removed the Vaccaria and Squama Manitis, and added Radix Rubrus Paeoniae Lactiflorae (*Chi Shao*), 9g, Cortex Radicis Moutan (*Dan Pi*), 9g, Feces Trogopterori Seu Pteromi (*Wu Ling Zhi*), 9g, Pollen Typhae (*Pu Huang*), 9g, Herba Leonuri Heterophylli (*Yi Mu Cao*), 15g, and Herba Agromoniae Pilosae (*Xian He Cao*), 15g. These additions were to quicken the blood and dispel stasis, stop pain and stop flooding. After this menstruation, the patient reported that her menses had been without cramps and that there had been no excessively heavy bleeding.

Key patterns to memorize	
1. Repletion patterns	**A. Qi stagnation** **B. Blood stasis** **C. Liver depression, fire effulgence** **D. Cold damp congelation & stagnation**
2. Vacuity patterns	**A. Qi & blood vacuity** **B. Liver-kidney yin vacuity** **C. Vacuity heat** **D. Uterine vacuity cold**
3. Mixed repletion/vacuity pattern	**Hot & cold, repletion & vacuity**

Addendum: Endometriosis

Below are summaries of a number of recently published Chinese TCM journal articles on the treatment of endometriosis. Each of these are included in order to exemplify one or more key points in the modern TCM treatment of this disease. In general, the protocols used in TCM journal articles more closely resemble real-life clinical practice than do those given in standard textbooks. The authors of these articles all assume that real-life clinical practice is made up of patients with complicated patterns.

(From "The Treatment of 48 Cases of Endometriosis by the Methods of Quickening the Blood & Transforming Stasis" by Hu Guo-zhen, *Shang Hai Zhong Yi Yao Za Zhi [Shanghai Journal of Chinese Medicine & Medicinals]*, #2, 1995, p. 38-40)

The clinical manifestations of endometriosis consist of painful menstruation, menstrual irregularity, dyspareunia, infertility, lower abdominal sagging and distention, anal sagging and pain, etc. In TCM, it is categorized as *tong jing*, painful menstruation, and *zheng jia*, concretions and conglomerations. Since August 1992, Prof. Li Xiang-yun has treated 48 cases of endometriosis with very good results in the gynecology department at the Lung Hua Hospital associated with the Shanghai College of TCM. Eight of these women were between 40 and 48 years of age, 30 between 30 and 39, and 10 between 24 and 29 years of age. The duration of their disease had lasted from as short as six months to as long as 18 years. Twenty-eight women had severe abdominal pain and menstrual pain. Twelve women had such severe pain when their periods came that they had to take *Zhi Tong Pian* (Stop Pain Tablets). Eight women had dyspareunia, 16 menstrual irregularity, 14 infertility, and 16 low back soreness.

Pattern discrimination

1. Cold damp congelation and stagnation (5 cases): During menstruation, parturition, or in general, if one does not take sufficient care of their health, cold evils may invade. These yin cold evils then lodge in the *bao gong*. There they bind internally, cold and blood binding, obstructing, and stagnating in the vessels and network vessels. The symptoms of this are abdominal pain when the menstruation moves, fear of cold, chilled limbs, a sensation of downward dragging in the lower abdomen, blood clots in the menstrual movement, static spots on the tongue edges and tip, thin, white fur, and a deep, fine pulse.

2. Qi stagnation, blood stasis (16 cases): If there is emotional depression, the qi mechanism will not be smoothly flowing. The *chong* and *ren* qi and blood will be depressed and stagnant. The menstrual blood will not be able to flow normally, smoothly, or freely. Blood becomes static internally and this obstructs the vessels and network vessels. The manifestations of this are abdominal pain worse than distention. This may also involve breast and lateral costal distention and pain, and abdominal pain which gets worse one to two days before menstruation, abdominal pain at the time of menstruation which is piercing and refuses pressure, pain affecting the lumbosacral region and causing a sensation of sagging and distention in the anus, static spots on the edges and tip of the tongue which has thin fur, and a bowstring pulse.

3. Stasis heat internally obstructing (8 cases): Due to damp heat smoldering internally and flowing and pouring into the *chong* and *ren*, qi and blood are obstructed and become stagnant. It is also possible for damp heat toxins to invade at the time of menstruation or postpartum which are then retained in the *chong* and *ren*. These then smolder and bind within the uterus. The symptoms of this condition are lower abdominal aching and pain, a sensation of burning heat in the abdominal region, heart vexation, easy anger, a constant low-grade fever or fever during the menstrual movement, dry, bound stools, early menstruation, red colored menses, a red tongue with thin, yellow fur, and a fine, rapid pulse.

4. Qi vacuity & blood stasis (6 cases): Due to constitutional spleen qi vacuity weakness or consumption and damage of the qi and blood after surgery, qi and blood are insufficient. Qi vacuity leads to blood movement lacking force and the constructive and blood becoming vacuous and stagnant. It is also possible for a qi stagnation, blood stasis repletion pattern which endures for a long time to become a qi vacuity, blood stasis vacuity pattern. The manifestations of this are a sallow yellow facial complexion, lassitude of the spirit, lack of strength, dizziness, menstrual movement abdominal pain which desires pressure and warmth, anal sagging and distention, scanty menstruation which is colored a pale red, a pale, fat tongue with teeth marks on its edges, and a fine, weak pulse.

5. Kidney vacuity, stasis and obstruction (13 cases): Due to bedroom, *i.e.*, sexual, taxation and excessive births, there may be kidney qi vacuity weakness. If there is kidney vacuity and insufficiency of the essence and blood, the *chong* and *ren* qi and blood movement will be inhibited. This then results in kidney vacuity and blood stasis. The symptoms of this are abdominal pain at the time of menstruation, sagging and distention of the anus, pain affecting the lumbosacral area, scanty menstruation which is a pale red color, lassitude of the spirit, lack of strength, dizziness, tinnitus, lumbar soreness, diminished sexual desire, a slightly dark tongue with thin, white fur, and a fine pulse.

Treatment method

Self-composed *Yi Wei Zhu Yu Fang* (Abnormal Sites Dispelling Stasis Formula) was the root formula which was then modified with additions and subtractions: Rhizoma Sparganii (*San Leng*), 9g, Rhizoma Curcumae Zedoariae (*E Zhu*), 9g, Squama Manitis Pentadactylis (*Chuan Shan Jia*), 12g, Hirudo (*Shui Zhi*), 9g, Lignum Sappan (*Su Mu*), 12g, Eupoly-phaga Seu Ophistoplatia (*Di Bie Chong*), 12g, Fructus Liquidambaris Taiwaniae (*Lu Lu Tong*), 9g, Spica Prunellae Vulgaris (*Xia Ku Cao*), 12g.

If categorized as cold damp congelation, stagnation, stasis, and obstruction, Radix Lateralis Praeparatus Aconiti Carmichaeli (*Fu Zi*), 9g, and Ramulus Cinnamomi Cassiae

(*Gui Zhi*), 4.5g, were added. If the menses did not come smoothly, Radix Angelicae Sinensis (*Dang Gui*), 9g, and Flos Carthami Tinctorii (*Hong Hua*), 9g, were added. If there was severe abdominal pain, Rhizoma Corydalis Yanhusuo (*Yan Hu Suo*), 12g, *Shi Xiao San* (Sudden Smile Powder), 12g, Radix Aconiti (*Chuan Wu*), 9g, and Radix Angelicae Dahuricae (*Bai Zhi*), 9g, were added.

If there was qi stagnation and blood stasis, Fructus Meliae Toosendan (*Chuan Lian Zi*), 9g, Guangdong Tuber Curcumae (*Guang Yu Jin*), 9g, and Radix Linderae Strychnifoliae (*Wu Yao*), 9g, were added. If there was breast distention and pain, Fructus Akebiae Trifoliatae (*Ba Yue Zha*), 9g, Semen Citri Reticulatae & Folium Citri Reticulatae (*Ju He Ye*), 10g @, and Pericarpium Citri Reticulatae Viride (*Qing Pi*), 9g, were added. If there was abdominal distention which was not soothed, Fructus Citri Aurantii (*Zhi Ke*), 9g, and Pericarpium Arecae Catechu (*Da Fu Pi*), 12g, were added. If there was anal sagging and distention, Radix Bupleuri (*Chai Hu*), 9g, and Rhizoma Cimicifugae (*Sheng Ma*), 9g, were added.

If there was stasis heat internally obstructing, uncooked Radix Et Rhizoma Rhei (*Da Huang*), 4.5-9g, and Cortex Phellodendri (*Huang Bai*), 9g, were added. If damp heat was heavy, Caulis Sargentodoxae (*Hong Teng*), 30g, and Herba Patriniae Heterophylli Cum Radice (*Bai Jiang Cao*), 30g, were added.

If there was qi vacuity and blood stasis, Radix Codonopsitis Pilosulae (*Dang Shen*), 15g, Radix Astragali Membranacei (*Huang Qi*), 15g, and Radix Dioscoreae Oppositae (*Huai Shan Yao*), 15g, were added. If there was dizziness, Fructus Mori Albi (*Sang Shen Zi*), 9g, and Fructus Lycii Chinensis (*Gou Qi Zi*), 12g, were added. If the menses were excessive, Herba Agrimoniae Pilosae (*Xian He Cao*), 12g, and Gelatinum Corii Asini (*E Jiao*), 9g, were added.

If there was kidney vacuity and blood stasis obstruction tending to kidney yang vacuity, Rhizoma Curculiginis Orchioidis (*Xian Mao*), 9g, and Herba Epimedii (*Xian Ling Pi*), 12g, Fructus Trigonellae Foeni-graeci (*Hu Lu Ba*), 12g, and Cornu Cervi (*Lu Jiao Pian*), 9g, were added. If it tended towards kidney yin vacuity, then Fructus Corni Officinalis (*Shan Yu Rou*), 9g, Fructus Ligustri Lucidi (*Nu Zhen Zi*), 12g, and uncooked Radix Rehmanniae (*Sheng Di*), 12g, were added. If lumbar soreness was severe, Cortex Eucommiae Ulmoidis (*Du Zhong*), 15g, Ramulus Loranthi Seu Visci (*Sang Ji Sheng*), 12g, and processed Rhizoma Cibotti Barometsis (*Gou Ji*), 12g, were added.

In addition to the internally administered medicinals, if there were obvious lumps, a retention enema formula was used: Rhizoma Sparganii (*San Leng*), 9g, Rhizoma

Curcumae Zedoariae (*E Zhu*), 9g, Nidus Vespae (*Feng Fang*), 12g, Radix Rubrus Paeoniae Lactiflorae (*Chi Shao*), 9g, Spina Gelditschiae Sinensis (*Zao Jiao Ci*), 12g. These were soaked and decocted in water until they produced 150ml. Each evening, after expelling the stools, this was administered as a retention enema. This was stopped during the menstruation. This is suitable for those with intense abdominal pain during the menstrual movement, those with lumps within the abdomen, or those whose posterior fornix has nodules which are markedly painful when touched. If the menstrual movement abdominal pain was intense or if the woman commonly took *Zhi Tong Pian* (Stop Pain Tablets), then ear point press plasters were used. Typically, each month one or two days before the period came, press plasters were applied to *Zi Gong* (Uterus), *Luan Chao* (Ovaries), *Jiao Gan* (Sympathetic), and other such points.

Treatment outcomes

Ten women were cured with this protocol. This meant that 10 of the 14 women who suffered from infertility conceived after being treated. Five women experienced marked improvement, 28 women got some improvement, and five women got no results. Thus the total amelioration rate was 89.5%.

Endometriosis & static blood

Endometriosis is not a disease category in TCM. However, the *Jin Gui Yao Lue (Essentials from the Golden Cabinet)*, "Women's Miscellaneous Diseases' Pulse, Pattern & Treatment" chapter has this description: "The menstrual water is inhibited and there is lower abdominal fullness and pain." The *Jing Yue Quan Shu ([Zhang] Jing-yue's Complete Book)*, "Women's Regulation: Blood Conglomerations" chapter states:

> Static blood which is retained and stagnates eventually becomes concretions. Only women have this. This pattern may be caused during the period or postpartum and may be due to internal damage engendering chill, external invasion of wind cold, rage and anger damaging the liver, qi counterflow and blood stagnation, long-standing taxation, long-standing weakness, and qi weakness not moving [the blood]. Therefore, sometimes the blood stirs and sometimes it has almost nothing. It may also counterflow, thus leading to retention and stagnation which accumulates for days, gradually becoming concretions.

The *Zheng Zhi Zheng Sheng (Patterns & Treatments Proven Restraint)*, "Blood Conglomerations" chapter states:

> If there is gathering of blood conglomeration, there will be low back pain and inability to bend, accumulation of qi below the transverse bone [*i.e.*, pubic bone], hardness like stone, tension inside the lower abdomen, bitter pain, upper back spine pain penetrating to and reaching the

low back and abdomen, spasms within the vagina, if there is contraction of wind chill, a secluded child gate [*i.e.*, vaginal meatus], menstrual water not on time, sometimes coming and sometimes not. This disease is found in people without children [*i.e.*, with infertility]. If treatment precipitates the conglomerations, it can be cured.

The above literary cites and endometriosis all share the same symptoms. In endometriosis there is the production of nodulations and lumps within the body. In TCM this is related to blood gathering becoming stasis, and stasis accumulation becoming concretions and conglomerations. Therefore, the great method for treating endometriosis is to quicken the blood and transform stasis.

Experience in the use of worm type medicinals

Based on the theories that enduring disease enters the network vessels and that worms and insects can search and pick out, Prof. Li has found out that worm type medicinals are relatively good for breaking the blood and scattering stasis in the treatment of endometriosis. Therefore, he commonly uses worm type medicinals such as Hirudo (*Shui Zhi*), Scolopendra Subspinipes (*Wu Gong*), Eupolyphaga Seu Ophistoplatia (*Di Bie Chong*), Squama Manitis Pentadactylis (*Chuan Shan Jia*), and Lumbricus (*Di Long*). The *Ben Cao Gang Mu (Great Outline of the Materia Medica)*, states:

> Leech's flavor is salty and bitter and it is neutral. It has toxins. It is mainly for dispelling malign blood, static blood, blocked menstruation, breaking blood conglomerations, accumulations, and gatherings, infertility, and disinhibiting the water passageways.

The *Bie Lu (Divergent Records)* says that Centipede has the ability to "treat heart and abdomen cold and heat, accumulations and gatherings, and falling fetus; it removes malign blood and treats concretions and conglomerations." In addition, Squama Manitis, Eupolyphaga, and Earthworm also have the ability to attack congelation and scatter nodulation. Because worm type medicinals have a good ability to search wind and resolve toxins, quicken the blood and transform stasis, attack the hard and break accumulations, open the channels and extend the network vessels, they get a good effect in clinical practice in the treatment of this disease.

(From "Lai Chun-mao's Treatment of 38 Cases of Endometriosis" by Cao Dong *et al.*, *Yun Nan Zhong Yi Za Zhi [Yunnan Journal of Chinese Medicine]*, #5, 1994, p. 7)

In TCM, endometriosis is categorized as menstrual movement abdominal pain. According to elder Lai, this disease is mostly due to external contraction of chill and coolness, internal smoldering of dampness and heat, and lack of emotional ease. This leads to dampness and heat mutally binding in the *bao gong* or uterus and viscera and bowels. Therefore, if there is stasis and heat, using a heat-clearing, dampness-disinhibiting formula with additions and subtractions following the pattern achieves a good result.

From August 1988 to March, 1994, elder Lai treated 38 cases of this disease. Their ages ranged from 28-46 years old. There were 29 cases between 28-38 and 9 cases between 39-46 years old. Clinically, they presented with severe, difficult to bear lower abdominal pain when their menses came. This was accompanied by heart vexation and chaotic thought, oral thirst, dry lips, sweating and a damp exterior, fleshy blood clots when their menses came with diminishment of their pain after the expulsion of these clots. They were diagnosed with endometriosis through ultrasound examination.

Treatment method

Based on the saying, "If there is free flow, there is no pain", the treatment principles were to remove stasis and engender new (tissue). Therefore, the patients were given: Hirudo (*Shui Zhi*), Eupolyphaga Seu Ophistoplatia (*Tu Bie Chong*), Semen Pruni Persicae (*Tao Ren*), uncooked Radix Et Rhizoma Rhei (*Da Huang*), Fructus Meliae Toosendan (*Jin Ling Zi*), Rhizoma Corydalis Yanhusuo (*Yan Hu*), Talcum (*Hua Shi*), Semen Plantaginis (*Che Qian Zi*), Caulis Akebiae Mutong (*Mu Tong*), Resina Myrrhae (*Mo Yao*), Pollen Typhae (*Pu Huang*), and Feces Trogopterori Seu Pteromi (*Wu Ling Zhi*) with additions and subtractions following each patient's pattern. This treatment is based on the *Shang Han Lun (Treatise on Cold Damage)*'s treatment of amassed blood resulting in mania through the use of *Di Dang Tang* (Resistance Decoction). However, since in this case there was dampness and heat mutually binding in the lower burner, Talcum, Akebia, and Plantago were added in order to free and disinhibit dampness and heat. One *ji* was given per day decocted in water and administered in three divided doses. Twelve days equalled one course of treatment. During treatment with the above Chinese medicinals, these patients did not take any Western medication.

Treatment outcomes

Of the 38 women treated with this protocol, 26 were cured. This meant that their symptoms disappeared and their ultrasound was normal. Another five cases experienced some improvement, while seven cases got no result. Treatment lasted from as short as one course to as long as six courses. The cure rate was 68.4% and the total amelioration rate was 81.6%.

Discussion

Endometriosis is a commonly seen gynecological disease for which *Di Dang Tang* with added flavors is effective. According to Zhang Zhong-jing, this formula is one of several which breaks the blood and dispels stasis. It mainly treates amassed blood resulting in mania, lower abominal hardness and fullness, spontaneously disinhibited urination but hard stools which are black in color, and a deep, bound pulse. It also treats women's inhibition of menstrual water, lower abdominal hardness and fullness which refuses pressure, and amassed blood conditions for which other formulas composed only of grass and woods are not effective. This is because it uses worm type medicinals which enter the blood network vessels. Thus this formula is able to move stasis and break binding.

Within this formula, Hirudo is salty and bitter and has a neutral nature. It enters the two channels of the liver and urinary bladder. It has a strong power to dispel malign blood and static blood. It breaks the blood in concretions and conglomerations, accumulations and gatherings, and it breaks stasis without damaging the fresh or new blood. Tabanus (*Meng Chong,* which is not mentioned in the above enumeration of medicinals used in this formula but which is part of *Di Dang Tang*) also has a strong power to break the blood and dispel stasis. However, when these two medicinals are used together, they can be too violently draining. Therefore Eupolyphaga is used instead. Its functions are the same as Hirudo's. Rhubarb sweeps away filth and evil heat. It abducts stasis to move downward. Persica breaks the blood and moves stasis. The ingredients in *Shi Xiao San* (Loose a Smile Powder) are added to quicken the blood and transform stasis, scatter nodulation and stop pain. Melia and Corydalis course the liver and discharge heat, move the qi and stop pain. Myrrh quickens the blood, scatters stasis, and stops pain. These are aided by Talcum, Plantago, and Akebia which clear and disinhibit dampness and heat. Thus, taken as a whole, this formula is very effective for stasis and heat with putrid flesh mutually binding resulting in severe lower abdominal pain which refuses pressure with hardness and fullness and amassed blood resulting in mania.

(From "Experiences in the Chinese Medical Treatment of Endometriosis" by Sha Ming-rong, *Zhong Yi Za Zhi [Journal of Chinese Medicine],* # 4, 1995, p. 213)

Endometriosis is a commonly seen disease in the gynecological department. Typically, severe abdominal pain during the menstrual period, sagging and distention of the anus, excessive menstruation, prolonged menstruation, and infertility are its common manifestations. The author has treated this disease with Chinese medicinals for a number of years with very good results.

According to the author, the cause of the onset of this disease is, in most cases, loss of regularity of the *chong* and *ren* resulting in the menstrual blood obstructing and stagnating the *bao mai*. This may, in turn, be due to loss of care and regulation during the menstrual period or postpartum or damage and detriment caused by surgery. Hence malign blood is retained and stagnates and the movement of blood suffers obstruction. Lack of free flow then leads to pain. If static blood is retained and stagnates for days on end, this will gradually lead to the formation of conglomerations. The *chong* and *ren* are not smoothly flowing and blood cannot abide in the channels. Therefore, they are not able to restrain the essence which thus forms pregnancy.

This disease is located in the lower burner and its course is enduring. There is excessive menstruation and thus "poverty must reach the kidneys." This means that this disease is a combination of repletion and vacuity. Repletion refers to the static blood which is retained and accumulates. The vacuity is vacuity of the spleen and kidneys or, in other words, qi and yin dual vacuity. Hence the treatment principles are mainly to quicken the blood and transform stasis while simultaneously attending to the spleen and kidneys. For these purposes, the author commonly uses self-composed *Tuo Mo Tang* (Cast Off the Membrane Decoction).

Treatment method

Tuo Mo Tang is comprised of: Radix Bupleuri (*Chai Hu*), 10g, Radix Angelicae Sinensis (*Dang Gui*), Radix Albus Paeoniae Lactiflorae (*Bai Shao*), Radix Rubrus Paeoniae Lactiflorae (*Chi Shao*), 15g @, Cortex Radicis Moutan (*Dan Pi*), 10g, Rhizoma Cyperi Rotundi (*Xiang Fu*), 15g, Tuber Curcumae (*Yu Jin*), 12g, Semen Sinapis Albae (*Bai Jie Zi*), 10g, bile-processed Rhizoma Arisaematis (*Dan Xing*), 10g, Pericarpium Citri Reticulatae (*Chen Pi*), 10g, Radix Et Rhizoma Rhei (*Da Huang*), 9g, Squama Manitis Pentadactylis (*Shan Jia*), 15g, Sanguis Draconis (*Xue Jie*), 6g, Aspongopus (*Jiu Xiang Chong*), 10g, Rhizoma Sparganii (*San Leng*), Rhizoma Curcumae Zedoariae (*E Zhu*), 10g @, Rhizoma Atractylodis Macrocephalae (*Bai Zhu*), 10g, Fructus Corni Officinalis (*Shan Zhu Yu*), 12g, Radix Glycyrrhizae (*Gan Cao*), 10g.

Discussion

Within this formula, Red Peony, Dragon's Blood, Aspongopus, Sparganium, Zedoaria, Bupleurum, Cyperus, and Curcuma quicken the blood and transform stasis, soothe the liver and rectify the qi, scatter nodulation and stop pain while simultaneously dispersing concretions. Dang Gui and White Peony nourish the blood and soften the liver, regulate and supplement the *chong* and *ren*. Moutan clears and discharges depressive heat in the liver channel. The bitterness of Rhubarb severely precipitates, promoting the elimination of the old and, therefore, the arrival of the new. It precipitates stasis and opens blockage. Squama Manitis enters the *jue yin* and can soften the hard and scatter nodulation. When added to Mustard Seed, bile-processed Arisaema, and Orange Peel, these disinhibit the qi and transform stasis, free the flow of menstruation and stop pain. The combination of Atractylodes and Cornus fortifies the spleen and boosts the kidneys, thus supplementing vacuity. While the combination of Licorice and Peony relax cramping and stop pain. Taken as a whole, therefore, this formula quickens the blood and transforms stasis, soothes the liver and rectifies the qi, scatters nodulation and stops pain. If liver depression obtains resolution, depressive heat obtains elimination, stasis obtains transformation, and qi and blood flow freely and smoothly, then the effect is that "free flow leads to the absence of pain."

If there is also blazing and accumulation of liver heat, add Radix Scutellariae Baicalensis (*Huang Qin*), Fructus Gardeniae Jasminoidis (*Shan Zhi*), and Spica Prunellae Vulgaris (*Xia Ku Cao*). If there is marked qi stagnation, use double amounts of Cyperus and Curcuma and add Radix Auklandiae Lappae (*Mu Xiang*). If there is qi and blood vacuity weakness, add Radix Codonopsitis Pilosulae (*Dang Shen*), Radix Astragali Membranacei (*Huang Qi*), and Gelatinum Corii Asini (*E Jiao*). If there is dual vacuity of the qi and yin, add *Sheng Mai San* (Engender the Pulse Powder). If there is liver-kidney vacuity with loss of regulation of the *chong* and *ren*, add Radix Morindae Officinalis (*Ba Ji Tian*) and Semen Cuscutae (*Tu Si Zi*). And if there is cold lodged in the uterus, remove Moutan and add Folium Artemisiae Argyii (*Ai Ye*), blast-fried Rhizoma Zingiberis (*Pao Jiang*), and Cortex Cinnamomi Cassiae (*Rou Gui*).

(From "The Treatment of 40 Cases of Endometriosis by Boosting the Qi & Transforming Stasis" by He Shu-ying, *Si Chuan Zhong Yi [Sichuan Chinese Medicine]*, #9, 1993, p. 41)

All 40 women in this study suffered from endometriosis as diagnosed by gynecological examination and other modern Western medical procedures. Their ages ranged from 24-48 years old, the course of their disease ranged from as short as one year to as long as 18 years. Among these 40 women, 25 were infertile. Thirty-one had had previous surgery for ectopic pregnancies, artificial abortions, and other such surgical procedures. Thirty-seven cases experienced occasionally intense abdominal and menstrual pain. Twelve had pain with intercourse. Twenty-eight had pelvic pain. Eighteen had a heavy, distended, pulling and tugging feeling in their anus.

Treatment method

The formula with which these women were treated consisted of: Radix Codonopsitis Pilosulae (*Dang Shen*) and Radix Astragali Membranacei (*Huang Qi*), 20g @, Radix Bupleuri (*Chai Hu*), Pericarpium Citri Reticulatae (*Chen Pi*), Fructus Liquidambaris Taiwaniae (*Lu Lu Tong*), and Rhizoma Corydalis Yanhusuo (*Yan Hu*), 10g @, Rhizoma Cimicifugae (*Sheng Ma*), 6g, uncooked Radix Rehmanniae (*Sheng Di*), Pollen Typhae (*Pu Huang*), Radix Rubrus Paeoniae Lactiflorae (*Chi Shao*), Resina Olibani (*Ru*), and Resina Myrrhae (*Mo*), 10g @, and Rhizoma Sparganii (*San Leng*) and Rhizoma Curcumae Zedoariae (*E Zhu*), 20g @.

If there was yang vacuity, Radix Lateralis Praeparatus Aconiti Carmichaeli (*Fu Pian*), 10g, and Cortex Cinnamomi Cassiae (*Rou Gui*), 6g, were added. If there was severe tugging and pulling aching and pain of the anus, Fructus Foeniculi Vulgaris (*Xiao Hui Xiang*) and Fructus Meliae Toosendan (*Chuan Lian Zi*), 10g @, were added. If there was blood vacuity, Gelatinum Corii Asini (*E Jiao*) and Radix Polygoni Multiflori (*Shou Wu*), 10g @, were added. If there was constipation, uncooked Radix Et Rhizoma Rhei (*Sheng Jun*), 8g, was added. If the menses were profuse and like a rush, Herba Agrimoniae Pilosae (*Xian He Cao*), 20g, carbonized Radix Scutellariae Baicalensis (*Huang Qin*), 10g, and carbonized Cacumen Biotae Orientalis (*Ce Bai Ye*), 12g, were added. If there was lumbar ache, Cortex Eucommiae Ulmoidis (*Du Zhong*), Ramulus Loranthi Seu Visci (*Sang Ji Sheng*), and Herba Cistanchis Deserticolae (*Cong Rong*), 10g @, were added. If there were cystic lumps or chocolate cysts, Spina Gleditschiae Sinensis (*Zao Jiao Ci*) and Lignum Sappan (*Su Mu*), 10g @, were added.

Treatment outcomes

Marked improvement was defined as disappearance of the main symptoms and obvious reduction in the nodulations within the pelvis. Some improvement was defined as a reduction in the symptoms and a reduction in the nodulations. Based on these criteria, 33 women experienced marked improvement and seven conceived afterwards. Four cases experienced some improvement, and three cases got no result. Thus the combined amelioration rate was 92.5%.

Discussion

The author relates this condition primarily to binding of static malign blood. This may be due to either cold congelation or qi stagnation leading to blood stasis. If, however, there is excessive menstrual bleeding like a rush, this is due to insufficient qi and blood. In this case, qi is unable to contain or to move the blood. Thus qi vacuity changes into blood stagnation. If the qi is vacuous, central qi may fall downward resulting in anal heaviness and distention with tugging and pulling aching and pain. Therefore, in this protocol, Codonopsis, Astragalus, Bupleurum, and Cimicifuga upbear the central qi. These are then combined with medicinals to quicken the blood and transform stasis.

(From "An Analysis of the Treatment of 35 Cases of Endometriosis Using the Transforming Stasis, Supplementing the Kidneys Method" by Yin Xiu-lan, *Shang Hai Zhong Yi Yao Za Zhi [Shanghai Journal of Traditional Chinese Medicine & Medicinals]*, #11, 1993, p. 21-22)

After defining this condition in Western medical terms, the author says that in Chinese medicine it is categorized as painful menstruation and conglomerations and concretions and its main associated conditions are menstrual pain, menstrual irregularities, and infertility. The 35 women treated in this study ranged in age from 21-53 years old, with the average being 36.9 years of age. Thirty-four of the cases had painful menstruation and menstrual irregularity. Seven women were infertile. Twenty-seven of the women had so-called chocolate ovarian cysts. Gynecologic examination found obviously painful nodulations in 20 cases and 1/3 of the women had retroverted uteri.

Treatment method

This study used a staged protocol involving two different formulas. Formula 1 consisted of: Uncooked Radix Astragali Membranacei (*Huang Qi*) and Radix Salviae Miltiorrhizae (*Dan Shen*), 30g @, whole Radix Angelicae Sinensis (*Quan Dang Gui*) and Herba Epimedii (*Yin Yang Huo*), 12g @, Radix Rubrus Paeoniae Lactiflorae (*Chi Shao*) and Spica Prunellae Vulgaris (*Xia Ku Cao*), 20g @, Rhizoma Sparganii (*San Leng*), Rhizoma Curcumae Zedoariae (*E Zhu*), and Fructus Ligustri Lucidi (*Nu Zhen Zi*), 10g @, Radix Dipsaci (*Xu Duan*), 15g, uncooked Radix Et Rhizoma Rhei (*Da Huang*) and Feces Trogopterori Seu Pteromi (*Wu Ling Zhi*), 6g @, and Sanguis Draconis (*Xue Jie*), 0.3g (ground into powder and swallowed down with the other decocted medicinals).

Formula 2 consisted of: Uncooked Radix Astragali Membranacei (*Huang Qi*), 30g, Radix Angelicae Sinensis (*Dang Gui*), 9g, Radix Rubrus Paeoniae Lactiflorae (*Chi Shao*), Radix Salviae Miltiorrhizae (*Dan Shen*), Herba Ecliptae Prostratae (*Han Lian Cao*), and uncooked Radix Rehmanniae (*Sheng Di*), 20g @, uncooked and stir-fried Pollen Typhae (*Pu Huang*), 12g @ (wrapped), Radix Rubiae Cordifoliae (*Qian Cao*), Cortex Radicis Lycii (*Di Gu Pi*), and Radix Dipsaci (*Xu Duan*), 15g @, Fructus Ligustri Lucidi (*Nu Zhen Zi*), 10g, Feces Trogopterori Seu Pteromi (*Wu Ling Zhi*), 6g, processed Radix Et Rhizoma Rhei (*Zhi Jun*), 9g, Resina Olibani (*Ru Xiang*) and Resina Myrrhae (*Mo Yao*), 3g @.

Formula 1 was administered from the cessation of the menstruation till after the next menses began, one *ji* per day. Then formula 2 was administered. (In other words, formula 2 was administered only during the menstruation itself.) This was continued for three to six months.

If, after taking the Sanguis Draconis, the patient became nauseous, it was removed and Eupolyphaga Seu Opisthoplatia (*Di Bie Chong*), 12g, was added. If the menstrual pain was categorized as cold, Eclipta, Agrimonia, Cortex Lycii, and uncooked Rehmannia were removed and aged Folium Artemisiae Argyii (*Chen Ai*), 10g, and Fructus Evodiae Rutecarpae (*Wu Zhu Yu*), 3g, were added to warm the channels (or menses), scatter cold, and stop pain. If the menstruate was profuse like a downpour and was colored purple and dark with large amounts of blood clots, Ophicalcitum (*Hua Ru Shi*), 30g, was added to dispel stasis and stop pain.

Treatment outcomes

Complete cure consisted of disappearance of the symptoms and the infertile patients becoming pregnant. Marked improvement consisted of disappearance of the symptoms with the cysts or nodules reduced in size by half or more. Also, those who were infertile conceived. Some improvement meant that the symptoms were stabilized somewhat but the majority of symptoms were not eliminated. And no result meant that there was no change in the condition or it got worse. Based on these criteria, four cases or 11.4% were cured, 20 or 57.15% were markedly improved, and eight or 22.9% got some improvement. Thus, the combined amelioration rate was 91.4%.

Discussion

The author bases this approach on the sayings that "The kidneys govern reproduction" and that "The *bao tai* is fastened to the kidneys." Because this condition is often accompanied by infertility, tinnitus, low back and knee soreness and weakness, diminished sexual desire, and other such symptoms corresponding to essence qi debility, this condition commonly involves kidney vacuity. Therefore, within this protocol, Epimedium, Dipsacus, and Ligustrum warm the kidneys and invigorate yang, enrich and supplement the liver and kidneys, while Astragalus supplements the qi. Then, because many of the other symptoms of endometriosis correspond to blood stasis, these supplementing medicinals are combined with blood-quickening and stasis-transforming ingredients. In this case, kidney vacuity is the root and blood stasis is the branch, and, although transforming stasis is the main principle, it should be accompanied by simultaneous supplementation.

(From "A Clinical Study of the Treatment of 68 Cases of Endometriosis by the Methods of Transforming Stasis & Softening the Hard" by Chang Nuan & Ma Ping-chong, *Tian Jin Zhong Yi [Tianjin Chinese Medicine]*, #5, 1995, p. 11-12)

The authors of this article begin by saying that endometriosis is a commonly seen disease in gynecology departments and is one of the knotty, difficult diseases. In Chinese medicine it is categorized as painful menstruation, menstrual irregularity, infertility, and concretions and conglomerations. Its disease mechanism is primarily static blood. Therefore, most Chinese doctors treat this disease by the methods of quickening the blood and transforming stasis. However, based on their more than 30 years of clinical experience, Han Bing believes that the disease mechanisms are enduring stasis producing concretions. These are mixed with phlegm and with dampness. Therefore, Dr. Han uses transforming stasis and softening the hard, dispersing phlegm and scattering nodulation as the methods to treat this disease. This article describes the treatment of 68 women with endometriosis using these methods.

All 68 of these women's diagnoses were confirmed by ultrasound and corresponded to the criteria established at the Second National Conference on Integrated Chinese-Western Medicine Gynecology as published in the *Zhong Xi Yi Jie He Za Zhi (The Journal of Integrated Chinese-Western Medicine)*, #5, 1987, p. 317. These women ranged in age from 27-43 with a median age of 35.3 years. All were married and the course of their disease had lasted from six months to 12 years with a median duration of 3.8 years. Twenty-eight of these patients had had abortions and four had had ectopic pregnancies. Twenty cases had been treated with hormone therapy in the prior six months and 16 cases had been treated with surgical decollement but, after surgical excision, the disease recurred.

Fifty-six cases (82.4%) suffered from painful menstruation, 41 (60.3%) from pelvic pain, and 24 (35.3%) from lumbar soreness and pain. Twenty-nine cases (42.6%) suffered from sagging pain in the anus, 36 (52.9%) from menstrual irregularity, and 10 (14.7%) from infertility. Thirty-eight cases (55.9%) had pelvic adhesions and lumps, while 32 cases (47.1%) had chocolate ovarian cysts. Of these, five had bilateral cysts. Most of these patients had dark red tongues and a number had static spots and static macules on their tongue edges or tips. Their pulses were mostly fine and choppy or bowstring, fine, and choppy.

Treatment method

The formula used consisted of: Sanguis Draconis (*Xue Jie*), 3g, Rhizoma Curcumae Zedoariae (*E Zhu*), 10g, Squama Manitis Pentadactylis (*Chuan Shan Jia*), 10g, Carapax Amydae Sinensis (*Bie Jia*), 15g, Spina Gleditschiae Sinensis (*Zao Jiao Ci*), 15g, Herba Sargassii (*Hai Zao*), 10g, Thallus Algae (*Kun Bu*), 10g, Semen Coicis Lachryma-jobi (*Yi*

Yi Ren), 15g. If there was menstrual pain, before menstruation, Radix Linderae Strychni-foliae (*Wu Yao*), Ramulus Cinnamomi Cassiae (*Gui Zhi*), Radix Achyranthis Bidentatae (*Niu Xi*), and Fructus Liquidambaris Taiwaniae (*Lu Lu Tong*) were added to free the flow of menstruation and stabilize pain. If menstruation was profuse, before and during menstruation, Pollen Typhae (*Pu Huang*), Ophicalcitum (*Hua Rui Shi*), and Radix Pseudoginseng (*San Qi*) were added. If the menstruation was irregular or if there was infertility, Chinese medicinals were combined with the above protocol based on artificially regulating the menstrual cycle. Once the symptoms remitted, patients were administered the soluble granules, *Fu Tong Ning* (Women's Pain Tranquilizer). If the symptoms recurred, the previous methods were resumed and continued as regulating therapy. Medicinals were continued for three months which constituted one course of treatment.

Definition of treatment outcomes

The criteria for treatment efficacy was based on the above-mentioned Second National Conference on Integrated Chinese-Western Medicine Gynecology. Marked effect meant that the symptoms basically disappeared and that the physical masses decreased in size by 1/3 or more. If there was infertility, the woman was able to conceive. Some effect was defined as marked decrease in the symptoms and some decrease in the size of the physical masses. No effect meant that there was no marked or obvious change in either the symptoms or the size of the masses or that they got worse.

Treatment outcomes

Based on the above criteria, 38 cases (55.9%) got marked effect, 26 cases (38.2%) got some effect, and four cases (5.9%) got no effect. Thus the total effectiveness rate for this protocol was 94.1%. The effectiveness rates for remission of painful menstruation, pelvic pain, lumbar pain, and anal sagging pain were 92.9% (52 out of 56 cases), 78.2% (32 out of 41 cases), 62.5% (15 out of 24 cases), and 93.1% (27 out of 29 cases) respectively. The effectiveness rate for normalizing menstrual irregularity was 88.9% (32 out of 36 cases). The conception rate for those who were previously infertile was 40% (four out of 10 cases). The effectiveness rate for decrease in size of pelvic adhesions and lumps was 86.8% (33 out of 38 cases). And the effectiveness rate for disappearance or decrease in ovarian cysts was 81.3% (26 out of 32 cases).

Discussion

According to the authors, Dragon's Blood is the ruler of this formula. It breaks concretions and accumulations and long-standing blood, stops bleeding and stabilizes pain. Therefore, it addresses the two great symptoms of endometriosis — menstrual pain and bleeding. It is assisted by Zedoaria which breaks the blood and disperses concretions and by Squama Manitis and Spina Gleditschiae which transform stasis and free the flow of the channels and/or menses. Carapax Amydae softens the hard, Sargassium disperses phlegm, and Coix seeps dampness. Thus the production of both phlegm and stasis are equally dispersed.

(From "Clinical Experiences in the Treatment of 89 Cases of Endometriosis with the Methods of Quickening the Blood & Freeing the Flow of the Bowels" by Li Ying, *Xin Zhong Yi [New Chinese Medicine]*, #3, 1996, p. 24-26)

From October 1992 to December 1994, the author treated 89 cases of endometriosis. These women ranged in age between 23 and 46. Ten cases were between 23-30, 63 were 31-40, and 16 were 41-46. Their disease course had lasted from three months to 11 years. Eighty-two were married and seven were unmarried. Seventy-four cases had had artificial abortions, 12 had had dilations (meaning the insertion of IUDs), and only three had primary onset dysmenorrhea. Fifty-eight cases had been previously treated with Western and Chinese medicinals for one half year or more with no result. These women were diagnosed using standards set at the Third Chinese National Integrated Chinese-Western Medicine Gynecology Conference. They included:

1. Before or after menstruation lower abdominal or lumbosacral discomfort or pain which gradually became more severe
2. Pathological lumps and nodulations in the pelvic cavity
3. A purple tongue or static macules or static spots on the tongue body
4. A choppy or bound, regularly irregular pulse
5. Fixed, piercing pain or (pain) which refuses pressure
6. Blood vessel abnormalities, such as engorged, tortuous veins under the tongue, blood vessel spasm, tongue or limb tips purple or dark purple, blood vessel obstruction and blockage
7. Subdermal static macules

All the women in this study had criteria #1 and #2 combined with at least one of criteria #3-7.

Symptom analysis

Seventy-seven cases or 86.5% had gradually increasing menstrual pain. Twenty-four cases or 26.9% had pain with sexual intercourse. Thirty-nine cases or 43.8% had pelvic pain. Forty-two cases or 47.2% had anal region sagging, distented pain. Forty-four cases or 49.4% had chocolate ovarian cysts. And 30 cases or 33.7% had pelvic nodulations.

Analysis of pattern discrimination

Twenty-eight cases or 31.5% were categorized as qi stagnation blood stasis pattern. Twenty cases or 22.5% were categorized as depressive heat blood stasis pattern. Twenty-four cases or 26.9% were categorized as cold congelation blood stasis pattern. And 17 cases or 19.1% were categorized as kidney vacuity and blood stasis pattern.

Treatment method

All the members of this group were treated with the methods of quickening the blood and freeing the flow of the bowels. The basic formula was *Tao He Cheng Qi Tang* (Persica Seed Order the Qi Decoction). This was then modified depending upon the menstrual cycle phase and the pattern. The formula was composed of: Semen Pruni Persica (*Tao Ren*), 12g, Ramulus Cinnamomi Cassiae (*Gui Zhi*), Fructus Aurantii (*Zhi Ke*), Mirabilitum (*Mang Xiao*), 9g @, Carapax Amydae Sinensis (*Bie Jia*), 15g, powdered Radix Pseudoginseng (*San Qi Fen*, swallowed with the decoction), Eupolyphaga Seu Opisthoplatia (*Tu Bie*), 10g @, Radix Et Rhizoma Rhei (*Da Huang*), Radix Glycyrrhizae (*Gan Cao*), 6g @, and Herba Leonuri Hetrophylli (*Yi Mu Cao*), 20g.

Additions & subtractions: For the qi stagnation blood stasis pattern, Rhizoma Sparganii (*San Leng*), Rhizoma Curcumae Zedoariae (*E Zhu*), and Rhizoma Cyperi Rotundi (*Xiang Fu*) were added. For the depressive heat blood stasis pattern, Herba Patriniae Heterophyllae Cum Radice (*Bai Jiang Cao*) was added and up to 10g of Radix Et Rhizoma Rhei (*Da Huang*) was used. For the cold congelation blood stasis pattern, Ramulus Cinnamomi was changed to Cortex Cinnamomi Cassiae (*Rou Gui*), Mirabilitum was deleted, and dry Rhizoma Zingiberis (*Gan Jiang*) and Fructus Evodiae Rutecarpae (*Wu Zhu Yu*) were added. For the kidney vacuity and blood stasis pattern, Mirabilitum was deleted and Cortex Eucommiae Ulmoidis (*Du Zhong*) and Radix Dipsaci (*Xu Duan*) or Fructus Ligustri Lucidi (*Nu Zhen Zi*) were added.

Method of use: The medicinals were commenced seven to ten days before menstruation. They were administered until day 5 of the cycle and then stopped. Each day, one *ji* was decocted in water and taken in two divided doses, morning and evening. Successive administration for two menstrual cycles equalled one course of treatment.

Methods for determining outcomes

There were three methods for determining the outcomes:

1. Clinical and generalized signs and symptoms: These included changes in the menstrual cycle and the color, consistency, and amount of the menstruate as well as changes in menstrual period pain, accompanying signs and symptoms, and tongue and pulse changes. In addition, gynecological and ultrasound examination.
2. Changes in blood circulation and flow
3. Determination of menstrual period blood serum prostaglandin content

Criteria for establishing outcomes

The criteria for establishing outcomes were set by the Third Chinese National Integrated Chinese-Western Medicine Gynecology Conference. Clinical cure meant that all the symptoms disappeared, all lumps in the plevic cavity basically disappeared, and conception or birth within three years in those who were infertile. Marked effect meant that the symptoms basically disappeared and pelvic lumps got smaller. However, in those with infertility, there was still no conception. Some effect meant that the symptoms diminished, there was either no increase in size in the pelvic lumps or some slight decrease, and there was no worsening in the condition within three months of stopping the medicinals. No effect meant that there was no change or a change for the worse in the symptoms and a change for the worse in the areas of disease.

Analysis of outcomes

After one to three courses of treatment, 31 cases or 34.8% were cured. Thirty-seven cases or 41.6% got marked effect. Sixteen cases or 17.9% got some effect. And five cases or 5.6% experienced no effect. Thus 76.4% got a marked effect or better and the total effectiveness rate was 94.4%.

Of the 77 cases with menstrual pain, treatment was effective in 65 cases. Of the 24 cases of painful sexual intercourse, treatment was effective in 19 cases. Of the 39 cases with pelvic cavity pain, treatment was effective in 30 cases. Of the 42 cases with anal region sagging and distented pain, treatment was effective in 40 cases. Of the 44 cases of cysts, treatment was effective in 39 cases. And of the 30 cases with nodulations, treatment was effective in 22 cases. Thus the treatment cure rate was relatively high for anal region sagging and distended pain, ovarian cysts, painful menstruation, and pain during sexual intercourse.

Of the 28 cases with qi stagnation blood stasis pattern, 12 were cured, 14 got marked effect, two got some effect, and none got no effect. Of the 20 cases with depressive heat blood stasis pattern, nine were cured, 10 got marked effect, one got some effect, and none got no effect. Of the 24 cases with cold congelation pattern, seven were cured, eight got marked effect, seven got some effect, and two got no effect. And of the 17 cases with kidney vacuity and blood stasis pattern, three were cured, five got marked effect, six got some effect, and three got no effect. Thus this treatment was more effective for the two interior repletion patterns of depressive heat blood stasis and qi stagnation blood stasis.

In terms of blood circulation and flow, the blood of 36 patients was examined both before and after treatment. In all those 36 patients, red blood cell agglutination, blood sedimentation, blood serum viscosity, etc. all marked improved as compared to normal women (P <0.05). In 41 cases, menstrual period serum prostagandins were measured before and after treatment. Before treatment, PGE_2 and PGF_2 were all markedly higher than in normal women and after treatment these were markedly reduced (P <0.05).

Discussion

The author of this study says that the main clinical manifestations of this disease are secondary onset dysmenorrhea, painful intercourse, pelvic cavity pain, menstrual abnormality, and infertility. In Chinese medicine, this disease is categorized as painful menstruation and concretions and conglomerations or "lower burner static blood." In Chinese medicine, the uterus is in the lower burner and is called an "extraordinary bowel." Typically the menstrual period pain is severe. Therefore, this treatment protocol is based on the following Chinese medical statements: "Use dispelling for extreme (situations)", "When the bowels are free-flowing, they can function", and "Free flow leads to absence of pain." Based on the treatment methods of quickening the blood and freeing the flow of the bowels, (Zhang) Zhong-jing's *Tao He Cheng Qi Tang* was selected as the basic formula with additions and subtractions.

(From *Zhong Yi Zi Xue Cong Shu* [*The Chinese Medical Self-study Series*], *Vol. II*, *"Gynecology"*, Hebei Science & Technology Press, Shijiazhuang, 1987)

THE TREATMENT OF PAINFUL MENSTRUATION

PATTERNS	TREATMENT METHOD		MEDICINAL SUBSTANCES
Qi Stagnation, Blood Stasis	Free	*Dang Gui,*	*Tao Ren, Hong Hua, Yuan Hu, Wu Yao, E Zhu*
Cold Damp Congelation & Stagnation	and	*Bai Shao,*	*Wu Zhu Yu, Rou Gui, Fu Ling, Ban Xia*
Damp Heat Brewing & Binding	Regulate the	*Chuan Xiong,*	*Huang Lian, Huang Bai, Chun Gen Pi, Dan Pi, Lian Qiao, Yin Hua*
Qi & Blood Vacuity Weakness	Qi and		*Ren Shen, Huang Qi, Dan Shen, Ai Ye*
Liver-Kidney Insufficiency	Blood	*Xiang Fu*	*Shan Yu Rou, Ba Ji Tian, Shan Yao, Du Zhong, Chuan Duan*

9

Menstrual Movement Diseases

Premenstrual syndrome or PMS is a recent addition to TCM menstrual disease categories. In Chinese, premenstrual syndrome is frequently translated as *jing xing qian qi zhu zheng*. *Jing xing* means menstrual movement. *Qian qi* means before the period. And *zhu zheng* means various pathoconditions or syndromes. This is a modern Chinese attempt to literally translate PMS into Chinese. This new category is now beginning to show up in Chinese gynecology texts and articles. However, if one looks, for instance, at the table of contents of the gynecology section of the *Yi Zong Jin Jian (The Golden Mirror of Ancestral Medicine)* — the famous Qing dynasty compendium of medicine published in 1749— under the subheading of regulating menstruation, one finds a group of conditions each prefixed by the words *jing xing*. As stated above, these words mean menstrual movement. The implication in Chinese is that these conditions all in some way have to do with pathological mechanisms occurring when the menses are moving to and out of the uterus. Thus, in the older Chinese medical literature, these *jing xing* diseases refer to what we now group as the various conditions constituting premenstrual syndrome.

The list of such menstrual movement conditions is in no way categorically finite. Some Chinese gynecology texts only give one or two menstrual movement diseases, while others give dozens. In fact, we can say that any complaint or pathological condition occurring during the premenstruum or the menses themselves can be prefixed with the words menstrual movement. Therefore, there are some commonly seen menstrual movement diseases and there can be some pretty unusual ones. Common ones would include menstrual movement breast distention and pain, menstrual movement diarrhea, and menstrual movement low back pain. More unusual one might include menstrual movement pneumothorax and menstrual movement lip swelling and pain. The only criteria for a complaint to be labelled as a menstrual movement disease is that it must occur on a semi-regular basis before or during the menses.

This means that PMS in modern Chinese gynecology is actually no one thing. The actual complaints that any given patient may present are highly variable and idiosyncratic.

Nonetheless, it is my clinical experience that Chinese gynecology can diagnose and successfully treat just about every possible premenstrual complaint any woman can present. The reader should remember that premenstrual or menstrual movement headache is nothing other than a headache occurring before or during menstruation. Therefore, it is not some totally other disease. Hence, its diagnosis and treatment are essentially the same as for headaches in general. The exception is that certain patterns of headache are more likely to occur before or during menstruation due to the mechanisms of the menstrual cycle and menstruation itself. So to begin with, in order to understand how and to be able to treat menstrual movement diseases, one must first have a good grasp of the TCM pattern discrimination and treatment of internal or *nei ke* diseases in general since these are what make up the various conditions that constitute premenstrual syndrome.

That being said, let me first discuss the common textbook patterns associated with PMS in the contemporary Chinese gynecology textbook literature. Both Sun Jiu-ling, author of *Fu Ke Zheng Zhi (Gynecological Patterns & Treatments)*, and Zhu Cheng-han, author of *Zhong Yi Fu Ke (Chinese Medical Gynecology)*, list PMS as a disease category similar to modern Western medicine. Sun discusses three patterns in the TCM treatment of PMS. To these same three, Zhu adds a fourth. Understanding these four basic patterns will enable the practitioner to understand the mechanisms behind most of the various signs and symptoms associated with PMS. However, after discussing these four patterns, I will add several more in an attempt to achieve categorical completeness.

Disease causes, disease mechanisms

The root cause of PMS is almost always a disharmony between the liver and spleen. Due to emotional stress and frustration, the liver becomes depressed and the qi becomes stagnant. Due to worry, lack of exercise, overtaxation, or improper diet, the spleen may become vacuous and weak. Because the liver controls the spleen, if the liver becomes replete this itself can cause or worsen spleen vacuity. Conversely, if the spleen is vacuous, this may allow the liver to become or become even more replete. As we have seen above, liver depression tends to worsen or arise during the premenstruum because the blood that was emolliating, nourishing, and harmonizing the liver is now being sent down to nourish the uterus. If there is not sufficient blood for both these purposes, the liver may not receive sufficient nourishment so that it can perform its duty of controlling coursing and discharge. If the liver does not course and discharge, the qi does not move freely and becomes stagnant.

It is the spleen which is the latter heaven root of qi and blood engenderment and transformation. If the spleen is vacuous, then it may not engender and transform qi and blood sufficiently. If the spleen does not engender blood sufficiently, then, as we have just seen above, liver blood may become insufficient to allow the liver to perform its function of coursing and discharging the qi. On the other hand, if the spleen does not engender the qi sufficiently, the qi will lack its motivating force to move. Thus it is easy to see how closely these two viscera are related in terms of the free flow of the qi. The liver allows the qi to flow freely, but it is the spleen which is the latter heaven source of the qi's power to move. Hence liver depression and spleen vacuity typically occur together in clinical practice. In addition, we should remember that women's spleens must work harder at producing blood then men's spleens must. This also predisposes them towards spleen vacuity. In my experience, liver depression-spleen vacuity is usually the root mechanism behind PMS. I have never seen a single case of PMS in 16 years of clinical practice without liver depression.

If the liver becomes depressed and qi stagnant, this may transform into evil heat. Over time, this evil heat will consume kidney yin. Since yin controls yang, if kidney yin becomes vacuous, liver yang may become effulgent. Since fire burns upward, this evil heat may also accumulate in the heart. Also since heat rises, evil heat may accumulate in the lungs, disturbing the lungs' ability to control the qi by diffusing and downbearing it.

As mentioned above, since the spleen is the latter heaven root of the engenderment and transformation of blood, if the spleen becomes weak, the blood may also become vacuous. Since blood and essence share a common source, enduring blood vacuity may lead to insufficiency of kidney essence. This may aggravate any tendency to kidney yin vacuity already caused by damage due to enduring heat.

Because the spleen is also in charge of moving and transforming liquids, if the spleen becomes weak, water dampness may accumulate. This yin evil may further block the free flow of qi, aggravating liver depression. Water dampness may also transform into phlegm turbidity. This phlegm even further impedes the free flow of qi and may lodge between the skin and flesh, in the channels and network vessels, and in the clear orifices of the heart and head.

Further, if the spleen remains chronically weak, since kidney yang is the source of the righteous warmth of the middle burner, true yang or kidney yang may also become weak. Since kidney essence is the material basis of both kidney yin and yang, this process can be accelerated if there is long-term blood vacuity. On the other hand, enduring kidney yang vacuity and weakness will also impair blood production as well.

As we will see below, there are a few other mechanisms which may occur as ramifications of these main disease mechanisms. However, these mechanisms are the root of most premenstrual signs and symptoms. If one understands these mechanisms and has a sound grasp of the basic theories of TCM discussed in the first part of this book, one can figure out a rational explanation for any sign or symptom any woman may experience before her menses.

Treatment based on pattern discrimination

Liver depression qi stagnation

Main symptoms: Premenstrual breast and nipple distention and pain, chest and rib-side secret anguish, lower abdominal distention and pain, discomfort of the stomach and epigastrium, diminished appetite, possible delayed menstruation, amount either scanty or profuse, clots within the menstrual blood, menses unable to come easily, a normal or slightly dark tongue with thin, white fur, and a bowstring, fine pulse

Treatment principles: Course the liver and rectify the qi, rectify the blood and regulate the menses

Guiding formulas:

1. Zhu Cheng-han's *Xiao Yao San Jia Jian* (Rambling Powder with Additions & Subtractions)

Ingredients: Stir-fried Radix Bupleuri (*Chai Hu*), whole Radix Angelicae Sinensis (*Dang Gui*), Radix Albus Paeoniae Lactiflorae (*Bai Shao*), Rhizoma Atractylodis Macrocephalae (*Bai Zhu*), Sclerotium Poriae Cocos (*Fu Ling*), mix-fried Radix Glycyrrhizae (*Gan Cao*), processed Rhizoma Cyperi Rotundi (*Xiang Fu*), Pericarpium Citri Reticulatae Viride (*Qing Pi*), Sichuan Tuber Curcumae (*Yu Jin*), Pericarpium Trichosanthis Kirlowii (*Gua Lou Pi*)

Like most Chinese authors, Zhu Cheng-han uses *Xiao Yao San* as his main guiding formula for this pattern of PMS. This formula not only courses the liver and rectifies the qi but also fortifies the spleen and disinhibits dampness, nourishes the blood and soothes the liver.

Additions & subtractions: If the patient is easily angered and the amount of her menstruate is excessive due to liver depression transforming into fire, add Fructus Gardeniae Jasminoidis (*Zhi Zi*) and Cortex Radicis Moutan (*Dan Pi*) to clear the liver and discharge fire. If the breasts are swollen and lumpy, add Herba Taraxaci Mongolici Cum Radice (*Pu Gong Ying*) and Fructus Liquidambaris Taiwaniae (*Lu Lu Tong*) to scatter nodulation and free the flow of the network vessels. It is interesting to note that Zhu recommends Taraxacum without any signs of heat. This corresponds to the Western herbal use of Dandelion for breast problems in general. If the amount of the menstruate is scanty but with

390

comparatively a lot of blood clots, delete Atractylodes Macrocephala and Licorice and add Flos Carthami Tinctorii (*Hong Hua*), processed Resina Olibani (*Ru Xiang*), and *Shi Xiao San* (Loose a Smile Powder), *i.e.*, Feces Trogopterori Seu Pteromi (*Wu Ling Zhi*) and uncooked Pollen Typhae (*Pu Huang*), to quicken the blood and transform stasis.

2. Sun Jiu-ling's *Xiao Yao San Jia Jian* (Rambling Powder with Additions & Subtractions)

Ingredients: Radix Bupleuri (*Chai Hu*), Radix Angelicae Sinensis (*Dang Gui*), Rhizoma Atractylodis Macrocephalae (*Bai Zhu*), Radix Albus Paeoniae Lactiflorae (*Bai Shao*), Sclerotium Poriae Cocos (*Fu Ling*), roasted Rhizoma Zingiberis (*Wei Jiang*), Herba Menthae Haplocalycis (*Bo He*), Fructus Meliae Toosendan (*Chuan Lian Zi*), Tuber Curcumae (*Yu Jin*), Pericarpium Citri Reticulatae Viride (*Qing Pi*), Fructus Trichosanthis Kirlowii (*Gua Lou*)

Additions & subtractions: If there is premenstrual fever, headache, a bitter taste in the mouth, dry mouth, and vexation and agitation, delete the roasted Ginger and add Cortex Radicis Moutan (*Dan Pi*), Fructus Gardeniae Jasminoidis (*Zhi Zi*), and Radix Ligustici Wallichii (*Chuan Xiong*). If there is edema, add Rhizoma Alismatis (*Ze Xie*) and Semen Plantaginis (*Che Qian Zi*).

3. *Qi Zhi Xiang Fu Wan* (Qi Stagnation Cyperus Pills)

Ingredients: Rhizoma Cyperi Rotundi (*Xiang Fu*), Radix Angelicae Sinensis (*Dang Gui*), Rhizoma Curcumae Zedoariae (*E Zhu*), Radix Linderae Strychnifoliae (*Wu Yao*), Cortex Radicis Moutan (*Dan Pi*), Folium Artemisiae Argyii (*Ai Ye*), Radix Ligustici Wallichii (*Chuan Xiong*), Rhizoma Corydalis Yanhusuo (*Yan Hu Suo*), Fructus Crataegi (*Shan Zha*), Radix Bupleuri (*Chai Hu*), Flos Carthami Tinctorii (*Hong Hua*), Fructus Pruni Mume (*Wu Mei*)

Zhu Cheng-han suggests this formula for the treatment of a menstrual discharge which is dry at the end. If the menses are also scanty in amount, he suggests taking *Shi Xiao San* (Loose a Smile Powder) or Feces Trogopterori Seu Pteromi (*Wu Ling Zhi*) and Pollen Typhae (*Sheng Pu Huang*) along with this.

4. *Xiao Chai Hu Tang Jia Wei* (Minor Bupleurum Decoction with Added Flavors)

Ingredients: Radix Bupleuri (*Chai Hu*), Radix Codonopsitis Pilosulae (*Dang Shen*), Radix Scutellariae Baicalensis (*Huang Qin*), Rhizoma Pinelliae Ternatae (*Ban Xia*), Rhizoma Cyperi Rotundi (*Xiang Fu*), Radix Albus Paeoniae Lactiflorae (*Bai Shao*), uncooked Rhizoma

Zingiberis (*Sheng Jiang*), Fructus Zizyphi Jujubae (*Da Zao*), mix-fried Radix Glycyrrhizae (*Gan Cao*)

This formula is for the treatment of premenstrual syndrome due to liver qi, a vacuous but not excessively damp spleen, and heat in the stomach and lungs. In this case, there is no significant blood vacuity.

5. *Chai Hu Gui Zhi Tang Jia Wei* (Bupleurum & Cinnamon Twig Decoction with Added Flavors)

Ingredients: Radix Bupleuri (*Chai Hu*), Radix Scutellariae Baicalensis (*Huang Qin*), Radix Codonopsitis Pilosulae (*Dang Shen*), mix-fried Radix Glycyrrhizae (*Gan Cao*), Rhizoma Pinelliae Ternatae (*Ban Xia*), Radix Albus Paeoniae Lactiflorae (*Bai Shao*), Ramulus Cinnamomi Cassiae (*Gui Zhi*), Fructus Zizyphi Jujubae (*Da Zao*), uncooked Rhizoma Zingiberis (*Sheng Jiang*)

This formula is the same as the above except for the addition of Cinnamon Twigs. This formula is for the same basic pattern but in a weaker, more vacuous patient with more obvious counterflow chilling of the extremities.

Additions: For upper back and neck tension and pain, add Radix Puerariae (*Ge Gen*) and Radix Ledebouriellae Divaricatae (*Fang Feng*). For headache behind the eyes, add Flos Chrysanthemi Morifolii (*Ju Hua*). For premenstrual diarrhea or loose stools, add Rhizoma Atractylodis Macrocephalae (*Bai Zhu*) and Sclerotium Poriae Cocos (*Fu Ling*). If there is constipation, add a small amount of Radix Et Rhizoma Rhei (*Da Huang*).

Spleen-kidney yang vacuity

Main symptoms: Edema either before or after the menses, dizziness, lumbar soreness and weary extremities, reduced appetite, loose stools or diarrhea before the menses, stomach and epigastric distention and fullness, lack of warmth in the hands and feet, a pale facial complexion, menses scanty in amount, a fat tongue with thin, white or slimy, white fur, and a deep, fine, weak pulse

In actual clinical fact, this pattern never presents in this simple, discreet manner in PMS. But spleen qi and kidney yang vacuity do typically complicate most women's PMS in their late 30s and 40s. According to my clinical experience, there will also be liver depression as well in all cases. Therefore, in clinical practice, one would choose one of the guiding formulas below only if spleen vacuity was the predominant disease mechanism. If liver depression is the dominant pattern, then one would choose one of the above formulas and modify that accordingly.

Treatment principles: Warm the kidneys, fortify the spleen, and disinhibit water

Guiding formulas:

1. Sun Jiu-ling's *Jian Gu Tang Jia Wei* (Fortifying & Securing Decoction with Added Flavors)

Ingredients: Radix Codonopsitis Pilosulae (*Dang Shen*), Rhizoma Atractylodis Macrocephalae (*Bai Zhu*), Sclerotium Poriae Cocos (*Fu Ling*), Semen Coicis Lachryma-jobi (*Yi Yi Ren*), Radix Morindae Officinalis (*Ba Ji Tian*), Radix Lateralis Praeparatus Aconiti Carmichaeli (*Fu Zi*), Cortex Cinnamomi Cassiae (*Rou Gui*), Rhizoma Alismatis (*Ze Xie*), Semen Plantaginis (*Che Qian Zi*)

2. Zhu Cheng-han's *Jian Gu Tang Jia Jian* (Fortifying & Securing Decoction with Additions & Subtractions)

Ingredients: Stir-fried Radix Codonopsitis Pilosulae (*Dang Shen*), stir-fried Rhizoma Atractylodis Macrocephalae (*Bai Zhu*), mix-fried Radix Glycyrrhizae (*Gan Cao*), Sclerotium Poriae Cocos (*Fu Ling*), dry Rhizoma Zingiberis (*Gan Jiang*), Herba Epimedii (*Xian Ling Pi*), stir-fried Semen Coicis Lachryma-jobi (*Yi Yi Ren*)

3. *Shen Ling Bai Zhu San* (Ginseng, Atractylodes & Poria Powder)

Ingredients: Radix Panacis Ginseng (*Ren Shen*), Semen Nelumbinis Nuciferae (*Lian Zi Rou*), Radix Dioscoreae Oppositae (*Shan Yao*), Rhizoma Atractylodis Macrocephalae (*Bai Zhu*), Sclerotium Poriae Cocos (*Fu Ling*), Semen Dolichoris Lablab (*Bai Bian Dou*), Semen Coicis Lachryma-jobi (*Yi Yi Ren*), Fructus Amomi (*Sha Ren*), Radix Platycodi Grandiflori (*Jie Geng*), mix-fried Radix Glycyrrhizae (*Gan Cao*)

Zhu Cheng-han recommends this formula if the menses become dry at the end after treating with the above formula.

Heart-spleen dual vacuity

Main symptoms: Heart palpitations either before or after the menses, loss of sleep, lassitude of the spirit, lack of strength, face slightly puffy, amount of menses either profuse or scant but color pale, a pale tongue with thin, white fur, and a soggy, small or fine, weak pulse

Heart-spleen dual vacuity means heart blood vacuity and spleen qi vacuity. If heart blood is more vacuous, the amount of the menstruate is scanty. If spleen qi vacuity is more prominent, the amount of discharge is profuse. However, in both cases, the color of the menstruate is pale. Likewise, if the spleen is vacuous and, therefore, also damp, the pulse will be soggy. But if blood is vacuous, the pulse will be fine. As with the above pattern, this one also is rarely if ever seen in its simple, discreet form in clinical practice. Commonly, if there is heart blood vacuity, this merely complicates liver depression and spleen vacuity. If the liver depression is secondary in importance, then one would choose the guiding formula given below. If liver depression is primary, then one would modify a formula from under that pattern.

Treatment principles: Supplement and nourish heart and spleen qi and blood

Guiding formula: *Gui Pi Tang* **(Restore the Spleen Decoction)**

Ingredients: Radix Codonopsitis Pilosulae (*Dang Shen*), Radix Astragali Membranacei (*Huang Qi*), Radix Angelicae Sinensis (*Dang Gui*), Arillus Euphoriae Longanae (*Long Yan Rou*), Rhizoma Atractylodis Macrocephalae (*Bai Zhu*), Radix Auklandiae Lappae (*Mu Xiang*), Sclerotium Poriae Cocos (*Fu Ling*), Radix Polygalae Tenuifoliae (*Yuan Zhi*), Semen Zizyphi Spinosae (*Suan Zao Ren*), mix-fried Radix Glycyrrhizae (*Gan Cao*), uncooked Rhizoma Zingiberis (*Sheng Jiang*), Fructus Zizyphi Jujubae (*Da Zao*)

Additions & subtractions: To enhance this formula's blood-nourishing effect, add cooked Radix Rehmanniae (*Shu Di*). For menstrual irregularity with increased volume but pale in color, add Gelatinum Corii Asini (*E Jiao*), Ramulus Loranthi Seu Visci (*Sang Ji Sheng*), and Radix Polygoni Multiflori (*He Shou Wu*). Zhu Cheng-han suggests removing Arillus Euphoriae Longanae (*Long Yan Rou*) and Semen Zizyphi Spinosae (*Suan Zao Ren*) and adding instead Semen Biotae Orientalis (*Bai Zi Ren*) and Radix Albus Paeoniae Lactiflorae (*Bai Shao*). In addition, Zhu suggests stir-frying Codonopsis, Atractylodes Macrocephala, and Dang Gui, while mix-frying Astagalus and Polygala. He also says that, if the menstrual discharge is dry at the end, keep on treating with *Gui Pi Wan*, the patent pill form of this basic formula.

Kidney vacuity, liver effulgence

Main symptoms: Menstruation either early or late, lumbar soreness, numb extremities, one-sided headache, tinnitus, blurred vision, distention and pain feels as if it stretches from the lower abdomen to the chest and breasts, frequent, short urination, length of menstruation short and amount profuse, tongue fur shiny and peeled with a fat tongue and purple edges, and a deep, small, bowstring pulse

Although not stated in the Chinese title of this pattern, liver qi depression and stagnation are a part of this scenario. This is evidenced by the feeling of lower abdominal distention and pain reaching to the chest and breasts and also by the bowstring pulse. In this case, liver depression transforms into fire and causes the blood to move frenetically. Therefore, the amount of menses is profuse. But because liver blood is relatively vacuity, the length of the menses is short.

Treatment principles: Boost the kidneys and regulate the liver

Guiding formulas:

1. *Yi Shen Tiao Gan Tang* (Boost the Kidneys & Regulate the Liver Decoction)

Ingredients: Carapax Amydae Sinensis (*Bie Jia*), uncooked Concha Ostreae (*Mu Li*), Fructus Lycii Chinensis (*Gou Qi Zi*), stir-fried sweet Flos Chrysanthemi Morifolii (*Gan Ju*), Radix Dioscoreae Oppositae (*Huai Shan Yao*), Radix Albus Paeoniae Lactiflorae (*Bai Shao*), whole Radix Angelicae Sinensis (*Quan Dang Gui*), large uncooked Radix Rehmanniae (*Sheng Di*), aged Fructus Corni Officinalis (*Zhu Rou*), Cortex Radicis Moutan (*Dan Pi*), stir-fried Rhizoma Alismatis (*Ze Xie*)

Additions & subtractions: If the tongue is shiny and peeled with a red tongue and dry mouth and throat, delete Dioscorea and add Tuber Ophiopogonis Japonici (*Mai Dong*) and Radix Glehniae Littoralis (*Sha Shen*).

2. *Qi Ju Di Huang Wan* (Lycium & Chrysanthemum Rehmannia Pills)

Ingredients: Flos Chrysanthemi Morifolii (*Ju Hua*), Fructus Lycii Chinensis (*Gou Qi Zi*), cooked Radix Rehmanniae (*Shu Di*), Fructus Corni Officinalis (*Shan Zhu Yu*), Radix Dioscoreae Oppositae (*Shan Yao*), Cortex Radicis Moutan (*Dan Pi*), Sclerotium Poriae Cocos (*Fu Ling*), Rhizoma Alismatis (*Ze Xie*)

Zhu Cheng-han says that if the menses are dry at the end, continue treating with the above patent pills after having treated with the first formula.

Discussion

Although textbook discriminations such as this make it seem like all the practitioner has to do is match up their patient's symptoms with one of the afore-mentioned patterns and then prescribe the recommended guiding formula, in actual clinical practice, one usually encounters combinations of the above discreet patterns and their related disease mechanisms or progressions. In trying to identify all the mechanisms I have encountered in women with PMS, I have come up with a list of 20.

These are:

Liver depression qi stagnation
Depressive heat
Spleen qi vacuity
Spleen dampness
Liver blood vacuity
Kidney yin vacuity
Spleen-kidney yang vacuity
Replete heat in the heart, lungs, and/or stomach
Vacuity heat in the heart, lungs, and/or stomach
Heart qi and/or blood vacuity
Liver yang hyperactivity
Liver fire flaring above
Stirring of liver wind
Food stagnation
Phlegm confounding the orifices
Phlegm fire
Damp heat accumulating below
Blood stasis
External invasion
Retained evils or deep-lying warm evils

In all cases of PMS, liver qi plays a central role. This is because, the premenstruum and the menstrual movement are about yang reaching its apogee and transforming into yin just as ovulation is about yin reaching its apogee and transforming into yang. Such transformation can only proceed freely and correctly if the qi mechanism is free-flowing and uninhibited. This qi mechanisms free and uninhibited flow is dependent on the liver's coursing and discharge. Therefore, liver depression and qi stagnation are at the heart of every woman's PMS. No matter what other disease mechanisms are at work, the presence and degree of premenstrual complaints are directly proportional to the presence of liver qi.

However, because of the interrelationships between the liver and all the other viscera and bowels of Chinese medicine and between the qi, blood, fluids, and essence, liver depression qi stagnation may be complicated or evolve into a number of other patterns. Therefore, in clinical practice, one must identify the main disease mechanism currently at work and choose a guiding formula based on rebalancing that imbalance. Then this guiding formula should be modified to address all of the patient's associated disease mechanisms and signs and symptoms. However, if a mechanism or symptom will disappear by merely rebalancing some more fundamental mechanism, such secondary or dependent mechanisms and symptoms need not be addressed specifically.

If one understands the interrelationships between the above 20 mechanisms, they should be able to diagnose and understand *any* premenstrual symptom of *any* woman. These 20 mechanisms or patterns are not just a random collection of patterns. There is an underlying logic to this list. We have already discussed the relationships between the first seven mechanisms above. If liver depression transforms into depressive heat, that heat may counterflow upward and harass the heart, lungs, and/or stomach. On the other hand, if liver blood-kidney vacuity gives rise to vacuity heat, this vacuity heat may also counterflow upward to harass the heart, lungs, and/or stomach and damage their yin fluids. Because both heart qi and blood have their source in the spleen's engenderment and transformation of water and grains, if the spleen is vacuous and weak, this may easily give rise to either heart blood or heart qi vacuity. If depressive heat damages yin, yang will become effulgent and give rise to liver yang hyperactivity. If such liver yang hyperactivity becomes even worse, it may become liver fire flaring above, while liver fire and/or liver blood vacuity may engender internal stirring of liver wind.

Because of the interrelationships between Zhu Dan-xi's six depressions, if qi becomes stagnant and the spleen becomes weak, food stagnation is easily engendered. Such food stagnation may also transform depressive heat. If dampness due to spleen not moving and transporting gathers and endures, it may congeal into phlegm. However, phlegm may also be due to intense heat steaming and fuming the fluids, congealing them into phlegm. In either case, phlegm, being a yin depression, obstructs the free and uninhibited flow of qi and blood. It may gather and obstruct the area between the skin and muscles or flesh, within the viscera and bowels, and within the channels and network vessels. It may also confound and block the clear orifices, *i.e.*, the sensory organs of the head, or the orifices of the heart. If there clear orifices are blocked, there will be diminished or loss of sensual acuity of the associated orifice. If the orifices of the heart are confounded, there will be disturbed or diminshed mental-emotional function.

However, dampness, being heavy and turbid, tends to precolate and pour downward. Because it too is a yin depression, it obstructs the free flow of qi, blood, and fluids. If damp depression gives rise to depressive heat, then dampness may become damp heat. It is also possible for liver depression-transformative heat to stew the juices and give rise to damp heat. If qi stagnation fails to move the blood, the blood will stop and become static. Thus, if liver depression is bad enough or lasts long enough, it may give rise to blood stasis.

Because the spleen and stomach are the latter heaven source of the defensive qi, if the spleen becomes vacuous and weak premenstrually, there may be defensive qi vacuity. Such a defensive qi vacuity premenstrually is often aggravated by blood vacuity. Because the blood is downborne to the uterus before menstruation, this leaves the upper body relatively blood vacuous and insufficient in women whose blood engenderment tends to be poor. The blood and constructive are closely related. Therefore, such a blood and constructive vacuity in the upper body leads to a defensive and constructive disharmony which easily allows for external evils to take advantage of this vacuity and enter.

It is also possible that either retained evils or deep-lying warm evils may become active during the premenstruum. Retained evils are evils that have invaded the body at some previous time. Due to lack of or erroneous treatment, these evils are not all eliminated from the body at the time of their invasion and subsequent disease. If some of these evils linger, they may be relatively latent. However, given the proper internal environment, they may become active again. Hidden or deep-lying warm evils are warm or damp heat evils which enter the body but do not cause disease at that time. Rather, they lie latent until the internal environment is conducive to their exuberance and activity. Because dampness tends to accumulate premenstrually and because there is often depressive heat premenstrually at the same time as there is a righteous qi vacuity affecting the spleen and/or kidneys, either retained or deep-lying warm evils often find the premenstruum at a time when the internal environment is conducive to their exuberance and activity.

All signs and symptoms of PMS can be diagnosed and treated according to TCM based on various combinations of the above disease mechanisms and patterns. In order to make this work, one must have a firm grasp of the defining or main symptoms of each pattern. These can be found in Daniel Finney's and my, *Compendium of TCM Patterns & Treatments* published by Blue Poppy Press. One first determines what mechanisms are at work in a given woman's PMS, then prioritizes the order of these mechanisms. Next one states ones treatment principles for all the mechanisms at work. From there, one chooses a guiding formula from the category of formulas which corresponds to the first element in the pattern discrimination as stated in the first of the treatment principles. And finally, one modifies that guiding formula in the light of the complicating patterns and their subsequent treatment principles.

That being said, below I give the pattern discrimination treatments of a number of menstrual movement diseases. These are not necessarily categorically complete. Therefore, one must still be careful to do an individualized pattern discrimination and base treatment accordingly. However, these treatments should help provide a starting place and general pattern for how one goes about diagnosing and treating any woman's PMS.

Because the spleen and kidneys both tend to become weak and the blood tends to become scanty in the majority of women in their late 30s and 40s, it is no wonder that PMS tends to worsen in women of those ages. There are three viscera primarily involved in the free flow of the qi. The liver courses and discharges. This means it opens and allows the qi to flow. The spleen is the main source for providing the power behind the qi's movement. And the kidneys provide the warmth that promotes the qi to flow freely. Thus one should typically look for liver depression, blood and yin vacuity, and spleen qi-kidney vacuity at work in women with PMS who are this age. At this point in time, it is these women who make up the overwhelming bulk of my patient population.

Menstrual Movement Breast Distention & Pain

As women move into their 30s, many experience increased breast distention and pain before menstruation. This may begin only a few days before the expected onset of the menses or may occur even before mid-cycle. Usually, this distention and pain disappear or becomes markedly reduced a day or so before or right after the start of menstruation. In some cases, breast distention and pain may persist even through the menstruation. Besides distention and pain, some women also experience lumps in their breasts. These lumps may come and go with their menses. They may also persist throughout the cycle and merely enlarge and grow smaller with the coming and going of menstruation.

Premenstrual breast distention, pain, and lumpiness are a common part of many women's PMS complaints. Some women with this complaint are diagnosed by modern Western medicine as suffering from fibrocystic breast disease (FBD). Many Western MDs now recognize that so-called FBD is not a disease *per se* but part of aging in women. This certainly agrees with the TCM mechanisms associated with these changes in the breast tissue. Happily, Chinese medicine actively tries to slow and reverse the aging process, including the aging of the breast tissue.

In the Chinese medical literature, premenstrual breast distention and pain are often discussed in relationship to infertility. Chinese doctors have recognized that many women with fertility problems also complain of premenstrual breast problems. Since such premenstrual breast complaints tend to occur in the late 20s and early 30s and then worsen through the late 30s and into the 40s, this connection with decreasing fertility also makes sense from a Western medical perspective. The incidence of premenstrual breast complaints does seem to be inversely proportional to the natural decline in fertility with age.

Besides infertility, TCM gynecology texts also say that if premenstrual breast distention and pain are left untreated and persist, they can evolve into breast neoplasms. Therefore, the treatment of premenstrual breast distention and pain has far-reaching consequences on a woman's systemic health and happiness.

Disease causes, disease mechanisms

To understand the disease causes and mechanisms of premenstrual breast problems according to TCM, one must first consider the channels and network vessels which traverse the breast. In TCM it is said that the foot *yang ming* stomach channel canalizes the breasts in general but that an internal branch of the foot *jue yin* liver channel homes to the nipples. Although most TCM gynecology texts do not mention it, the breast tissue is also traversed by the foot *shao yang* gallbladder channel and the hand *jue yin* pericardium channel on the breasts' lateral sides. Perhaps this is not mentioned in Chinese gynecology texts since, in terms of disease mechanisms, pathological changes in these two channels are closely related to changes in the liver in any case.

As we have seen in previous discussions of menstrual disease mechanisms, the liver tends to become depressed prior to the onset of the menses. If there is a tendency to liver qi, this typically becomes exacerbated leading up to the onset of menstruation. Since qi is yang, when it accumulates, it tends to do either or both of two things. First, it may counterflow upward and, secondly, it may transform into heat. It is said in Chinese medicine that the liver is responsible for the path of qi circulation in the intercostal spaces. Therefore, it is easy to understand how stagnation and accumulation of liver qi might accumulate in the chest in general and the ribs and breasts in particular. In Chinese, this is called liver qi counterflowing horizontally. TCM theory also recognizes the close reciprocal relationship between the liver and stomach. When one becomes pathologically replete, the other tends to as well. If the stomach becomes hot and replete, its qi often counterflows upward along the course of its channel and thus may add to distention and pain in the breast.

As mentioned previously, premenstrual liver qi is mostly due to stress and frustration causing a tightening of the sinews and, therefore, a general impediment to the free flow of qi throughout the body. If that stress and frustration are more serious, it may transform into depressive heat. This can be aggravated by overeating hot, spicy, peppery, oily, or greasy foods and by drinking alcohol.

If the spleen becomes vacuous and damp, dampness may transform into phlegm and be drafted upwards by counterflow qi to lodge in the breasts. This may create phlegm nodules or lumps in the breast. In addition, enduring liver qi may result in the formation of blood stasis. Therefore, breast lumps are often a combination of phlegm, stagnant blood, stagnant heat, and liver qi. If the lumps come and go with the menses, they are mostly stagnant qi. If they remain throughout the cycle and are fixed in a single location, these lumps are mostly a combination of phlegm nodulation and blood stasis. If there is a burning pain in the breast or itching and hypersensitivity in the nipple, this denotes more evil heat.

As a woman moves into her late 30s and 40s, it is also possible for breast distention, pain, and especially lumps to be due to a more systemic separation of yin and yang. As yin becomes consumed and relatively exhausted, yang may come apart and float upward. Because yang loses its root in the lower burner, the root of yang also becomes relatively weak and vacuous . In TCM, this is referred to as breast distention, pain, and lumps due to loss of regulation or harmony between the *chong* and *ren*. Typically, this breast pain, distention, and lumps are accompanied by night sweats, hot flashes, and other premenopausal signs and symptoms. In this case, vacuity heat drafts upwards dampness and congeals it into phlegm nodules which lodge in the chest. This scenario is mostly an evolution from the preceding disease mechanisms and is distinguished, in part, by the age of the patient.

If a woman develops premenstrual breast distention and lumps due to either liver qi or vacuous yin-floating yang with phlegm nodulation, and this distention and lumps persist even after the menses are over, this may be due to blood loss during the menstruation leaving the woman with a qi and blood dual vacuity. In this case, the lumps usually do not arise because of qi and blood vacuity, but they may persist or become aggravated because of insufficient qi to move and transform blood and fluids.

Treatment based on pattern discrimination

Liver depression qi stagnation

Main symptoms: Breast distention or pain before menstruation, pain radiating to the chest and rib-sides, lower abdominal distention and pain, mental-emotional depression or irritability, possible painful menstruation, possible infertility, a somewhat darkish tongue with thin fur, and a bowstring pulse

Treatment principles: Course the liver, rectify the qi, and free the flow of the network vessels

Guiding formulas:

1. *Xiao Yao San Jia Wei* (Rambling Powder with Added Flavors)

Ingredients: Radix Bupleuri (*Chai Hu*), Radix Angelicae Sinensis (*Dang Gui*), Radix Albus Paeoniae Lactiflorae (*Bai Shao*), Rhizoma Atractylodis Macrocephalae (*Bai Zhu*), mix-fried Radix Glycyrrhizae (*Gan Cao*), Herba Menthae Haplocalycis (*Bo He*), uncooked Rhizoma Zingiberis (*Sheng Jiang*), Pericarpium Citri Reticulatae Viride (*Qing Pi*), Pericarpium Citri Reticulatae (*Chen Pi*), Folium Citri Reticulatae (*Ju Ye*), Fructus Liquidambaris Taiwaniae (*Lu Lu Tong*), Semen Citri Reticulatae (*Ju He*)

Additions: If the pain is severe, add Resina Olibani (*Ru Xiang*), Resina Myrrhae (*Mo Yao*), and Rhizoma Corydalis Yanhusuo (*Yan Hu Suo*). If there are sore, aching lumps within the breasts, add Squama Manitis Pentadactylae (*Chuan Shan Jia*) and Semen Vaccariae Segetalis (*Wang Bu Liu Xing*). If the breast is obviously enlarged, add Caulis Aristolochiae (*Tian Xian Teng*).

2. *Xiao Yao San Jia Gua Lou Qiang Huo* (Rambling Powder plus Trichosanthes & Notopterygium)

Ingredients: Radix Bupleuri (*Chai Hu*), Radix Angelicae Sinensis (*Dang Gui*), Radix Albus Paeoniae Lactiflorae (*Bai Shao*), Rhizoma Atractylodis Macrocephalae (*Bai Zhu*), Sclerotium Poriae Cocos (*Fu Ling*), Herba Menthae Haplocalycis (*Bo He*), uncooked Rhizoma Zingiberis (*Sheng Jiang*), mix-fried Radix Glycyrrhizae (*Gan Cao*), Fructus Trichosanthis Kirlowii (*Gua Lou*), Radix Et Rhizoma Notopterygii (*Qiang Huo*)

This formula is for premenstrual breast distention and pain with qi stagnating in the liver and stomach channels.

3. *Xiao Yao San Jia Jian* (Rambling Powder with Additions & Subtractions)

Ingredients: Radix Bupleuri (*Chai Hu*), Rhizoma Atractylodis Macrocephalae (*Bai Zhu*), Sclerotium Poriae Cocos (*Fu Ling*), Radix Angelicae Sinensis (*Dang Gui*), Radix Albus Paeoniae Lactiflorae (*Bai Shao*), Herba Menthae Haplocalycis (*Bo He*), uncooked Rhizoma Zingiberis (*Sheng Jiang*), Semen Vaccariae Segetalis (*Wang Bu Liu Xin*), Caulis Milletiae Seu Spatholobi (*Ji Xue Teng*), Radix Salviae Miltiorrhizae (*Dan Shen*), Rhizoma Cyperi Rotundi (*Xiang Fu*)

4. Unnamed formula composed by Zhu Xiao-nan appearing in *Shang Hai Lao Zhong Yi Jing Yan Xuan Bian (A Collection of Shanghai Old Doctors' Clinical Experiences)*

Ingredients: Rhizoma Cyperi Rotundi (*Xiang Fu*), Cortex Albizziae Julibrissin (*He Huan Pi*), Fructus Perillae Frutescentis (*Su Zi*), Fructus Liquidambaris Taiwaniae (*Lu Lu Tong*), Tuber Curcumae (*Yu Jin*), Rhizoma Atractylodis Macrocephalae (*Bai Zhu*), Radix Linderae Strychnifoliae (*Wu Yao*), Pericarpium Citri Reticulatae (*Chen Pi*), Fructus Immaturus Citri Aurantii (*Zhi Shi*)

Additions: For more prominent breast distention, add Semen Citri Reticulatae (*Ju He*) and Folium Citri Reticulatae (*Ju Ye*). For breast pain and distention, add Fructus Meliae Toosendan (*Chuan Lian Zi*) and Herba Taraxaci Mongolici Cum Radice (*Pu Gong Ying*). For breast distention with lumps, add Semen Vaccariae Segetalis (*Wang Bu Liu Xing*) and Squama Manitis Pentadactylis (*Chuan Shan Jia*). For kidney vacuity and lumbar pain, add

Cortex Eucommiae Ulmoidis (*Du Zhong*) and Radix Dipsaci (*Chuan Duan*). For blood vacuity, add Radix Angelicae Sinensis (*Dang Gui*) and cooked Radix Rehmanniae (*Shu Di*). For vacuity cold of the *chong* and *ren*, add Gelatinum Cornu Cervi (*Lu Jiao Jiao*) and Cortex Cinnamomi Cassiae (*Rou Gui*).

5. *Chai Hu Shu Gan Tang Jia Jian* (Bupleurum Soothe the Liver Decoction with Additions & Subtractions)

Ingredients: Radix Bupleuri (*Chai Hu*), Radix Angelicae Sinensis (*Dang Gui*), Radix Albus Paeoniae Lactiflorae (*Bai Shao*), Tuber Curcumae (*Yu Jin*), Fructus Immaturus Citri Aurantii (*Zhi Shi*), Rhizoma Cyperi Rotundi (*Xiang Fu*), Pericarpium Citri Reticulatae Viride (*Qing Pi*), Folium Citri Reticulatae (*Ju Ye*), Fructus Liquidambaris Taiwaniae (*Lu Lu Tong*)

This formula appears in an article by Xu Sheng-yang in *Qian Jia Miao Fang (A Thousand Practitioners' Wondrous Formulas)*.

Additions: If there is vexatious heat, add Cortex Radicis Moutan (*Dan Pi*) and Cortex Radicis Lycii Chinensis (*Di Gu Pi*). If there are lumps in the breast, add Semen Vaccariae Segetalis (*Wang Bu Liu Xing*), Semen Citri Reticulatae (*Ju He*), and Melo Pediculus (*Gua Di*). For accompanying headache, select from and add Fructus Viticis (*Man Jing Zi*), Flos Chrysanthemi Morifolii (*Ju Hua*), Herba Menthae Haplocalycis (*Bo He*), Radix Angelicae (*Bai Zhi*), or Radix Puerariae (*Ge Gen*). For edema, select from and add, Rhizoma Atractylodis (*Cang Zhu*), Sclerotium Poriae Cocos (*Fu Ling*), or Semen Plantaginis (*Che Qian Zi*). For nipple itchiness and hypersensitivity, select from and add Ramulus Uncariae Cum Uncis (*Gou Teng*), Herba Schizonepetae Tenuifoliae (*Jing Jie*), or Radix Ledebouriellae Divaricatae (*Fang Feng*). For nausea and vomiting, select from and add Caulis Bambusae In Taeniis (*Zhu Ru*), Rhizoma Pinelliae Ternatae (*Ban Xia*), or Fructus Citri Aurantii (*Zhi Ke*). For plum seed qi, add Cortex Magnoliae Officinalis (*Hou Bu*), Rhizoma Pinelliae Ternatae (*Ban Xia*), and Folium Perillae Frutescentis (*Su Ye*).

Liver depression, phlegm stasis

Main symptoms: This condition is usually found in younger women, *i.e.*, in their 20s and 30s, who are easily angered or agitated, who tend to be depressed and repressed, or whose psyche is not free and uninhibited. There is distention and pain in the breast or piercing pain which gets worse as the menses approach and which disappears after menstruation. There is swelling and lumps in the breast or nodules of various sizes which may grow or shrink depending both on the menstrual cycle and the patient's mood and stress. The tongue is pale red with thin, white fur and the pulse is bowstring and slippery.

Treatment principles: Course the liver and resolve depression, transform phlegm and free the flow of the network vessels

Guiding formula: *Xiao Yao Gua Lou San* **(Rambling Trichosanthes Powder)**

Ingredients: Radix Bupleuri (*Chai Hu*), Radix Angelicae Sinensis (*Dang Gui*), Radix Albus Paeoniae Lactiflorae (*Bai Shao*), Rhizoma Atractylodis Macrocephalae (*Bai Zhu*), Sclerotium Poriae Cocos (*Fu Ling*), Bulbus Fritillariae (*Bei Mu*), Rhizoma Pinelliae Ternatae (*Ban Xia*), Rhizoma Arisaematis (*Nan Xing*), Rhizoma Shancigu (*Shan Ci Gu*), Fructus Trichosanthis Kirlowii (*Gua Lou*), Concha Ostreae (*Mu Li*)

Additions: For more pronounced distention and pain before the menses or painful menstruation, add uncooked Pollen Typhae (*Pu Huang*), Feces Trogopterori Seu Pteromi (*Wu Ling Zhi*), Flos Carthami Tinctorii (*Hong Hua*), and Herba Artemisiae Anomalae (*Liu Ji Nu*). During the menses, add Herba Leonuri Heterophylli (*Yi Mu Cao*). For those with blood vacuity after menstruation with a pale tongue, add Radix Salviae Miltiorrhizae (*Dan Shen*), cooked Radix Rehmanniae (*Shu Di*), and Caulis Milletiae Seu Spatholobi (*Ji Xue Teng*). For those who are easily angered and agitated, add Fructus Gardeniae Jasminoidis (*Zhi Zi*) and Cortex Radicis Moutan (*Dan Pi*). For those with breast distention who are psychologically depressed, add Tuber Curcumae (*Yu Jin*), Fructus Meliae Toosendan (*Chuan Lian Zi*), Pericarpium Citri Reticulatae Viride (*Qing Pi*), and Rhizoma Cyperi Rotundi (*Xiang Fu*).

Liver-stomach depressive fire

Main symptoms: Menstrual movement piercing pain in the breast, nipple itchy or hypersensitive or a yellow, watery discharge, scorching heat in the breasts, heart vexation, easily angered, dry mouth, chest and rib-side distention and pain, dizziness and tinnitus, possible infertility, possible abnormal vaginal discharge, a red tongue with yellow, dry fur, and a bowstring, rapid pulse

Treatment principles: Clear heat, discharge fire, and resolve depression

Guiding formula: *Dan Zhi Xiao Yao San Jia Jian* **(Moutan & Gardenia Rambling Powder with Additions & Subtractions)**

Ingredients: Radix Bupleuri (*Chai Hu*), Radix Angelicae Sinensis (*Dang Gui*), Radix Albus Paeoniae Lactiflorae (*Bai Shao*), Fructus Gardeniae Jasminoidis (*Zhi Zi*), Cortex Radicis Moutan (*Dan Pi*), mix-fried Radix Glycyrrhizae (*Gan Cao*), Spica Prunellae Vulgaris (*Xia Ku Cao*), Radix Scutellariae Baicalensis (*Huang Qin*), Fructus Trichosanthis Kirlowii (*Gua*

Lou), Herba Taraxaci Mongolici Cum Radice (*Pu Gong Ying*), uncooked Radix Rehmanniae (*Sheng Di*)

Additions: If there is heart vexation and loss of sleep, add Cortex Albizziae Julibrissin (*He Huan Pi*). If there is profuse vaginal discharge, add Cortex Phellodendri (*Huang Bai*), Cortex Toonae (*Chun Bai Pi*), and Rhizoma Smilacis Glabrae (*Tu Fu Ling*). For hard lumps in the breast which do not disperse, add Thallus Algae (*Kun Bu*) and Herba Sargassii (*Hai Zao*).

Qi stagnation blood stasis

Main symptoms: Enduring lumps in the breast, chest oppression, rib-side distention, chest and rib-side pain aggravated just before or after the menses, pain worse due to emotional stress, breast lumps moderately hard and painful to palpation, possible pale red or blood-streaked discharge from the nipples, a red tongue with static spots or macules and thin, white fur, and a bowstring, fine pulse

Treatment principles: Move the qi and quicken the blood, dispel stasis and scatter nodulation

Guiding formula: *Xiao He San* (Disperse Kernels Powder)

Ingredients: Radix Bupleuri (*Chai Hu*), Radix Rubrus Paeoniae Lactiflorae (*Chi Shao*), Radix Albus Paeoniae Lactiflorae (*Bai Shao*), Radix Salviae Miltiorrhizae (*Dan Shen*), Pericarpium Citri Reticulatae Viride (*Qing Pi*), Radix Linderae Strychnifoliae (*Wu Yao*), Semen Sinapis Albae (*Bai Jie Zi*), Herba Scutellariae Barbatae (*Ban Zhi Lian*), Bulbus Shancigu (*Shan Ci Gu*), Concha Ostreae (*Mu Li*), Herba Oldenlandiae Diffusae (*Bai Hua She She Cao*), Radix Glycyrrhizae (*Gan Cao*)

Chong & ren disharmony

Main symptoms: This condition is mostly seen in older women in their late 30s and 40s who have had breast problems for a long time. There may be bodily emaciation, lassitude of the spirit, possible low-grade fever in the afternoon, vacuity vexation and diminished sleep, headache and dizziness, or they may be easily excited and angered. There may be either menstrual irregularities or blocked menstruation. There are swollen lumps in the breast or swelling and nodulation. There may also be secretion coming from the nipples. The tongue is slightly red with white fur and the pulse is mostly deep and fine or floating and vacuous.

Treatment principles: Nourish yin and supplement yang, discharge fire and regulate *chong* and *ren*, soften the hard and scatter nodulation

Guiding formulas:

1. *Er Xian Tang* (Two Immortals Decoction)

Ingredients: Rhizoma Curculiginis Orchioidis (*Xian Mao*), Herba Epimedii (*Yin Yang Huo*), Radix Morindae Officinalis (*Ba Ji Tian*), Radix Angelicae Sinensis (*Dang Gui*), Rhizoma Anemarrhenae Aspheloidis (*Zhi Mu*), Cortex Phellodendri (*Huang Bai*)

Additions & subtractions: If there are no signs or symptoms of heat, delete Anemarrhena and Phellodendri. For lumbar soreness and chilly lower abdominal pain, add Cortex Eucommiae Ulmoidis (*Du Zhong*), Radix Achyranthis Bidentatae (*Niu Xi*), blast-fried Rhizoma Zingiberis (*Pao Jiang*), and Radix Linderae Strychnifoliae (*Wu Yao*). For chest oppression and dry stools, add Fructus Trichosanthis Kirlowii (*Gua Lou*), Radix Bupleuri (*Chai Hu*), Radix Albus Paeoniae Lactiflorae (*Bai Shao*), and Tuber Curcumae (*Yu Jin*). For obvious swelling and lumps in the breast, add Radix Scrophulariae Ningpoensis (*Yuan Shen*), uncooked Concha Ostreae (*Mu Li*), Bulbus Fritillariae Thunbergii (*Bei Mu*), Semen Citri Reticulatae (*Ju He*), Semen Vaccariae Segetalis (*Wang Bu Liu Xing*), and Spica Prunellae Vulgaris (*Xia Ku Cao*).

2. *Da Bu Yin Wan Jia Jian* (Greatly Supplementing Yin Pills with Additions & Subtractions)

Ingredients: Rhizoma Anemarrhenae Aspheloidis (*Zhi Mu*), Cortex Phellodendri (*Huang Bai*), cooked Radix Rehmanniae (*Shu Di*), Plastrum Testudinis (*Gui Ban*), Radix Scrophulariae Ningpoensis (*Yuan Shen*), Spica Prunellae Vulgaris (*Xia Ku Cao*), Herba Sargassii (*Hai Zao*), Thallus Algae (*Kun Bu*), Concha Ostreae (*Mu Li*), Bulbus Fritillariae (*Bei Mu*), Semen Citri Reticulatae (*Ju He*)

This formula treats yin vacuity, internal heat, and phlegm nodulation. Although the mechanism in this case is quite similar to the preceding formula and involves loss of regulation between the *chong* and *ren*, there is no complicating yang vacuity.

3. *Tiao Chong Hua Jian Tang* (Regulate the *Chong* & Transform the Hard Decoction)

Ingredients: Cortex Eucommiae Ulmoidis (*Du Zhong*), Fructus Lycii Chinensis (*Gou Qi Zi*), Radix Angelicae Sinensis (*Dang Gui*), Spica Prunellae Vulgaris (*Xia Ku Cao*), Radix Salviae Miltiorrhizae (*Dan Shen*), Herba Lycopi Lucidi (*Ze Lan*), Pericarpium Citri Reticulatae Viride (*Qing Pi*), Concha Ostreae (*Mu Li*), Radix Ligustici Wallichii (*Chuan*

Xiong), Radix Rubrus Paeoniae Lactiflorae (*Chi Shao*), Radix Albus Paeoniae Lactiflorae (*Bai Shao*), Radix Glycyrrhizae (*Gan Cao*)

This formula treats yin and blood vacuity with blood stasis and nodulation.

4. *Wen Bu Pi Shen Tang Jia Jian* (Warmly Supplement the Spleen & Kidneys Decoction with Additions & Subtractions)

Ingredients: Semen Cuscutae (*Tu Si Zi*), Fructus Psoraleae Corylifoliae (*Bu Gu Zhi*), Sclerotium Poriae Cocos (*Fu Ling*), Fructus Trichosanthis Kirlowii (*Gua Lou*), Pericarpium Citri Reticulatae (*Chen Pi*), Tuber Curcumae (*Yu Jin*), Semen Sinapis Albae (*Bai Jie Zi*), Rhizoma Atractylodis Macrocephalae (*Bai Zhu*), Rhizoma Cyperi Rotundi (*Xiang Fu*), Radix Dioscoreae Oppositae (*Huai Shan Yao*), Fructus Amomi (*Sha Ren*), Radix Glycyrrhizae (*Gan Cao*)

This formula is primarily for spleen-kidney vacuity with no yin vacuity or vacuity heat.

Qi & blood dual vacuity

Main symptoms: Persistent lumps in the breasts, lack of strength in the four limbs, a pale white facial complexion, dizziness, blurred vision, emaciation, fatigue, lassitude of the spirit, appetite diminished, shortness of breath on moving, thin, slimy tongue fur, and a fine, forceless pulse

Treatment principles: Supplement the qi and blood, transform phlegm and scatter nodulation

Guiding formulas:

1. *Xiang Bei Yang Ying Wan Jia Jian* (Cyperus & Fritillaria Nourish the Constructive Pills with Additions & Subtractions)

Ingredients: Cooked Radix Rehmanniae (*Shu Di*), Radix Angelicae Sinensis (*Dang Gui*), Radix Albus Paeoniae Lactiflorae (*Bai Shao*), Radix Ligustici Wallichii (*Chuan Xiong*), Radix Panacis Ginseng (*Ren Shen*), Rhizoma Atractylodis Macrocephalae (*Bai Zhu*), Sclerotium Poriae Cocos (*Fu Ling*), mix-fried Radix Glycyrrhizae (*Gan Cao*), Rhizoma Cyperi Rotundi (*Xiang Fu*), Bulbus Fritillariae (*Bei Mu*), Rhizoma Dioscoreae Bulbiferae (*Huang Yao Zi*), Herba Sargassii (*Hai Zao*), calcined Concha Ostreae (*Mu Li*), Pericarpium Citri Reticulatae (*Chen Pi*), uncooked Rhizoma Zingiberis (*Sheng Jiang*), Fructus Zizyphi Jujubae (*Da Zao*)

2. *Ba Zhen Tang Jia Jian* (Eight Pearls Decoction with Additions & Subtractions)

Ingredients: Radix Astragali Membranacei (*Huang Qi*), Radix Codonopsitis Piosulae (*Dang Shen*), Caulis Milletiae Seu Spatholobi (*Ji Xue Teng*), Tuber Dioscoreae Bulbiferae (*Huang Yao Zi*), Radix Angelicae Sinensis (*Dang Gui*), Sclerotium Poriae Cocos (*Fu Ling*), cooked Radix Rehmanniae (*Shu Di*), Radix Albus Paeoniae Lactiflorae (*Bai Shao*), Rhizoma Atractylodis Macrocephalae (*Bai Zhu*), Pericarpium Citri Reticulatae (*Chen Pi*), Fructus Trichosanthis Kirlowii (*Gua Lou*), Radix Glycyrrhizae (*Gan Cao*)

Discussion

Many modern women are not aware that breast distention preceding the menses is a pathological symptom. Many women think that it is a normal experience. TCM does not believe so nor does my clinical experience suggest that premenstrual distention and discomfort are normal. Chinese medicine can reduce or eliminate most premenstrual breast swelling and pain.

Lumps, on the other hand, can be a different story. Lumps which are due to phlegm nodulation plus heat will often shrink and become less tender but may remain as a benign sequela. The discrimination between malignant and benign lumps is one which TCM is not good at making. Therefore, if there is any question about a lump being either fibrocystic and benign or a potential malignancy, the patient should be referred to a Western MD. In actual fact, most of my patients with fibrocystic breasts already come to me with that Western medical diagnosis from their Western MD.

It is said in Chinese medicine that new breast diseases or breast diseases in young women are mainly due to the liver, while enduring breast diseases or breast diseases in older women are mainly due to the *chong mai*. In both cases there is liver depression. The difference is that, with loss of harmony or regulation of the *chong* and *ren*, there is also kidney vacuity, whether that be yin vacuity, yang vacuity, or both. Most women with breast distention and pain or fibrocystic lumps who are in their 40s will typically have elements of both spleen vacuity and kidney yang vacuity. Therefore, even if their main pattern is liver depression, depressive heat, or blood stasis, the guiding formulas for these patterns usually need to be modified by the addition of appropriate supplements. If there is fatigue due to spleen vacuity, I recommend adding Radix Astragali Membranacei (*Huang Qi*), Radix Panacis Ginseng (*Ren Shen*), and Rhizoma Atractylodis Macrocephalae (*Bai Zhu*). If there is kidney vacuity with lumbar pain, I recommend adding Cortex Eucommiae Ulmoidis (*Du Zhong*) and Radix Dipsaci (*Xu Duan*).

Acupuncture & moxibustion

Based on both Chinese and my own clinical experience, I believe that acupuncture is an important adjunctive therapy in the treatment of premenstrual breast distention and pain and fibrocystic breasts. Often, premenstrual breast distention and pain respond to acupuncture by the time the woman gets up off the treatment couch. When there are fibrocystic lumps in the breasts, internal Chinese medicinals alone may not provide totally effective relief on their own. Acupuncture then makes the treatment much more effective. Generally, treatments should be begun each month as soon as there is any breast swelling or pain. Treatments spaced every other day get the best results and one should only have to provide such intensive acupuncture treatment for the first one or two cycles.

Compresses, poultices & plasters

If there is just swelling and distention, some relief can be afforded by ginger compresses applied at home. If there are lumps, treatment efficacy can be improved by using various compresses and plasters.

1. *Shen Xian Tai Yi Gao* (Divine Immortal Supreme Medicinal Plaster)

Ingredients: Radix Scrophulariae Ningpoensis (*Yuan Shen*), Radix Angelicae Dahuricae (*Bai Zhi*), Radix Angelicae Sinensis (*Dang Gui*), Cortex Cinnamomi Cassiae (*Rou Gui*), uncooked Radix Rehmanniae (*Sheng Di*), Radix Rubrus Paeoniae Lactiflorae (*Chi Shao*), Radix Et Rhizoma Rhei (*Da Huang*)

Method of preparation & administration: Take one *liang* of each of the above ingredients and fry in two *jin* of sesame oil until the medicinals turn black. Remove the dregs and filter the oil after it has cooled. Then reheat this oil and add 12 *liang* of powdered Minium (*Qian Dan*). Mix until thoroughly blended. Next, pour the contents into cold water and let stand 10-15 days changing the water twice per day to remove the fire toxins. Remove the paste from the water and reheat until the mass becomes pliable. Shape as desired and apply to the affected area. Change this plaster every few days and remove if it causes skin irritation and blistering.

Alternative method: One can also grind the above ingredients into powder and then mix these with vinegar. Form into a flat cake and apply to the affected area. Change this once per day and discontinue if it causes a rash or irritation.

2. *Xiang Fu Bing* (Cyperus Pancake)

Ingredients: Rhizoma Cyperi Rotundi (*Xiang Fu*), Secretio Moschi Moschiferi (*She Xiang*), Herba Taraxaci Mongolici Cum Radice (*Pu Gong Ying*), rice wine

Method of preparation & administration: Grind one *liang* of Rhizoma Cyperi Rotundi (*Xiang Fu*) with two *fen* of Secretio Moschi Moschiferi (*She Xiang*). Decoct two *liang* of Herba Taraxaci Mongolici Cum Radice (*Pu Gong Ying*) in rice wine. Remove the dregs and use the remaining liquid to mix with the above powdered medicinals. Apply to the affected area while hot. Repeat daily as needed.

Chinese self-massage

Chinese self-massage is a very effective preventive and remedial adjunctive therapy for breast diseases. For more information about specific such self-massage protocols, see Fan Ya-li's *Chinese Self-massage, The Easy Way to Health*, Blue Poppy Press, 1996.

Dietary therapy

It is extremely important that women with breast distention, pain, and lumps avoid drinking coffee. This applies especially to caffeinated coffee but to decaff as well. Coffee is a bitter, acrid, exterior-relieving medicinal according to TCM theory and, therefore, tends to cause or aggravate loss of balance between the *chong* and *ren*.

Women with breast lumps associated with phlegm nodulation should take care to avoid uncooked and chilled foods as well as foods which engender fluids very strongly. Such fluid-engendering foods include sugars and sweets, dairy products, greasy, oily foods, tomatoes, oranges, and fruit juices in general. These foods will cause dampness and aggravate phlegm production and accumulation.

Prognosis

Premenstrual breast distention and pain respond quite well to TCM therapy. Once again, however, because one of their common root disease mechanisms is liver qi due to emotional stress and frustration, these conditions can return if one does not learn better relaxation skills and modify their lifestyle.

When breast lumps come and go with the period without leaving a nodule behind during the rest of the cycle, these are qi stagnations and respond very well to TCM therapy. When lumps are associated with pain, swelling, and inflammation, these three accompanying conditions can almost always be alleviated.

When treating otherwise asymptomatic breast lumps that are firm and persisting, one should use more Thallus Algae (*Kun Bu*) and Herba Sargassii (*Hai Zao*) to soften the hard and scatter nodulation. It is especially important not to overuse blood-quickening, stasis-breaking ingredients in women who are yin or qi and blood vacuous and debilitated.

Addendum: Fibrocystic breasts

The following functional translations help to exemplify the contemporary Chinese treatment of premenstrual breast distention and pain and fibrocystic breasts. The first describes more complicated patterns than the above typical textbook discussion. The second discusses the role of the *chong mai* in enduring breast diseases or breast diseases in older women.

(From "The Pattern Discrimination Treatment of 90 Cases of Menstrual Movement Breast Distention" by Wang Fa-chang & Wang Qu-an, *Shan Dong Zhong Yi Za Zhi [Shandong Journal of Chinese Medicine]*, #5, 1993, p. 24-25)

Menstrual movement breast distention and pain is one of the most commonly seen complaints in gynecology departments. The authors of this clinical audit have treated 90 cases of this condition based on pattern discrimination. Of these 90 women, four were between 16-20 years old, 11 between 21-25, 20 between 26-30, 21 between 31-35, 20 between 36-40, five between 41-45, seven between 46-50, and two cases were more than 50 years old. The course of these women's disease was from one half year to 20 years.

1. Simultaneous liver depression with damp heat pattern

The main symptoms of this pattern were premenstrual chest oppression, heart vexation and easy anger, breast distention and pain, a dry mouth, vexatious heat of the chest and epigastrium, lower abdominal aching and pain, possible vaginal itching or excessive, yellow-colored vaginal discharge, a bowstring, rapid pulse, and red tongue with thin, yellow fur. The treatment principles were to course the liver and resolve depression, clear heat and disinhibit dampness. The formula consisted of a combination of *Dan Zhi Xiao Yao San* (Moutan & Gardenia Rambling Powder), *Yi Huang Tang* (Change Yellow [Discharge] Decoction), and *San Miao San* (Three Wonders Powder) plus Rhizoma Cyperi Rotundi (*Xiang Fu*).

2. Simultaneous liver depression with blood stasis pattern

The main symptoms of this pattern were premenstrual heart vexation and easy anger, breast distention and pain, occasional nodulation, lower abdominal distention and pain disliking pressure, possible scanty menstruation which does not come smoothly, a dark, purplish menstruate containing clots, a bowstring, slippery pulse, and a purplish, dark tongue with static spots or patches and thin, white fur. The treatment principles were to course the liver and resolve depression, quicken the blood, transform stasis, and stop pain. The formula consisted of *Dan Zhi Xiao Yao San* (Moutan & Gardenia Rambling Powder) combined with *Tao Hong Si Wu Tang* (Persica & Carthamus Four Materials Decoction) plus Pericarpium Citri Reticulatae Viride (*Qing Pi*), Rhizoma Corydalis Yanhusuo (*Yan Hu Suo*), and Tuber Curcumae (*Yu Jin*).

3. Simultaneous liver depression with heart-spleen dual vacuity pattern

The main symptoms of this pattern were premenstrual chest oppression, heart vexation and chaotic thoughts, mild, insidious breast pain or small sensations of distention, heart palpitations, dizziness, loss of sleep, profuse dreams, lack of strength of the entire body, lassitude of the spirit, diminished appetite, excessive, pasty, white vaginal discharge, a bowstring, fine pulse, and a pale tongue with teeth marks on its border and thin, white fur. The treatment principles were to course the liver and resolve depression, fortify the spleen and harmonize the stomach, nourish the heart and quiet the spirit. The formula consisted of *Dan Shen Gui Pi Tang* (Salvia Restore the Spleen Decoction) plus Rhizoma Cyperi Rotundi (*Xiang Fu*) and Tuber Curcumae (*Yu Jin*).

4. Liver-kidney insufficiency pattern

The main symptoms of this pattern were premenstrual chest oppression, heart vexation and chaotic thoughts, mild, insidious breast pain, dizziness, tinnitus, lumbar pain, weakness of the extremities, lack of strength, a deep, bowstring pulse, and a pale tongue with scant fur. The treatment principles were to course the liver and fortify the spleen, supplement and boost the liver and kidneys. The formula consisted of *Dan Zhi Xiao Yao San* (Moutan & Gardenia Rambling Powder) plus Cortex Eucommiae Ulmoidis (*Du Zhong*), Radix Dipsaci (*Chuan Xu Duan*), Ramulus Loranthi Seu Visci (*Sang Ji Sheng*), Cornu Degelatinum Cervi (*Lu Jiao Shuang*), Fructus Corni Officinalis (*Shan Zhu Yu*), and Semen Cuscutae Chinensis (*Tu Si Zi*).

5. Simultaneous liver depression with *chong* & *ren* vacuity cold pattern

The main symptoms of this pattern were premenstrual heart vexation and chaotic thoughts, lassitude of the spirit, breast distention and pain, insidious lower abdominal pain with a cool sensation, a fine, slow pulse, and a pale tongue with thin, white fur. The treatment principles were to course the liver and resolve depression, cherish the palace (*i.e.*, uterus) and scatter cold. The formula consisted of *Dan Zhi Xiao Yao San* (Moutan & Gardenia Rambling Powder) plus Radix Linderae Strychnifoliae (*Wu Yao*), Rhizoma Cyperi Rotundi (*Xiang Fu*), stir-fried Fructus Foeniculi Vulgaris (*Xiao Hui*), and stir-fried Folium Artemisiae Argyii (*Ai Ye*).

One course of treatment was comprised of three *ji* of the appropriate Chinese medicinals being given during the premenstruum. Complete cure was defined as disappearance of such symptoms as premenstrual chest oppression, heart vexation and chaotic thoughts, breast distention and pain, etc. with reduction or disappearance of nodulations and lumps in the breasts within three courses of treatment. Marked improvement consisted of reduction in such symptoms as premenstrual chest oppression, heart vexation and chaotic thoughts, breast distention and pain, etc. within three courses of treatment. Good improvement consisted of reduction in the same sorts of symptoms as above in three courses of treatment but recurrence or worsening of these symptoms due to emotional stress. Of the 90 women treated in this study, 57 were cured, 23 were markedly improved, eight experienced good improvement, and two got no result. Thus the total amelioration rate using this protocol was 97.8%.

(From "Lu De-ming's Experiences Treating Mammary Hyperplasia Disease" by Que Hua-fa, *Shang Hai Zhong Yi Yao Za Zhi [Shanghai Journal of Chinese Medicine & Medicinals]*, #2, 1994, p. 6-7)

Mammary hyperplasia disease is categorized as *ru pi* or mammary aggregation in Chinese medical theory. According to the *Sheng Ji Zong Lu (General Collection for Sage-like Relief)* [published between 1111-1117 CE, a medical encyclopedia in 200 volumes], loss of regularity of the *chong* and *ren* is the main disease mechanism in breast disease:

> In women, the *chong* and *ren* are the root. If there is loss of command or authority and orderly management, the *chong* and *ren* may become disharmonious, there may be heat in the *yang ming* channel, or wind evils may settle therein. This then leads to qi congestion which is not scattered and thence to binding and accumulation within the breast with possible hardness and swelling, aching, pain, and the presence of kernels [*i.e.*, lumps].

The *Feng Shi Jin Nang (Master Feng's Instructions)* states, "In women, if there is disharmony and lack of regulation and nourishment, the *chong* and *ren* will be damaged." Further, the *Wai Ke Yi An Hui Bian (A Collection of Case Histories in External Medicine)*, says:

> The *chong* and *ren* are the sea of qi and blood. They move above and become the breast [milk]. They move below and become the menses.

Thus it is evident that, in ancient times, it was believed that loss of regulation of the *chong* and *ren* was the disease cause of breast disease. Fifty years ago, Gu Bo-hua taught that to treat mammary hyperplasia one should regulate and harmonize the *chong* and *ren* and for this purpose to use medicinals such as *Xiao Yao San* (Rambling Powder) plus medicinals to warm yang. This method has achieved comparatively good results in clinical practice. Lu De-ming, based on Prof.

Gu Bo-hua's teachings and his own clinical experience, has found that the cause of mammary hyperplasia disease is indeed loss of regulation of the *chong* and *ren* and that regulating and containing (*i.e.*, conserving the health of) the *chong* and *ren* should be the method for treating the root of this disease.

According to Master Lu, if viscera and bowel function loses normalcy, qi and blood will also lose normalcy. This results in the *chong* and *ren* losing normalcy and the engenderment of breast disease. Thus the onset of mammary hyperplasia is related to the two vessels, the *chong* and *ren*. The *chong* is the sea of blood and the *ren* rules the *bao tai* (*i.e.*, uterus and fetus). The *bao mai* is tied to the kidneys. The *chong mai* and kidney vessel mutually merge and move together and require kidney yin to enrich and nourish them. In addition, the kidney qi transforms and engenders the *tian gui*. The *tian gui's* origin is in the former heaven which is stored in the kidneys. It is able to be set off (referring to menarche and each successive menstruation) only when the *chong* and *ren* are free-flowing and exuberant. Below, the *chong* and *ren* rise up from the *bao gong*. Above, they link with the breasts. If qi and blood are sufficient, this makes the *bao gong* and the breasts capable of conceiving and functioning actively. Thus the kidney qi, *tian gui*, and the *chong* and *ren* are all mutually interconnected.

If kidney qi is insufficient, this leads to the *tian gui* not being full and the two vessels, the *chong* and *ren* not being exuberant. The connection between the *bao gong* and the breasts is troubled or inconvenienced (on account of this) and thus disease arises. In addition, the liver and kidneys share a common source, and the ability of the liver to store the blood and govern coursing and discharge is dependent on the warming and steaming of the kidney qi. If kidney qi is insufficient, this may lead to the liver losing its nourishment. In that case, the liver's coursing and discharging function may lose normalcy and the liver qi may become depressed and bound. This then may result in the *chong* and *ren* losing their regulation. Qi stagnation brings on phlegm stasis congelation and accumulation and this becomes breast elusive mass. Therefore, kidney qi insufficiency resulting in loss of regulation of the *chong* and *ren* is the root of the onset of this disease, while liver qi depression and knotting, phlegm stasis congelation and stagnation are the branches of the onset of this disease.

Based on the above theory, Lu De-ming's treatment of mammary hyperplasia is founded on the principles of supplementing and boosting the kidney qi, regulating and containing (*i.e.*, conserving the health of) the *chong* and *ren*. These are the methods for treating the root of this disease. However, because the *chong* and *ren* are not rooted in a single viscus, one is not able to move only a single channel. The *chong* and *ren* pertain to the vessels of the two viscera, the liver and kidneys. And as Ye Gui [a.k.a. Ye Tian-shi, 1667-1746 CE] also said, "The *chong* and *ren* are subordinate to (or serve) the *yang ming*." Therefore, in clinical practice, one must differentiate between the *chong* and *ren* and their connection with the kidneys, liver, spleen-stomach, and the qi and blood. Thus, there are altogether three different but related sets of treatment principles for this condition:

1. Supplement the kidneys and reinforce yang in order to regulate the *chong* & *ren*. It is said, "The *chong* and *ren* are rooted in the kidneys." The kidneys also command the two yin (*i.e.*, the anus and urethra/vagina). If kidney qi is exuberant, the *chong* and *ren* are sufficient. Therefore, supplementing the kidneys and reinforcing yang also supplements and boosts the *chong* and *ren*.

2. Course the liver and quicken the blood in order to regulate the *chong* & *ren*. It is also said, "The liver is the former heaven in women." The liver stores the blood and rules coursing and discharge. Therefore, the liver also regulates and adjusts the *chong* and *ren*/sea of blood's waxing and waning. The liver is yin in form and yang in function and it easily becomes depressed. Worry, anxiety, depression, and anger can result in restraint, depression, and lack of joy (or vigor). This may lead to liver depression not out-thrusting and hence to qi stagnation, blood stasis. This then causes the two vessels, the *chong* and *ren*, to lose their orderly reaching. The breasts then lose their nourishment, and breast disease is engendered. The qi is the commander of the blood and the blood is the mother of the qi. The qi and blood are mutually rooted. Movement of qi leads to movement of blood. If the qi flows normally, the blood flows normally. Then the qi and blood are open and flowing normally. This leads to the *chong* and *ren* automatically being regulated. Therefore, coursing the liver and quickening the blood also is able to regulate the *chong* and *ren*.

3. Nourish the blood and harmonize the constructive in order to regulate the *chong* & *ren*. In many women, the liver is depressed and the blood is vacuous. "The *chong mai* is subservient to the *yang ming*" and "the *chong* and *ren* are the sea of qi and blood." The blood of the viscera and bowels all gather in the *chong mai*. And the spleen and stomach are the source of the engenderment and transformation of the qi and blood. Therefore, the waxing and waning of the *chong* and *ren*/sea of blood is also related to the spleen and stomach. If there is vacuity detriment of the spleen and stomach, the source of the engenderment of blood will be insufficient and unable to warm and nourish the liver and kidneys or to moisten and nourish the *chong* and *ren*. Thus, the *chong* and *ren* will lose their regulation. Therefore, Xu Ling-tai [a.k.a. Xu Da-chun, 1693-1771 CE] said:

> The method to treat the *chong* and *ren* resides completely in nourishing the blood. Hence the ancients always founded this method on mainly blood medicinals.

Based on the above, one can see that Master Lu's treatment of mammary hyperplasia consists of supplementing the kidneys, reinforcing yang, and regulating the *chong* and *ren* as the major method. This is then combined with coursing the liver and quickening the blood, nourishing the blood and harmonizing the constructive, transforming phlegm and softening the hard, etc. to also regulate and contain the *chong* and *ren*. The ingredients he commonly uses for supplementing the kidneys and reinforcing yang, regulating and supplementing the *chong* and *ren* are: Rhizoma Curculiginis Orchioidis (*Xian Mao*), Herba Epimedii (*Xian Ling Pi*), Herba Cistanchis Deserticolae (*Rou Cong Rong*), Herba Cynomorii Songarici (*Suo Yang*), etc. Because there is often concomitant yin vacuity, he uses warm but not hot natured medicinals and moist not drying medicinals, such as Epimedium, Cistanches, Cynomorium, and Semen Cuscutae (*Tu Si Zi*), etc., combined with nourishing blood, enriching yin medicinals, such as Radix Angelicae Sinensis (*Dang Gui*), Radix Albus Paeoniae Lactiflorae (*Bai Shao*), Radix Salviae Miltiorrhizae (*Dan Shen*), uncooked Radix Polygoni Multiflori (*Shou Wu*), Tuber Asparagi Cochinensis (*Tian Dong*), etc. Thus, as yang is engendered, yin grows and yin and yang are mutually engendered.

For quickening the blood and transforming stasis, Master Lu mainly uses qi within the blood medicinals such as Rhizoma Curcumae Zedoariae (*E Zhu*), Tuber Curcumae (*Yu Jin*), Rhizoma Corydalis Yanhusuo (*Xuan Hu*), Radix Ligustici Wallichii (*Chuan Xiong*), etc. and blood within the qi division medicinals, such as Rhizoma Cyperi Rotundi (*Xiang Fu*) and Radix Bupleuri (*Chai Hu*). If the course of the disease is prolonged and there are swollen, hard, tough lumps which are difficult to disperse, he commonly adds to the formula Cornu Cervi (*Lu Jiao Pian*) and Squama Manitis Pentadactylis (*Chuan Shan Jia*), bloody, meaty natured ingredients to fill and supplement the essence blood of the extraordinary channels in order to construct and nourish the *chong* and *ren*. At the same time, these are combined with breaking stasis, scattering nodulation ingredients, such as Rhizoma Sparganii (*San Leng*), Rhizoma Curcumae Zedoariae (*E Zhu*), Herba Sargassii (*Hai Zao*), etc.

Thus Master Lu's basic formula for regulating and containing the *chong* and *ren*, coursing the liver and quickening the blood consists of: Rhizoma Curculiginis Orchioidis (*Xian Mao*), Herba Epimedii (*Xian Ling Pi*), Herba Cistanchis Deserticolae (*Rou Cong Rong*), Rhizoma Curcumae Zedoariae (*E Zhu*), Semen Pruni Persicae (*Tao Ren*), Herba Lycopi Lucidi (*Ze Lan*), processed Rhizoma Cyperi Rotundi (*Xiang Fu*), Rhizoma Corydalis Yanhusuo (*Xuan Hu*), Tuber Curcumae (*Yu Jin*), etc. This then is added to and subtracted from following the symptoms. Using this method, Master Lu usually gets very good results.

Menstrual Movement Diarrhea and/or Vomiting

Diarrhea either directly before or with the onset of menstruation is commonly met in women complaining of PMS. Often, there is first a period of constipation in the week before the menses, followed by loose stools or diarrhea the day of the onset of menstruation. Vomiting or nausea before or during menstruation is not as commonly encountered. In my experience, if vomiting is seen, it often presents along with extreme painful menstruation.

Disease causes, disease mechanisms

Wu Qian *et al.*, the authors of the *Yi Zong Jin Jian (The Golden Mirror of Ancestral Medicine)*, say that menstrual movement diarrhea and vomiting are basically due to spleen vacuity, and Han Bai-ling in his discussion of menstrual movement diarrhea echoes this opinion. However, if the spleen becomes vacuous premenstrually, it is mostly because the liver becomes stagnant and, therefore, replete. A replete liver thus invades spleen earth based on the control cycle with the spleen becoming vacuous and weak. This vacuity may also be aggravated by heart blood having a tendency to become relatively vacuous before the menstruation due to the heart's sending blood and qi down to the uterus. Therefore, the mother may fail to nourish the child according to the engenderment cycle. If spleen vacuity endures, because of the relationship between spleen and kidney yang, kidney yang may also become weak.

Due to spleen vacuity, it is also possible for cold dampness to accumulate in the middle. This can cause watery, clear diarrhea with pain. If the stomach is weak and excessive fluids accumulate in the stomach, this may cause vomiting. Likewise, food stagnation may also contribute to vomiting. In the first case, there will be vomiting of fluids, and in the second, vomiting of food. And finally, if the liver becomes depressed and this depression transforms into heat, dampness from the spleen may join with this heat and cause damp heat diarrhea.

The factors contributing to or causing spleen weakness include chilled, uncooked foods, drinking too many or cold liquids with meals, overeating sugary, sweet foods, overeating fluid-engendering foods, such as dairy products and fruit juices, excessive worry and anxiety, lack of exercise, or excessive fatigue. The main factors leading to liver depression qi stagnation are stress and frustration. Damp heat may be aggravated by spicy, hot foods, alcohol, greasy foods, and orange juice which is both damp and warm.

Treatment based on pattern discrimination

Spleen vacuity, dampness retained

Main symptoms: Diarrhea and borborygmus during the menses, stomach not transforming, appetite diminished, bodily emaciation, muscles and flesh withered, edema of the eyelids and four extremities, a scanty amount of menstruate which is pale in color, continuous vaginal discharge, abdominal pain, a sallow yellow facial complexion, a pale, moist tongue, and a vacuous, relaxed (retarded) pulse

Treatment principles: Fortify the spleen, boost the qi, and percolate dampness

Guiding formulas:

1. *Shen Ling Bai Zhu San* (Ginseng, Atractylodes & Poria Powder)

Ingredients: Radix Panacis Ginseng (*Ren Shen*), Rhizoma Atractylodis Macrocephalae (*Bai Zhu*), Sclerotium Poriae Cocos (*Fu Ling*), Semen Dolichoris Lablab (*Bian Dou*), Radix Dioscoreae Oppositae (*Shan Yao*), Fructus Amomi (*Sha Ren*), Radix Glycyrrhizae (*Gan Cao*), Semen Nelumbinis Nuciferae (*Lian Rou*), Pericarpium Citri Reticulatae (*Chen Pi*), Radix Platycodi Grandiflori (*Jie Geng*), Semen Coicis Lachryma-jobi (*Yi Yi Ren*)

Additions & subtractions: Han Bai-ling suggests adding Radix Albus Paeoniae Lactiflorae (*Bai Shao*) to constrain yin and level the liver. The authors of *Zhong Yi Fu Ke (A Study of Chinese Medical Gynecology)* suggest adding Radix Puerariae (*Ge Gen*), Radix Albus Paeoniae Lactiflorae (*Bai Shao*), and Rhizoma Cimicifugae (*Sheng Ma*). Guo Yuan deletes Amomum, Licorice, Semen Nelumbinis, Orange Peel, Platycodon, and Coix and adds Radix Angelicae Sinensis (*Dang Gui*), Radix Albus Paeoniae Lactiflorae (*Bai Shao*), Radix Ligustici Wallichii (*Chuan Xiong*), Fructus Perillae Frutescentis (*Zi Su*), and Herba Agastachis Seu Pogostemi (*Huo Xiang*). In addition, Guo says to use stir-fried Atractylodes Macrocephala, Dioscorea, and Dolichos. Guo Yuan gives this formula for menstrual movement diarrhea with a watery discharge which does not stop accompanied by abdominal distention. This is obviously diarrhea due to liver-spleen disharmony.

2. *Xiang Sha Liu Jun Zi Tang* (Auklandia & Amomum Six Gentlemen Decoction)

Ingredients: Radix Panacis Ginseng (*Ren Shen*), Rhizoma Atractylodis Macrocephalae (*Bai Zhu*), Sclerotium Poriae Cocos (*Fu Ling*), mix-fried Radix Glycyrrhizae (*Gan Cao*), Rhizoma Pinelliae Ternatae (*Ban Xia*), Pericarpium Citri Reticulatae (*Chen Pi*), Fructus Amomi (*Sha Ren*), Radix Auklandiae Lappae (*Mu Xiang*)

Wu Qian *et al.* suggest this formula for the treatment of vomiting fluids due to phlegm water.

3. *Qi Wei Bai Zhu San* (Seven Flavors Atractylodes Macrocephala Powder)

Ingredients: Radix Panacis Ginseng (*Ren Shen*), Rhizoma Atractylodis Macrocephalae (*Bai Zhu*), Sclerotium Poriae Cocos (*Fu Ling*), mix-fried Radix Glycyrrhizae (*Gan Cao*), Radix Auklandiae Lappae (*Mu Xiang*), Herba Agastachis Seu Pogostemi (*Huo Xiang*), Radix Puerariae (*Ge Gen*)

Wu Qian *et al.* suggest this formula for the treatment of loose stools associated with vacuity heat, "muscles hot, thirst, diarrhea." The loose stools are, however, primarily due to spleen vacuity and dampness and these are this formula's main targets.

Phlegm rheum hidden in the stomach

Main symptoms: At the time of menstruation, there is vomiting of phlegm drool like clear water. At the same time there is stomach and epigastric glomus and fullness, a sticky mouth, torpid intake, vomiting provoked by drinking water, possible dizziness and vertigo, delayed menstruation which is pale in color and scanty in amount, slimy, white tongue fur, and a slippery or bowstring pulse.

Treatment principles: Warm and transform phlegm rheum, harmonize the stomach and downbear counterflow

Guiding formula: *Xuan Fu Hua Dai Zhe Shi Tang Jia Wei* (Inula & Hematite Decoction with Added Flavors)

Ingredients: Flos Inulae (*Xuan Fu Hua*), Haemititum (*Dai Zhe Shi*), Radix Panacis Ginseng (*Ren Shen*), Rhizoma Pinelliae Ternatae (*Ban Xia*), uncooked Rhizoma Zingiberis (*Sheng Jiang*), mix-fried Radix Glycyrrhizae (*Zhi Gan Cao*), Fructus Zizyphi Jujubae (*Da Zao*)

Within this formula, Inula, Hematite, and Pinellia downbear counterflow and transform phlegm, harmonize the stomach and stop vomiting. Uncooked Ginger warms the middle and stops vomiting. Ginseng boosts the qi and fortifies the spleen.

Additions: One can also add Fructus Evodiae Rutecarpae (*Wu Zhu Yu*) to increase the power of warming of the middle and downbearing counterflow. If there is the sound of water in the stomach or there is intestinal noises, this is due to phlegm rheum being exuberant in the stomach. Therefore, to the above formula add *Ling Gui Zhu Gan Tang* (Poria, Cinnamon, Atractylodes & Licorice Decoction) in order to warm and transform phlegm rheum: Sclerotium Poriae Cocos (*Fu Ling*), Ramulus Cinnamomi (*Gui Zhi*), Rhizoma Atractylodis Macrocephalae (*Bai Zhu*), mix-fried Radix Glycyrrhizae (*Gan Cao*).

Spleen yang vacuity

Main symptoms: Menstrual movement diarrhea like duck droppings, borborygmus and chilly pain desiring warmth and pressure, counterflow chilling of the four limbs, a greenish white or bluish-greenish, pale facial complexion, a pale tongue with white fur, and a deep, slow, forceless pulse

I rarely see this as a discreet pattern in Western patients although I often saw it in Chinese patients when I was an intern in Shanghai. When it occurs in Western patients, it is usually only a part of a more complicated pattern.

Treatment principles: Supplement yang, warm the center, and boost the qi

Guiding formula: *Li Zhong Tang* **(Rectify the Center Decoction)**

Ingredients: Radix Panacis Ginseng (*Ren Shen*), Rhizoma Atractylodis Macrocephalae (*Bai Zhu*), Radix Glycyrrhizae (*Gan Cao*), dry Rhizoma Zingiberis (*Gan Jiang*)

Additions: Han Bai-ling suggests adding Radix Lateralis Praeparatus Aconiti Carmichaeli (*Fu Zi*) and Ramulus Cinnamomi Cassiae (*Gui Zhi*) to warm the center and scatter cold. For vomiting, add uncooked Rhizoma Zingiberis (*Sheng Jiang*).

Liver attacking the stomach, liver fire harassing above

Main symptoms: Several days before menstruation there is nausea, vomiting, and acid eructation. The facial region is flooded with heat and there is dizziness, profuse dreaming, a red tongue with thick, slimy, slightly yellow fur, and a bowstring, rapid pulse.

Treatment principles: Clear the liver and harmonize the stomach

Guiding formulas:

1. *Huang Lian Wen Dan Tang Jia Wei* (Coptis Warm the Gallbladder Decoction with Added Flavors)

Ingredients: Sclerotium Poriae Cocos (*Fu Ling*), Pericarpium Citri Reticulatae (*Chen Pi*), lime-processed Rhizoma Pinelliae Ternatae (*Fa Xia*), Radix Glycyrrhizae (*Gan Cao*), Caulis In Taeniis Bambusae (*Zhu Ru*), Fructus Citri Aurantii (*Zhi Ke*), Rhizoma Coptidis Chinensis (*Huang Lian*), Concha Ostreae (*Mu Li*), Concha Arcae Inflatae (*Wa Leng Zi*)

2. *Si Qi Tang Jia Zuo Jin Wan* (Four Seven Decoction plus (Left Gold Pills)

Ingredients: Processed Rhizoma Pinelliae Ternatae (*Zhi Ban Xia*), Cortex Magnoliae Officinalis (*Hou Po*), Folium Perillae Frutescentis (*Zi Su Ye*), uncooked Rhizoma Zingiberis (*Sheng Jiang*), Fructus Zizyphi Jujubae (*Da Zao*), Rhizoma Coptidis Chinensis (*Huang Lian*), Fructus Evodiae Rutecarpae (*Wu Zhu Yu*)

The formula *Si Qi Tang* moves the qi, resolves depression, and transforms phlegm. *Zuo Jin Wan* acirdly opens and bitterly downbears. It courses the liver and harmonizes the stomach.

Additions: If phlegm heat is relatively heavy, add Fructus Citri Aurantii (*Zhi Ke*), Caulis Bambusae In Taeniis (*Zhu Ru*), Pericarpium Citri Erythrocarpae (*Ju Pi*), etc. to clear heat and transform phlegm, downbear the qi and stop vomiting. If there is simultaneous obvious liver depression, combine with *Dan Zhi Xiao Yao San* (Moutan & Gardenia Rambling Powder).

Liver wood exploiting the spleen

Main symptoms: Chest oppression and rib-side distention, belching, decreased food intake, abdominal pain preceding or occurring with diarrhea and with both aggravated by tension and emotional upset, a pale red tongue with thin, white fur, and a bowstring, possibly fine pulse

As discussed above under spleen vacuity and *Shen Ling Bai Zhu San*, often premenstrual or menstrual diarrhea is due to the liver becoming replete just before the menses and then counterflowing onto or attacking the spleen via the control cycle. Although spleen vacuity is the direct mechanism causing the diarrhea, *i.e.*, the spleen is insufficient to move and transform water and grains properly, this spleen vacuity most often occurs due to exploitation by a replete and stagnant liver. Chinese gynecology texts do not list this as a separate pattern. I believe it is useful, especially for beginners, to do so since menstrual movement diarrhea is rarely a Western woman's major complaint. Therefore, the guiding formula is probably going to be picked based on some other criteria besides, but nonetheless taking into account, menstrual movement diarrhea.

Treatment principles: Course the liver and rectify the qi, fortify the spleen and stop diarrhea

Guiding formulas:

1. *Tong Xie Yao Fang* (Painful Diarrhea Essential Formula)

Ingredients: Radix Albus Praeparatus Paeoniae Lactiflorae (*Chao Bai Shao*), stir-fried Rhizoma Atractylodis Macrocephalae (*Bai Zhu*), stir-fried Pericarpium Citri Reticulatae (*Chen Pi*), Radix Ledebouriellae Divaricatae (*Fang Feng*)

Additions & subtractions: For watery diarrhea, add Semen Plantaginis (*Che Qian Zi*), Sclerotium Poriae Cocos (*Fu Ling*), and dry Rhizoma Zingiberis (*Gan Jiang*). For porridge-like diarrhea, add Rhizoma Atractylodis (*Cang Zhu*). For severe abdominal pain, double the amount of Peony and add Pericarpium Citri Reticulatae Viride (*Qing Pi*) and Rhizoma Cyperi Rotundi (*Xiang Fu*). For diarrhea associated with hypothyroidism and an enlarged thyroid, delete Ledebouriellae, double the amount of Peony, and add Radix Puerariae (*Ge*

Gen), Concha Ostreae (*Mu Li*), and Spica Prunellae Vulgaris (*Xia Ku Cao*). If spleen qi is pronouncedly vacuous, add Radix Codonopsitis Pilosulae (*Dang Shen*) and mix-fried Radix Glycyrrhizae (*Gan Cao*). If chest oppression and abdominal distention are more pronounced due to more severe liver depression, add the ingredients of *Si Mo Tang* (Four Milled [Medicinals] Decoction): Radix Panacis Ginseng (*Ren Shen*), Semen Arecae Catechu (*Bing Lang*), Lignum Aquillariae Agallochae (*Chen Xiang*), and Radix Linderae Strychnifoliae (*Wu Yao*).

2. *Xiao Yao San Jia Wei* (Rambling Powder with Added Flavors)

Ingredients: Radix Bupleuri (*Chai Hu*), Rhizoma Atractylodis Macrocephalae (*Bai Zhu*), Sclerotium Poriae Cocos (*Fu Ling*), Radix Angelicae Sinensis (*Dang Gui*), Radix Albus Paeoniae Lactiflorae (*Bai Shao*), Herba Menthae Haplocalycis (*Bo He*), mix-fried Radix Glycyrrhizae (*Zhi Gan Cao*), uncooked Rhizoma Zingiberis (*Sheng Jiang*), Exocarpium Citri Rubri (*Ju Hong*), Bulbus Fritillariae (*Bei Mu*), Rhizoma Pinelliae Ternatae (*Ban Xia*)

This formula is for premenstrual depression, cough, and vomiting due to liver qi and phlegm dampness attacking the lungs and/or stomach.

3. *Xiao Yao San Jia Jian* (Rambling Powder with Additions & Subtractions)

Ingredients: Mix-fried Radix Astragali Membranacei (*Huang Qi*), Radix Bupleuri (*Chai Hu*), Radix Angelicae Sinensis (*Dang Gui*), Radix Albus Paeoniae Lactiflorae (*Bai Shao*), Rhizoma Atractylodis Macrocephalae (*Bai Zhu*), Sclerotium Poriae Cocos (*Fu Ling*), mix-fried Radix Glycyrrhizae (*Gan Cao*), Rhizoma Cimicifugae (*Sheng Ma*), Pericarpium Citri Reticulatae (*Chen Pi*), uncooked Rhizoma Zingiberis (*Sheng Jiang*)

This formula is for diarrhea and loose stools due to liver attacking the spleen accompanied by borborygmus but no abdominal pain.

Liver channel damp heat

Main symptoms: Yellowish diarrhea at the menstrual period, lower abdominal pain, reddish urine, perianal burning and heat, menses colored dark red, amount scant, heart palpitations, easily angered, chest and rib-side distention and oppression, a bitter taste in the mouth, dry throat, a red facial complexion, yellow, dry tongue fur, and a bowstring, slippery, rapid pulse

Treatment principles: Regulate the liver, clear heat, and stop diarrhea

Guiding formula: *Long Dan Xie Gan Tang* **(Gentiana Drain the Liver Decoction)**

Ingredients: Radix Gentianae Scabrae (*Long Dan Cao*), Radix Scutellariae Baicalensis (*Huang Qin*), Fructus Gardeniae Jasminoidis (*Zhi Zi*), Rhizoma Alismatis (*Ze Xie*), Caulis Akebiae Mutong (*Mu Tong*), Semen Plantaginis (*Che Qian Zi*), Radix Angelicae Sinensis (*Dang Gui*), Radix Bupleuri (*Chai Hu*), uncooked Radix Rehmanniae (*Sheng Di*), Radix Glycyrrhizae (*Gan Cao*)

Additions: Han Bai-ling suggests adding Radix Albus Paeoniae Lactiflorae (*Bai Shao*) to constrain the liver and stop diarrhea.

Damp heat with spleen vacuity

Main symptoms: Nausea, vomiting, or diarrhea before the menses. As with liver wood exploiting the spleen, there may be constipation leading up to and then diarrhea just before or accompanying the onset of menstruation. If there is diarrhea, it tends to be yellow or mustard color and there is perianal burning. Often there are cravings for sweets. The patient may complain of cold hands and feet or chills if the discomfort is severe. This is mostly due to the four counterflows, *i.e.*, counterflow of the qi and heat trapped in the interior. If not severe, there are more obvious signs of heat. The tongue may be red with slimy, yellow fur or there may be a peeled, geographic, dry, turbid or slimy, yellow fur. In other cases, there may be thick, white, dryish fur. The pulse tends to be bowstring, slippery, and rapid.

Although this pattern shares many similarities with the preceding pattern, this is the damp heat menstrual movement diarrhea pattern I typically see in Western women.

Treatment principles: Clear heat and eliminate dampness, fortify the spleen and boost the qi

Guiding formulas:

1. *Ban Xia Xie Xin Tang* (Pinelliae Drain the Heart Decoction)

Ingredients: Rhizoma Pinelliae Ternatae (*Ban Xia*), Radix Panacis Ginseng (*Ren Shen*), mix-fried Radix Glycyrrhizae (*Gan Cao*), Rhizoma Coptidis Chinensis (*Huang Lian*), Radix Scutellariae Baicalensis (*Huang Qin*), Fructus Zizyphi Jujubae (*Da Zao*), dry Rhizoma Zingiberis (*Gan Jiang*)

This formula is made up of medicinals which fortify and warm the spleen and transform dampness with medicinals which clear heat and eliminate dampness. When the spleen becomes vacuous and damp, the stomach and intestines often become damp and hot. In Western patients, one does not often see true spleen-stomach vacuity weakness.

Additions: If there is more pronounced spleen vacuity manifesting as fatigue, add Radix Astragali Membranacei (*Huang Qi*). If there is more pronounced spleen vacuity causing indigestion and loose stools, add Rhizoma Atractylodis Macrocephalae (*Bai Zhu*) and Sclerotium Poriae Cocos (*Fu Ling*). If heat has damaged stomach fluids, add Tuber Ophiopogonis Japonici (*Mai Dong*). To help stop diarrhea, one can also add Radix Puerariae (*Ge Gen*).

2. *Sheng Jiang Xie Xin Tang* (Uncooked Ginger Drain the Heart Decoction)

Ingredients: Same as above. However, substitute uncooked Rhizoma Zingiberis (*Sheng Jiang*) for dry Ginger.

This formula treats more conspicuous spleen dampness and less spleen cold.

3. *Gan Cao Xie Xin Tang* (Licorice Drain the Heart Decoction)

Ingredients: Same as *Ban Xia Xie Xin Tang* above but with a higher dosage of mix-fried Licorice.

This formula is for more marked qi vacuity affecting the heart. Typically there is a relaxed (retarded) pulse.

4. *Xiao Chai Hu Tang* (Minor Bupleurum Decoction)

Ingredients: Radix Bupleuri (*Chai Hu*), Radix Panacis Ginseng (*Ren Shen*), mix-fried Radix Glycyrrhizae (*Gan Cao*), Rhizoma Pinelliae Ternatae (*Ban Xia*), Radix Scutellariae Baicalensis (*Huang Qin*), Fructus Zizyphi Jujubae (*Da Zao*), uncooked Rhizoma Zingiberis (*Sheng Jiang*)

This formula is useful for the treatment of damp heat diarrhea complicated by spleen vacuity and liver depression, a commonly seen pattern in clinical practice.

Additions & subtractions: For more pronounced spleen vacuity, add Rhizoma Atractylodis Macrocephalae (*Bai Zhu*) and Sclerotium Poriae Cocos (*Fu Ling*). For more pronounced damp heat, add Rhizoma Coptidis Chinensis (*Huang Lian*), Cortex Phellodendri (*Huang Bai*), and/or Radix Pulsatillae Chinensis (*Bai Tou Weng*). For concomitant cold, replace fresh Ginger with dry Rhizoma Zingiberis (*Gan Jiang*) and/or Ramulus Cinnamomi Cassiae (*Gui Zhi*). In order to stop diarrhea and protect stomach fluids, add Radix Puerarae (*Ge*

Gen). If there are more pronounced symptoms of stomach dryness, add Tuber Ophiopogonis Japonici (*Mai Dong*). For more marked qi stagnation, add Rhizoma Cyperi Rotundi (*Xiang Fu*) and Fructus Amomi (*Sha Ren*). If qi stagnation causes tenesmus, add Radix Auklandiae Lappae (*Mu Xiang*).

5. *Wu Mei Wan* (Mume Pills)

Ingredients: Fructus Pruni Mume (*Wu Mei*), Herba Asari Cum Radice (*Xi Xin*), dry Rhizoma Zingiberis (*Gan Jiang*), Fructus Zanthoxyli Bungeani (*Chuan Jiao*), Ramulus Cinnamomi Cassiae (*Gui Zhi*), Radix Lateralis Praeparatus Aconiti Carmichaeli (*Fu Zi*), Rhizoma Coptidis Chinensis (*Huang Lian*), Cortex Phellodendri (*Huang Bai*), Radix Panacis Ginseng (*Ren Shen*), Radix Angelicae Sinensis (*Dang Gui*)

Additions & subtractions: If there are no signs of cold or chilling of the extremities, delete Aconite and Cinnamon. If cold is more prominent, substitute Cortex Cinnamomi Cassiae (*Rou Gui*) for Cinnamon Twigs. If there are no signs of qi and/or blood vacuity, delete Radix Panacis Ginseng and/or Radix Angelicae Sinensis. If nausea and vomiting are severe, add Fructus Evodiae Rutecarpae (*Wu Zhu Yu*) and Rhizoma Pinelliae Ternatae (*Ban Xia*). If there is abdominal pain, including menstrual pain, add Fructus Meliae Toosendan (*Chuan Lian Zi*), Radix Auuklandiae Lappae (*Mu Xiang*), and/or Radix Albus Paeoniae Lactiflorae (*Bai Shao*). If one is quite sure of a diagnosis of candidiasis and this formula provokes diarrhea, vomiting, nausea, and headache, this is due to yeast die-off or a Herxheimer reaction. In this case, add Radix Et Rhizoma Rhei (*Da Huang*) and Mirabilitum (*Mang Xiao*) to precipitate the stools, thus eliminating the parasites from the body more quickly.

Kidney yang vacuity

Main symptoms: Watery, thin stools associated with the menses, inhibited urination, menses scanty in amount, color thin and watery, lower abdominal pain desiring pressure, low back and knee soreness and weakness, frequent urination, lack of warmth in the four extremities, a dark facial complexion, a pale, moist tongue with thin, white fur, and a deep, weak pulse

That being said, this pattern really only complicates spleen qi vacuity and does not present all by itself premenstrually.

Treatment principles: Warm the kidneys and support yang, fortify the spleen and stop diarrhea

Guiding formulas:

1. *Ba Wei Di Huang Wan* (Eight Flavors Rehmannia Pills)

Ingredients: Cooked Radix Rehmanniae (*Shu Di*), Fructus Corni Officinalis (*Shan Zhu Yu*), Radix Dioscoreae Oppositae (*Shan Yao*), Cortex Radicis Moutan (*Dan Pi*), Rhizoma Alismatis (*Ze Xie*), Sclerotium Poriae Cocos (*Fu Ling*), Cortex Cinnamomi Cassiae (*Rou Gui*), Radix Lateralis Praeparatus Aconiti Carmichaeli (*Fu Zi*)

Additions: Han Bai-ling says to add Rhizoma Atractylodis Macrocephalae (*Bai Zhu*) and Semen Euryalis Ferocis (*Qian Shi*) to fortify the spleen and percolate dampness.

2. *Si Shen Wan* (Four Divine [*i.e.*, Magic, Medicinals] Pills)

Ingredients: Fructus Schisandrae Chinensis (*Wu Wei Zi*), Fructus Evodiae Rutecarpae (*Wu Zhu Yu*), Semen Myristicae Fragrantis (*Rou Dou Kou*), Fructus Psoraleae Corylifoliae (*Bu Gu Zhi*), Fructus Zizyphi Jujubae (*Da Zao*), uncooked Rhizoma Zingiberis (*Sheng Jiang*)

In clinical practice, the first four of these ingredients are usually added to other formulas when there is diarrhea due, in part, to complicating kidney yang vacuity.

Additions: Han Bai-ling suggests adding Semen Euryalis Ferocis (*Qian Shi*) and Radix Dioscoreae Oppositae (*Shan Yao*) to boost yang and percolate dampness at the same time as supplementing the spleen and kidneys.

3. *Jian Gu Tang* (Fortifying & Securing Decoction)

Ingredients: Radix Panacis Ginseng (*Ren Shen*), Rhizoma Atractylodis Macrocephalae (*Bai Zhu*), Sclerotium Poriae Cocos (*Fu Ling*), Semen Coicis Lachryma-jobi (*Yi Yi Ren*), Radix Morindae Officinalis (*Ba Ji Tian*)

This formula from *Fu Qing Zhu Nu Ke (Fu Qing-zhu's Gynecology)* can be combined with *Si Shen Wan* above for the treatment of menstrual movement diarrhea due to kidney vacuity.

Discussion

Many women with PMS experience loose stools or diarrhea just before or at the onset of their menstruation. These same women will also tend to crave sweets. This craving for sweets and carbohydrates is a symptom of spleen vacuity. Often the spleen is vacuous and damp but the stomach is replete and hot or hot and dry. In this case, there is often excessive hunger in general. If the spleen is vacuous and the liver depressed, such excessive eating may lead to food stagnation. In this case, one should modify the appropriate guiding formulas above with ingredients which disperse food.

Prognosis

Premenstrual diarrhea is well treated by TCM. Patients must be taught, however, how and why to avoid uncooked, chilled foods and excessively sweet and fluid-engendering foods if the treatment is going to be effective long-term. The TCM teachings on diet are, I believe, extremely wise and clinically efficacious. Unfortunately, most modern patients' diets are quite different from that which TCM recommends. This makes knowledge of and attention to TCM dietary therapy all the more important. I have written *Arisal of the Clear: A Simple Guide to Healthy Eating According to Traditional Chinese Medicine,* also available from Blue Poppy Press, specifically to explain Chinese dietary wisdom to patients and laypersons.

Menstrual Movement Body Pain

Many women complain of body aches and pains before their menses. Sometimes this is associated with other signs and symptoms suggesting a common cold. In other instances, the pain and soreness is more suggestive of chronic muscular tension which becomes aggravated preceding the menses.

Disease causes, disease mechanisms

The authors of the *Yi Zong Jin Jian (The Golden Mirror of Ancestral Medicine)* discuss menstrual movement body pain under the heading of menstrual movement cold and hot body pain. They say that if the menses arrive and there is cold and hot body pain, fear of cold, fever, sweating, but no distention, this is due to insufficiency of the constructive and defensive. If, on the other hand, there is fever, fear of cold, an absence of sweating, and bodily distention and pain, this is due to repletion of the constructive and defensive leading to surplus.

Using this basic discrimination as one's guide, one can understand that body pain may be due to insufficiency of defensive yang which allows external invasion. The constructive is the mother or root of the defensive qi and the constructive is associated with the blood. When the blood accumulates in the lower part of the body, if there is insufficient blood production, this may leave the upper body relatively vacuous. The defensive qi thus tends to disperse away from the body too rapidly leaving the external defensive permeable to attack.

Secondly, if liver qi becomes stagnant, qi, being yang, has a tendency to rise. This may be aggravated again by the blood being sent down and accumulating below. Liver qi may counterflow upward accumulating in the upper back and neck, while the blood may be insufficient to properly nourish and moisten the sinews. This scenario causes chronic upper back and neck tension and tightness. Its cause is a combination of liver qi due to stress and frustration and spleen vacuity not engendering and transforming sufficient blood, in turn due to faulty diet, lack of exercise, excessive fatigue, or worry and anxiety.

Third, dampness and heat may be engendered by faulty diet and/or internal injury due to excesses of the seven affects transforming into heat. In either case, this damp heat tends to percolate down and heat impediment in the lower half of the body. This then may result in lumbosacral pain, sciatic pain, and swelling and pain of the lower extremities.

Fourth, if there is insufficient blood and yin to both create the menstruate and nourish and moisten the rest of the body, this may cause drying of the sinews prior to, during, or after the menses. When the sinews are malnourished, they become dry, stiff, and tight. Such insufficiency of blood and yin may be due to congenital insufficiency, aging, enduring disease, or any excessive stimulation and activity which consumes and exhausts true yin.

Fifth, premenstrual body pain may also be due to blood stasis. If the blood is stagnant and static, it may not be able to flow freely as the menstruate when and as it should. This then may cause a general plethora and stasis of blood throughout the entire body or may affect a particular part of the body where stasis is already present.

Treatment according to pattern discrimination

External invasion, defensive vacuity

Main symptoms: Alternating fever and chills, fear of cold, sweating, stuffy nose, sore throat, body aches and pain, typically a lack of appetite, white or slightly yellow tongue fur, and a floating, fine, possibly rapid pulse

Treatment principle: Harmonize the constructive and defensive

Guiding formulas:

1. *Xiao Chai Hu Tang He Si Wu Tang* (Minor Bupleurum Decoction plus Four Materials Decoction)

Ingredients: Radix Bupleuri (*Chai Hu*), Rhizoma Pinelliae Ternatae (*Ban Xia*), Radix Codonopsitis Pilosulae (*Dang Shen*), mix-fried Radix Glycyrrhizae (*Gan Cao*), Radix

Scutellariae Baicalensis (*Huang Qin*), Fructus Zizyphi Jujubae (*Da Zao*), uncooked Rhizoma Zingiberis (*Sheng Jiang*), Radix Angelicae Sinensis (*Dang Gui*), cooked Radix Rehmanniae (*Shu Di*), Radix Albus Paeoniae Lactiflorae (*Bai Shao*), Radix Ligustici Wallichii (*Chuan Xiong*)

2. *Ma Huang Si Wu Tang* (Ephedra Four Materials Decoction)

Ingredients: Herba Ephedrae (*Ma Huang*), Radix Angelicae Sinensis (*Dang Gui*), Radix Albus Paeoniae Lactiflorae (*Bai Shao*), cooked Radix Rehmanniae (*Shu Di*), Radix Ligustici Wallichii (*Chuan Xiong*)

This formula nourishes the blood and resolves the exterior. Although the authors of the *Yi Zong Jin Jian (The Golden Mirror of Ancestral Medicine)* list it under menstrual movement body pain, it is most appropriate where the lungs have lost their depurative downbearing and where there is an absence of sweating. However, because external invasion prior to or accompanying the menses is almost always due to evils taking advantage of vacuity and Ephedra is strongly draining, I have never had occasion to use this formula.

3. *Gui Zhi Si Wu Tang* (Cinnamon Twig Four Materials Decoction)

Ingredients: Ramulus Cinnamomi Cassiae (*Gui Zhi*), Radix Angelicae Sinensis (*Dang Gui*), Radix Albus Paeoniae Lactiflorae (*Bai Shao*), cooked Radix Rehmanniae (*Shu Di*), Radix Ligustici Wallichii (*Chuan Xiong*), Radix Glycyrrhizae (*Gan Cao*)

This formula is also recommended by the authors of the *Yi Zong Jin Jian (The Golden Mirror of Ancestral Medicine)*. It is likewise for menstrual movement body pain where there is more obvious chill and fear of cold.

4. *Ge Qi Si Wu Tang* (Pueraria & Astragalus Four Materials Decoction)

Ingredients: Radix Puerariae (*Ge Gen*), Radix Astragali Membranacei (*Huang Qi*), Radix Angelicae Sinensis (*Dang Gui*), Radix Albus Paeoniae Lactiflorae (*Bai Shao*), Radix Ligustici Wallichii (*Chuan Xiong*), uncooked Radix Rehmanniae (*Sheng Di*), Folium Perillae Frutescentis (*Zi Su*), Pericarpium Citri Reticulatae (*Chen Pi*)

This formula is given by Guo Yuan under the heading menstrual movement common cold. Guo gives this formula's indications as stuffy nose, runny nose, sneezing, headache, fever, and body pain occurring before or during each menstruation.

Yang qi counterflowing upward

Main symptoms: Premenstrual breast, rib-side, and abdominal distention, chest oppression, upper back and neck tension and tightness, possible hiccup or belching, cold hands and feet due to counterflow chilling, delayed and/or scanty menstruation, possible painful menstruation, possible premenstrual headache, a darkish, red, or orangy brown tongue with possible inflated rims and white or yellow fur, and a bowstring, fine pulse

Tongue and pulse signs will depend on how much internal heat there is, if any, and how much blood vacuity.

Treatment principles: Course the liver and rectify the qi, nourish the blood and soothe the sinews

Guiding formulas:

1. *Chai Hu Gui Zhi Tang Jia Ge Gen* (Bupleurum & Cinnamon Twig Decoction plus Pueraria)

Ingredients: Radix Bupleuri (*Chai Hu*), Radix Codonopsitis Pilosulae (*Dang Shen*), Radix Scutellariae Baicalensis (*Huang Qin*), Rhizoma Pinelliae Ternatae (*Ban Xia*), Radix Albus Paeoniae Lactiflorae (*Bai Shao*), Ramulus Cinnamomi Cassiae (*Gui Zhi*), Radix Puerariae (*Ge Gen*), mix-fried Radix Glycyrrhizae (*Gan Cao*), Fructus Zizyphi Jujubae (*Da Zao*), uncooked Rhizoma Zingiberis (*Sheng Jiang*)

2. *Si Ni San Jia Wei* (Four Counterflows Powder with Added Flavors)

Ingredients: Radix Bupleuri (*Chai Hu*), Radix Albus Paeoniae Lactiflorae (*Bai Shao*), Fructus Immaturus Citri Aurantii (*Zhi Shi*), Cortex Radicis Moutan (*Dan Pi*), Fructus Gardeniae Jasminoidis (*Zhi Zi*), Radix Glycyrrhizae (*Gan Cao*)

This formula is for body pain preceding or accompanying menstruation due to depressive heat and blood vacuity. In this case, there will be definite signs of heat, such as heart vexation, a bitter taste in the mouth, a red tongue and/or inflated rims, and a fine, bowstring, rapid pulse. If there are cold hands and feet but the tongue is red and the pulse is rapid, this means that heat has counterflowed internally. It should not be mistaken for a true cold condition.

Damp heat impediment

Main symptoms: Pain in the low back and extremities with red, hot, swollen joints preceding or accompanying the menses, profuse, thick, foul-smelling, possibly yellow vaginal discharge, possible burning urination or vaginitis, a red tongue with greasy yellow fur to the rear, and a slippery, rapid, possibly bowstring or soggy and rapid pulse

Treatment principles: Clear heat and disinhibit dampness

Guiding formula: *San Miao Wan Jia Wei* **(Three Wonders Pills with Added Flavors)**

Ingredients: Cortex Phellodendri (*Huang Bai*), Rhizoma Atractylodis (*Cang Zhu*), Radix Achyranthis Bidentatae (*Niu Xi*), Fructus Chaenomelis Lagenariae (*Mu Gua*), Cortex Radicis Acanthopanacis (*Wu Jia Pi*)

This formula is based on Zhu Dan-xi's *Er Miao Wan* (Two Wonders Pills). This guiding formula is for the treatment of damp heat in the lower burner and may be modified with various additions to treat a wide range of problems.

Additions: If there is pronounced swelling and edema of the lower extremities, add Semen Coicis Lachryma-jobi (*Yi Yi Ren*). If there are sores on the lower extremities, such as herpes lesions on the thighs, hips, or buttocks, add Semen Coicis Lachryma-jobi (*Yi Ren*), Radix Gentianae Scabrae (*Long Dan Cao*), and Semen Phaseoli Calcarati (*Chi Xiao Dou*). If there is liver depression qi stagnation, add Radix Bupleuri (*Chai Hu*) and Fructus Meliae Toosendan (*Chuan Lian Zi*). If there is concomitant spleen vacuity, add Rhizoma Atractylodis (*Bai Zhu*), Sclerotium Poriae Cocos (*Fu Ling*), Radix Astragali Membranacei (*Huang Qi*), and/or Radix Panacis Ginseng (*Ren Shen*). If there is concomitant blood stasis, add Herba Patriniae Heterophyllae Cum Radice (*Bai Jiang Cao*) and/or Caulis Sargentodoxae (*Hong Teng*). If there is heat impediment, add Caulis Lonicerae Japonicae (*Ren Dong Teng*).

Yin & blood vacuity, sinews not nourished

Main symptoms: Before, during, or after menstruation, pain and stiffness in the joints and especially in the hands and feet which are the reunion of the sinews, worse after immobility with a tendency to improve with use, possible flushing of the cheeks, heart vexation and agitation, heat in the centers of the hands, feet, and heart, possible tidal fever and/or night sweats, blurred vision or night blindness, a red tongue with scanty fur, and a fine, rapid pulse

Treatment principles: Supplement the liver and kidneys and enrich yin, nourish the blood and moisten the sinews

Guiding formulas:

1. *Qin Jiao Si Wu Tang Jia Wei* (Gentiana Macrophylla Four Materials Decoction with Added Flavors)

Ingredients: Radix Angelicae Sinensis (*Dang Gui*), cooked Radix Rehmanniae (*Shu Di*), Radix Albus Paeoniae Lactiflorae (*Bai Shao*), Radix Ligustici Wallichii (*Chuan Xiong*), Radix Gentianae Macrophyllae (*Qin Jiao*), Fructus Chaenomelis Lagenariae (*Mu Gua*), Semen Coicis Lachryma-jobi (*Yi Yi Ren*), Excrementum Bombycis Mori (*Can Sha*), Herba Cistanchis Desertocilae (*Rou Cong Rong*), Radix Glycyrrhizae (*Gan Cao*)

2. *Si Wu Tang Jia Duan Gua Yang* (Four Materials Decoction plus Dipsacus, Chaenomeles & Cynomorium)

Ingredients: Radix Angelicae Sinensis (*Dang Gui*), Radix Albus Paeoniae Lactiflorae (*Bai Shao*), cooked Radix Rehmanniae (*Shu Di*), Radix Ligustici Wallichii (*Chuan Xiong*), Radix Dipsaci (*Chuan Duan*), Fructus Chaenomelis Lagenariae (*Mu Gua*), Herba Cynomorii Songarici (*Suo Yang*)

3. *Huang Qi Jian Zhong Tang* (Astragalus Fortify the Center Decoction)

Ingredients: Radix Astragali Membranacei (*Huang Qi*), Ramulus Cinnamomi Cassiae (*Gui Zhi*), Radix Albus Paeoniae Lactiflorae (*Bai Shao*), Radix Glycyrrhizae (*Gan Cao*), uncooked Rhizoma Zingiberis (*Sheng Jiang*), Fructus Zizyphi Jujubae (*Da Zao*), Maltose (*Yi Tang*)

This formula is suggested by the authors of the *Yi Zong Jin Jian (The Golden Mirror of Ancestral Medicine)* for the treatment of menstrual movement body pain due to blood vacuity not nourishing (the sinews). Wu Qian *et al.* say that, in this case, the menses will either be late or the amount of blood discharged will be profuse. This formula addresses itself to the spleen as the latter heaven root of blood engenderment and transformation. By fortifying the spleen, blood production is automatically benefitted. Therefore, this formula does not contain the slimy ingredients of *Si Wu Tang* (Four Materials Decoction) which are rich with flavor such as the preceding formulas.

Blood stasis

Main symptoms: Pain and/or numbness in the extremities or low back, purplish, congested veins in the affected area, typically a long history of trauma or pain in the area, painful menstruation and/or clots in the menstrual discharge, pain worse at night, a purplish, dark tongue or ecchymotic spots or macules on the tongue, and a deep, choppy pulse

Treatment principles: Quicken the blood, transform stasis, and free the flow of the network vessels

Guiding formulas:

1. *Tao Hong Si Wu Tang Jia Wei* (Persica & Carthamus Four Materials Decoction with Added Flavors)

Ingredients: Radix Angelicae Sinensis (*Dang Gui*), Radix Albus Paeoniae Lactiflorae (*Bai Shao*), cooked Radix Rehmanniae (*Shu Di*), Radix Ligustici Wallichii (*Chuan Xiong*), Flos Carthami Tinctorii (*Hong Hua*), Semen Pruni Persicae (*Tao Ren*), Radix Salviae Miltiorrhizae (*Dan Shen*), Radix Dipsaci (*Chuan Duan*)

2. *Qiang Gui Si Wu Tang* (Notopterygium & Cinnamon Four Materials Decoction)

Ingredients: Radix Et Rhizoma Notopterygii (*Qiang Huo*), Ramulus Cinnamomi Cassiae (*Gui Zhi*), Radix Angelicae Sinensis (*Dang Gui*), Radix Albus Paeoniae Lactiflorae (*Bai Shao*), cooked Radix Rehmanniae (*Shu Di*), Radix Ligustici Wallichii (*Chuan Xiong*)

This formula, contained in the *Yi Zong Jin Jian (The Golden Mirror of Ancestral Medicine)*, is suggested by Wu Qian *et al.* for the treatment of menstrual movement body pain due to obstruction of the blood vessels. It unfolds and frees the flow of the channels and network vessels.

Discussion

Body pain either before, during, or after menstruation is again rarely a woman's major complaint but is an often heard complicating complaint when taking the PMS patient's history. Because the alleviation of pain is accorded primary branch treatment, it should be specifically addressed even if the patient's main complaints are seemingly more psychological in nature. Every emotional feeling is simultaneously a bodily sensation. Therefore, by alleviating body discomfort, we automatically relieve mental-emotional suffering as well.

Acupuncture & moxibustion

Acupuncture and moxibustion are especially effective for relieving bodily aches and pains. Even if one only treats *a shi* points, this can provide immediate relief. The key to treating pain with acupuncture and moxibustion is to identify the affected channels and network vessels and then pick appropriate points on those channels and vessels. If the pain is chronic and recurrent, burning small, thread-like cones of moxa directly over the points of pain is very effective. If the pain is associated with blood stasis, *luo ci* or network vessel puncturing, *i.e.,* bleeding any small, visibly engorged and purplish veins in the affected area, is also very effective. Acupuncture for malnourishment of the sinews is less effective, and for those cases I recommend primarily internal Chinese medicinal therapy to nourish the blood and enrich yin.

Menstrual Movement Headache

Many women experience headaches before, during, or immediately after their menses. These may be categorized by modern Western medicine as either muscular tension or neurovascular headaches. Some women develop menstrual migraines at puberty which then continue until menopause and then cease. Other women may develop migraines at menopause itself. Menstrual movement headaches can be a female patient's major complaint. If they come before or right at the onset of the menses, they are usually only one of a number of PMS signs and symptoms. In some women, they may be so intense as to cause nausea, sweating, chills, diarrhea, vomiting, and extreme sensitivity to sound and/or light. Pain may last for hours or even for days and may be so incapacitating as to force the woman home from work to take to her bed in a darkened room.

Disease causes, disease mechanisms

In general, pathoconditions manifesting before menstruation tend to be due to repletion. While pathoconditions manifesting after the menses tend to be due to vacuity. This rule of thumb also holds true for most menstrual movement headaches. Because headache is merely a subspecies of body pain, its disease causes and mechanisms are generally similar to those discussed above.

If there is disharmony between constructive and defensive, the wind gates on the upper body may not be tightly shut and impermeable to external invasion. In this case, wind evils may lodge in the grandchild network vessels, thus obstructing the free and uninhibited flow of qi, blood, and fluids. This obstruction may then result in pain. In this case, there will be other signs and symptoms of external invasion.

Because of stress and frustration, liver qi may become depressed and stagnant. It may then either counterflow upward until it reaches the bottleneck of the neck and the bony box of the cranium. As it jams into these tight spaces, it obstructs the free and uninhibited flow of righteous qi, blood, and fluids and thus causes pain. If liver qi is enduring or severe, it may transform into fire which may flare upward to the head. Or, if there is insufficient blood, the qi may come apart from its more material basis and counterflow upwards as wind. Likewise, if there is insufficient yin, yang may become effulgent and become hyperactive above. These are all variations on a single theme which begins as liver depression qi stagnation mostly due to tension in turn due to stress.

If the spleen is vacuous and damp, dampness and phlegm may be engendered. Because the spleen tends to become vacuous as the menses approach, this dampness and phlegm may become more pronounced during the premenstruum. Although dampness and phlegm are heavy and tend to descend, if there is counterflow qi moving upward, this dampness and phlegm may be drafted upward also to lodge in and obstruct the channels, network vessels, and clear orifices like soot in a flue-pipe. Such phlegm and dampness obstructing the free flow of qi and blood in the head may result in pain. Because the spleen is the root of phlegm engenderment, anything which weakens or disturbs spleen function *vis à vis* its moving and transforming of liquids may result in the accumulation of phlegm and dampness. This includes faulty diet, lack of exercise, excessive fatigue, worry, and anxiety.

The brain is also referred to as the sea of marrow in Chinese medicine. Marrow is associated with essence and blood. If there is insufficient blood and yin above, the sea of marrow may be vacuous and, therefore, there may be a dull headache. This type of headache is more commonly met with towards the latter part of the menses in women who are either blood or yin vacuous. If it is simple blood vacuity, this is most often due to faulty diet, lack of exercise, and poor spleen function. If this persists, the heart may also become involved. If it is more yin vacuity, this is either due to aging, congenital insufficiency, enduring disease, or excessive and prolonged exhaustion due to any stimuli or stressor.

Although the brain as an anatomical entity is referred to as the sea of marrow, functionally it is the reunion of all yang. It is the arisal of clear yang which is responsible for our consciousness and sentience. Clear yang is derived from kidney yang or the life gate fire prenatally, but its postnatal or latter heaven source is the spleen. If the spleen becomes too weak to separate clear from turbid and upbear the clear yang, there may not be sufficient yang qi to keep the qi and blood flowing through the brain and the clear orifices open and sentient. This mechanism of headache is usually associated with factors, such as faulty diet, which cause chronic spleen vacuity. Because the blood is the mother of the qi, when the blood is lost through the menstrual discharge, qi may become weak. Typically, this type of menstrual movement headache occurs towards the end of or after menstruation.

As in menstrual movement body pain, menstrual movement headache may also be due, at least in part, to blood stasis. If there is blood stasis in the uterus, it may cause a general lack of patency and free flow throughout all the blood vessels of the body. On the other hand, because of enduring damage to the network vessels by liver yang, fire, wind, dampness, phlegm, or even insufficiency, blood may become static and stagnant in the network vessels of the head itself. It is said in TCM that enduring disease eventually causes stasis in the network vessels. Therefore, anything which may cause blood stasis in the uterus may contribute to a blood stasis menstrual movement headache, and any disease cause which persists long enough may also cause blood stasis as a complicating factor.

Treatment according to pattern discrimination

External invasion

Main symptoms: Headache, body aches and pains, fear of cold, fever, sweating, stuffy nose, sneezing, and possible cough which tends to recur before or at the onset of menstruation, a pale, perhaps fat tongue, possibly with teeth prints on the lingual edges, thin, white or possibly light yellow fur, and a fine, bowstring pulse which is floating in the inch position

Treatment principles: Harmonize constructive and defensive, expel wind and stop pain

Guiding formula: *Xiao Chai Hu Tang He Si Wu Tang* (Minor Bupleurum Decoction plus Four Materials Decoction)

Ingredients: Radix Bupleuri (*Chai Hu*), Radix Codonopsitis Pilosulae (*Dang Shen*), Rhizoma Pinelliae Ternatae (*Ban Xia*), Radix Scutellariae Baicalensis (*Huang Qin*), Radix Angelicae Sinensis (*Dang Gui*), Radix Albus Paeoniae Lactiflorae (*Bai Shao*), cooked Radix Rehmanniae (*Shu Di*), Radix Ligustici Wallichii (*Chuan Xiong*), Fructus Zizyphi Jujubae (*Da Zao*), mix-fried Radix Glycyrrhizae (*Gan Cao*), uncooked Rhizoma Zingiberis (*Sheng Jiang*)

Additions: Depending upon where the headache is on the head, one can add any of several ingredients. If the headache is on the sides of the head, increase the amount of Radix Ligustici Wallichii (*Chuan Xiong*). If the headache is in the forehead, add Radix Angelicae Dahruicae (*Bai Zhi*). If the headache is in the nape of the neck, add a large amount of Radix Puerariae (*Ge Gen*). If the headache is centered behind the eyes and the eyes are red and painful, add Semen Cassiae Torae (*Jue Ming Zi*), Scapus Eriocaulonis Buergeriani (*Gu Jing Cao*), and Spica Prunellae Vulgaris (*Xia Ku Cao*). If there is headache and generalized body, back, and shoulder pain, add Fructus Viticis (*Man Jing Zi*) and Radix Ledebouriellae Divaricatae (*Fang Feng*). And, if there is headache at the crown of the head, add Fructus Evodiae Rutecarpae (*Wu Zhu Yu*).

Liver depression qi stagnation

Main symptoms: Either before, during, or after menstruation, there is distention and pain on both sides of the head. There is also chest and rib-side pain and oppression and possible hiccup, belching, or sighing. The menstrual movement is not freely flowing and its color is dark. The tongue is normal with thin fur, and the pulse is bowstring.

Treatment principles: Soothe the liver and resolve depression, rectify the qi and harmonize the blood

Guiding formulas:

1. *Chai Hu Shu Gan Tang Jia Wei* (Bupleurum Soothe the Liver Decoction with Added Flavors)

Ingredients: Radix Bupleuri (*Chai Hu*), Radix Albus Paeoniae Lactiflorae (*Bai Shao*), Fructus Citri Aurantii (*Zhi Ke*), Radix Ligustici Wallichii (*Chuan Xiong*), Rhizoma Cyperi Rotundi (*Xiang Fu*), Pericarpium Citri Reticulatae (*Chen Pi*), Radix Glycyrrhizae (*Gan Cao*), Herba Menthae Haplocalycis (*Bo He*)

2. *Xiao Yao San Jia Wei* (Rambling Powder with Added Flavors)

Ingredients: Radix Bupleuri (*Chai Hu*), Radix Ligustici Wallichii (*Chuan Xiong*), Radix Angelicae Sinensis (*Dang Gui*), Radix Albus Paeoniae Lactiflorae (*Bai Shao*), Rhizoma Atractylodis Macrocephalae (*Bai Zhu*), Sclerotium Poriae Cocos (*Fu Ling*), mix-fried Radix Glycyrrhizae (*Gan Cao*), Herba Menthae Haplocalycis (*Bo He*), uncooked Rhizoma Zingiberis (*Sheng Jiang*), Radix Puerariae (*Ge Gen*), Ramulus Uncariae Cum Uncis (*Gou Teng*)

Liver yang ascendant hyperactivity

Main symptoms: One-sided headache or pain on the top of the head preceding or accompanying the onset of the menses, splitting headache, red eyes, insomnia, vexation, easily angered, distention and pain in the chest, rib-sides, and breast, dizziness and tinnitus, a bitter taste in the mouth, dry mouth, a red facial complexion, a red tongue and/or inflated tongue rims, and a bowstring pulse

Treatment principles: Level or calm the liver and subdue yang, extinguish wind and stop pain

Guiding formulas:

1. *Tian Ma Gou Teng Yin* (Gastrodia & Uncaria Drink)

Ingredients: Rhizoma Gastrodiae Elatae (*Tian Ma*), Ramulus Uncariae Cum Uncis (*Gou Teng*), Concha Haliotidis (*Shi Jue Ming*), Ramulus Loranthi Seu Visci (*Sang Ji Sheng*), Cortex Eucommiae Ulmoidis (*Du Zhong*), Radix Cyathulae Officinalis (*Chuan Niu Xi*), Fructus Gardeniae Jasminoidis (*Zhi Zi*), Radix Scutellariae Baicalensis (*Huang Qin*), Herba Leonuri Heterophylli (*Yi Mu Cao*), Caulis Polygoni Multiflori (*Ye Jiao Teng*), Sclerotium Parardicis Poriae Cocos (*Fu Shen*)

This formula clears heat from the liver, extinguishes wind, heavily subdues liver yang, leads ministerial fire back to its lower source, and also nourishes liver blood and kidney yin. Therefore, it is very useful for treating the changeable mixture of these elements causing headache and dizziness.

2. Unnamed formula from Ou-yang Yi's *A Handbook of Differential Diagnosis with Key Signs & Symptoms, Therapeutic Principles, and Guiding Prescriptions*

Ingredients: Uncooked Radix Rehmanniae (*Sheng Di*), Radix Albus Paeoniae Lactiflorae (*Bai Shao*), Cortex Radicis Moutan (*Dan Pi*), Ramulus Uncariae Cum Uncis (*Gou Teng*), Concha Haliotidis (*Shi Jue Ming*), Folium Ilicis Latifoliae (*Ku Ding Cha*)

This formula clears heat and cools the blood, heavily subdues yang and extinguishes wind.

3. *Si Wu Tang Jia Wei* (Four Materials Decoction with Added Flavors)

Ingredients: Radix Angelicae Sinensis (*Dang Gui*), Radix Albus Paeoniae Lactiflorae (*Bai Shao*), cooked Radix Rehmanniae (*Shu Di*), Radix Ligustici Wallichii (*Chuan Xiong*), Fructus Mori Albi (*Sang Shen*), Fructus Viticis (*Man Jing Zi*), Scapus Eriocaulonis Buergeriani (*Gu Jing Zi*)

This formula supplements liver blood at the same time as it clears liver heat.

4. *Zhen Gan Xi Feng Tang Jia Jian* (Settle the Liver & Extinguish Wind Decoction with Additions & Subtractions)

Ingredients: Radix Achyranthis Bidentatae (*Huai Niu Xi*), Haemititum (*Dai Zhe Shi*), Os Draconis (*Long Gu*), Concha Ostreae (*Mu Li*), Plastrum Testudinis (*Gui Ban*), Radix Albus Paeoniae Lactiflorae (*Bai Shao*), Radix Scrophulariae Ningpoensis (*Xuan Shen*), Tuber Asparagi Cochinensis (*Tian Dong*), Fructus Meliae Toosendan (*Chuan Lian Zi*), Fructus

Germinatus Hordei Vulgaris (*Mai Ya*), Herba Artemisiae Capillaris (*Yin Chen Hao*), Radix Glycyrrhizae (*Gan Cao*)

This formula subdues yang and drains fire.

Additions: For headache, add Spica Prunellae Vulgaris (*Xia Ku Cao*) and Flos Chrysanthemi Morifolii (*Ju Hua*). For profuse phlegm, add Rhizoma Arisaematis (*Tian Nan Xing*) and Bulbus Fritillariae (*Bei Mu*). If there is concomitant yin vacuity, add cooked Radix Rehmanniae (*Shu Di*) and Fructus Corni Officinalis (*Shan Zhu Yu*). And if there is concomitant heat in the heart, add uncooked Gypsum Fibrosum (*Shi Gao*).

Phlegm turbidity harassing above

Main symptoms: Headache before or during menstruation with dizziness, a heavy sensation in the eyes, inability to open the eyes, nausea, chest oppression, profuse phlegm, white, slimy tongue fur, and a bowstring, slippery pulse

Treatment principles: Fortify the spleen and disinhibit dampness, transform phlegm and extinguish wind

Guiding formulas:

1. *Ban Xia Bai Zhu Tian Ma Wan* (Pinellia, Atractylodes & Gastrodia Pills)

Ingredients: Rhizoma Pinelliae Ternatae (*Ban Xia*), Rhizoma Gastrodiae Elatae (*Tian Ma*), Rhizoma Atractylodis Macrocephalae (*Bai Zhu*), Exocarpium Citri Rubri (*Ju Hong*), Sclerotium Poriae Cocos (*Fu Ling*), Radix Glycyrrhizae (*Gan Cao*), uncooked Rhizoma Zingiberis (*Sheng Jiang*), Fructus Zizyphi Jujubae (*Da Zao*)

Additions: For severe headache, add Fructus Viticis (*Man Jing Zi*). For severe dizziness, add Bombyx Batryaticus (*Jiang Can*) and bile-processed Rhizoma Arisaematis (*Dan Nan Xing*). For fatigue, add Radix Codonopsitis Pilosulae (*Dang Shen*) and Radix Astragali Membranacei (*Huang Qi*).

2. *Ban Xia Bai Zhu Tian Ma Tang Jia Wei* (Pinellia, Atractylodes & Gastrodia Decoction with Added Flavors)

Ingredients: Rhizoma Pinelliae Ternatae (*Ban Xia*), Sclerotium Poriae Cocos (*Fu Ling*), Exocarpium Citri Rubri (*Ju Hong*), Rhizoma Atractylodis Macrocephalae (*Bai Zhu*), Rhizoma Gastrodiae Elatae (*Tian Ma*), Fructus Gardeniae Jasminodis (*Shan Zhi*), Radix Ligustici Wallichii (*Chuan Xiong*), Radix Glycyrrhizae (*Gan Cao*), uncooked Rhizoma Zingiberis (*Sheng Jiang*), Fructus Zizyphi Jujubae (*Da Zao*)

This formula clears depressive heat in the liver as a minor element and quickens the blood in the head.

Depressive heat ascends phlegm

Main symptoms: Intolerable headache and dizziness preceding or at the onset of menstruation, red eyes, tinnitus, a bitter taste in the mouth, vexatious heat, insomnia, chest oppression, yellow, slimy tongue fur, and a slippery, bowstring, rapid pulse

This pattern is the same as the above except complicated by depressive heat.

Treatment principles: Clear heat and resolve depression, downbear counterflow and transform phlegm

Guiding formula: *Huang Lian Wen Dan Tang* (Coptis Warm the Gallbladder Decoction)

Ingredients: Rhizoma Coptidis Chinensis (*Huang Lian*), Rhizoma Pinelliae Ternatae (*Ban Xia*), Caulis Bambusae In Taeniis (*Zhu Ru*), Fructus Immaturus Citri Aurantii (*Zhi Shi*), Pericarpium Citri Reticulatae (*Chen Pi*), Sclerotium Poriae Cocos (*Fu Ling*), Radix Glycyrrhizae (*Gan Cao*), uncooked Rhizoma Zingiberis (*Sheng Jiang*)

Qi & blood vacuity

Main symptoms: Headache which begins towards the latter part of the menses or directly afterward, pain not too intense but persistent, unrelieved, and worsened by fatigue, a sallow, yellow or pale facial complexion, dizziness, generalized fatigue, shortness of breath, heart palpitations, possible loss of appetite, a pale tongue with teeth marks on its edges and thin, white fur, and a fine, weak or big, weak pulse

In this pattern, the headache is caused by blood vacuity not nourishing the sea of marrow. However, the pattern is called qi and blood vacuity because a number of the other, generalized signs and symptoms have to do with qi vacuity, not blood vacuity.

Treatment principles: Supplement the qi and nourish the blood

Guiding formulas:

1. *Ba Zhen Tang* (Eight Pearls Decoction)

Ingredients: Radix Panacis Ginseng (*Ren Shen*), Rhizoma Atractylodis Macrocephalae (*Bai Zhu*), Sclerotium Poriae Cocos (*Fu Ling*), mix-fried Radix Glycyrrhizae (*Gan Cao*), cooked Radix Rehmanniae (*Shu Di*), Radix Angelicae Sinensis (*Dang Gui*), Radix Albus Paeoniae

Lactiflorae (*Bai Shao*), Radix Ligustici Wallichii (*Chuan Xiong*), uncooked Rhizoma Zingiberis (*Sheng Jiang*), Fructus Zizyphi Jujubae (*Da Zao*)

2. *Ba Zhen Tang Jia Wei* (Eight Pearls Decoction with Added Flavors)

Ingredients: Radix Angelicae Sinensis (*Dang Gui*), Radix Ligustici Wallichii (*Chuan Xiong*), cooked Radix Rehmanniae (*Shu Di*), Radix Albus Paeoniae Lactiflorae (*Bai Shao*), Radix Codonopsitis Pilosulae (*Dang Shen*), Sclerotium Poriae Cocos (*Fu Ling*), Rhizoma Atractylodis Macrocephalae (*Bai Zhu*), Radix Glycyrrhizae (*Gan Cao*), Fructus Lycii Chinensis (*Gou Qi Zi*), Ramulus Uncariae Cum Uncis (*Gou Teng*)

3. *Gui Pi Tang* (Restore the Spleen Decoction)

Ingredients: Radix Panacis Ginseng (*Ren Shen*), Radix Astragali Membranacei (*Huang Qi*), Arillus Euphoriae Longanae (*Long Yan Rou*), Radix Angelicae Sinensis (*Dang Gui*), Rhizoma Atractylodis Macrocephalae (*Bai Zhu*), Radix Auklandiae Lappae (*Mu Xiang*), Sclerotium Poriae Cocos (*Fu Ling*), Radix Polygalae Tenuifoliae (*Yuan Zhi*), Semen Zizyphi Spinosae (*Suan Zao Ren*), Fructus Zizyphi Jujubae (*Da Zao*), mix-fried Radix Glycyrrhizae (*Gan Cao*), uncooked Rhizoma Zingiberis (*Sheng Jiang*)

This formula should be used instead of the preceding one when qi and blood vacuity affect the heart as well as the spleen.

Central qi vacuity

Main symptoms: Dull, persistent headache towards the end of the menses or directly after, orthostatic hypotension, general fatigue, a dragging sensation in the lower abdomen, shortness of breath, heart palpitations, alleviation of symptoms with rest and aggravation with prolonged standing or fatigue, a pale tongue with thin, white fur, and a short or large, weak pulse

This pattern is different from the preceding one in that there are no prominent signs and symptoms of blood vacuity, only qi vacuity.

Treatment principles: Supplement the spleen and boost the qi

Guiding formula: *Bu Zhong Yi Qi Tang* (Supplement the Center & Boost the Qi Decoction)

Ingredients: Radix Astragali Membranacei (*Huang Qi*), Radix Panacis Ginseng (*Ren Shen*), Rhizoma Atractylodis Macrocephalae (*Bai Zhu*), Radix Angelicae Sinensis (*Dang*

Gui), Rhizoma Cimicifugae (*Sheng Ma*), Radix Bupleuri (*Chai Hu*), Pericarpium Citri Reticulatae (*Chen Pi*), mix-fried Radix Glycyrrhizae (*Gan Cao*)

Additions: For headache, add Radix Et Rhizoma Ligustici Sinensis (*Gao Ben*). For heaviness of the head, add Fructus Viticis (*Man Jing Zi*).

Liver-kidney yin vacuity

Main symptoms: Headache at the end of menstruation in yin vacuous women or before or after the menses in premenopausal women, dizziness, tinnitus, low back and knees soreness and weakness, soreness and pain in the supraorbital region, heat in the center of the hands, feet, and heart, tidal fever, night sweats, flushing of the cheeks, poor memory, heart vexation, insomnia, a red tongue with scanty fur, and a fine, bowstring, possibly rapid pulse

Treatment principles: Supplement the kidneys and nourish yin

Guiding formulas:

1. *Liu Wei Di Huang Wan Jia Wei Yi Hao* (Six Flavors Rehmannia Pills with Added Flavors No. 1)

Ingredients: Cooked Radix Rehmanniae (*Shu Di*), Radix Dioscoreae Oppositae (*Shan Yao*), Fructus Corni Officinalis (*Shan Zhu Yu*), Sclerotium Poriae Cocos (*Fu Ling*), Rhizoma Alismatis (*Ze Xie*), Cortex Radicis Moutan (*Dan Pi*), Radix Albus Paeoniae Lactiflorae (*Bai Shao*), Fructus Ligustri Lucidi (*Nu Zhen Zi*), Fructus Mori Albi (*Sang Shen*)

This formula clears vacuity heat at the same time as it supplements the liver and kidneys and nourishes the blood.

2. *Liu Wei Di Huang Wan Jia Wei Er Hao* (Six Flavors Rehmannia Pills with Added Flavors No. 2)

Ingredients: Cooked Radix Rehmanniae (*Shu Di*), Fructus Corni Officinalis (*Shan Zhu Yu*), Radix Dioscoreae Oppositae (*Shan Yao*), Sclerotium Poriae Cocos (*Fu Ling*), Cortex Radicis Moutan (*Dan Pi*), Rhizoma Alismatis (*Ze Xie*), Flos Chrysanthemi Morifolii (*Ju Hua*), Fructus Tribuli Terrestris (*Bai Ji Li*)

This formula clears specifically liver heat at the same time as it nourishes yin. As a minor motif, it also courses the liver.

3. *Da Bu Yuan Jian* (Greatly Supplement the Source Decoction)

Ingredients: Radix Panacis Ginseng (*Ren Shen*), Radix Dioscoreae Oppositae (*Shan Yao*), cooked Radix Rehmanniae (*Shu Di*), Cortex Eucommiae Ulmoidis (*Du Zhong*), Radix Angelicae Sinensis (*Dang Gui*), Fructus Corni Officinalis (*Shan Zhu Yu*), Fructus Lycii Chinensis (*Gou Qi*), mix-fried Radix Glycyrrhizae (*Gan Cao*)

This formula, from Zhang Jing-yue's *Jing Yue Quan Shu ([Zhang] Jing-yue's Complete Book),* supplements the liver and kidneys. It does not directly clear heat. However, if yin is nourished, vacuity heat is automatically controlled.

Blood stasis

Main symptoms: Headache with localized pricking or sharp pain, tends to be worse at night, possible history of trauma in the affected area, begins typically before or at the onset of the menses. If there is blood stasis in the uterus, there will also tend to be painful menstruation, dark, clotty blood, possible purplish, engorged veins on the abdomen, low back, or back of the legs, a purplish or darkish tongue or static spots or macules on the tongue, and a deep, bowstring, choppy pulse

Treatment principles: Quicken the blood and transform stasis, free the flow of the network vessels and stop pain

Guiding formulas:

1. *Xue Fu Zhu Yu Tang* (Blood Mansion Dispel Stasis Decoction)

Ingredients: Semen Pruni Persicae (*Tao Ren*), Flos Carthami Tinctorii (*Hong Hua*), Radix Angelicae Sinensis (*Dang Gui*), Radix Ligustici Wallichii (*Chuan Xiong*), Radix Rubrus Paeoniae Lactiflorae (*Chi Shao*), Radix Cyathulae Officinalis (*Chuan Niu Xi*), Radix Bupleuri (*Chai Hu*), Radix Platycodi Grandiflori (*Jie Geng*), Fructus Citri Aurantii (*Zhi Ke*), uncooked Radix Rehmanniae (*Sheng Di*), Radix Glycyrrhizae (*Gan Cao*)

This formula is built upon the basis of *Tao Ren Si Wu Tang* (Persica & Carthamus Four Materials Decoction).

Additions: If there is blood stasis in the network vessels, add Lumbricus (*Di Long*) and Buthus Martensi (*Quan Xie*) to free the flow of the network vessels and extinguish wind.

443

2. *Tao He Cheng Qi Tang* (Persica Order the Qi Decoction)

Ingredients: Semen Pruni Persicae (*Tao Ren*), Ramulus Cinnamomi Cassiae (*Gui Zhi*), Radix Et Rhizoma Rhei (*Da Huang*), Mirabilitum (*Mang Xiao*), mix-fried Radix - Glycyrrhizae (*Gan Cao*)

This formula is appropriate for blood stasis accompanied by constipation. It can downbear ascendant yang by freeing the flow of the stools.

Additions: If there is pronounced qi stagnation, add Rhizoma Cyperi Rotundi (*Xiang Fu*) and Pericarpium Citri Reticulatae Viride (*Qing Pi*). If there is more severe or persistent blood stasis, add Flos Carthami Tinctorii (*Hong Hua*) and Radix Angelicae Sinensis (*Dang Gui*). If there is menstrual pain, add Rhizoma Corydalis Yanhusuo (*Yan Hu Suo*), Pollen Typhae (*Sheng Pu Huang*), and Feces Trogopterori Seu Pteromi (*Wu Ling Zhi*).

3. *Tao Hong Si Wu Tang Jia Wei* (Persica & Carthamus Four Materials Decoction with Added Flavors)

Ingredients: Semen Pruni Persicae (*Tao Ren*), Flos Carthami Tinctorii (*Hong Hua*), Radix Angelicae Sinensis (*Dang Gui*), Radix Ligustici Wallichii (*Chuan Xiong*), uncooked Radix Rehmanniae (*Sheng Di*), Radix Rubrus & Albus Paeoniae Lactiflorae (*Chi Bai Shao*), Radix Achyranthis Bidentatae (*Niu Xi*), Fructus Citri Aurantii (*Zhi Ke*), Radix Bupleuri (*Chai Hu*), Radix Puerariae (*Ge Gen*)

Discussion

The main cause of headache before or at the onset of menstruation is ascension of liver yang. Although other patterns are discriminated and treatment principles and guiding formulas given for these, most often in clinical practice, liver yang/fire/wind is complicated by phlegm, dampness, and/or blood stasis. Therefore, formulas for the treatment of real life patients tend to be highly modified. These modifications can be made based on discrimination of qi and blood patterns, discrimination of fluids and humors patterns, discrimination of disease causation patterns, and discrimination of channel and network vessel patterns.

In particular, one should add ingredients to a guiding formula which lead the other medicinals into the affected channel. For instance, for *tai yang* headache where the pain is occipital and nuchal, add Radix Et Rhizoma Ligustici Sinensis (*Gao Ben*). For pain in the *yang ming*, add Radix Angelicae Dahuricae (*Bai Zhi*). For pain in the temples or *shao yang*, add either or both Radix Ligustici Wallichii (*Chuan Xiong*) and Radix Bupleuri (*Chai Hu*). Some practitioners believe that if the pain is left-sided one should add Bupleurum, while if the pain is on the right side, one should add Ligusticum.

Root & branch

There are two phases in the treatment of menstrual movement headache. There is the first aid or branch treatment of the headache itself during its occurrence at the time of menstruation. There is also the preventive, root treatment of the disease mechanisms causing the headache. This treatment is given prior to the expected time of the headache in order to head it off or diminish its intensity. In some cases, such as phlegm dampness, blood stasis, qi and/or blood vacuity, and yin vacuity, the same formula may be used during both phases of treatment. In other cases, one may choose to employ certain treatment principles at one stage of the cycle and others at another stage. For instance, in cases where there is both blood vacuity and liver heat, one might primarily nourish the blood in the week after the menses and then emphasize resolving depression and clearing heat in the week before menstruation.

There are two formulas for first aid use which can be used for migrainous headaches which are particularly effective. The first is *Chuan Xiong Cha Tiao San* (Ligusticum & Tea Regulating Powder).[28] This formula comes as a patent medicine in the form of pills. It is composed of a number of exterior-resolving medicinals which each relieve a different channel traversing the head. This formula specifically resolves the exterior and attempts to out-thrust yang qi rising up into the bony box of the cranium. These pills are taken with tea (*Camellia thea*) to increase their dispersing ability. Women suffering from a replete species of migraine or menstrual movement headache in turn due to an accumulation and then up-flushing of yang qi can take these pills at the first sign of an impending headache.

If, however, the woman is prone to nausea and vomiting during a migrainous attack, I suggest using *Wu Zhu Yu Tang Jia Wei* (Evodia Decoction with Added Flavors). This formula is composed of Fructus Evodiae Rutecarpae (*Wu Zhu Yu*), Radix Panacis Ginseng (*Ren Shen*) or Radix Codonopsitis Pilosulae (*Dang Shen*), uncooked Rhizoma Zingiberis (*Sheng Jiang*), Fructus Zizyphi Jujubae (*Da Zao*), Radix Et Rhizoma Ligustici Sinensis (*Gao Ben*), Radix Angelicae Dahiricae (*Bai Zhi*), Radix Ligustici Wallichii (*Chuan Xiong*), and Radix Angelicae Sinensis (*Dang Gui*). A packet of this formula can be kept by the patient and made up in 20 minutes if she feels a headache coming on accompanied by nau-

---

[28] The ingredients in these pills are: Radix Ligustici Wallichii (*Chuan Xiong*), Radix Et Rhizoma Notopterygii (*Qiang Huo*), Radix Angelicae Dahuricae (*Bai Zhu*), Herba Asari Cum Radice (*Xi Xin*), Herba Schizonepetae Tenuifoliae (*Jing Jie*), Radix Ledebouriellae Divaricatae (*Fang Feng*), Herba Menthae Haplicalycis (*Bo He*), Radix Glycyrrhizae (*Gan Cao*), Folium Camelliae Theae (*Cha Ye*).

sea. In women whose headaches are diminished by the catharsis of vomiting, this formula is quite effective. This formula is meant to allay nausea but may cause vomiting if a large amount is drunk. This typically ends the migraine at that point.

Acupuncture & moxibustion

Acupuncture can be very effective as a first aid therapy in menstrual movement headaches due to hyperactivity of liver yang. Most replete liver headaches will begin to diminish within 10-15 minutes of insertion of the needles. If there is marked blood stasis, bleeding the affected area with seven star needle is effective. If there is marked dampness and phlegm, yin or blood vacuity, I have not found acupuncture to be particularly effective in terms of the first aid treatment of menstrual movement headache. However, for central qi vacuity headache, moxaing indirectly *Bai Hui* (GV 20) can almost immediately relieve this pain.

Prognosis

Chinese medicine treats most types of menstrual movement headaches quite well. Hyperactive liver yang headaches can usually be eliminated after only one to two menstrual cycles. However, because the etiology of this condition is basically characterological, unless the patient learns more effective coping and relaxation techniques, recidivism is to be expected. Qi and blood vacuity varieties of perimenstrual headaches respond very well to internal Chinese medicinal therapy, and, as long as the patient understands proper diet and gets enough rest, such headaches should not recur after successful treatment. Even phlegm turbidity headaches respond well to TCM treatment. Perimenstrual headaches, however, due to kidney yin insufficiency mixed with phlegm can be recalcitrant to treatment if the cause is congenital. But hyperactive yang-yin vacuity migraines which occur preceding or at menopause are usually quite easily remedied.

If blood stasis complicates a perimenstrual headache and the stasis is not eliminated, this may be the cause of otherwise unexplained failure to respond to therapy. Static blood can be either relatively easy or recalcitrant to treatment depending upon where the stasis is and how deeply it has insinuated itself into the network vessels. If a woman has suffered from migraines on a regular basis for more than six years, a complete cure may not be possible due to damage to the network vessels. Nonetheless, some degree of relief should be expected.

Menstrual Movement Fever

Some women experience fever, flushing, and hot flashes prior to or along with their menses. This is known as menstrual movement fever in Chinese medicine. When it occurs before or at the onset of the menses, it is rarely a modern woman's major complaint but frequently is a component of some women's PMS. When it occurs after menstruation it may be simply referred to as hot flashes which may be a premenopausal woman's major complaint.

Disease causes, disease mechanisms

Wu Qian *et al.* divide menstrual movement fever into external and internal varieties and repletion and vacuity varieties. If the exterior is invaded by an external evil, this can congest the flow of the defensive qi, resulting in fever. As above in discussing both menstrual movement body pain and headache, some women are prone to catching a cold prior to or at the onset of their menses due to the fact that their blood is concentrated in their lower burner. This leaves the upper burner relatively vacuous and open to easy invasion. Han Bai-ling adds that such external invasion may be either a wind cold or wind heat pattern.

If external evils are not successfully expelled from the body, they may lodge internally or half inside/half outside. In this case, they may transform into heat and wither and consume yin. Such retained pathogens may correspond to chronic viral syndromes as described by modern Western medicine. This type of premenstrual fever is often found in women suffering from chronic fatigue immune deficiency syndrome or CFIDS.

If depressive liver heat builds up before menstruation, this may also cause menstrual movement fever. Mostly this is due to emotional stress and frustration which transform into heat. Wu Qian *et al.* also mention that, in such cases, the spleen is also vacuous, but it is not clear from the cryptic lines of the *Yi Zong Jin Jian (The Golden Mirror of Ancestral Medicine)* whether they saw this spleen vacuity as playing a part in this disease mechanism.

The fourth mechanism resulting in menstrual movement fever is vacuity heat due to blood vacuity occurring after the menses. This may be due to excessive blood loss, enduring disease, faulty diet, as in inappropriate and prolonged vegetarianism, and age. If this is found in a premenopausal woman in her late 30s or 40s, it is due to exhaustion and consumption of liver blood and kidney yin. If this is not treated but allowed to persist, this may also become complicated by kidney yang vacuity and upward floating of vacuous yang. In the Chinese literature, the term *chao re* literally means tidal heat or fever and is found in descriptions of yin vacuity often corresponding to perimenopausal syndrome.

447

Han Bai-ling also says that if yang becomes insufficient, this may lead to floating yang or qi vacuity fever. This is due to blood vacuity after the menses and the relationship between the qi and blood. It was Li Dong-yuan in the Yuan dynasty who first emphasized the possibility of a qi vacuity fever.

Further, Han Bai-ling says that menstrual movement fever may be due to food stagnation. If the spleen becomes vacuous prior to the onset of menstruation, it may result in food stagnation. This can be aggravated if the spleen is weak but the stomach hot, in which case the patient may have an excessive appetite and eat too much. Because of the interrelationship between the six depressions and transformative heat, food stagnation often tends to transform into heat.

Yet another cause and mechanism of menstrual movement fever identified by Han Bai-ling is blood stasis. This is also based on the stasis and stagnation tending to cause evil heat. According to Dr. Han, heat in the *yang ming* can cause constipation and this can cause or accompany menstrual movement fever. And finally, Dr. Han says that long-standing water accumulation may also cause menstrual movement fever. In this case, water dampness impedes the free flow of qi before menstruation and this transforms into damp heat.

Treatment based on pattern discrimination

Cold damage

Main symptoms: Fever just before or at the onset of menstruation, fear of cold, no sweating, body aches, cough, sneezing, stuffy nose, clear, thin nasal discharge, greenish-bluish white facial complexion, thin, white tongue fur, and a floating, tight pulse

Treatment principles: Dispel wind, scatter cold, and resolve the exterior

Guiding formulas:

1. *Gui Zhi Si Wu Tang* (Cinnamon Twigs Four Materials Decoction)

Ingredients: Ramulus Cinnamomi Cassiae (*Gui Zhi*), Radix Angelicae Sinensis (*Dang Gui*), Radix Albus Paeoniae Lactiflorae (*Bai Shao*), cooked Radix Rehmanniae (*Shu Di*), Radix Ligustici Wallichii (*Chuan Xiong*), Radix Glycyrrhizae (*Gan Cao*)

Additions: One may also add uncooked Rhizoma Zingiberis (*Sheng Jiang*) and Fructus Zizyphi Jujubae (*Da Zao*) to further harmonize the constructive and defensive.

2. *Xing Su Si Wu Tang* (Armeniaca & Perilla Four Materials Decoction)

Ingredients: Radix Angelicae Sinensis (*Dang Gui*), Radix Albus Paeoniae Lactiflorae (*Bai Shao*), uncooked Radix Rehmanniae (*Sheng Di*), Radix Ligustici Wallichii (*Chuan Xiong*), Semen Pruni Armeniacae (*Xing Ren*), Folium Perillae Frutescentis (*Su Ye*), Fructus Zizyphi Jujubae (*Da Zao*), uncooked Rhizoma Zingiberis (*Sheng Jiang*)

Wind heat

Main symptoms: Fever, fear of cold, sweating, head and nape of the neck achy and painful, a sore, dry throat, a pale red facial complexion, yellowish white tongue fur, and a floating, rapid pulse

Treatment principles: Clear heat and resolve the exterior

Guiding formula: *Jing Fang Si Wu Tang* (Schizonepeta & Ledebouriella Four Materials Decoction)

Ingredients: Radix Angelicae Sinensis (*Dang Gui*), Radix Albus Paeoniae Lactiflorae (*Bai Shao*), Radix Ligustici Wallichii (*Chuan Xiong*), uncooked Radix Rehmanniae (*Sheng Di*), Herba Schizonepetae Tenuifoliae (*Jing Jie*), Radix Ledebouriellae Divaricatae (*Fang Feng*)

Retained evils, internal heat

Main symptoms: Fever before the menses, tidal fever, night sweats, menstruation ahead of schedule, heat in the center of the hands, feet, and heart, flushed cheeks, heart palpitations and vexation, tinnitus, dizziness, lumbar soreness, a red tongue with scanty fur, and a fine, bowstring, rapid or surging, rapid pulse

Treatment principles: Clear heat and cool the blood, nourish yin and recede fever

Guiding formulas:

1. *Jia Wei Di Gu Pi Yin* (Added Flavors Cortex Lycii Drink)

Ingredients: Radix Angelicae Sinensis (*Dang Gui*), Radix Albus Paeoniae Lactiflorae (*Bai Shao*), cooked Radix Rehmanniae (*Shu Di*), Radix Ligustici Wallichii (*Chuan Xiong*), Cortex Radicis Moutan (*Dan Pi*), Cortex Radicis Lycii Chinensis (*Di Gu Pi*), Rhizoma Picrorrhizae (*Hu Huang Lian*)

This is the version of *Di Gu Pi Yin* suggested by Wu Qian *et al.* in the *Yi Zong Jin Jian (The Golden Mirror of Ancestral Medicine)*.

2. *Di Gu Pi Yin* (Cortex Lycii Drink)

Ingredients: Cortex Radicis Lycii Chinensis (*Di Gu Pi*), Radix Bupleuri (*Chai Hu*), Rhizoma Anemarrhenae Aspheloidis (*Zhi Mu*), mix-fried Radix Glycyrrhizae (*Gan Cao*), Carapax Amydae Sinensis (*Bie Jia*), Radix Scutellariae Baicalensis (*Huang Qin*), Radix Panacis Ginseng (*Ren Shen*), Sclerotium Poriae Cocos (*Fu Ling*)

This is another *Di Gu Pi Yin* found in *Shen Shi Zun Sheng Shu (Master Shen's Book on Revering Life)*. I have found this formula to be quite useful in treating fever before the menses in women with chronic viral infections. If deep-lying warm evils are lurking in the blood division in a person with a complicating liver qi condition or in the *shao yang* in a person who is yin vacuous, heat accumulating in the liver prior to the onset of menstruation may create an environment conducive to the flourishing of such retained or deep-lying evils.

Additions: For chronic viral infections, add Radix Isatidis Seu Baphicacanthi (*Ban Lan Geng*) and Folium Daqingye (*Da Qing Ye*). For swollen glands and sore throat, add Spica Prunellae Vulgaris (*Xia Ku Cao*), Bulbus Fritillariae (*Bei Mu*), and Radix Scrophulariae Ningpoensis (*Yuan Shen*).

Liver depression transforming heat

Main symptoms: Vexatious heat preceding the menses, red eyes, a red facial complexion, a bitter taste in the mouth, dry throat, breast, rib-side, and abdominal distention and pain, chest oppression, easily angered, possible early or painful menstruation, a red tongue with yellow fur and possible swollen rims, and a bowstring, rapid pulse. If the spleen is also vacuous and there is blood vacuity as well, the tongue may not be particularly red. In this case, the tongue may be a light orangy, brownish red or only the tips and front edges may be red. There may also be teeth marks on the lingual edges and the pulse may also be fine.

Treatment principles: Course the liver and rectify the qi, clear heat and resolve depression

Guiding formula: *Dan Zhi Xiao Yao San* (Moutan & Gardenia Rambling Powder)

Ingredients: Radix Bupleuri (*Chai Hu*), Cortex Radicis Moutan (*Dan Pi*), Fructus Gardeniae Jasminoidis (*Zhi Zi*), Radix Angelicae Sinensis (*Dang Gui*), Radix Albus Paeoniae Lactiflorae (*Bai Shao*), Rhizoma Atractylodis Macrocephalae (*Bai Zhu*), Sclerotium Poriae Cocos (*Fu Ling*), mix-fried Radix Glycyrrhizae (*Zhi Gan Cao*)

Blood vacuity, internal heat

Main symptoms: Feverish feelings after menstruation and especially after excessive blood loss, dry mouth and throat with a desire to drink, night sweats, tidal fever, flushing of the cheeks, dizziness, blurred vision, night blindness, possible heart palpitations, a light red tongue with dry, white fur or lack of moisture, and a fine, rapid; big, weak, and rapid; or surging and rapid pulse

Treatment principles: Nourish the blood and clear vacuity heat

Guiding formulas:

1. *Liu Shen Tang* (Six Divine [*i.e.*, Magic, Medicinals] Decoction)

Ingredients: Radix Astragali Membranacei (*Huang Qi*), Cortex Radicis Lycii Chinensis (*Di Gu Pi*), Radix Angelicae Sinensis (*Dang Gui*), Radix Albus Paeoniae Lactiflorae (*Bai Shao*), cooked Radix Rehmanniae (*Shu Di*), Radix Ligustici Wallichii (*Chuan Xiong*)

This formula is recommended by Wu Qian *et al.* in the *Yi Zong Jin Jian (The Golden Mirror of Ancestral Medicine)* for blood vacuity after menstruation with internal heat.

2. *Liu Wei Di Huang Wan Jia Wei* (Six Flavors Rehmannia Pills with Added Flavors)

Ingredients: Cooked Radix Rehmanniae (*Shu Di*), Radix Angelicae Sinensis (*Dang Gui*), Radix Albus Paeoniae Lactiflorae (*Bai Shao*), Cortex Radicis Moutan (*Dan Pi*), Sclerotium Poriae Cocos (*Fu Ling*), Radix Dioscoreae Oppositae (*Shan Yao*), Fructus Corni Officinalis (*Shan Zhu Yu*), Rhizoma Alismatis (*Ze Xie*), salt-processed Cortex Phellodendri (*Huang Bai*)

Han Bai-ling gives this formula for the treatment of fever after the menses due to yin and blood insufficiency.

Yang qi insufficiency

Main symptoms: Fever and sweating, a puffy, red face, a pale, moist tongue, no thirst, white, slimy tongue fur, loose stools, clear, white urination, and a floating, large, forceless pulse

Treatment principles: Boost the qi and supplement yang, lead fire back to gather at its origin

Guiding formulas:

1. *Ba Wei Di Huang Wan* (Eight Flavors Rehmannia Pills)

Ingredients: Cooked Radix Rehmanniae (*Shu Di*), Radix Dioscoreae Oppositae (*Shan Yao*), Fructus Corni Officinalis (*Shan Zhu Yu*), Sclerotium Poriae Cocos (*Fu Ling*), Cortex Radicis Moutan (*Dan Pi*), Rhizoma Alismatis (*Ze Xie*), Cortex Cinnamomi Cassiae (*Rou Gui*), Radix Lateralis Praeparatus Aconiti Carmichaeli (*Fu Zi*)

Han Bai-ling says this formula is for the treatment of kidney yang blocked menstruation. In this case, yang floats upward instead of descending to promote the menstruation. This is met with in premenopausal women and those suffering from congenital insufficiency.

2. *Ren Shen Yang Rong Tang* (Ginseng Nourish the Constructive Decoction)

Ingredients: Radix Panacis Ginseng (*Ren Shen*), cooked Radix Rehmanniae (*Shu Di*), Rhizoma Atractylodis Macrocephalae (*Bai Zhu*), Radix Angelicae Sinensis (*Dang Gui*), Radix Albus Paeoniae Lactiflorae (*Bai Shao*), Radix Astragali Membranacei (*Huang Qi*), Cortex Cinnamomi Cassiae (*Rou Gui*), Fructus Schisandrae Chinensis (*Wu Wei Zi*), Radix Polygalae Tenuifoliae (*Yuan Zhi*), Pericarpium Citri Reticulatae (*Chen Pi*), mix-fried Radix Glycyrrhizae (*Zhi Gan Cao*), uncooked Rhizoma Zingiberis (*Sheng Jiang*), Fructus Zizyphi Jujubae (*Da Zao*)

Han Bai-ling recommends this formula for the treatment of blood vacuity leading to qi vacuity fever after menstruation.

Food stagnation

Main symptoms: Chest and epigastric vexation and oppression, sour eructations, bad breath, burping and belching, fever and sweating, dry throat with a desire to drink, a yellow face and emaciated flesh, glossy, slimy tongue fur, and a bowstring, slippery pulse

Treatment principles: Fortify the spleen and harmonize the stomach, clear heat and disperse and conduct

Guiding formula: *Xiang Sha Liu Jun Zi Tang* (Auklandia & Amomum Six Gentlemen Decoction)

Ingredients: Radix Auklandiae Lappae (*Mu Xiang*), Fructus Amomi (*Sha Ren*), Radix Codonopsitis Pilosulae (*Dang Shen*), Sclerotium Poriae Cocos (*Fu Ling*), Rhizoma Atractylodis Macrocephalae (*Bai Zhu*), Pericarpium Citri Reticulatae (*Chen Pi*), Rhizoma Pinelliae Ternatae (*Qing Ban Xia*), Radix Glycyrrhizae (*Gan Cao*)

Additions: Han Bai-ling suggests adding a small amount of Radix Et Rhizoma Rhei (*Da Huang*) to clear the intestines.

Blood stasis

Main symptoms: Fever, dizziness, heart vexation, agitation, and disquietude, worse at night, menstruation astringent and scanty, color dark red, lower abdominal pain resisting pressure, a red facial complexion, yellow, dry tongue fur, a bitter taste in the mouth and dry throat, desire for chilled drinks, and a bowstring, slippery pulse

These symptoms indicate heat as well as blood stasis.

Treatment principles: Clear heat and quicken the blood

Guiding formula: *Xue Fu Zhu Yu Tang* **(Blood Mansion Dispel Stasis Decoction)**

Ingredients: Semen Pruni Persicae (*Tao Ren*), Flos Carthami Tinctorii (*Hong Hua*), Radix Angelicae Sinensis (*Dang Gui*), Radix Rubrus Paeoniae Lactiflorae (*Chi Shao*), Radix Ligustici Wallichii (*Chuan Xiong*), uncooked Radix Rehmanniae (*Sheng Di*), Radix Cyathulae Officinalis (*Chuan Niu Xi*), Radix Bupleuri (*Chai Hu*), Fructus Citri Aurantii (*Zhi Ke*), Radix Platycodi Grandiflori (*Jie Geng*), Radix Glycyrrhizae (*Gan Cao*)

As Han Bai-ling remarks, this type of menstrual movement fever typically goes along with qi stagnation and blood stasis painful menstruation.

Stools dry & replete

Main symptoms: Fever and steaming perspiration, abdominal pain and constipation, scanty, reddish urination, profuse, clotty menstruation, color dark red, oral thirst and a desire for chilled drinks, a red facial complexion, yellow tongue fur, and a bowstring, surging, and slippery pulse

Treatment principles: Clear heat and free the flow of the stools

Guiding formula: *Yu Zhu San* **(Stasis-dispelling Powder)**

Ingredients: Radix Angelicae Sinensis (*Dang Gui*), uncooked Radix Rehmanniae (*Sheng Di*), Radix Albus Paeoniae Lactiflorae (*Bai Shao*), Radix Ligustici Wallichii (*Chuan Xiong*), Radix Et Rhizoma Rhei (*Da Huang*), Mirabilitum (*Mang Xiao*), Radix Glycyrrhizae (*Gan Cao*)

Long-standing water

Main symptoms: Heart vexation, fever, oral thirst, inhibited urination, abdominal disten-tion, scanty menstruation, color clear and watery, a pale white facial complexion, a pale, moist tongue, and a bowstring, relaxed (retarded) pulse

Treatment principles: Move water and disinhibit urination

Guiding formula: *Wu Ling San* **(Five [Ingredients] Poria Powder)**

Ingredients: Ramulus Cinnamomi Cassiae (*Gui Zhi*), Sclerotium Poriae Cocos (*Fu Ling*), Rhizoma Alismatis (*Ze Xie*), Rhizoma Atractylodis Macrocephalae (*Bai Zhu*), Sclerotium Polypori Umbellati (*Zhu Ling*)

Additions: Han Bai-ling suggests adding Semen Plantaginis (*Che Qian Zi*) and Talcum (*Hua Shi*) to aid in disinhibiting urination.

Discussion

Modern TCM gynecology texts do not list menstrual movement fever as a disease category. However, with the growing incidence of chronic viral infections in the modern world, some knowledge of this disease category is important. Many women suffering from CFIDS experience a worsening or aggravation of their signs and symptoms before or during their menstruation. In treating women with CFIDS, I find it very important to regulate the menses and treat any TCM categories of menstrual disease. If one is able to regulate the menses and eliminate any menstrual disease, this means that the woman's endocrine system has been brought back into balance.

Prognosis

If a woman experiences fever due to the common cold accompanying her menstruation as an episodic complaint and if the pulse in the inch position is floating, this should be treated as one would a common cold normally but with the addition of *Si Wu Tang* (Four Materials Decoction) to nourish the constructive and blood and support the righteous. This may not mean necessarily using *Gui Zhi Si Wu Tang* (Cinnamon Twig Four Materials Decoction), *Ma Huang Si Wu Tang* (Ephedra Four Materials Decoction), etc. However, there should be little difficulty in controlling and speeding up the course of the cold.

If, on the other hand, the woman develops feverish symptoms before each menstruation and has a history of chronic fatigue, a retained evil should be suspected. Even though the symptoms may look like a common cold and that may be how the patient herself describes her condition, usually in this case there are attendant signs and symptoms pointing to yin vacuity and internal heat accompanied by qi stagnation. In this case, one should try to harmonize the *shao yang* division while simultaneously clearing heat and nourishing yin as necessary. TCM can definitely help shorten the course of chronic viral infections, such as CFIDS, but still the course of treatment will be relatively protracted with ups and downs. Typically, there will be periods of improvement followed by acute exacerbations and regressions. However, when one looks at several months of treatment, overall improvement should be noted.

Depressive heat causing vexatious heat, red eyes, and flushing is sometimes difficult to distinguish from the foregoing viral condition. Nonetheless its course and progress are different. In the case of retained evils, there are usually such symptoms of immune activity as swollen glands and lymph node enlargement. Also, the feverish sensations tend to precede every menses regardless of the patient's mood or stress. In the case of depressive heat, this is usually caused by stress and frustration and, therefore, women tend to experience this only in months when they are under special stress. If the woman can recognize and change the stressors in her life as well as learn how to relax around those which she cannot change, depressive heat can usually be eliminated quickly by TCM therapy. In this case, a tendency to liver qi will typically persist, but this does not have to transform into evil heat.

Blood vacuity, internal heat after menstruation is most often encountered in women in their late 30s and 40s who are moving towards menopause. If such vacuity heat is not treated, it will only consume yin essence all the more quickly, thus hastening menopause itself. By treating vacuity heat symptoms after the menses, liver blood and kidney yin are supplemented. Since aging is primarily the consumption of yin substance by yang function, such supplementation of true yin is equivalent to slowing down the aging process. This cannot but have a beneficial effect on the woman's entire health and well being. Typically, such vacuity heat symptoms after the menses can be brought under control with Chinese medicinals within one to two cycles.

Qi and/or yang vacuity fever is mostly seen in premenopausal women or in women who have lost an excessive amount of blood. In both cases, treatment with Chinese medicinals is very effective. Qi vacuity fever responds to treatment almost immediately.

Food stagnation menstrual movement fever is easy to treat. Likewise, blood stasis menstrual movement fever is also usually easy to treat and responds very quickly to therapy. With heat in the *yang ming* causing constipation, all one has to do is free the flow of the stools with cold precipitation to recede this fever. And long-standing accumulation of water dampness also tends to respond quickly to therapy as soon as urination is disinhibited. All of these last four types of menstrual movement fever are species of transformative heat from various of the six depressions. If one resolves the depression and disperses the stagnation, the root of evil heat transformation is cut.

Menstrual Movement Vertigo & Dizziness

Some women experience dizziness and vertigo during their premenstruum. This is referred to as menstrual movement dizziness and vertigo in the Chinese gynecological literature.

Disease causes, disease mechanisms

If the spleen becomes weak during the premenstruum due to any reason, qi vacuity may fall downward and fail to upbear clear yang. Conversely, blood vacuity may not be able to construct and nourish the brain. If blood vacuity is more severe or due to congenital insufficiency, there may be liver-kidney yin vacuity not filling the sea of marrow. Any of the foregoing insufficiencies may result in dizziness and vertigo. In addition, spleen vacuity preceding or accompanying the menstruation may give rise to the engenderment of phlegm. This phlegm may then block the clear orifices, causing dizziness and vertigo.

Treatment according to pattern discrimination

Central qi fall

Main symptoms: Premenstrual dizziness, lassitude of the spirit, fatigue, lack of strength, a pale tongue with thin fur, and a fine, relaxed (retarded) pulse

Treatment principles: Boost the qi and nourish the blood

Guiding formula: *Sheng Yu Tang Jia Wei* (Sage-like Curing Decoction with Added Flavors)

Ingredients: Radix Astragali Membranacei (*Huang Qi*), Radix Codonopsitis Pilosulae (*Dang Shen*), Radix Angelicae Sinensis (*Dang Gui*), Radix Ligustici Wallichii (*Chuan Xiong*), cooked Radix Rehmanniae (*Shu Di*), Radix Albus Paeoniae Lactiflorae (*Bai Shao*), Fructus Corni Officinalis (*Shan Yu Rou*), Flos Chrysanthemi Morifolii (*Ju Hua*), Radix Salviae Miltiorrhizae (*Dan Shen*), Rhizoma Gastrodiae Elatae (*Tian Ma*)

Blood Vacuity

Main symptoms: During or after menstruation, there is dizziness and vertigo. The menses are scanty, pale colored, and watery. The facial complexion is sallow yellow or somber white and without luster. There is loss of sleep and insomnia, a pale tongue with thin, white fur, and a fine, weak pulse

Treatment principles: Boost the spleen and nourish the blood

Although these treatment principles appear the same as those for the pattern above, the signs and symptoms in this pattern primarily have to do with blood vacuity. In this case, the spleen is supplemented because it is the latter heaven source of blood engenderment.

Guiding formulas:

1. *Gui Pi Tang Jia Jian* (Restore the Spleen Decoction with Additions & Subtractions)

Ingredients: Radix Panacis Ginseng (*Ren Shen*), Radix Astragali Membranacei (*Huang Qi*), Radix Angelicae Sinensis (*Dang Gui*), Rhizoma Atractylodis Macrocephalae (*Bai Zhu*), Sclerotium Poriae Cocos (*Fu Ling*), Arillus Euphoriae Longanae (*Long Yan Rou*), Radix Polygalae Tenuifoliae (*Yuan Zhi*), Semen Zizyphi Spinosae (*Suan Zao Ren*), Radix Auklandiae Lappae (*Mu Xiang*)

Additions: If there is simultaneous lack of strength of the body, shortness of breath, and disinclination to speak, add stir-fried Radix Dioscoreae Oppositae (*Shan Yao*), Rhizoma Cimicifugae (*Sheng Ma*), Radix Bupleuri (*Chai Hu*), and Semen Dolichoris Lablab (*Bai Bian Dou*) to fortify the spleen and boost the qi. If the amount of the menses is scanty and there are heart palpitations and scanty sleep, add Fructus Lycii Chinensis (*Gou Qi*) and processed Radix Polygoni Multiflori (*Shou Wu*) to supplement the blood and nourish the heart.

2. Unnamed formula from *Zhong Yi Fu Ke Zhi Liao Shou Ce (A Handbook of Chinese Medical Gynecological Treatments)*

Ingredients: Radix Astragali Membranacei (*Huang Qi*), Radix Codonopsitis Pilosulae (*Dang Shen*), stir-fried Radix Dioscoreae Oppositae (*Shan Yao*), Radix Angelicae Sinensis (*Dang Gui*), Radix Ligustici Wallichii (*Chuan Xiong*), Radix Albus Paeoniae Lactiflorae (*Bai Shao*), Radix Bupleuri (*Chai Hu*), mix-fried Radix Glycyrrhizae (*Gan Cao*), Fructus Zizyphi Jujubae (*Da Zao*)

Liver-kidney yin vacuity

Main symptoms: Menstrual movement dizziness and vertigo, amount of the menses is excessive, their color is fresh red, vexation and agitation, easy anger, mouth dry, throat parched, possible vexatious heat in the five hearts, steaming bones, tidal fever, a red tongue with yellow fur, and a fine, rapid pulse

Treatment principles: Enrich and supplement the liver and kidneys

Guiding formulas:

1. *Qi Ju Di Huang Tang Jia Wei* (Lycium & Chrysanthemum Rehmannia Decoction with Added Flavors)

Ingredients: Fructus Lycii Chinensis (*Gou Qi Zi*), Flos Chrysanthemi Morifolii (*Ju Hua*), cooked Radix Rehmanniae (*Shu Di*), Fructus Corni Officinalis (*Shan Zhu Yu*), Radix Dioscoreae Oppositae (*Shan Tao*), Sclerotium Poriae Cocos (*Fu Ling*), Cortex Radicis Moutan (*Dan Pi*), Rhizoma Alismatis (*Ze Xie*), Radix Angelicae Sinensis (*Dang Gui*), Radix Albus Paeoniae Lactiflorae (*Bai Shao*), Folium Mori Albi (*Sang Ye*)

2. *Zhen Gan Xi Feng Tang Jia Wei* (Settle the Liver & Extinguish Wind Decoction with Added Flavors)

Ingredients: Radix Achyranthis Bidentatae (*Niu Xi*), uncooked Haemititum (*Zhe Shi*), uncooked Os Draconis (*Long Gu*), uncooked Concha Ostreae (*Mu Li*), uncooked Plastrum Testudinis (*Gui Ban*), uncooked Radix Albus Paeoniae Lactiflorae (*Bai Shao*), Radix Scrophulariae Ningpoensis (*Yuan Shen*), Tuber Asparagai Cochinensis (*Tian Dong*), Fructus Meliae Toosendan (*Chuan Lian Zi*), uncooked Fructus Germinatus Hordei Vulgaris (*Mai Ya*), Herba Artemisiae Capillaris (*Yin Chen*), Radix Glcyyrrhizae (*Gan Cao*), Spica Prunellae Vulgaris (*Xia Ku Cao*), Flos Chrysanthemi Morifolii (*Ju Hua*)

3. Unnamed formula from *Zhong Yi Fu Ke Zhi Liao Shou Ce (A Handbook of Chinese Medical Gynecological Treatments)*

Ingredients: Radix Angelicae Sinensis (*Dang Gui*), cooked Radix Rehmanniae (*Shu Di*), Fructus Lycii Chinensis (*Gou Qi*), Radix Scrophulariae Ningpoensis (*Yuan Shen*), Fructus Corni Officinalis (*Shan Zhu Rou*), Plastrum Testudinis (*Gui Ban*), Rhizoma Anemarrhenae Aspheloidis (*Zhi Mu*), Cortex Radicis Lycii Chinensis (*Di Gu Pi*), Radix Achyranthis Bidentatae (*Niu Xi*), mix-fried Radix Glycyrrhizae (*Gan Cao*)

4. Unnamed formula from *Zhong Yi Fu Ke Zhi Liao Shou Ce (A Handbook of Chinese Medical Gynecological Treatments)*

Ingredients: Cooked Radix Rehmanniae (*Shu Di*), Radix Angelicae Sinensis (*Dang Gui*), Radix Ligustici Wallichii (*Chuan Xiong*), Radix Albus Paeoniae Lactiflorae (*Bai Shao*), Rhizoma Gastrodiae Elatae (*Tian Ma*), Ramulus Uncariae Cum Uncis (*Gou Teng*), Folium Mori Albi (*Sang Ye*), Flos Chrysanthemi Morifolii (*Ju Hua*), uncooked Radix Glycyrrhizae (*Gan Cao*)

Spleen vacuity mixed with phlegm

Main symptoms: Before, during, or after menstruation, there is dizziness and a heavy head, chest oppression, nausea, scanty appetite, excessive sleep, inhibited menstrual movement which is thick and pasty, pale colored or darkish red, slimy, white tongue fur, and a slippery, soggy pulse

Treatment principles: Fortify the spleen, transform dampness, and eliminate phlegm

Guiding formulas:

1. *Ban Xia Bai Zhu Tian Ma Tang Jia Wei* (Pinellia, Atractylodes & Gastrodia Decoction with Added Flavors)

Ingredients: Rhizoma Pinelliae Ternatae (*Ban Xia*), Rhizoma Atractylodis Macrocephalae (*Bai Zhu*), Rhizoma Gastrodiae Elatae (*Tian Ma*), Pericarpium Citri Reticulatae (*Chen Pi*), Sclerotium Poriae Cocos (*Fu Ling*), Radix Glycyrrhizae (*Gan Cao*), uncooked Rhizoma Zingiberis (*Sheng Jiang*), Fructus Zizyphi Jujubae (*Da Zao*), Fructus Viticis (*Man Jing Zi*), Radix Salviae Miltiorrhizae (*Dan Shen*), Herba Leonuri Heterophylli (*Yi Mu Cao*), Semen Coicis Lachryma-jobi (*Yi Yi Ren*)

2. Unnamed formula from *Zhong Yi Fu Ke Zhi Liao Shou Ce* (*A Handbook of Chinese Medical Gynecological Treatments*)

Ingredients: Rhizoma Atractylodis (*Cang Zhu*), Pericarpium Citri Reticulatae (*Chen Pi*), Rhizoma Pinelliae Ternatae (*Ban Xia*), Rhizoma Gastrodiae Elatae (*Tian Ma*), Ramulus Uncariae Cum Uncis (*Gou Teng*), Radix Ligustici Wallichii (*Chuan Xiong*), Radix Achyranthis Bidentatae (*Niu Xi*), Fructus Cardomomi (*Bai Kou Ren*), Semen Raphani Sativi (*Lai Fu Zi*)

3. Unnamed formula from *Zhong Yi Fu Ke Zhi Liao Shou Ce* (*A Handbook of Chinese Medical Gynecological Treatments*)

Ingredients: Talcum (*Hua Shi*), Sclerotium Poriae Cocos (*Fu Ling*), Sclerotium Polypori Umbellati (*Zhu Ling*), Rhizoma Pinelliae Ternatae (*Ban Xia*), Rhizoma Atractylodis (*Cang Zhu*), Semen Pruni Persicae (*Tao Ren*), Herba Leonuri Heterophylli (*Yi Mu Cao*)

Menstrual Movement Edema

Edematous swelling of the hands, feet, and/or face before menstruation is called menstrual movement superficial or floating edema. In Chinese medicine, breast abdominal distention during the premenstruum are not considered species of edema but are seen as symptoms of distention, *i.e.*, qi stagnation and accumulation.

Disease causes, disease mechanisms

Devitalized spleen yang may result in loss of normalcy of movement and transformation. Thus water dampness spills over into the muscles and skin. Commonly, spleen vacuity premenstrually presents with or is due to liver depression. In theory, external invasion taking advantage of premenstrual vacuity and thus disturbing the lungs' diffusion and downbearing and governance of the water passageways might cause premenstrual edema, but I have never seen this in clinical practice.

Treatment based on pattern discrimination

Devitalized spleen yang

Main symptoms: Several days before the menses, there is superficial edema of the face reaching to the four limbs. There is also lassitude of the spirit, fatigue, lack of strength, scanty urination, slimy, glossy, white tongue fur, and a bowstring, fine or deep, weak pulse.

Treatment principles: Fortify the spleen, transform the qi, and move water

Guiding formula: *Wu Ling San Jia Wu Pi Yin Jia Jian* **(Five [Ingredients] Poriae Powder plus Five Skins Drink with Additions & Subtractions)**

Ingredients: Ramulus Cinnamomi Cassiae (*Gui Zhi*), Fructus Amomi (*Sha Ren*), Rhizoma Atractylodis Macrocephalae (*Bai Zhu*), Sclerotium Polypori Umbellati (*Zhu Ling*), Cortex Sclerotii Poriae Cocos (*Fu Ling Pi*), Semen Plantaginis (*Che Qian Zi*), Pericarpium Citri Reticulatae (*Chen Pi*), Cortex Rhizomatis Zingiberis (*Jiang Pi*), Pericarpium Arecae Catechu (*Da Fu Pi*), Rhizoma Sparganii (*San Leng*), Rhizoma Dioscoreae Hypoglaucae (*Bi Xie*)

Due to its inclusion of Sparganium, this formula appears to assume there is severe blood stasis complicating such menstrual movement edema. If there are no signs and symptoms of such blood stasis, this ingredient should be removed so as not to damage the correct qi.

Additions: For edema of the upper body, add Radix Ledebouriellae Divaricatae (*Fang Feng*) and Radix Et Rhzioma Notopterygium (*Qiang Huo*). For edema of the lower body, add Radix Stephaniae Tetrandrae (*Fang Ji*) and Rhizoma Alismatis (*Ze Xie*).

Spleen vacuity-liver depression

Main symptoms: A sallow yellow facial complexion, swollen and distended four extremities, possible generalized edema, chest and rib-side propping distention, epigastric and abdominal fullness and oppression, non-freely flowing menstrual movement, a normal tongue with thin, slimy fur, and a deep, bowstring pulse

Treatment principles: Fortify the spleen and regulate the liver, disinhibit the qi and eliminate dampness

Guiding formula: *Dao Zhi Tong Jing Tang Jia Wei* **(Abduct Stagnation & Free the Flow of the Channels [or Menses] Decoction with Added Flavors)**

Ingredients: Radix Angelicae Sinensis (*Dang Gui*), Radix Ligustici Wallichii (*Chuan Xiong*), Rhizoma Cyperi Rotundi (*Xiang Fu*), Radix Auklandiae Lappae (*Mu Xiang*), Pericarpium Citri Reticulatae (*Chen Pi*), Rhizoma Atractylodis Macrocephalae (*Bai Zhu*), Sclerotium Poriae Cocos (*Fu Ling*), Cortex Radicis Mori Albi (*Sang Bai Pi*)

Additions: If there is inhibited urination with lower limb heaviness, add Semen Benincasae Hispidae (*Dong Kui Zi*) and Semen Plantiginis (*Che Qian Zi*). If distention of the limbs and body is severe, add Caulis Aristolochiae Debilis (*Tian Xian Teng*), Pericarpium Citri Reticulatae Viride (*Qing Pi*), and Pericarpium Arecae Catechu (*Da Fu Pi*). If the menstrual movement is not freely flowing and there is lower abdominal distention, add Herba Leonuri Heterophylli (*Yi Mu Cao*), Radix Rubrus Paeoniae Lactiflorae (*Chi Shao*), and Radix Linderae Strychnifoliae (*Wu Yao*).

Menstrual Movement Oral *Gan*

Canker sores and sores on the tongue occurring prior to menstruation are called menstrual movement oral *gan*. This includes recurrent cold sores during the premenstruum.

Disease causes, disease mechanisms

Before the menses, yin blood pours downward to the *chong* and *ren*. This results in the penetrating vessel becoming effulgent and hot. Since the *chong* connects with the foot *yang ming* at *Qi Ji* (St 30), *chong mai* effulgence can mutually give rise to stomach fire which can then mutually engender heart fire. Thus heart-stomach fire accumulates and becomes exuberant, flaming upward.

Treatment based on pattern discrimination

Heart-stomach fire flaring

Main symptoms: Several days before each menstruation comes like a tide, there appears oral *gan*, lingual *gan*, or tongue ulcers. Blisters may arise on the lips and the gums may become swollen and painful. The stools are constipated, and the urine is short and red. The mouth is dry and thirsty and there is heart vexation and insomnia. The tongue is red with scanty fluids and thin, slimy or slimy, yellow fur, and the pulse is bowstring and fine or fine and rapid.

Treatment principles: Clear heart fire, drain stomach fire, and enrich kidney yin

Guiding formula: *Yu Nu Jian Jia Xie Xin Tang Jia Jian* (Jade Maiden Decoction plus Drain the Heart Decoction with Additions & Subtractions)

Ingredients: Gypsum Fibrosum (*Shi Gao*), cooked Radix Rehmanniae (*Shu Di*), Tuber Ophiopogonis Japonici (*Mai Dong*), Rhizoma Anemarrhenae Aspheloidis (*Zhi Mu*), Radix Achyranthis Bidentatae (*Niu Xi*), Radix Et Rhizoma Rhei (*Da Huang*), Rhizoma Coptidis Chinensis (*Huang Lian*), Radix Scutellariae Baicalensis (*Huang Qin*)

Additions & subtractions: If the stool is dry and bound, use a heavy amount of Rhubarb. If yin is vacuous and there is internal heat with vacuity fire harassing above, add *Zhi Bai Di Huang Wan* (Anemarrhena & Phellodendron Rehmannia Pills). If there is damp heat internally smoldering with a slimy, yellow tongue coating, add *Er Miao Wan* (Two Wonders Pills). If there are ulcers on the tongue, remove uncooked Gypsum and add Plumula Nelumbinis Nuciferae (*Lian Zi Xin*) and Sichuan Rhizoma Coptidis Chinensis (*Chuan Lian*).

Menstrual Movement Loss of Sleep

Before or during menstruation there is insomnia. If severe, one may not sleep all night. After the menstruation is over, sleep becomes normal again.

Disease causes, disease mechanisms

Again because of blood accumulating in the uterus prior to the menstruation, there may be insufficient blood and yin to nourish the rest of the body and to control yang. If this blood and yin vacuity gives rise to internal or vacuity heat, heat may counterflow upward and harass the heart spirit at the same time that the heart spirit is not nourished by yin blood. Thus there is disturbed or lost sleep. Likewise, if there is a heart blood-spleen qi vacuity, because the heart sends the blood down to the uterus to accumulate there prior to menstruation, the heart spirit may lack sufficient nourishment. Thus the heart spirit becomes disquieted and there may be disturbed or loss of sleep. It is also possible for depressive heat engendered due to liver depression in turn due to emotional stress and frustration to counterflow upward and give rise to depressive heat in the heart. Once again this heat disturbs the heart spirit causing it to be disquieted and thus disturbing sleep.

Treatment based on pattern discrimination

Yin vacuity-fire effulgence

Main symptoms: For several nights before menstruation there is insomnia. If severe, one may not sleep the whole night. This is accompanied by a dry mouth and parched throat, heart vexation, despondency, a red tongue tip with thin, yellow fur, and a fine, rapid pulse.

Treatment principles: Nourish the blood, clear the heart, and quiet the spirit

Guiding formula: *Huang Lian E Jiao Tang Jia Wei* (Coptis & Donkey Skin Glue Decoction with Added Flavors)

Ingredients: Rhizoma Coptidis Chinensis (*Huang Lian*), Gelatinum Corii Asini (*E Jiao*), Radix Scutellariae Baicalensis (*Huang Qin*), Radix Paeoniae Lactiflorae (*Shao Yao*), Egg Yolk (*Ji Zi Huang*), Caulis Polygoni Multiflori (*Shou Wu Teng*), Sclerotium Polypori Umbellati & Poriae Cocos (*Zhu Fu Ling*), Fructus Schisandrae Chinensis (*Wu Wei Zi*), Cortex Albizziae Julibrissin (*He Huan Pi*), Fructus Rubi Chingii (*Sang Zhi Zi*), Fructus Lycii Chinensis (*Gou Qi Zi*)

Heart-spleen dual vacuity

Main symptoms: Insomnia before or after the menstruation, profuse dreaming, confusion, amount of the menses scanty or normal, lack of flavor for food eaten, dizziness, lassitude of the spirit, fatigue, lumbar soreness, limb pain, a pale, fat tongue with thin, slimy fur, and a fine, weak pulse

Treatment principles: Fortify the spleen and nourish the blood, calm the heart and quiet the spirit

Guiding formula: *Gui Pi Tang Jia Jian* **(Restore the Spleen Decoction with Additions & Subtractions)**

Ingredients: Radix Astragali Membranacei (*Huang Qi*), Radix Codonopsitis Pilosulae (*Dang Shen*), Rhizoma Atractylodis Macrocephalae (*Bai Zhu*), Sclerotium Poriae Cocos (*Fu Ling*), Semen Zizyphi Spinosae (*Zao Ren*), Radix Auklandiae Lappae (*Mu Xiang*), Radix Angelicae Sinensis (*Dang Gui*), Radix Polygalae Tenuifoliae (*Yuan Zhi*), Arillus Euphoriae Longanae (*Long Yan Rou*), Fructus Zizyphi Jujubae (*Da Zao*), uncooked Rhizoma Zingiberis (*Sheng Jiang*), Radix Glycyrrhizae (*Gan Cao*)

Heart-liver fire effulgence

Main symptoms: Premenstrual insomnia, if severe, no sleep the entire night, a bitter taste in the mouth, dry throat, heart vexation, easy anger, headache, dizziness, nipple distention and pain, a red tongue tip arising like thorns with thin, slimy fur, and a bowstring, rapid pulse

Treatment principles: Clear the liver, drain heat, and quiet the spirit

Guiding formulas:

1. *Long Dan Xie Gan Tang Jia Jian* **(Gentiana Drain the Liver Decoction with Additions & Subtractions)**

Ingredients: Radix Gentianae Scabrae (*Long Dan Cao*), Semen Plantaginis (*Che Qian Zi*), uncooked Radix Rehmanniae (*Sheng Di*), Fructus Gardeniae Jasminoidis (*Shan Zhi*), Radix Scutellariae Baicalensis (*Huang Qin*), Radix Glycyrrhizae (*Gan Cao*), Ramulus Uncariae Cum Uncis (*Gou Teng*), Rhizoma Anemarrhenae Aspheloidis (*Zhi Mu*), Cortex Phellodendri (*Huang Bai*), Sclerotium Polypori Umbellati & Poriae Cocos (*Zhu Fu Ling*), Semen Zizyphi Spinosae (*Suan Zao Ren*)

Although this may be a textbook standard formula for clearing replete heat from the liver, I personally find this formula too draining for Western women who almost always have an element of spleen vacuity in their case.

2. *Dan Zhi Xiao Yao San Jia Wei* (Moutan & Gardenia Rambling Powder with Added Flavors)

Ingredients: Cortex Radicis Moutan (*Dan Pi*), Fructus Gardeniae Jasminoidis (*Zhi Zi*), Radix Bupleuri (*Chai Hu*), Radix Angelicae Sinensis (*Dang Gui*), Radix Albus Paeoniae Lactiflorae (*Bai Shao*), Rhizoma Atractylodis Macrocephalae (*Bai Zhu*), Sclerotium Poriae Cocos (*Fu Ling*), mix-fried Radix Glycyrrhizae (*Gan Cao*), Ramulus Uncariae Cum Uncis (*Gou Teng*), Cortex Albizzinae Julibrissin (*He Huan Pi*), Rhizoma Coptidis Chinensis (*Huang Lian*)

3. *Chai Hu Jia Long Gu Mu Li Tang Jia Wei* (Bupleurum Plus Dragon Bone & Oyster Shell Decoction with Added Flavors)

Ingredients: Radix Bupleuri (*Chai Hu*), Radix Panacis Ginseng (*Ren Shen*), Rhizoma Pinelliae Terantae (*Ban Xia*), Sclerotium Poriae Cocos (*Fu Ling*), Radix Scutellariae Baicalensis (*Huang Qin*), Os Draconis (*Long Gu*), Concha Ostreae (*Mu Li*), Ramulus Cinnamomi Cassiae (*Gui Zhi*), Radix Et Rhizoma Rhei (*Da Huang*), uncooked Rhizoma Zingiberis (*Sheng Jiang*), Fructus Zizyphi Jujubae (*Da Zao*)

4. *Suan Zao Ren Tang Jia Wei* (Zizyphus Spinosa Decoction with Added Flavors)

Ingredients: Semen Zizyphi Spinosae (*Suan Zao Ren*), Sclerotium Poriae Cocos (*Fu Ling*), Radix Ligustici Wallichii (*Chuan Xiong*), Rhizoma Anemarrhenae Aspheloidis (*Zhi Mu*), Radix Glycyrrhizae (*Gan Cao*), Rhizoma Coptidis Chinensis (*Huang Lian*), Fructus Gardeniae Jasminoidis (*Shan Zhi*), Cortex Albizzinae Julibrissin (*He Huan Pi*), Caulis Polygoni Multiflori (*Ye Jiao Teng*)

Menstrual Movement Acne

Many women get pimples on their face during their premenstruum. In Chinese gynecology, this is called menstrual movement acne. Although it is not usually the patient's main complaint, it is often an important secondary symptom and it can help the practitioner understand the total premenstrual pattern.

Disease causes, disease mechanisms

Although overeating acrid, peppery foods, oily, fried foods, and drinking too much alcohol can cause damp heat in the liver and spleen, the most common cause of premenstrual acne is liver depression transforming into depressive heat. This heat counterflows upward to accumulate in the lungs. At the same time, premenstrual spleen vacuity may result in the spleen's failure to move and transport fluids properly. In that case, fluids gather and accumulate and may transform into dampness and/or phlegm. If heat endures for a long time or becomes very intense, it may engender heat toxins. Because depressive and/or toxic heat obstructs the free flow in the network vessels of the face, they can also give rise to blood stasis. Finally, if premenstrually there is blood and yin vacuity giving rise to vacuity heat, this vacuity heat may counterflow upward and steam the lungs, thus also causing acne. In clinical practice, most women present with a combination of heat and phlegm dampness with blood stasis usually complicating severe heat and/or phlegm nodulation.

Treatment according to pattern discrimination

Liver-spleen damp heat

Main symptoms: Before menstruation there appear on the face small, round pimples which may itch and even be painful. Also before the menstruation, there may be either white or yellow colored vaginal discharge, a dry, sticky, slimy mouth, white, slimy or yellow, slimy tongue fur, and a soggy, fine pulse.

This is a replete heat pattern usually associated with overeating acrid, peppery foods, oily, greasy foods, and drinking too much alcohol.

Treatment principles: Clear heat and disinhibit dampness

Guiding formula: *Long Dan Xie Gan Tang Jia Jian* (Gentiana Drain the Liver Decoction with Additions & Subtractions)

Ingredients: Radix Gentianae Scabrae (*Long Dan Cao*), Semen Plantaginis (*Che Qian Zi*), uncooked Radix Rehmanniae (*Sheng Di*), Fructus Gardeniae Jasminoidis (*Shan Zhi*), Radix Scutellariae Baicalensis (*Huang Qin*), Radix Glycyrrhizae (*Gan Cao*), Radix Rubrus Paeoniae Lactiflorae (*Chi Shao*), Herba Artemisiae Capillaris (*Yin Chen*), Rhizoma Smilacis Glabrae (*Tu Fu Ling*), Semen Coicis Lachryma-jobi (*Yi Yi Ren*)

Liver depression transforms heat

Main symptoms: Acne before menstruation is accompanied by a dry mouth and parched throat, emotional vexation and agitation, a tendency to cry for little reason, breast distention and pain, scanty menstruation which is not freely flowing, dry, bound stools, a red tongue with thin, yellow fur, and a bowstring, fine, rapid pulse.

This is the most commonly seen pattern of premenstrual acne. Typically, there are only one or two pimples located somewhere on the course of the *yang ming* channels on the face.

Treatment principles: Course the liver and rectify the qi, clear heat and resolve depression

Guiding formulas:

1. *Dan Zhi Xiao Yao San Jia Jian* (Moutan & Gardenia Rambling Powder with Additions & Subtractions)

Ingredients: Cortex Radicis Moutan (*Dan Pi*), Fructus Gardeniae Jasminoidis (*Zhi Ren*), Radix Albus Paeoniae Lactiflorae (*Bai Shao*), Radix Bupleuri (*Chai Hu*), uncooked Rhizoma Zingiberis (*Sheng Jiang*), Fructus Meliae Toosendan (*Chuan Lian Zi*), Tuber Curcumae (*Yu Jin*), Cortex Albizzinae Julibrissin (*He Huan Pi*), Radix Achyranthis Bidentatae (*Niu Xi*), Radix Et Rhizoma Rhei (*Da Huang*)

Additions & subtractions: If there is no constipation, delete the Rhubarb. In order to clear heat more effectively from the skin, one may add Flos Chrysanthemi Indici (*Ye Ju Hua*), Herba Taraxaci Mongolici Cum Radice (*Pu Gong Ying*), and/or Herba Violae Yedoensitis Cum Radice (*Zi Hua Di Ding*).

2. *Xiao Chai Hu Tang* (Minor Bupleurum Decoction)

Ingredients: Radix Bupleuri (*Chai Hu*), Radix Panacis Ginseng (*Ren Shen*), Rhizoma Pinelliae Ternatae (*Ban Xia*), Radix Scutellariae Baicalensis (*Huang Qin*), mix-fried Radix Glycyrrhizae (*Gan Cao*), Fructus Zizyphi Jujubae (*Da Zao*), uncooked Rhizoma Zingiberis (*Sheng Jiang*)

Because I find Scutellaria a very effective medicinal for clearing depressive heat from the stomach and liver, I usually use this formula as my base for treating women with mild premenstrual acne. This formula can then be modified with additions to rectify the qi or the blood more, clear heat more, eliminate dampness more, scatter nodulation more, or resolve toxins as necessary.

Spleen vacuity, phlegm dampness

Main symptoms: Pus-filled lesions, excessively oily skin, nodules or cysts under the skin with little or no reddening of the skin, torpid intake, loose stools, slimy tongue fur, and a slippery pulse

Treatment principles: Fortify the spleen and transform phlegm, soften the hard and scatter nodulation

Guiding formula: *Si Jun Zi Tang He Er Chen Tang Jia Wei* (Four Gentlemen Decoction plus Two Aged [Ingredients] Decoction with Added Flavors)

Ingredients: Radix Codonopsitis Pilosulae (*Dang Shen*), Rhizoma Atractylodis Macrocephalae (*Bai Zhu*), Sclerotium Poriae Cocos (*Fu Ling*), Rhizoma Pinelliae Ternatae (*Ban Xia*), Pericarpium Citri Reticulatae (*Chen Pi*), mix-fried Radix Glycyrrhizae (*Gan Cao*), Fructus Zizyphi Jujubae (*Da Zao*), Bulbus Fritillariae (*Bei Mu*)

Additions: If there are cystic nodulations, add Spica Prunellae Vulgaris (*Xia Ku Gao*), Herba Sargassii (*Hai Zao*), and Concha Ostreae (*Mu Li*). If the skin is greasy, add Rhizoma Alismatis (*Ze Xie*) and Semen Coicis Lachryma-jobi (*Yi Yi Ren*).

Blood stasis

Main symptoms: Acne which worsens during the premenstruum and menses, purple red lesions, purplish scars from past lesions, possible painful menstruation which is dark in color and contains clots, menstrual irregularities, a purplish tongue or static spots or macules on the tongue, and a bowstring, choppy pulse

Treatment principles: Quicken the blood and transform stasis

Guiding formula: *Tao Hong Si Wu Tang Jia Wei* (Persica & Carthamus Four Materials Decoction with Added Flavors)

Ingredients: Semen Pruni Persicae (*Tao Ren*), Flos Carthami Tinctorii (*Hong Hua*), Radix Angelicae Sinensis (*Dang Gui*), uncooked Radix Rehmanniae (*Sheng Di*), Radix Rubrus Paeoniae Lactiflorae (*Chi Shao*), Radix Ligustici Wallichii (*Chuan Xiong*), Herba Leonuri Heterophylli (*Yi Mu Cao*)

Additions: If stasis is mixed with heat toxins as it often is, add Flos Chrysanthemi Indici (*Ye Ju Hua*), Herba Taraxaci Mongolici Cum Radice (*Pu Gong Ying*), and/or Herba Violae Yedoensitis Cum Radice (*Zi Hua Di Ding*). If there are cystic lumps, add the same medicinals as added above under spleen vacuity, phlegm dampness. If the face is flushed red for days on end accompanied by oral thirst and a desire for cold drinks, add Gypsum Fibrosum (*Shi Gao*) and Rhizoma Anemarrhenae Aspheloidis (*Zhi Mu*). If the mouth is dry and the lips are chapped, add Tuber Ophiopogonis Japinici (*Mai Dong*), Tuber Asparagi Cochinensis (*Tian Dong*), and Radix Scrophulariae Ningpoensis (*Xuan Shen*). If there are dry, bound stools, add Radix Et Rhizoma Rhei (*Da Huang*).

Vacuity heat fuming the lungs

Main symptoms: Premenstrual acne which is light red in color and shaped like a scattering of small papules over the forehead. This may be accompanied by a dry cough with no phlegm, a dry mouth and sore throat, flushed red cheeks, a red tongue with thin, yellow fur and scanty fluids, and a fine, rapid pulse.

Treatment principles: Supplement the kidneys and enrich yin, clear heat and drain the lungs

Guiding formula: *Si Wu Tang Jia Xie Bai San Jia Wei* (Four Materials Decoction plus Drain the White Powder with Added Flavors)

Ingredients: Cooked Radix Rehmanniae (*Shu Di*), uncooked Radix Rehmanniae (*Sheng Di*), Radix Angelicae Sinensis (*Dang Gui*), Radix Rubrus Paeoniae Lactiflorae (*Chi Shao*), Radix Lugustici Wallichii (*Chuan Xiong*), Cortex Radicis Mori Albi (*Sang Bai Pi*), Cortex Radicis Lycii Chinensis (*Di Gu Pi*), Radix Glycyrrhizae (*Gan Cao*), Radix Scutellariae Baicalensis (*Huang Qin*), Radix Platycodi Grandiflori (*Jie Geng*), uncooked Semen Coicis Lachryma-jobi (*Yi Ren*), Fructus Forsythiae Suspensae (*Lian Qiao*)

Menstrual Movement Raving & Confused Vision

Three to seven days before menstruation, raving speech, confused vision, and essence spirit abnormality appear. After the menses, these disappear. However, with the next menstruation, they return again. This disease category refers to premenstrual tension and emotional lability. It most definitely is many Western women's major complaint even if the Chinese name is not very felicitous.

Disease causes, disease mechanisms

Due to constitutional yin vacuity, because of the accumulation of yin blood in the uterus before menstruation, the heart may lose its moistening nourishment and the blood becomes insufficient to construct the brain. Thus the spirit becomes disquieted. It is also possible for liver depression to transform into fire, hence the liver cannot treasure the ethereal soul and the ethereal soul is, therefore, not calm. If liver qi becomes depressed and binds with phlegm turbidity, it may confound the clear portals or orifices above causing disturbances in consciousness.

Treatment based on pattern discrimination

Heart blood insufficiency

Main symptoms: Several days before the menses, there is sadness and desire to cry, sudden essence spirit abstraction, inability to control oneself, restless sleep at night, heart palpitations, racing heart, deep silence, scanty speech, excessive worry and anxiety, and scanty menstruation. The tongue is pale with thin fur, and the pulse is fine, relaxed (*i.e.,* retarded), and forceless.

Treatment principles: Nourish the heart and quiet the spirit

Guiding formula: *Gan Mai Da Zao Tang Jia Bai He Di Huang Tang* **(Licorice, Triticus & Red Dates Decoction plus Lily & Rehmannia Decoction)**

Ingredients: Fructus Levis Tritici Aestivi (*Fu Xiao Mai*), Radix Glycyrrhizae (*Gan Cao*), Fructus Zizyphi Jujubae (*Da Zao*), Bulbus Lilii (*Bai He*), uncooked Radix Rehmanniae (*Sheng Di*), Semen Zizyphi Spinosae (*Zao Ren*), Radix Polygalae Tenuifoliae (*Yuan Zhi*)

Liver depression-fire effulgence

Main symptoms: Three to seven days or more before the menses, the emotions become agitated. There is heart vexation and easy anger or mania, agitation, and restlessness. If severe, one may climb on high and sing or shed their clothes. The tongue is red with thick, slimy, yellow fur, and the pulse is bowstring, fine, and rapid.

Climbing naked on high and singing is a cultural norm or expectation for mania in Asia. Interestingly, I have met an Asian who did just this during a nervous breakdown.

Treatment principles: Clear the liver and resolve depression, drain fire and quiet the spirit

Guiding formulas:

1. *Long Dan Xie Gan Tang Jia Jian* **(Gentiana Drain the Liver Decoction with Additions & Subtractions)**

Ingredients: Radix Gentianae Scabrae (*Long Dan Cao*), Rhizoma Alismatis (*Ze Xie*), Semen Plantaginis (*Che Qian Zi*), uncooked Radix Rehmanniae (*Sheng Di*), Radix Angelicae Sinensis (*Dang Gui*), Fructus Gardeniae Jasminoidis (*Shan Zhi*), Radix Scutellariae Baicalensis (*Huang Qin*), Radix Glycyrrhizae (*Gan Cao*), Cortex Radicis Moutan (*Dan Pi*), Rhizoma Coptidis Chinensis (*Huang Lian*), Ramulus Uncariae Cum Uncis (*Gou Teng*), Os Draconis (*Long Gu*), Concha Ostreae (*Mu Li*)

This formula is for strong replete heat. It is usually too strong for most Western women unless it is used short-term in cases of severe fire effulgence mania.

2. *Dan Zhi Xiao Yao San Jia Wei* (Moutan & Gardenia Rambling Powder with Added Flavors)

Ingredients: Cortex Radicis Moutan (*Dan Pi*), Fructus Gardeniae Jasminoidis (*Shan Zhi*), Radix Bupleuri (*Chai Hu*), Radix Angelicae Sinensis (*Dang Gui*), Radix Albus Paeoniae Lactiflorae (*Bai Shao*), Rhizoma Atractylodis Macrocephalae (*Bai Zhu*), Sclerotium Poriae Cocos (*Fu Ling*), mix-fried Radix Glycyrrhizae (*Gan Cao*), Herba Menthae Haplocalycis (*Bo He*), Caulis Polygoni Multiflori (*Ye Jiao Teng*), Cortex Albizziae Julibrissin (*He Huan Pi*)

Additions: If there is more severe agitation, add Dens Draconis (*Long Chi*) and Concha Ostreae (*Mu Li*).

3. *Chai Hu Jia Long Gu Mu Li Tang Jia Wei* (Bupleurum Plus Dragon Bone & Oyster Shell Decoction with Added Flavors)

Ingredients: Radix Bupleuri (*Chai Hu*), Radix Panacis Ginseng (*Ren Shen*), Rhizoma Pinelliae Terantae (*Ban Xia*), Sclerotium Poriae Cocos (*Fu Ling*), Radix Scutellariae Baicalensis (*Huang Qin*), Os Draconis (*Long Gu*), Concha Ostreae (*Mu Li*), Ramulus Cinnamomi Cassiae (*Gui Zhi*), Radix Et Rhizoma Rhei (*Da Huang*), uncooked Rhizoma Zingiberis (*Sheng Jiang*), Fructus Zizyphi Jujubae (*Da Zao*)

Phlegm qi depression & binding

Main symptoms: Premenstrual emotional depression, dizziness as if one's head were covered in a bag, profuse, sticky phlegm, fatigue, somnolence, if severe, spontaneous sadness and spontaneous weeping, crying out as if in pain, or deep silence, an anxious heart laden with cares, thin, white, slimy tongue fur, and a soggy, fine or bowstring, slippery pulse

Treatment principles: Rectify the qi and resolve depression, transform phlegm and open the orifices

Guiding formulas:

1. *Sheng Tie Luo Yin Jia Jian* **(Uncooked Iron Filings Drink with Additions & Subtractions)**

Ingredients: Pericarpium Citri Reticulatae (*Chen Pi*), Sclerotium Poriae Cocos (*Fu Ling*), lime-processed Rhizoma Pinelliae Ternatae (*Fa Xia*), Fructus Citri Aurantii (*Zhi Ke*), Caulis Bambusae In Taeniis (*Zhu Ru*), uncooked Iron Filings (*Tie Luo*), Ramulus Uncariae Cum Uncis (*Gou Teng*), Radix Salviae Miltiorrhizae (*Dan Shen*), Fructus Forsythiae Suspensae (*Lian Qiao*), Tuber Ophiopogonis Japonici (*Mai Dong*), Bulbus Fritillariae (*Bei Mu*), Radix Scrophulariae Ningpoensis (*Xuan Shen*), bile-processed Rhizoma Arisaematis (*Dan Nan Xing*), Radix Polygalae Tenuifoliae (*Yuan Zhi*), Rhizoma Acori Graminei (*Shi Chang Pu*)

Although neither the above listed signs and symptoms nor the name of the pattern indicate heat, the ingredients in this formula do suggest phlegm heat.

Additions & subtractions: If the stools are constipated, add uncooked Radix Et Rhizoma Rhei (*Da Huang*) and Lapis Chloriti (*Meng Shi*). If there is profuse phlegm, add Secretio Silicea Bambusae (*Tian Zhu Huang*) and *Bai Jin Wan* (White Metal Pills). If there is chest oppression and qi depression, add Rhizoma Nardostachytis (*Gan Song Xiang*) and Pericarpium Citri Reticulatae (*Chen Pi*).

2. *Huang Lian Wen Dan Tang* **(Coptis Warm the Gallbladder Decoction)**

Ingredients: Rhizoma Coptidis Chinensis (*Huang Lian*), Rhizoma Pinelliae Ternatae (*Ban Xia*), Sclerotium Poriae Cocos (*Fu Ling*), mix-fried Radix Glycyrrhizae (*Gan Cao*), Pericarpium Citri Reticulatae (*Chen Pi*), Fructus Immaturus Citri Aurantii (*Zhi Shi*), Caulis Bambusae In Taeniis (*Zhu Ru*), uncooked Rhizoma Zingiberis (*Sheng Jiang*)

This formula also addresses phlegm fire, not just phlegm confounding the orifices. It is an extremely useful and effective formula. When phlegm causes mental-emotional disturbances, it is usually phlegm fire, not just phlegm.

Menstrual Movement Dull-wittedness & Stupidity

This refers to feeling as if one's intelligence was diminished or incapacitated during the premenstruum. Many women also say they feel clumsy during this same time.

Disease causes, disease mechanisms

In the Chinese gynecological literature, the main cause of this menstrual disease is kidney yang vacuity mixed with blood vacuity and stasis.

Treatment according to pattern discrimination

Kidney yang insufficiency & stasis

Main symptoms: Several days before each menstruation, the essence spirit is wanting. There is fatigue, worry, and somnolence. When questioned, there is no response. There is also no thought for food or drink, movement is slow and there is the appearance of fear and fright at the appearance of outside people. There may also be lumbar and abdominal aching and pain. When the menses come, there are blood clots. The tongue tip is slightly red and there is thin, white fur. The pulse is deep, fine, and weak.

Some of the symptoms above are pretty severe. Usually in Western women, these symptoms are only secondary complaints and are not so severe.

Treatment principles: Warm and supplement kidney yang, nourish the blood and dispel stasis

Guiding formula: _Si Ni Tang Jia Wei_ (Four Counterflows Decoction with Added Flavors)

Ingredients: Radix Lateralis Praeparatus Aconiti Carmichaeli (_Fu Pian_), Radix Angelicae Sinensis (_Dang Gui_), cooked Radix Rehmanniae (_Shu Di_), Herba Epimedii (_Yin Yang Huo_), Rhizoma Curcumae Zedoariae (_E Zhu_), Radix Rubrus Paeoniae Lactiflorae (_Chi Shao_), Radix Et Rhizoma Rhei (_Da Huang_), Rhizoma Sparganii (_San Leng_), Rhizoma Zingiberis (_Gan Jiang_), Radix Ligustici Wallichii (_Chuan Xiong_)

Menstrual Movement Addictive Papules

Menstrual movement addictive papules refer to premenstrual or menstrual hives or urticaria. They are called addictive papules since the patient is addicted to scrating them. Three to seven days or so before the menses, a nettle rash appears over the entire body. This disappears after the menstruation is over.

Disease causes, disease mechanisms

Because the liver stores the blood, if liver depression gives rise to depressive heat, this heat may be transferred to the blood division. This blood heat may smolder and obstruct the muscles and skin, thus becoming mixed with dampness. This then may result in raised, red wheals. If premenstrually, there is insufficient constructive and blood, blood vacuity may engender wind. This results in itching. In addition, blood stasis in the uterus may also result in blood vacuity. In this case, old blood prevents the engenderment of new blood.

Treatment according to pattern discrimination

Liver effulgence, blood heat

Main symptoms: Several days before menstruation, various sized urticaria wheals appear all over the body. These are bright red and burning hot. If these meet heat, their number increases. The menses are profuse in amount and they come early. There is also headache, constipated stools, red lips, a red tongue with thin, yellow fur, and a bowstring, fine, rapid pulse.

Treatment principles: Clear heat and cool the blood, level or calm the liver and course wind

Guiding formulas:

1. *Xiao Feng San* (Disperse Wind Powder)

Ingredients: Herba Schizonepetae Tenuifoliae (*Jing Jie*), Radix Ledebouriellae Divaricatae (*Fang Feng*), Periostracum Cicadae (*Chan Yi*), Radix Angelicae Sinensis (*Dang Gui*), uncooked Radix Rehmanniae (*Sheng Di*), Semen Sesami Indici (*Hu Ma Ren*), Radix Sophorae Flavescentis (*Ku Shen*), Rhizoma Atractylodis (*Cang Zhu*), Rhizoma Anemarrhenae Aspheloidis (*Zhi Mu*), Gypsum Fibrosum (*Shi Gao*), Caulis Akebiae Mutong (*Mu Tong*), uncooked Radix Glycyrrhizae (*Gan Cao*), Fructus Arctii (*Niu Bang Zi*)

2. *Xiao Feng San Jia Long Dan Xie Gan Tang Jia Jian* (Disperse Wind Powder plus Gentiana Drain the Liver Decoction with Additions & Subtractions)

Ingredients: Herba Schizonepetae Tenuifoliae (*Jing Jie*), Radix Ledebouriellae Divaricatae (*Fang Feng*), Periostracum Cicadae (*Chan Yi*), Fructus Arctii (*Niu Bang Zi*), uncooked Radix Rehmanniae (*Sheng Di*), Semen Sesami Indici (*Hu Ma Ren*), Radix Angelicae Sinensis (*Dang Gui*), Rhizoma Anemarrhenae Aspheloidis (*Zhi Mu*), Radix Gentianae

Scabrae (*Long Dan Cao*), Fructus Gardeniae Jasminoidis (*Zhi Ren*), Radix Scutellariae Baicalensis (*Huang Qin*), Radix Bupleuri (*Chai Hu*), Semen Plantaginis (*Che Qian Zi*)

Additions & subtractions: If menstruation is profuse, add processed carbonized Radix Et Rhizoma Rhei (*Jun*), *Shi Hui Wan* (Ten Ashes Pills), and carbonized Schizonepeta. If heat endures for days and severely damages yin, add Tuber Ophiopogonis Japonici (*Mai Dong*). If there is simultaneous damp heat, add uncooked Semen Coicis Lachryma-jobi (*Yi Yi Ren*) and Rhizoma Atractylodis (*Cang Zhu*). If there is concomitant spleen vacuity, delete Gentiana and add Rhizoma Atractylodis Macrocephalae (*Bai Zhu*) and Sclerotium Poriae Cocos (*Fu Ling*).

Blood vacuity engendering wind

Main symptoms: Urticaria before the menses, pale, flat, not very raised lesions, dry, parched skin, formication, profuse menstruation but pale in color, lassitude of the spirit, fatigue, lack of strength, heart palpitations, shortness of breath, a sallow yellow facial complexion, a fat tongue with thin fur, and a fine, soft pulse

Treatment principles: Nourish the blood and dispel wind

Guiding formula: *Si Wu Tang Jia Wei* (Four Materials Decoction with Added Flavors)

Ingredients: Radix Astragali Membranacei (*Huang Qi*), Radix Angelicae Sinensis (*Dang Gui*), Radix Polygoni Multiflori (*He Shou Wu*), cooked Radix Rehmanniae (*Shu Di*), Radix Albus Paeoniae Lactiflorae (*Bai Shao*), Radix Ligustici Wallichii (*Chuan Xiong*), Fructus Tribuli Terrestris (*Bai Ji Li*), Radix Ledebouriellae Divaricatae (*Fang Feng*), Herba Schizonepetae Tenuifoliae (*Jing Jie*), uncooked Radix Glycyrrhizae (*Gan Cao*)

Additions: If menstruation is profuse, add Herba Agrimoniae Pilosae (*He Xian Cao*) and *Gui Pi Wan* (Restore the Spleen Pills).

Blood stasis obstructing & stagnating

Main symptoms: Premenstrually there are hives appearing over the entire body. The rash is shaped like static patches or macules. The menses are scanty and there is lower abdominal pain, a static, dark tongue, and a bowstring, fine pulse.

Treatment principles: Quicken the blood and dispel wind

Guiding formula: *Tao Hong Si Wu Tang Jia Wei* **(Persica & Carthamus Four Materials Decoction with Added Flavors)**

Ingredients: Semen Pruni Persicae (*Tao Ren*), Flos Carthami Tinctorii (*Hong Hua*), Radix Angelicae Sinensis (*Dang Gui*), Radix Ligustici Wallichii (*Chuan Xiong*), cooked Radix Rehmanniae (*Shu Di*), Radix Rubrus Paeoniae Lactiflorae (*Chi Shao*), Cortex Radicis Moutan (*Dan Pi*), whole Fructus Trichosanthis Kirlowii (*Quan Gua Lou*), Radix Achyranthis Bidentatae (*Niu Xi*), Radix Lithospermi Seu Arnebiae (*Zi Cao Gen*)

Additions: If stasis is not precipitated smoothly and lower abdominal pain is severe, add Rhizoma Corydalis Yanhusuo (*Xuan Hu Suo*).

Menstrual Movement Flowing Drool

Premenstrually, the woman may find that she has excessive saliva in her mouth. This is called menstrual movement flowing drool. In my experience, this is not a common complaint even though the disease mechanism given below is extremely common.

Disease causes, disease mechanisms

If spleen qi is consitutionally vacuous and liver qi is depressed and bound, over time, this may lead to blockage and stagnation of spleen earth. This results in water dampness being retained in the center which then flows upward to spill over as drool.

Treatment according to pattern discrimination

Liver wood exploiting the spleen

Main symptoms: Each time the menses come, excessive watery drool is discharged from the mouth. When the menses cease, this drool spontaneously stops. This is accompanied by breast distention, occasional hiccup, diminished appetite, nausea, bodily emaciation, a lusterless facial complexion, tension and agitation, easy anger, a dry mouth but no desire to drink, a fine, bowstring pulse, and a pale red tongue with scanty fur.

Treatment principles: Course the liver and resolve dperession, fortify the spleen and transform dampness

Guiding formula: *Xiao Yao San Jia Wei* **(Rambling Powder with Added Flavors)**

Ingredients: Radix Angelicae Sinensis (*Dang Gui*), Radix Albus Paeoniae Lactiflorae (*Bai Shao*), Radix Bupleuri (*Chai Hu*), Sclerotium Poriae Cocos (*Fu Ling*), Rhizoma Atractylodis Macrocephalae (*Bai Zhu*), Fructus Alpiniae Oxyphyllae (*Yi Zhi Ren*), Tuber Curcumae (*Yu Jin*), Herba Menthae Haplocalycis (*Bo He*), mix-fried Radix Glycyrrhizae (*Gan Cao*), uncooked Rhizoma Zingiberis (*Sheng Jiang*)

Menstrual Movement Oral Thirst

If a woman experiences an increase in thirst and oral dryness, this is called menstrual movement oral thirst.

Disease causes, disease mechanisms

Premenstrual oral thirst may be due to depressive heat damaging stomach fluids. It may also be due to qi and blood stasis and stagnation. In this latter case, the qi is unable to upbear fluids to the mouth and blood stasis hinders the engenderment of blood. This results in oral thirst since the blood and fluids share a common source. Once the blood stasis is eliminated, then new blood and, therefore, new fluids can be engendered.

Treatment according to pattern discrimination

Stomach heat

Main symptoms: When the menses come there is oral thirst. When the menses cease, this thirst stops. The tongue is red with yellow fur, and the pulse is rapid.

Treatment principles: Clear stomach fire and enrich yin

Guiding formulas:

1. Unnamed formula from *Fu Ke San Bai Zheng (Three Hundred Gynecological Conditions)*

Ingredients: Radix Trichosanthis Kirlowii (*Hua Fen*), Rhizoma Coptidis Chinensis (*Huang Lian*), Tuber Ophiopogonis Japonicae (*Mai Dong*), Fructus Schisandrae Chinensis (*Wu Wei Zi*), Gypsum Fibrosum (*Shi Gao*), dry Radix Puerariae (*Gan Ge*)

2. *Xiao Chai Hu Tang Jia Wei* **(Minor Bupleurum Decoction with Added Flavors)**

Ingredients: Radix Bupleuri (*Chai Hu*), Radix Codonopsitis Pilosulae (*Dang Shen*), Rhizoma Pinelliae Ternatae (*Ban Xia*), mix-fried Radix Glycyrrhizae (*Gan Cao*), Fructus Zizyphi Jujubae (*Da Zao*), uncooked Rhizoma Zingiberis (*Sheng Jiang*), Radix Angelicae Sinensis (*Dang Gui*), Tuber Ophiopogonis Japonici (*Mai Dong*), Radix Trichosanthis Kirlowii (*Tian Hua Fen*)

Since heat damaging stomach fluids premenstrually is mostly depressive heat stemming from the liver, I prefer to use a harmonizing formula which contains medicinals to clear stomach heat and additions to enrich stomach fluids.

Stasis & stagnation

Main symptoms: Dry mouth but drinking not too much water when the menses come, a dark red tongue, and a choppy pulse

Treatment principles: Quicken the blood, move stasis, and regulate the menses

Guiding formula: Unnamed formula from *Fu Ke San Bai Zheng (Three Hundred Gynecological Conditions)*

Ingredients: Rhizoma Sparganii (*San Leng*), Rhizoma Curcumae Zedoariae (*E Zhu*), Radix Achyranthis Bidentatae (*Niu Xi*), Lignum Sappanis (*Su Mu*), Flos Carthami Tinctorii (*Hong Hua*)

Since blood stasis causing or participating in oral dryness and thirst may complicate any number of other commonly seen premenstrual patterns, a selection of blood-quickening and stasis-dispelling medicinals may also be added to other guiding formulas for other patterns.

Menstrual Movement Hoarse Voice

If a woman experiences a dry throat and hoarse voice before or accompanying each menstruation, this is called menstrual movement hoarse voice.

Disease causes, disease mechanisms

If there is constitutional yin vacuity, this typically gets worse before, during, and just after menstruation due to blood and yin accumulating in and then being discharged from the uterus. In this case, there may not be sufficient yin fluids above in order to nourish the throat and engender the voice. In addition, yin fluids of the lungs may be damaged and consumed by excessive singing or speaking during menstruation. It is also possible that, due to early marriage, too many births, and too much breast-feeding or unrestrained sexual activity, each time the menses come, yin blood pours downward and essence and blood become more deficient. This may then give rise to vacuity fire becoming effulgent. This burns and damages lung fluids and this also results in hoarse voice. Because of liver depression and the liver and stomach's close mutual relationship, if one eats too much acrid, peppery, hot food, too much oily, greasy, fried food, or drinks too much alcohol, damp heat may accumulate in the stomach and intestines premenstrually. Although this damp heat may be located in the lower burner, heat travels upward and may damage the fluids of the lungs, while below, damp heat may damage the network vessels of the intestines, bladder, or uterus.

Treatment based on pattern discrimination

Lung dryness

Main symptoms: Loss of voice each menstruation, dry mouth, parched throat, occasional dry cough, heat in the hands, feet, and heart, vacuity vexation, scanty sleep, dry, bound stools, a tongue tending towards red with scanty fluids and thin fur, and a fine pulse

Treatment principles: Clear dryness, moisten the lungs, and free the flow of the voice

Guiding formulas:

1. *Qing Zao Jiu Fei Tang Jia Jian* (Clear Dryness & Rescue the Lungs Decoction with Additions & Subtractions)

Ingredients: Folium Mori Albi (*Sang Ye*), Gypsum Fibrosum (*Shi Gao*), Radix Glycyrrhizae (*Gan Cao*), Radix Glehniae Littoralis (*Bei Sha Shen*), Semen Sesami Indici (*Hu Ma Ren*), Gelatinum Corii Asini (*E Jiao*), Tuber Ophiopogonis Japonici (*Mai Dong*), Semen Pruni Armeniacae (*Xing Ren*), Folium Eriobotryae Japonicae (*Pi Pa Ye*), Rhizoma Polygonati Odorati (*Yu Zhu*), Radix Trichosanthis Kirlowii (*Tian Hua Fen*)

2. *Sha Shen Mai Dong Tang Jia Jian* (Glehnia & Ophiopogon Decoction with Additions & Subtractions)

Ingredients: Radix Glehniae Littoralis (*Bei Sha Shen*), Radix Adenophorae Strictae (*Nan Sha Shen*), Tuber Ophiopogonis Japonici (*Mai Dong*), Rhizoma Polygonati Odoarati (*Yu Zhu*), Radix Trichosanthis Kirlowii (*Tian Hua Fen*), Folium Mori Albi (*Sang Ye*), Radix

Platycodi Grandiflori (*Jie Geng*), Radix Scrophulariae Ningpoensis (*Xuan Shen*), Rhizoma Phragmitis Communis (*Lu Gen*), Radix Glycyrrhizae (*Gan Cao*)

This formula is stronger than the preceding one for nourishing yin and moistening dryness and it is weaker for clearing heat.

Kidney vacuity

Main symptoms: Loss of voice or unsmooth vocal sound with each menstrual movement, low back and knee soreness and weakness, dizziness, tinnitus, a pale tongue with thin, white fur, and a deep, fine pulse

Treatment principles: Supplement the qi and secure the kidneys, nourish yin and moisten dryness

Guiding formula: *Qi Wei Dou Qi Wan Jia Wei* (Seven Flavors All Qi Pills with Added Flavors)

Ingredients: Uncooked Radix Rehmanniae (*Sheng Di*), Sclerotium Poriae Cocos (*Fu Ling*), Fructus Corni Officinalis (*Shan Yu Rou*), Radix Dioscoreae Oppositae (*Shan Yao*), Cortex Radicis Moutan (*Dan Pi*), Rhizoma Alismatis (*Ze Xie*), Radix Tinosporae (*Jin Guo Lan*), Fructus Schisandrae Chinensis (*Wu Wei Zi*), Fructus Sterculiae Scaphageriae (*Pang Da Hai*), Rhizoma Atractylodis Macrocephalae (*Bai Zhu*), Herba Menthae Haplocalycis (*Bo He*), uncooked Rhizoma Zingiberis (*Sheng Jiang*), Fructus Pruni Mume (*Wu Mei*), stir-fried Herba Schizonepetae Tenuifoliae (*Jing Jie*)

Damp heat

Main symptoms: Before or during the menses, there is oral thirst and a dry throat and mouth. If damp heat is severe, this may be accompanied by precipitation of blood with defecation, hematuria, or early and/or profuse menstruation. Urination is short, scanty, and yellow-colored, while defecation may be burning hot, foul-smelling, and loose. The tongue has a thick, yellow coating, and the pulse is soggy and rapid; slippery and rapid; or slippery, bowstring, and rapid.

Treatment principles: Clear heat and eliminate dampness, nourish the blood and regulate the menses

Guiding formula: *Fen Li Wu Ling Tang Jia Wei* (Divide & Disinhibit Five [Ingredients] Poria Decoction with Added Flavors)

Ingredients: Radix Rubrus Paeoniae Lactiflorae (*Chi Shao*), Radix Angelicae Sinensis (*Dang Gui*), Radix Ligustici Wallichii (*Chuan Xiong*), Gelatinum Corii Asini (*E Jiao*), Sclerotium Poriae Cocos (*Fu Ling*), Sclerotium Polypori Umbellati (*Zhu Ling*), Rhizoma Alismatis (*Ze Xie*), Rhizoma Atractylodis Macrocephalae (*Bai Zhu*), Semen Phaseoli Calcarati (*Chi Xiao Dou*)

The above guiding formula is mostly for damp heat in the lower burner affecting urination with possible hematuria. Different guiding formulas may be chosen depending on the location of the damp heat. For instance, there may be damp heat in the intestines causing diarrhea. There may be damp heat in the liver channel causing abnormal vaginal discharge and vaginitis, etc. In all such cases, there will be oral dryness and thirst. On the one hand, this will automatically go away if the damp heat is cleared and eliminated. On the other, all dampness and heat clearing and eliminating formulas can be modified by the addition to stomach-nourishing medicinals, such as Tuber Ophiopogonis Japonici (*Mai Dong*).

Menstrual Movement Eye Pain

It is possible for a woman to experience eye pain before, during or after each menstruation. When this occurs, it is called menstrual movement eye pain.

Disease causes, disease mechanisms

If a woman's liver blood is insufficient for any reason, this insufficiency is aggravated before, during, and immediately after menstruation. This is because the blood is moved down to the uterus, leaving the upper body, especially blood, vacuous and insufficient. The liver opens into the orifices of the eyes. If the eyes lose their nourishment, there is pain.

Treatment based on pattern discrimination

Liver blood vacuity

Main symptoms: When the menses come, the eyes become itchy and painful, swollen, astringent, and difficult to open or slight corneal opacity may be engendered causing loss of visual acuity. There may also be headache, vertigo, dizziness, a pale red tongue, and a surging, large pulse which, when pressed, becomes empty and vacuous.

Treatment principles: Supplement the blood and nourish the liver

Guiding formula: *Dang Gui Bu Xue Tang Jia Qi Ju Di Huang Wan* **(Dang Gui Supplement the Blood Decoction plus Lycium & Chrysanthemum Rehmannia Pills)**

Ingredients: Radix Angelicae Sinensis (*Dang Gui*), Radix Astragali Membranacei (*Huang Qi*), Fructus Lycii Chinensis (*Gou Qi Zi*), Flos Chrysanthemi Morifolii (*Ju Hua*), cooked Radix Rehmanniae (*Shu Di*), Sclerotium Poriae Cocos (*Fu Ling*), Fructus Corni Officinalis (*Shan Zhu Yu*), Cortex Radicis Moutan (*Dan Pi*), Rhizoma Alismatis (*Ze Xie*), Radix Dioscoreae Oppositae (*Huai Shan Yao*)

Menstrual Movement Lumbar Pain

Low back pain preceding or accompanying the menses is extremely common. Its incidence goes up as women enter their mid to late 30s and 40s. By the late 40s, it is an almost universal complaint accompanying the menstrual movement in women who complain of PMS.

Disease causes, disease mechanisms

Lumbar pain either immediately preceding or accompanying menstruation is usually a kidney vacuity symptom. "The lumbus is the mansion of the kidneys." This may be either liver-kidney yin vacuity, kidney yang vacuity, or yin and yang vacuity. Liver-kidney yin vacuity either occurs or worsens premenstrually due to the accumulation of yin blood in the uterus prior to and during menstruation. This may leave the sinews malnourished. Kidney yang vacuity also includes blood vacuity. This is because, "The essence and blood share a common source." Thus kidney yang vacuity low back pain is also a species of malnourishment of the sinews. Yin and/or yang vacuity low back pain may either be due to insufficient natural endowment, enduring disease, sex, drugs, and rock 'n roll, or merely aging. However, as we have seen above under menstrual movement body pain, damp heat may also cause premenstrual lumbar pain.

Treatment based on pattern discrimination

Liver-kidney yin vacuity

Main symptoms: Premenstrual or menstrual low back soreness and stiffness, knee soreness and weakness, tinnitus and dizziness, frequent, scanty, yellow urination, night sweats, red cheeks, tidal fever, a red tongue with scanty fur or a pale tongue with red tip and thin, white fur, and a fine, bowstring, possibly rapid pulse

Treatment principles: Nourish the liver and enrich the kidneys, strengthen the sinews and bones and the low back

Guiding formula: *Qi Ju Di Huang Wan Jia Jian* **(Lycium & Chrysanthemum Rehmannia Pills with Additions & Subtractions)**

Ingredients: Cooked Radix Rehmanniae (*Shu Di*), Radix Angelicae Sinensis (*Dang Gui*), Radix Albus Paeoniae Lactiflorae (*Bai Shao*), Fructus Lycii Chinensis (*Gou Qi Zi*), Radix Achyranthis Bidentatae (*Niu Xi*), Ramulus Loranthi Seu Visci (*Sang Ji Sheng*), Fructus Corni Officinalis (*Shan Zhu Yu*), Radix Dioscoreae Oppositae (*Shan Yao*), Sclerotium Poriae Cocos (*Fu Ling*), Cortex Radicis Moutan (*Dan Pi*), Rhizoma Alismatis (*Ze Xie*)

Kidney yang vacuity

Main symptoms: When the menses come like a tide, there is aching and pain in the low back region, weak knees, and lack of strength which are made worse by overtaxation. Rest makes the pain diminish.

Treatment principles: Supplement the kidneys and invigorate yang, strengthen the sinews and bones and the low back

Guiding formula: *Gui Shen Wan Jia Wei* **(Restore the Kidneys Pills with Added Flavors)**

Ingredients: Radix Angelicae Sinensis (*Dang Gui*), Radix Ligustici Wallichii (*Chuan Xiong*), cooked Radix Rehmanniae (*Shu Di*), Radix Albus Paeoniae Lactiflorae (*Bai Shao*), Radix Astragali Membranacei (*Huang Qi*), mix-fried Radix Glycyrrhizae (*Gan Cao*), Fructus Corni Officinalis (*Shan Zhu Yu*), Sclerotium Poriae Cocos (*Fu Ling*), Cortex Radicis Moutan (*Dan Pi*), Cortex Eucommiae Ulmoidis (*Du Zhong*), Radix Dipsaci (*Xu Duan*), Radix Morindae Officinalis (*Ba Ji Rou*)

This formula includes qi-boosting spleen supplements as well as kidney-supplementing, yang-invigorating medicinals. This exemplifies the fact that premenstrual lumbar pain is mostly seen in older women where there is both spleen qi, kidney yang vacuity, and liver blood vacuity.

Menstrual Movement Suspended Vagina Pain

When the menses come like a tide, one may spontaneously feel two sinews within their vagina leading along to the front of the chest and the two breasts which are so aching and painful as to be difficult to bear. There may also be generalized fever. This is called suspended yin pain. I have yet to hear this complaint from a Western woman.

Disease causes, disease mechanisms

Menstrual movement suspended vagina pain is mostly due to cold congelation, damp heat due to liver depression, or qi binding. Cold congelation in this case is due to kidney yang vacuity cold. Cold causes constriction and congelation which impede free flow. Such kidney yang vacuity is typically part of a woman's aging process. If heat due to liver depression steams and fumes the fluids and humors, it may give rise to damp heat which pours downward to the liver channel. This damp heat obstructs the free and uninhibited flow of qi and blood in the lower burner, giving rise to pain. It is also possible for blood vacuity premenstrually to aggravate a tendency to liver qi depression and binding. Since the liver loses its control over coursing and discharging, the qi loses its free and smooth flow, resulting in pain along the internal course of the liver channel.

Treatment based on pattern discrimination

Cold congelation

Main symptoms: There is vaginal pain leading to both sides of the lower abdomen. If severe, the vaginal meatus is tight and shrunken. There is tetany and inversion counterflow of the hands and feet. The facial complexion is bluish and dark. There is a chilly sweat which spontaneously exits, a pale tongue which is not a live-looking red, and a minute, fine pulse.

Treatment principles: Warm the kidneys, scatter cold, and move stagnation

Guiding formula: *Dang Gui Si Ni Tang Jia Wei* (Dang Gui Four Counterflows Decoction with Added Flavors)

Ingredients: Radix Angelicae Sinensis (*Dang Gui*), Fructus Evodiae Rutecarpae (*Wu Zhu*), Ramulus Cinnamomi Cassiae (*Gui Zhi*), Radix Albus Paeoniae Lactiflorae (*Bai Shao*), Herba Asari Cum Radice (*Xi Xin*), Caulis Akebiae (*Mu Tong*), mix-fried Radix Glycyrrhizae (*Gan Cao*), Fructus Zizyphi Jujubae (*Da Zao*), uncooked Rhizoma Zingiberis (*Sheng Jiang*)

Damp heat in the liver channel

Main symptoms: Initially, there is a yellowish white vaginal discharge which may contain bloody threads. There is also lower abdominal piercing pain. This is followed by pain in the vaginal tract and vaginal discharge like pus. The tongue fur is yellow and slimy or yellow and thick, and the pulse is bowstring and rapid.

Treatment principles: Clear the liver and eliminate dampness

Guiding formula: *Long Dan Xie Gan Tang Jia Wei* **(Gentiana Drain the Liver Decoction with Added Flavors)**

Ingredients: Radix Gentianae Scabrae (*Long Dan Cao*), Rhizoma Alismatis (*Ze Xie*), Caulis Akebiae (*Mu Tong*), Semen Plantaginis (*Che Qian Zi*), uncooked Radix Rehmanniae (*Sheng Di*), Radix Bupleuri (*Chai Hu*), Radix Angelicae Sinensis (*Dang Gui*), Fructus Gardeniae Jasminoidis (*Shan Zhi*), Radix Scutellariae Baicalensis (*Huang Qin*), Ramulus Sophorae Japonicae (*Huai Zhi*), Rhizoma Atractylodis (*Cang Zhu*), Cortex Phellodendri (*Huang Bai*), Fructus Meliae Toosendan (*Chuan Lian Zi*)

Blood vacuity, qi binding

Main symptoms: There is typically a pulling, draining painful sensation in the vaginal tract. There is emotional depression, oppression, and discomfort. The pulse image is bowstring, fine, choppy, and stagnant.

Treatment principles: Soothe the liver and scatter depression

Guiding formula: *Gan Mai Da Zao Tang Jia Xiao Yao San Jia Wei* **(Licorice, Wheat & Red Dates Decoction plus Rambling Powder with Added Flavors)**

Ingredients: Radix Glycyrrhizae (*Gan Cao*), Fructus Levis Tritici Aestivi (*Fu Xiao Mai*), Fructus Zizyphi Jujubae (*Da Zao*), Radix Angelicae Sinensis (*Dang Gui*), Radix Albus Paeoninae Lactiflorae (*Bai Shao*), Radix Bupleuri (*Chai Hu*), Sclerotium Poriae Cocos (*Fu Ling*), Rhizoma Atractylodis Macrocephalae (*Bai Zhu*), Herba Menthae Haplocalycis (*Bo He*), uncooked Radix Rehmanniae (*Sheng Di*), Semen Zizyphi Spinosae (*Suan Zao Ren*), Tian Tai Radix Linderae Struchnifoliae (*Tai Wu*), Cortex Albizziae Julibrissin (*He Huan Pi*), Flos Rosae Rugosae (*Mei Gui Hua*)

Menstrual Movement Nosebleed

If a woman experiences a nosebleed either before or during her menstruation, this is referred to as menstrual movement nosebleed. It is one of several bleeding disorders associated with menstruation. Although these are not commonly seen in clinical practice, all Chinese gynecology texts discuss at least some of these. When these recur on a regular monthly basis, they are usually an indication of endometriosis. In this case, endometrial tissue has migrated outside the endometrium. This endometrial tissue grows and necroses along with the endometrial tissue in the uterus in response to the cyclic changes in hormone levels. Thus this misplaced endometrial tissue bleeds just like the uterine endometrium during menstruation. In premodern Chinese gynecology texts, this type of menstrual movement spontaneous ejection of blood was believed to be counterflowing menstruation. Although some modern Chinese authors have criticized this is what they believe to be a naive idea, it is, in fact, basically correct according to modern Western medicine.

Many Chinese gynecology books do not differentiate between menstrual movement nosebleed and menstrual movement coughing of blood. Rather, they use menstrual movement spontaneous ejection of blood as a disease category to cover both of these. Therefore, most of the formulas given below under this disease category can also be used under the following one as well.

Disease causes, disease mechanisms

This condition is basically due to heat damaging the network vessels and forcing the blood to move frenetically outside its pathways. This heat can have several sources and, therefore, be of different kinds. First of all, internal, usually depressive heat, may be aggravated by external invasion of heat evils before the menses. Such external evils take advantage of the defensive and constructive disharmony that commonly occurs premenstrually because of a constructive and blood vacuity. It is also possible for liver depression to transform into heat and for this heat to counterflow up to and accumulate in the lungs and stomach. Such depressive heat can cause menstrual movement nosebleed all by itself without necessarily there being any external invasion. Third, this heat may be due to overeating acrid, hot, peppery foods, oily, greasy, fried foods or drinking too much alcohol. This causes stomach fire to blaze upward. In actual clinical practice, this is not that commonly seen and, when it occurs, it is usually mixed with depressive heat. And fourth, this heat may be vacuity heat due to yin and blood vacuity premenstrually. Yin vacuity fails to control yang which counterflows upward as vacuity heat, damaging the network vessels above.

Treatment based on pattern discrimination

Heat in both the exterior & interior

Main symptoms: Premenstrual or menstrual nosebleed accompanied by high fever, vexatious thirst leading to drinking, constipated stools, abdominal pain refusing pressure, yellowish red, scanty urination, dry, yellow tongue fur, and a flooding, rapid pulse

Treatment principles: Clear heat and harmonize the blood

Guiding formula: *San Huang Si Wu Tang* **(Three Yellows Four Materials Decoction)**

Ingredients: Radix Scutellariae Baicalensis (*Huang Qi*), Rhizoma Coptidis Chinensis (*Huang Lian*), Radix Et Rhizoma Rhei (*Da Huang*), Radix Angelicae Sinensis (*Dang Gui*), Radix Ligustici Wallichii (*Chuan Xiong*), cooked Radix Rehmanniae (*Shu Di*), Radix Albus Paeoniae Lactiflorae (*Bai Shao*)

Liver channel depressive fire

Main symptoms: Premenstrual or menstrual epistaxis accompanied by moderately excessive blood which is colored red, heart vexation, easy anger, possible rib-side distention and pain, a bitter taste in the mouth, dry throat, dizziness, tinnitus, yellow urine, constipation, menstruation ahead of schedule which is scanty in amount, a red tongue with yellow fur, and a mostly bowstring, rapid pulse

Treatment principles: Course the liver and clear heat, downbear counterflow and stop bleeding

Guiding formulas:

1. *Qing Gan Yin Jing Tang Jia Jian* **(Clear the Liver & Conduct the Menses Decoction with Additions & Subtractions)**

Ingredients: Radix Angelicae Sinensis (*Dang Gui*), Radix Albus Paeoniae Lactiflorae (*Bai Shao*), uncooked Radix Rehmanniae (*Sheng Di*), Cortex Radicis Moutan (*Dan Pi*), Fructus Gardeniae Jasminoidis (*Zhi Ren*), Radix Scutellariae Baicalensis (*Huang Qin*), Fructus Meliae Toosendan (*Chuan Lian Zi*), Radix Rubiae Cordifoliae (*Qian Cao*), Rhizoma Imperatae Cyclindricae (*Bai Mao Gen*), Radix Achyranthis Bidentatae (*Niu Xi*), Radix Glycyrrhizae (*Gan Cao*)

2. *Shun Jing Tang* (Normalize the Flow of the Menses Decoction)

Ingredients: Radix Angelicae Sinensis (*Dang Gui*), Radix Albus Paeoniae Lactiflorae (*Bai Shao*), cooked Radix Rehmanniae (*Shu Di*), Cortex Radicis Moutan (*Dan Pi*), Radix Glehniae Littoralis (*Sha Shen*), Sclerotium Poriae Cocos (*Fu Ling*), blackened Herba Schizonepetae Tenuifoliae (*Jing Jie*)

3. *Qing Jing Si Wu Tang Jia Jian* (Clears the Menses Four Materials Decoction with Additions & Subtractions)

Ingredients: Radix Angelicae Sinensis (*Dang Gui*), Radix Albus Paeoniae Lactiflorae (*Bai Shao*), uncooked Radix Rehmanniae (*Sheng Di*), Radix Scutellariae Baicalensis (*Huang Qin*), Rhizoma Coptidis Chinensis (*Huang Lian*), Cortex Phellodendri (*Huang Bai*), Rhizoma Anemarrhenae Aspheloidis (*Zhi Mu*), Gelatinum Corii Asini (*E Jiao*), Rhizoma Cyperi Rotundi (*Xiang Fu*), Radix Glycyrrhizae (*Gan Cao*), Cortex Radicis Moutan (*Dan Pi*), Radix Achyranthis Bidentatae (*Niu Xi*)

Additions: If defecation is difficult, add a small amount of Radix Et Rhizoma Rhei (*Da Huang*).

4. Unnamed formula from *Concise Traditional Chinese Gynecology*

Ingredients: Flos Imperatae Cylindricae (*Bai Mao Hua*), Radix Cyathulae Officinalis (*Chuan Niu Xi*), Radix Rubiae Cordifoliae (*Qian Cao*), Herba Lycopi Lucidi (*Ze Lan*), carbonized Cortex Radicis Moutan (*Dan Pi*), Semen Leonuri Heterophylli (*Chong Wei Zi*), blackened Fructus Gardeniae Jasminoidis (*Shan Zi*)

Stomach fire blazing & exuberant

Main symptoms: Sudden onset of epistaxis or hemoptysis one or two days before or just at the onset of menstruation accompanied by reduced amount of the menstruate or the menses may halt or not come, lower abdominal pain, dry mouth and throat, a red facial complexion, a red tongue with yellow fur, and a surging, rapid or slippery, rapid pulse

Treatment principles: Clear heat, cool the blood, and stop bleeding

Guiding formulas:

1. *San Huang Si Wu Tang* (Three Yellows Four Materials Decoction)

Ingredients: Radix Angelicae Sinensis (*Dang Gui*), uncooked Radix Rehmanniae (*Sheng Di*), Radix Albus Paeoniae Lactiflorae (*Bai Shao*), Radix Ligustici Wallichii (*Chuan Xiong*),

Radix Scutellariae Baicalensis (*Huang Qin*), Rhizoma Coptidis Chinensis (*Huang Lian*), Radix Et Rhizoma Rhei (*Da Huang*)

This formula is from the *Yi Zong Jin Jian (The Golden Mirror of Ancestral Medicine)*. If there is no constipation, the amount of Radix Et Rhizoma Rhei can be reduced or deleted altogether.

Additions & subtractions: Yang Yi-ya says to remove Ligusticum and add Herba Cirsii Japonici & Herba Cephalanoploris Segeti (*Da Xiao Ji*), Nodus Nelumbinis Nuciferae (*Ou Jie*), Rhizoma Imperatae Cylindricae (*Bai Mao Gen*), and Radix Achyranthis Bidentatae (*Niu Xi*).

2. Sun Si-miao's *Xi Jiao Di Huang Tang* (Rhinoceros Horn & Rehmannia Decoction)

Ingredients: Cornu Rhinocerotis (*Xi Jiao,* substitute Cornu Bubali, *Shui Niu Jiao*), uncooked Radix Rehmanniae (*Sheng Di*), Radix Rubrus Paeoniae Lactiflorae (*Chi Shao*), Cortex Radicis Moutan (*Dan Pi*)

This formula is from Sun Si-miao's *Qian Jin Yao Fang (Prescriptions [Worth] 1,000 [Pieces of] Gold)*.

3. Ye Tian-shi's *Xi Jiao Di Huang Tang* (Rhinoceros Horn & Rehmannia Decoction)

Ingredients: Cornu Rhinocerotis (*Xi Jiao,* substitute Cornu Bubali, *Shui Niu Jiao*), Radix Albus Paeoniae Lactiflorae (*Bai Shao*), Cortex Radicis Moutan (*Dan Pi*), Fructus Citri Aurantii (*Zhi Qiao*), uncooked Radix Rehmanniae (*Sheng Di*), Radix Scutellariae Baicalensis (*Huang Qin*), Radix Platycodi Grandiflori (*Jie Geng*), Pericarpium Citri Reticulatae (*Chen Pi*), Pulvis Carbonisatus Fumi (*Bai Cao Shuang*)

This formula is from *Ye Tian Shi Nu Ke (Ye Tian-shi's Gynecology)*.

4. *Si Wu Liang Ge San* (Four Materials Cool the Diaphragm Powder)

Ingredients: Radix Angelicae Sinensis (*Dang Gui*), Radix Ligustici Wallichii (*Chuan Xiong*), Radix Rubrus Paeoniae Lactiflorae (*Chi Shao*), uncooked Radix Rehmanniae (*Sheng Di*), wine stir-fried Radix Scutellariae Baicalensis (*Huang Qin*), wine stir-fried Rhizoma Coptidis Chinensis (*Huang Lian*), stir-fried black Fructus Gardeniae Jasminoidis (*Shan Zhi*), Fructus Forsythiae Suspensae (*Lian Qiao*), Radix Platycodi Grandiflori (*Jie Geng*), uncooked Radix Glycyrrhizae (*Sheng Cao*), Herba Menthae Haplocalycis (*Bo He*), Folium Bambusae (*Zhu Ye*)

Wan Mi-zhai gives this formula for the treatment of menstrual blood frenetic movement with spontaneous ejection of blood, in which case, Master Wan says to add fresh, macerated Chinese chive juice and take.

Lung-kidney yin vacuity

Main symptoms: During or after the menses there is epistaxis. The amount of the menses is scanty and colored dark red. There is dizziness, tinnitus, heat in the hands, feet, and heart, both cheeks tidal red, a dry throat and parched mouth, the menses may come early and be scanty in amount, and there is a red or scarlet tongue with flowery, peeled or absent fur and a mostly fine, rapid pulse.

Treatment principles: Enrich yin and moisten the lungs, clear heat and cool the blood

Guiding formulas:

1. *Shun Jing Tang Jia Jian* (Normalize the Flow of the Menses Decoction with Additions & Subtractions)

Ingredients: Radix Angelicae Sinensis (*Dang Gui*), cooked Radix Rehmanniae (*Shu Di*), Radix Albus Paeoniae Lactiflorae (*Bai Shao*), Cortex Radicis Moutan (*Dan Pi*), Sclerotium Poriae Cocos (*Fu Ling*), Radix Glehniae Littoralis (*Sha Shen*), blackened Herba Schizonepetae Tenuifoliae (*Jing Jie Sui*), Cornu Rhinocerotis (*Xi Jiao*, substitute Cornu Bubali, *Shui Niu Jiao*)

2. *Bai He Gu Jin Tang Jia Wei* (Lily Secure Metal Decoction with Added Flavors)

Ingredients: Bulbus Lilii (*Bai He*), uncooked Radix Rehmanniae (*Sheng Di*), cooked Radix Rehmanniae (*Shu Di*), Radix Scrophulariae Ningpoensis (*Yuan Shen*), Bulbus Fritillariae (*Bei Mu*), Radix Platycodi Grandiflori (*Jie Geng*), Tuber Ophiopogonis Japonici (*Mai Dong*), Radix Albus Paeoniae Lactiflorae (*Bai Shao*), Radix Angelicae Sinensis (*Dang Gui*), Radix Glycyrrhizae (*Gan Cao*), Rhizoma Imperatae Cylindricae (*Bai Mao Gen*), Cornu Rhinocerotis (*Xi Jiao*, substitute Cornu Bubali, *Shui Niu Jiao*)

3. *Huo Xue Run Zao Sheng Jin Tang Jia Jian* (Quicken the Blood, Moisten Dryness & Engender Fluids Decoction with Additions & Subtractions)

Ingredients: Radix Angelicae Sinensis (*Dang Gui*), Radix Albus Paeoniae Lactiflorae (*Bai Shao*), uncooked Radix Rehmanniae (*Sheng Di*), Tuber Ophiopogonis Japonici (*Mai Dong*), Tuber Asparagi Cochinensis (*Tian Dong*), Radix Trichosanthis Kirlowii (*Tian Hua Fen*), Semen Pruni Persicae (*Tao Ren*), Flos Carthami Tinctorii (*Hong Hua*)

This formula, composed by Zhu Dan-xi, quickens the blood, moistens dryness, and engenders fluids as its name says. It is recommended by the authors of *Zhong Yi Fu Ke Xue (A Study of Chinese Medical Gynecology)* for the treatment of yin vacuity, lung dryness menstrual movement spontaneous ejection of blood.

4. Unnamed formula from *Concise Traditional Chinese Gynecology*

Ingredients: Uncooked Radix Rehmanniae (*Sheng Di*), Radix Scrophulariae Ningpoensis (*Yuan Shen*), Tuber Ophiopogonis Japonici (*Mai Dong*), Radix Rubiae Cordifoliae (*Qian Cao*), Cortex Radicis Lycii Chinensis (*Di Gu Pi*), Radix Salviae Miltiorrhizae (*Dan Shen*)

5. *Jia Wei Mai Men Dong Tang* (Added Flavors Ophiopogon Decoction)

Ingredients: Tuber Ophiopogonis Japonici (*Mai Dong*), Radix Panacis Ginseng (*Ren Shen*), Rhizoma Pinelliae Ternatae (*Ban Xia*), Radix Dioscoreae Oppositae (*Shan Yao*), Radix Albus Paeoniae Lactiflorae (*Bai Shao*), Radix Salviae Miltiorrhizae (*Dan Shen*), Radix Glycyrrhizae (*Gan Cao*), Semen Pruni Persicae (*Tao Ren*), Fructus Zizyphi Jujubae (*Da Zao*)

This formula is given in the *Yi Xue Zhong Zhong Can Xi Lu (Records of Heart-felt Experiences in Medicine with Reference to the West)* for the treatment of stomach vacuity menstrual movement spontaneous ejection of blood. However, because of the mother/child relationship between the stomach and lungs, fluid dryness of one will often precipitate or accompany yin and qi vacuity of the other. This formula is similar to Zhu Dan-xi's formula given above. It contains only a single heat-clearing ingredient, Ophiopogon, and its emphasis is on nourishing yin, engendering fluids, and supplementing the qi of the middle burner. It should be considered when there is recurrent perimenstrual epistaxis without signs of either prominent heat or liver qi but signs of fluid dryness of the lungs and stomach with qi vacuity.

Discussion

Menstrual movement epistaxis and spitting blood are not all that frequently encountered in clinical practice but one does see them. Often the patient has no idea the bleeding is related to her menstruation. Most typically, she thinks it is due to some other, unrelated cause.

The authors of the *Yi Zong Jin Jian (The Golden Mirror of Ancestral Medicine)* state that the main reason for menstrual movement spontaneous ejection of blood is heat damaging the network vessels. If heat damages the yin network vessels below, there will be flooding. But if heat damages the yang network vessels above, there will be epistaxis and spitting of blood. Wu Qian *et al.* also say that if the epistaxis and hemoptysis are due to heat and precede menstruation, to use precipitation and discharge with *San Huang Si Wu Tang* (Three Yellows Four Materials Decoction), but, if the bleeding occurs after menstruation, do not use precipitation. In that case one should use *Xi Jiao Di Huang Tang* (Rhinoceros Horn & Rehmannia Decoction).

The formulas given above are mostly for administration during the bleeding episodes. After the bleeding has stopped, one should delete the hemostatic and styptic ingredients so as not to cause blood stasis. After menstruation, the emphasis should be on supplementing the blood and nourishing yin. During the premenstruum, the emphasis should be on rectifying the qi and clearing heat. One should not use the above formulas unmodified if the patient reports that she experienced epistaxis or hemoptysis several days or a week previously. That would be like shutting the barn door after the horse has run away. Therefore, when treating menstrual movement spontaneous ejection of blood, one must distinguish between root and branch and treat accordingly.

Menstrual Movement Coughing Blood

Just as a women may experience premenstrual or menstrual epistaxis, so some women may experience premenstrual or menstrual hemoptysis. When this occurs, it may be due to endometriosis.

Disease causes, disease mechanisms

If liver fire becomes effulgent during the premenstruum due to liver depression transforming heat, it may flare upward and harass the lungs, damaging the lung network vessels and forcing the blood to move frenetically outside its pathways. Thus there is coughing of blood.

Treatment based on pattern discrimination

Liver fire attacking the lungs

Main symptoms: During the menstruation there is hemoptysis with rapid breathing, chest fullness, vexatious heat in the five hearts, a dry, red tongue with thin, yellow fur, and a fine, bowstring pulse

Treatment principles: Clear heat and stop bleeding

Guiding formula: *Wu Hu Tang Jia Wei* (Five Tigers Decoction with Added Flavors)

Ingredients: Pericarpium Citri Reticulatae (*Chen Pi*), Cortex Radicis Mori Albi (*Sang Bai Pi*), Radix Platycodi Grandiflori (*Jie Geng*), Fructus Perillae Frutescentis (*Su Zi*), Gypsum Fibrosum (*Shi Gao*), Rhizoma Anemarrhenae Aspheloidis (*Zhi Mu*), Fructus Citri Aurantii (*Zhi Ke*), Gelatinum Corii Asini (*E Jiao*), Radix Asteris Tatarici (*Zi Wan*), Fructus Schisandrae Chinensis (*Wu Wei Zi*), Semen Pruni Armeniacae (*Xing Ren*), Flos Tussilaginis Farfarae (*Kuan Dong Hua*), Bulbus Fritillariae (*Bei Mu*)

Menstrual Movement Bloody Stool

Before, during, or after menstruation there may be bleeding with defecation. In the Chinese gynecological literature, this is called menstrual movement bloody stool.

Disease causes, disease mechanisms

Mostly, menstrual movement bloody stool is associated with a preference for eating acrid, peppery, hot foods. Thus there is heat smoldering in the viscera. Over time, this heat accumulates and becomes depressed. It is also possible for there to be liver channel depressive heat or yin vacuity and internal heat. This heat harasses the *chong* and *ren*, forcing the blood to move frentically outside its pathways.

Treatment based on pattern discrimination

Liver-stomach depressive heat

Main symptoms: Hemafecia with menstruation, the amount of menstrual blood scanty and colored deep red, thick and sticky in consistency. There is heart vexation, easy anger, thin, yellow tongue fur, and a bowstring, rapid pulse.

Treatment principles: Clear heat and soothe the liver

Guiding formulas:

1. *Dan Zhi Xiao Yao San Jia Wei* (Moutan & Gardenia Rambling Powder with Added Flavors)

Ingredients: Cortex Radicis Moutan (*Dan Pi*), Fructus Gardeniae Jasminoidis (*Zhi Ren*), Radix Scutellariae Baicalensis (*Huang Qin*), Radix Angelicae Sinensis (*Dang Gui*), Radix Albus Paeoniae Lactiflorae (*Bai Shao*), Radix Bupleuri (*Chai Hu*), Rhizoma Atractylodis Macrocephalae (*Bai Zhu*), Sclerotium Poriae Cocos (*Fu Ling*), mix-fried Radix Glycyrrhizae (*Gan Cao*), uncooked Radix Rehmanniae (*Sheng Di*), Herba Ecliptae Prostratae (*Han Lian Cao*), Radix Rubiae Cordifoliae (*Qian Cao*), Radix Sanguisorbae (*Di Yu*)

2. Zhang Jing-yue's *Yue Ying Jian* (Restrain the Constructive Decoction)

Ingredients: Uncooked Radix Rehmanniae (*Sheng Di*), Radix Albus Paeoniae Lactiflorae (*Bai Shao*), Radix Glycyrrhizae (*Gan Cao*), Radix Sanguisorbae (*Di Yu*), Radix Scutellariae Baicalensis (*Huang Qin*), Flos Immaturus Sophorae Japonicae (*Huai Hua*), stir-fried Herba Schizonepetae Tenuifoliae (*Jie Sui*), Radix Dipsaci (*Chuan Duan*)

Additions: If there is constipation due to heat, add a small amount of Radix Et Rhizoma Rhei (*Da Huang*) to clear heat and free the flow of the stools.

3. *Qing Ying Jian Jia Jian* (Clear the Constructive Decoction with Additions & Subtractions)

Ingredients: Uncooked Radix Rehmanniae (*Sheng Di*), Radix Albus Paeoniae Lactiflorae (*Bai Shao*), Radix Glycyrrhizae (*Gan Cao*), Radix Dipsaci (*Xu Duan*), Radix Sanguisorbae (*Di Yu*), Flos Immaturus Sophorae Japonicae (*Huai Hua Mi*), stir-fried Herba Schizonepetae Tenuifoliae (*Jing Jie*), Radix Scutellariae Baicalensis (*Huang Qin*), Fructus Gardeniae Jasminoidis (*Shan Zhi*), Rhizoma Coptidis Chinensis (*Huang Lian*), Semen Pruni (*Yu Li*), Fructus Pruni Mume (*Wu Mei*)

Although the first word in the name of this formula is different, it appears to be the same basic prescription as the preceding one with additional ingredients.

Vacuity heat

Main symptoms: During menstruation there is precipitation of blood with defecation, dizziness, vertigo, lassitude of the spirit, fatigue, shortness of breath, low back and knee soreness and weakness, heart vexation, scanty sleep, a red tongue with thin fur, and a fine or fine, rapid pulse.

Treatment principles: Boost the qi and nourish the blood, contain the blood and return it to the channels

Guiding formula: *Shun Jing Liang An Tang* (Normalize the Flow of the Menses Two Quieting [Medicinals] Decoction)

Ingredients: Radix Angelicae Sinensis (*Dang Gui*), Radix Albus Paeoniae Lactiflorae (*Bai Shao*), cooked Radix Rehmanniae (*Shu Di*), Fructus Corni Officinalis (*Shan Yu Rou*), Radix

Codonopsitis Pilosulae (*Dang Shen*), Rhizoma Atractylodis Macrocephalae (*Bai Zhu*), Tuber Ophiopogonis Japonici (*Mai Dong*), blackened Herba Schizonepetae Tenuifoliae (*Jing Jie Sui*), Radix Morindae Officinalis (*Ba Ji Rou*), Rhizoma Cimicifugae (*Sheng Ma*)

This formula treats yin vacuity-vacuity heat complicated by spleen qi vacuity.

Menstrual Movement Bloody Urine

Some women may also experience hematuria each month either directly before or along with their menstruation. This is called menstrual movement bloody urine.

Disease causes, disease mechanisms

Because of mental-emotional stress, heart fire may blaze up internally. This heat may be transferred to the small intestine and thence to the bladder with which it is connected. There, this heat damages the yin network vessels. Heat in the heart may become excessive just before or at the onset of menstruation because depressive heat in the liver may be at its maximum just before the menses. Thus, urinary bleeding may occur at the beginning or along with menstruation.

It is also possible for ministerial fire to stir frenetically due to liver-kidney yin vacuity. This is mostly the case in premenopausal women whose liver blood and kidney yin have become relatively exhausted. This vacuity heat scorches the network vessels in the lower burner and may cause urinary bleeding directly after the menses when yin vacuity is at its greatest cyclically. Han Bai-ling says that although menstrual movement bloody stool is mostly categorized as a replete full disease, menstrual movement bloody urine may be either a replete or vacuity pattern.

Treatment based on pattern discrimination

Heart fire blazing internally

Main symptoms: Hematuria with the menstrual period which is colored dark red, dizziness, heart vexation, a bitter taste in the mouth, dry throat, constipation, heat and pain in the urinary tract, red lips and facial complexion, dry, yellow tongue fur, possible sores on the tip of the tongue, and a bowstring, slippery, rapid pulse

Treatment principles: Clear the heart, cool the blood, and stop bleeding

Guiding formula: *Ba Zheng San* **(Eight [Ingredients] Correcting Powder)**

Ingredients: Caulis Akebiae Mutong (*Mu Tong*), Talcum (*Hua Shi*), Semen Plantaginis (*Che Qian Zi*), Herba Dianthi (*Qu Mai*), Herba Polygoni Aviculari (*Bian Xu*), Fructus Gardeniae Jasminoidis (*Zhi Zi*), Medulla Junci Effusi (*Deng Xin Cao*), Radix Glycyrrhizae (*Gan Cao*)

Additions: Han Bai-ling suggests adding Folium Pyrrosiae (*Shi Wei*), Radix Achyranthis Bidentatae (*Niu Xi*), Cortex Radicis Moutan (*Dan Pi*), and Rhizoma Imperatae Cylindricae (*Mao Geng*) to cool the blood and stop bleeding. If there is constipation due to heat, Han Bai-ling says to add a small amount of Radix Et Rhizoma Rhei (*Da Huang*) to clear heat and free the bowels. However, it should be noted that Bensky and Barolet say that Radix Et Rhizoma Rhei (*Da Huang*) is a standard ingredient in *Ba Zheng San*. If this latter ingredient is regarded as standard in this formula, the formula's name, Eight (Ingredients) Correcting Powder, then makes no sense as there would be nine ingredients.

Liver-kidney yin vacuity

Main symptoms: Hematuria at the time of menstruation in premenopausal women, color pale, heart palpitations, insomnia, dry mouth but no desire to drink, a red facial complexion, flushed cheeks, tidal fever and/or night sweats, heat in the center of the hands, feet, and heart, and a bowstring, fine, rapid pulse

Treatment principles: Nourish yin, clear heat, and stop bleeding

Guiding formula: *Dao Chi San* **(Abduct the Red Powder)**

Ingredients: Uncooked Radix Rehmanniae (*Sheng Di*), Caulis Akebiae Mutong (*Mu Tong*), Folium Bambusae (*Zhu Ye*), Radix Glycyrrhizae (*Gan Cao*)

Additions: Han Bai-ling says to add Tuber Ophiopogonis Japonici (*Mai Dong*), Rhizoma Anemarrhenae Aspheloidis (*Zhi Mu*), Radix Achyranthis Bidentatae (*Niu Xi*), and Cortex Radicis Moutan (*Dan Pi*) to enrich yin and cool the blood.

MENSTRUAL MOVEMENT DISEASES

Disease	Pattern	Treatment Methods	Formula
Menstrual movement breast distention & pain	Liver qi depression & binding	course liver, resolve depression, rectify qi, stop pain	Chai Hu Shu Gan San Jia Fu Ling
	Liver-kidney yin vacuity	enrich kidneys, nourish yin	Yi Guan Jian
Menstrual movement fever	Blood heat internally exuberant	clear heat, cool blood	Qing Jing San Jia Wei
	Liver-kidney yin vacuity	nourish yin, clear heat	Liang Di Tan
	Qi & blood vacuity weakness	boost qi, secure exterior	Bu Zhong Yi Qi Tang
	Stasis heat blockage obstruction	transform stasis, clear heat	Xue Fu Zhu Yu Tang
Menstrual movement headache	Blood vacuity	nourish blood, boost the qi	Ba Zhen Tang Jia Wei
	Liver fire	nourish yin, clear heat, soften liver, extinguish wind	Qi Ju Di Huang Wan Jia Wei
	Blood stasis	regulate qi, quicken blood, transform stasis, free network vessels	Tong Qiao Huo Xue Tang
Menstrual movement body pain	Blood stasis	nourish blood, dispel wind, scatter cold, eliminate pain	Chen Tang San Jia Wei
	Blood vacuity	nourish blood, boost qi, soften sinews, stop pain	Dan Gui Bu Xue Tang Jia Wei
Menstrual movement diarrhea	Spleen vacuity	fortify spleen, boost qi, transform dampness	Shen Ling Bai Zhu San
	Kidney vacuity	warm kidneys, support yang, warm spleen	Jian Gu Tang plus Si Shen Wan

Menstrual movement hemoptysis & epistaxis	Liver channel depressive fire	course liver, clear heat, abduct blood to move downward	*Qing Gan Dao Jing Tang*
	Lung-kidney yin vacuity	enrich yin, moisten lungs, abduct blood to move downward	*Shun Jing Tang*
Menstrual movement mouth sores	Yin vacuity, fire effulgence	enrich yin, downbear fire	*Zhi Bai Di Huang Wan*
	Stomach fire smoldering & steaming	clear stomach, drain fire	*Liang Ge San*
Menstrual movement addictive papules	Blood vacuity	nourish blood, course wind	*Dang Gui Yin Zi*
	Wind heat	course wind, clear heat	*Qing Feng San*
Menstrual movement vertigo & dizziness	Blood vacuity	nourish blood, boost spleen	*Gui Pi Tang Jia Wei*
	Yin vacuity, yang hyperactive	enrich yin, subdue yang	*Tian Ma Gou Teng Yin*
	Spleen vacuity mixed w/ damp	fortify spleen, warm yang, transform damp, dispel phlegm	*Ban Xia Bai Zhu Tian Ma Tang*
Menstrual movement superficial edema	Spleen-kidney yang vacuity	warm kidneys, fortify spleen, disinhibit water	*Ling Gui Zhu Gan Tang Jia Wei*
	Qi stagnation, blood stasis	rectify qi, quicken blood	*Ba Wu Tang Jia Wei*
Menstrual movement emotional abnormality	Liver qi depression & binding	soothe liver, resolve depression	*Xiao Yao San*
	Phlegm fire harassing above	clear heat, wash away phlegm	*Sheng Tie Lou Yin*

10

Perimenopausal Syndrome

Menopausal syndrome is a relatively recent addition to the TCM list of menstrual diseases. Its addition reflects the influence of modern Western medicine. Just as the Chinese have translated premenstrual syndrome very literally into Chinese, they likewise have translated perimenopausal syndrome into *jing duan qian hou zhu zheng*. *Jing* once again refers to the menses. *Duan* means to cut off or stop as in stopping one's water supply. *Qian hou* means before and after. And *zhu zheng* literally means various pathoconditions but is more typically translated as syndrome. This syndrome is also referred to as *geng nian qi zong he zheng*. In that case, *geng* means change. *Nian* means age as in old age. *Qi* means at the time of. *Zong he* means composite and *zheng* means pathocondition. Therefore, this term may be translated loosely as climacteric syndrome. This second name is used more in Chinese Western medical texts and in integrated Chinese-Western medicine.

Menopause itself is called *jing duan* or the cessation of menstruation. This itself is not a disease. It is a naturally occurring event manifesting the body's great inherent wisdom. It is, as both the last Chinese name for it, *geng nian qi*, and the English, change in life, imply, a physiologic change. When this change proceeds smoothly and without a hitch, there are few, if any pathological signs or symptoms. The menses cease and the woman goes on about her business. However, increasingly in the West, this change does not proceed smoothly and uneventfully. Rather, various conditions manifest which may last from several weeks to decades after the cessation of the menses. It is these various pathoconditions which are classified as species of menstrual disease in TCM and not the menopause itself. These conditions include hot flashes, night sweats, insomnia, heart palpitations and racing heart, anxiety, irritability, dizziness and vertigo, tinnitus, migraine headaches, fatigue, emotional lability, forgetfulness, hypertension, lumbar soreness, and formication.

As Song and Yu say, these signs and symptoms occurring before, during, or after the menopause may be more or less severe and may last a longer or shorter period of time depending upon the case. Although many modern women consider these signs and symptoms to be a natural and unavoidable part of menopause, similar to many modern women's belief that PMS and dysmenorrhea are natural and inevitable, in fact, they are not. They are a sign of imbalance and they can and should be treated. In fact, treatment with internally administered Chinese medicinals is exceptionally effective for treating the full constellation of perimenopausal complaints and does so cost effectively and without iatrogenesis.

In my experience with Western patients, very commonly a woman may begin to experience shorter menstrual cycles with scantier flow in her early 40s. This is often due to depressive heat gradually transforming into empty heat compounded by a decline in kidney yang and spleen qi. After several years, there may be breakthrough bleeding or spotting, menorrhagia, or metrorrhagia. Then, after some time, the cycle may tend to become sometimes early and sometimes late or consistently late for several cycles and then suddenly stop.

Although TCM theory suggests that the normative age for menopause should be after 49 years of age, many Western women experience what Western MDs refer to as premature menopause. If the practitioner encounters hot flashes and night sweats in a woman in her mid to late 30s or early 40s, they should consider treating this woman as a case of incipient menopause. The patterns involved in such cases are the same as those involved in perimenopausal syndrome. We will discuss this further below after parsing out the various disease mechanisms and patterns responsible for perimenopausal complaints.

Disease causes, disease mechanisms

It is said in the opening chapters of the *Nei Jing Su Wen (Inner Classic Simple Questions)* that, at seven times seven or 49 years of age, kidney essence is exhausted in the female and thus the *tian gui* ceases. In other words, at approximately 50 years of age, the *ren mai* is vacuous and the *chong mai* is debilitated and its blood is scanty. This is based on the fact that both the *chong* and *ren* arise from the uterus and carry or are filled with primarily kidney qi and essence. However, this is not the whole story.

Just as the maturation of the spleen-stomach creating a superabundance of acquired or latter heaven essence plays a part in the initial arrival of the *tian gui* or menarche, so does the decline of the spleen-stomach and, therefore, a decline in the production and storage of acquired essence play an important part in the cessation of the *tian gui*. The *Nei Jing (Inner Classic)* also says that the *yang ming* begins to decline at the age of 35 in a woman and that this is why the facial skin develops wrinkles since it is no longer nourished by sufficient blood. As the spleen's ability to engender postnatally abundant blood and acquired essence declines, this places more of a burden on kidney essence if blood is to regularly fill to overflowing the *chong mai/bao gong*/uterus. If this burden were allowed to continue indefinitely, this would really exhaust the kidneys and lead to premature aging and debility.

But this is not the case. The body recognizes the drain that the kidneys' maintenance of regular menses is after the spleen and stomach have begun to decline and slack off in their participation in the engenderment and transformation of blood. Therefore, a change is initiated primarily in the relationship between the kidneys and heart via the uterus and *chong mai/bao mai*. Rather than sending blood down from the heart, the *bao mai* reverses the direction of its flow, sending essence up to nourish the spirit residing in the heart. Instead of preparing the uterus for the growth of a physical addition to the community of humankind, the blood focuses on the heart to nourish the woman's spirit. Thus the postmenopausal woman becomes the wise woman or *sage femme*, the mother of her community and a fountain of wisdom. From this point of view, menopause should not be seen as a loss of youth but rather as the potential gaining of wisdom and spiritual power.

However, this change is initiated by blood vacuity and insufficiency of yin and essence. As the *bao mai* reverses its flow, it is easy for yang to come out of control and to flush upwards. This may manifest as evil heat accumulating or counterflowing up above. This heat may accumulate in the liver, the lungs, or the heart causing symptoms of dysfunction in any of these viscera. Along with symptoms of vacuity heat, fire, and rising, rootless yang, such as migraine headaches, hypertension, tinnitus, dizziness, heart palpitations, insomnia, restlessness, anxiety, lability[29], and hot flashes, yin may be insufficient to nourish the structure of the body and, therefore, symptoms of dryness, atrophy, shrinkage, and malnourishment of the various tissues of the body may manifest. These include dry skin, lumbar soreness, vaginal dryness and atrophy[30], greying of the hair, and stiffness of the sinews. As yang rises upward, it may leave the lower body vacuous and cold with cold feet and polyuria, nocturia, and incontinence.

It is also interesting to note that those women who seem to have the worst and most prolonged difficulties with perimenopausal complaints are those women with a long history of liver depression qi stagnation. All transformations in the body are managed by the qi mechanism. The change in life in women is just such a transformation. If there is liver qi, the qi mechanism is not freely flowing and uninhibited. In my experience, liver qi is the *sine qua non* of perimenopausal syndrome. If this change in life is able to proceed quickly and smoothly without hinderance or obstruction, then there are few if any menopausal complaints.

---

[29] In TCM gynecology, anxiety and emotional lability are typically discussed under the heading *zang zao* or visceral agitation, sometimes translated as hysteria.

[30] In TCM, this is usually discussed not under perimenopausal syndrome but under the *wai ke* category of *lao nian xing yin dao yan* or senile vaginitis.

In other words, the weakening and decline of the spleen and kidneys by themselves are not sufficient to create the kinds of symptoms one finds in women with perimenopausal syndrome. Granted, symptoms such as night sweats and hot flashes mostly have to do with yin vacuity-vacuity heat or yin vacuity-yang hyperactivity. However, if the woman goes through her change in life and her menses cease, then she no longer loses yin blood every month. In that case, her spleen and kidneys can produce sufficient blood and latter heaven essence to keep her from having such yin vacuity signs and symptoms. On the other hand, if the woman suffers from liver depression qi stagnation and her qi mechanism is inhibited, even though her menses have ceased, her spleen and kidneys may still not be able to engender and transform sufficient yin blood to keep from manifesting symptoms of vacuity heat or depressive heat. This is because liver depression transforming heat continuously damages and consumes blood and yin fluids. Thus there is never a chance for the woman to recuperate her loses and, in some cases, menopausal complaints can go on for many years.

Most of the symptoms of perimenopausal syndrome either have to do with liver depression qi stagnation, counterflowing heat and yang qi, yin blood vacuity and fluid dryness, or spleen qi and kidney yang vacuity.

Treatment based on pattern discrimination

Liver-kidney yin vacuity

Main symptoms: Dizziness, headache, blurred vision, heart vexation, easy anger, emotional lability, menses sometimes profuse, sometimes scanty, possible spotting without cessation, pale red colored blood, tinnitus, tidal fever, *i.e.*, hot flashes and night sweats, heat in the center of the hands, feet, and heart, soreness and weakness in the low back and knees, constipation, insomnia, a red facial complexion and red cheeks, a dry mouth but no particular desire to drink, a dry, red tongue with no fur, and a bowstring, fine, rapid pulse

Treatment principles: Enrich yin and nourish the liver

Guiding formulas:

1. *Liu Wei Di Huang Wan Jia Wei* (Six Flavors Rehmannia Pills with Added Flavors)

Ingredients: Cooked Radix Rehmanniae (*Shu Di*), Radix Dioscoreae Oppositae (*Shan Yao*), Fructus Corni Officinalis (*Shan Zhu Rou*), Sclerotium Poriae Cocos (*Fu Ling*), Cortex Radicis Moutan (*Dan Pi*), Rhizoma Alismatis (*Ze Xie*), Radix Albus Paeoniae Lactiflorae (*Bai Shao*), Concha Ostreae (*Mu Li*), Dens Draconis (*Long Chi*), Plastrum Testudinis (*Gui Ban*), Concha Haliotidis (*Shi Jue Ming*), Fructus Tribuli Terrestris (*Suo Ji Li*)

Liu Yan-chi's version of this formula, in *The Essential Book of Traditional Chinese Medicine,* is composed of: cooked Radix Rehmanniae (*Shu Di*), Radix Dioscoreae Oppositae (*Shan Yao*), Fructus Corni Officinalis (*Shan Zhu Yu*), Sclerotium Poriae Cocos (*Fu Ling*), Cortex Radicis Moutan (*Dan Pi*), Radix Rubrus Paeoniae Lactiflorae (*Chi Shao*), Radix Albus Paeoniae Lactiflorae (*Bai Shao*), Fructus Ligustri Lucidi (*Nu Zhen Zi*), Concha Haliotidis (*Jue Ming Zi*), and Radix Scrophulariae Ningpoensis (*Yuan Shen*). If accompanied by flaring of vacuity fire, add Rhizoma Anemarrhenae Aspheloidis (*Zhi Niu*) and Cortex Phellodendri (*Huang Bai*). With profuse sweating, add Fructus Levis Tritici Aestivi (*Fu Xiao Mai*). If there is insomnia, add Caulis Polygoni Multiflori (*Ye Jiao Teng*) and Magnetitum (*Ci Shi*). And if there is lumbar pain, add Radix Dipsaci (*Xu Duan*), Ramulus Loranthi Seu Visci (*Sang Ji Sheng*), and Fructus Psoraleae Corylifoliae (*Bu Gu Zhi*).

2. *Bu Shen Di Huang Wan* (Supplement the Kidneys Rehmannia Pills)

Ingredients: Cooked Radix Rehmanniae (*Shu Di*), Rhizoma Anemarrhenae Aspheloidis (*Zhi Mu*), salt-processed Cortex Phellodendri (*Huang Bai*), Rhizoma Alismatis (*Ze Xie*), Radix Dioscoreae Oppositae (*Shan Yao*), Radix Polygalae Tenuifoliae (*Yuan Zhi*), Sclerotium Poriae Cocos (*Fu Ling*), Cortex Radicis Moutan (*Dan Pi*), Semen Zizyphi Spinosae (*Zao Ren*), Radix Scrophulariae Ningpoensis (*Yuan Shen*), Tuber Ophiopogonis Japonici (*Mai Dong*), Folium Bambusae (*Zhu Ye*), Plastrum Testudinis (*Gui Ban*), Ootheca Mantidis (*Sang Piao Xiao*), Fructus Corni Officinalis (*Shan Zhu Rou*)

3. *Zhi Bai Di Huang Wan Jia Wei* (Anemarrhena & Phellodendron Rehmannia Pills with Added Flavors)

Ingredients: Cooked Radix Rehmanniae (*Shu Di*), Fructus Corni Officinalis (*Shan Zhu Rou*), Radix Dioscoreae Oppositae (*Shan Yao*), Sclerotium Poriae Cocos (*Fu Ling*), Rhizoma Alismatis (*Ze Xie*), Cortex Radicis Moutan (*Dan Pi*), Cortex Phellodendri (*Huang Bai*), Rhizoma Anemarrhenae Aspheloidis (*Zhi Mu*), Concha Ostreae (*Mu Li*), Os Draconis (*Long Gu*)

This formula and the one above it are appropriate if there is vacuity heat, not just yin vacuity symptoms of malnourishment and dryness.

4. *Gui Shao Di Huang Wan* (Dang Gui & Peony Rehmannia Pills)

Ingredients: Radix Angelicae Sinensis (*Dang Gui*), Radix Albus Paeoniae Lactiflorae (*Bai Shao*), cooked Radix Rehmanniae (*Shu Di*), Radix Dioscoreae Oppositae (*Shan Yao*), Fructus Corni Officinalis (*Shan Zhu Rou*), Cortex Radicis Moutan (*Dan Pi*), Rhizoma Alismatis (*Ze Xie*), Sclerotium Poriae Cocos (*Fu Ling*)

This formula is for the treatment of uncomplicated and not too severe liver blood-kidney yin vacuity.

Additions: For dizziness and tinnitus, add Fructus Gardeniae Jasminoidis (*Zhi Zi*), Fructus Corni Officinalis (*Zhu Rou*), sweet Flos Chrysanthemi Morifolii (*Gan Ju*), and Concha Haliotidis (*Shi Jue Ming*). For excessive sweating add, Concha Ostreae (*Mu Li*) and Radix Et Rhizoma Oryzae Glutinosae (*Nuo Dao Geng*).

5. *Zuo Gui Yin Jia Jian* (Restore the Left [Kidney] Drink with Additions & Subtractions) according to Zhu Cheng-han

Ingredients: Cooked Radix Rehmanniae (*Da Shu Di*), Radix Dioscoreae Oppositae (*Huai Shan Yao*), sweet Fructus Lycii Chinensis (*Gan Qi Zi*), aged Fructus Corni Officinalis (*Zhu Rou*), Sclerotium Poriae Cocos (*Fu Ling*), mix-fried Radix Glycyrrhizae (*Gan Cao*), uncooked Concha Ostreae (*Mu Li*), scalded Carapax Amydae Sinensis (*Bie Jia*), Caulis Polygoni Multiflori (*Ye Jiao Teng*)

This formula includes two shells, Oyster Shell and Carapax Amydae. The first may be seen as a heavy, spirit-quieting medicinal, while the second may be seen as a heavy, yang-subduing ingredient. Therefore, the reader will find this formula also listed under yin vacuity-yang hyperactivity below. However, Oyster Shell can also be seen as a yin-restraining and securing astringent, and Carapax Amydae can be seen as a powerful, "bloody" yin-enriching medicinal. This is why I have included this formula under simple yin vacuity as well.

6. *Geng Nian An Tang* (Climacteric Quieting Decoction)

Ingredients: Uncooked & cooked Radix Rehmanniae (*Sheng Shu Di*), Radix Polygoni Multiflori (*He Shou Wu*), Rhizoma Alismatis (*Ze Xie*), Sclerotium Poriae Cocos (*Fu Ling*), Cortex Radicis Moutan (*Dan Pi*), Radix Scrophulariae Ningpoensis (*Xuan Shen*), Tuber Ophiopogonis Japonicae (*Mai Dong*), Fructus Schisandrae Chinensis (*Wu Wei Zi*), Fructus Corni Officinalis (*Shan Zhu Yu*)

Additions: If sweating is excessive, add Fructus Levis Tritici Aestivi (*Fu Xiao Mai*) and aged Semen Setariae Italicae (*Kang Gu Lao*). If there is heart vexation, add Fructus Gardeniae Jasminoidis (*Zhi Zi*) and Semen Praeparatus Sojae (*Dan Dou Chi*). If there is profuse dreaming, add Hangzhou Radix Albus Paeoniae Lactiflorae (*Hang Shao*) and Fructus Chaenomelis Lagenariae (*Mu Gua*). If there is insomnia, add Magnetitum (*Ci Shi*), Concha Margaritiferae (*Zhen Zhu Mu*), and Caulis Polygoni Multiflori (*Ye Jiao Teng*). If there is headache, add Fructus Viticis (*Man Jing Zi*), Radix Angelicae Dahuricae (*Bai Zhi*), and Flos Chrysanthemi Morifolii (*Ju Hua*). If there is dizziness, add Herba Dendrobii (*Shi*

Hu), Radix Platycodi Grandiflori (*Jie Geng*), and Radix Glycyrrhizae (*Gan Cao*). And if there is low back and leg pain, add Radix Dipsaci (*Chuan Duan*), Ramulus Loranthi Seu Visci (*Ji Sheng*), and Radix Achyranthis Bidentatae (*Niu Xi*).

Heart & kidneys not interacting

Main symptoms: Amount of menses scanty, color pale red, or blocked menstruation, dizziness, tinnitus, vacuity vexation, loss of sleep, heart palpitations, impaired memory, aching low back and weak knees, tidal fever, night sweats, constipation, short, reddish urination, a flushed red facial complexion, dry throat but no desire to drink, a red tongue with no fur, and a fine, rapid or fine, weak, rapid pulse

Many Chinese gynecology texts do not list this as a separate pattern under menopausal syndrome since it is just another variation on kidney yin vacuity with vacuity heat. In this case, vacuity is mostly harassing the spirit and disturbing heart function as opposed to symptoms of liver-kidney dysfunction.

Treatment principles: Enrich yin and tranquilize the heart, quiet the spirit and promote the interaction between the heart and kidneys

Guiding formulas:

1. *Tian Wang Bu Xin Dan* (Heavenly Emperor Supplement the Heart Elixir)

Ingredients: Uncooked Radix Rehmanniae (*Sheng Di*), Radix Scrophulariae Ningpoensis (*Xuan Shen*), Tuber Ophiopogonis Japonici (*Mai Dong*), Tuber Asparagi Cochinensis (*Tian Dong*), Radix Salviae Miltiorrhizae (*Dan Shen*), Radix Angelicae Sinensis (*Dang Gui*), Sclerotium Poriae Cocos (*Fu Ling*), Semen Biotae Orientalis (*Bai Ren*), Semen Zizyphi Spinosae (*Zao Ren*), Radix Polygalae Tenuifoliae (*Yuan Zhi*), Fructus Schisandrae Chinensis (*Wu Wei Zi*), Radix Platycodi Grandiflori (*Jie Geng*), Radix Panacis Ginseng (*Ren Shen*)

Han Bai-ling gives this formula if heart yin vacuity is more prominent.

Additions: Dr. Han says to add Concha Ostrae (*Mu Li*) and Caulis Polygoni Multiflori (*Ye Jiao Teng*). For dizziness and tinnitus, add Fructus Gardeniae Jasminoidis (*Zhi Zi*), Fructus Corni Officinalis (*Zhu Rou*), sweet Flos Chrysanthemi Morifolii (*Gan Ju*), and Concha Haliotidis (*Shi Jue Ming*). For excessive sweating add, Concha Ostreae (*Mu Li*) and Radix Et Rhizoma Oryzae Glutinosae (*Nuo Dao Gen*).

2. *Liu Wei Di Huang Wan Jia Wei* (Six Flavors Rehmannia Pills with Added Flavors)

Ingredients: Cooked Radix Rehmanniae (*Shu Di*), Fructus Corni Officinalis (*Shan Zhu Yu*), Radix Dioscoreae Oppositae (*Shan Yao*), Cortex Radicis Moutan (*Dan Pi*), Rhizoma Alismatis (*Ze Xie*), Sclerotium Poriae Cocos (*Fu Ling*), Fructus Ligustri Lucidi (*Nu Zhen Zi*), Plastrum Testudinis (*Gui Ban*)

Dr. Han says to use this formula if kidney yin vacuity is more prominent.

3. *Kan Li Ji Ji Wan* (*Kan* [Water] & *Li* [Fire] Foundation & Extreme Pills)

Ingredients: Radix Angelicae Sinensis (*Dang Gui*), cooked Radix Rehmanniae (*Shu Di*), uncooked Radix Rehmanniae (*Sheng Di*), Fructus Corni Officinalis (*Shan Zhu Yu*), Radix Achyranthis Bidenatae (*Niu Xi*), Tuber Ophiopogonis Japonici (*Mai Dong*), Tuber Asparagi Cochinensis (*Tian Dong*), Radix Albus Paeoniae Lactiflorae (*Bai Shao*), Radix Dioscoreae Oppositae (*Shan Yao*), Fructus Schisandrae Chinensis (*Wu Wei Zi*), Plastrum Testudinis (*Gui Ban*), Rhizoma Anemarrhenae Aspheloidis (*Zhi Mu*), Cortex Phellodendri (*Huang Bai*)

Du Jie-hui gives this formula for the treatment of heart and kidneys not interacting perimenopausal syndrome. It enriches the kidneys, supplements the heart, and promotes the interaction between the heart and kidneys.

4. *Liu Wei Di Huang Tang He Huang Lian E Jiao Tang* (Six Flavors Rehmannia Decoction plus Coptis & Donkey Skin Glue Decoction)

Ingredients: Cooked Radix Rehmanniae (*Shu Di*), Fructus Corni Officinalis (*Shan Zhu Yu*), Radix Dioscoreae Oppositae (*Shan Yao*), Sclerotium Poriae Cocos (*Fu Ling*), Cortex Radicis Moutan (*Dan Pi*), Rhizoma Alismatis (*Ze Xie*), Rhizoma Coptidis Chinensis (*Huang Lian*), Gelatinum Corii Asini (*E Jiao*), Radix Scutellariae Baicalensis (*Huang Qin*), Radix Albus Paeoniae Lactiflorae (*Bai Shao*), Egg Yolk (*Ji Zi Huang*)

Liver yang hyperactivity or liver wind stirrring internally

Main symptoms: Dizziness, vertigo, heart vexation, easy anger, hot sensations in the body and face especially in the afternoon, sweating, soreness and weakness of the low back and knees, profuse menstrual bleeding or lingering menstrual flow, a red tongue with scanty fur, and a fine, bowstring, rapid pulse

These signs and symptoms are almost identical to those given under kidney yin vacuity above. This category and these signs and symptoms are given by Prof. Qiu Mao-lian & Dr. Su Xin-ming in *The Nanjing Seminars Transcript*. In this case, liver yang is effulgent and ascends upwards because kidney yin is vacuous below. However, these same signs and symptoms are also characteristic of liver wind stirring internally. In the case of liver wind, dizziness, tics and spasms, headache, and tinnitus are more prominent. But, whether liver yang is effulgent and ascends hyperactively above or liver wind vents itself above, insufficient yin and blood below fail to keep yang under control. Therefore, all the formulas listed below include yin and blood supplements as well as heat-clearing, heavy, yang-subduing, and/or wind extinguishing ingredients. The reader should note that this pattern has the largest number of formulas listed under it because it is so commonly seen in clinical practice.

Treatment principles: Enrich yin and descend fire, level or calm the liver and extinguish wind

Guiding formulas:

1. *Tian Ma Gou Teng Yin* (Gastrodia & Uncaria Drink)

Ingredients: Rhizoma Gastrodiae Elatae (*Tian Ma*), Ramulus Uncariae Cum Uncis (*Gou Teng*), Concha Haliotidis (*Shi Jue Ming*), Ramulus Loranthi Seu Visci (*Sang Ji Sheng*), Cortex Eucommiae Ulmoidis (*Du Zhong*), Radix Cyathulae Officinalis (*Chuan Niu Xi*), Fructus Gardeniae Jasminoidis (*Zhi Zi*), Radix Scutellariae Baicalensis (*Huang Qin*), Herba Leonuri Heterophylli (*Yi Mu Cao*), Sclerotium Pararadicis Poriae Cocos (*Fu Shen*)

2. *Ling Yang Gou Teng Tang* (Antelope & Uncaria Decoction)

Ingredients: Cornu Antelopis Saigae Tataricae (*Ling Yang Jiao,* substitute Cornu Caprae, *Shan Yang Jiao*), Folium Mori Albi (*Sang Ye*), Bulbus Fritillariae Cirrhosae (*Chuan Bei Mu*), uncooked Radix Rehmanniae (*Sheng Di*), Ramulus Uncariae Cum Uncis (*Gou Teng*), Sclerotium Poriae Cocos (*Fu Ling*), Flos Chrysanthemi Morifolii (*Ju Hua*), Radix Glycyrrhizae (*Gan Cao*), Caulis Bambusae In Taeniis (*Zhu Ru*), Radix Albus Paeoniae Lactiflorae (*Bai Shao*)

Bensky and Barolet call this formula *Ling Jiao Gou Teng Tang* (Antelope Horn & Uncaria Decoction). Although they say that this formula is indicated for the treatment of persistent high fever, irritability, restlessness, dizziness, vertigo, twitching, and spasms due to evil heat entering the *jue yin*, it may also be used to cool the liver and extinguish wind in conditions due to ascendant liver yang, such as headache, dizziness, vertigo, tics, and spasms.

Additions: For hypertension, add Radix Achyranthis Bidentatae (*Huai Niu Xi*) and Fructus Tribuli Terrestris (*Bai Ji Li*).

3. *Zhen Gan Xi Feng Tang* (Settle the Liver & Extinguish Wind Decoction)

Ingredients: Radix Achyranthis Bidentatae (*Huai Niu Xi*), Haemititum (*Zhe Shi*), Os Draconis (*Long Gu*), Concha Ostreae (*Mu Li*), Plastrum Testudinis (*Gui Ban*), Radix Scrophulariae Ningpoensis (*Xuan Shen*), Tuber Asparagi Cochinensis (*Tian Dong*), Radix Albus Paeoniae Lactiflorae (*Bai Shao*), Herba Artemisiae Capillaris (*Yin Chen Hao*), Fructus Meliae Toosendan (*Chuan Lian Zi*), Fructus Germinatus Hordei Vulgaris (*Mai Ya*), Radix Glycyrrhizae (*Gan Cao*)

The ingredients in this formula heavily subdue ascendant liver yang and anchor yang to its root below. At the same time, they also nourish yin and blood, thus balancing yin and yang but also emolliating and soothing the liver. In addition, this formula contains ingredients which course the liver and rectify the qi.

Additions substractions: For headache and dizziness, add Spica Prunellae Vulgaris (*Xia Gu Cao*) and Flos Chrysanthemi Morifolii (*Ju Hua*). For hypertension, add the two above ingredients plus Ramulus Uncariae Cum Uncis (*Gou Teng*). If the stools are loose, delete Haemititum and Plastrum Testudinis and add Hallyositum Rubrum (*Chi Shi Zi*).

4. *Jian Ling Tang* (Sweeping Down Decoction)

Ingredients: Radix Dioscoreae Oppositae (*Shan Yao*), Radix Achyranthis Bidentatae (*Niu Xi*), Haemititum (*Dai Zhe Shi*), Os Draconis (*Long Gu*), Concha Ostreae (*Mu Li*), uncooked Radix Rehmanniae (*Sheng Di*), Radix Albus Paeoniae Lactiflorae (*Bai Shao*), Semen Biotae Orientalis (*Bai Zi Ren*)

This formula also levels the liver and extinguishes liver wind while it enriches yin. However, it also quiets the spirit and tranquilizes the heart. It is indicated for dizziness, tinnitus, heart palpitations, impaired memory, heart vexation, easy anger, loss of sleep, and profuse dreaming.

5. *San Jia Fu Mai Tang* (Three Shells Restore the Pulse Decoction)

Ingredients: Mix-fried Radix Glycyrrhizae (*Gan Cao*), uncooked Radix Rehmanniae (*Sheng Di*), Radix Albus Paeoniae Lactiflorae (*Bai Shao*), Tuber Ophiopogonis Japonici (*Mai Dong*), Semen Cannabis Sativae (*Huo Ma Ren*), Gelatinum Corii Asini (*E Jiao*), Concha Ostreae (*Mu Li*), Carapax Amydae Sinensis (*Bie Jia*), Plastrum Testudinis (*Gui Ban*)

This formula is indicated for the treatment of dizziness, vertigo, tinnitus, a dry throat, heart palpitations, bleeding symptoms, a dry, glossy tongue with peeled fur, and a fine, bowstring pulse due to yin vacuity and yang effulgence and ascension. Due to the inclusion of Cannabis, it is appropriate when chronic constipation with dry stools complicates the case.

6. *Zuo Gui Yin Jia Jian* (Restore the Left [Kidney] Drink with Additions & Subtractions) according to Zhu Cheng-han

Ingredients: Cooked Radix Rehmanniae (*Da Shu Di*), Radix Dioscoreae Oppositae (*Huai Shan Yao*), sweet Fructus Lycii Chinensis (*Gan Qi Zi*), aged Fructus Corni Officinalis (*Zhu Rou*), Sclerotium Poriae Cocos (*Fu Ling*), mix-fried Radix Glycyrrhizae (*Gan Cao*), uncooked Concha Ostreae (*Mu Li*), scalded Carapax Amydae Sinensis (*Bie Jia*), Caulis Polygoni Multiflori (*Ye Jiao Teng*)

7. *Zuo Gui Yin Jia Jian* (Restore the Left [Kidney] Drink with Additions & Subtractions) according to Zhang En-qin *et al.*

Ingredients: Cooked Radix Rehmanniae (*Shu Di*), Radix Dioscoreae Oppositae (*Shan Yao*), Fructus Lycii Chinensis (*Gou Qi*), Fructus Corni Officinalis (*Shan Zhu Rou*), stir-fried Radix Albus Paeoniae Lactiflorae (*Bai Shao*), Ramulus Uncariae Cum Uncis (*Gou Teng*), Plastrum Testudinis (*Gui Ban*), Placenta Hominis (*Zi He Che*), Fructus Ligustri Lucidi (*Nu Zhen Zi*), Herba Ecliptae Prostratae (*Han Lian Cao*)

8. *Qi Ju Di Huang Tang Jia Wei* (Lycium & Chrysanthemum Rehmannia Decoction with Added Flavors)

Ingredients: Cooked Radix Rehmanniae (*Shu Di*), Fructus Corni Officinalis (*Shan Zhu*), Cortex Radicis Moutan (*Dan Pi*), Sclerotium Poriae Cocos (*Fu Ling*), Radix Dioscoreae Oppositae (*Shan Yao*), Rhizoma Alismatis (*Ze Xie*), Radix Albus Paeoniae Lactiflorae (*Bai Shao*), Fructus Lycii Chinensis (*Gou Qi Zi*), Flos Chrysanthemi Morifolii (*Ju Hua*), Ramulus Uncariae Cum Uncis (*Gou Teng*), uncooked Os Draconis (*Long Gu*), uncooked Concha Ostreae (*Mu Li*)

Additions: If kidney yin is insufficient and is unable to nourish the heart above, this may lead to heart palpitations. In that case, add Concha Margaritaferae (*Zhen Zhu Mu*). If there is insomnia and profuse dreaming, add Caulis Polygoni Multiflori (*Ye Jiao Teng*).

9. Unnamed formula from *Concise Traditional Chinese Gynecology*

Ingredients: Ramulus Uncariae Cum Uncis (*Gou Teng*), Concha Mauritiae (*Zi Bei Chi*), uncooked Radix Rehmanniae (*Sheng Di*), cooked Radix Rehmanniae (*Shu Di*), mix-fried Plastrum Testudinis (*Gui Ban*), stir-fried Semen Zizyphi Spinosae (*Suan Zao Ren*), Sclerotium Poriae Cocos (*Fu Ling*), Sclerotium Pararadicis Poriae Cocos (*Fu Shen*)

10. Unnamed formula given by Shang Xian-ming *et al.*

Ingredients: Uncooked Radix Rehmanniae (*Sheng Di*), cooked Radix Rehmanniae (*Shu Di*), Fructus Lycii Chinensis (*Gou Qi Zi*), Radix Polygoni Multiflori (*He Shou Wu*), Fructus Mori Albi (*Sang Shen*), Fructus Ligustri Lucidi (*Nu Zhen Zi*), Gelatinum Plastri Testudinis (*Gui Ban Jiao*), Radix Albus Paeoniae Lactiflorae (*Bai Shao*), Os Draconis (*Long Gu*), Concha Ostreae (*Mu Li*)

Additions: For liver wind due to hyperactivity of yang manifesting as hypertension and spasms, add powdered Cornu Antelopis Saigae Tataricae (*Ling Yang Jiao*, substitute Cornu Capra, *Shan Yang Jiao*) and Ramulus Uncariae Cum Uncis (*Gou Teng*). For itching skin and formication due to blood vacuity and internal wind, add Radix Angelicae Sinensis (*Dang Gui*), Radix Salviae Miltiorrhizae (*Dan Shen*), Flos Campsitis (*Ling Xiao Hua*), and Buthus Martensis (*Quan Xie*).

11. Unnamed formula given by Shang Xian-min *et. al.*

Ingredients: Magnetitum (*Ci Shi*), Haemititum (*Dai Zhe Shi*), Fructus Mori Albi (*Sang Shen*), Radix Angelicae Sinensis (*Dang Gui*), Rhizoma Pinelliae Ternatae (*Ban Xia*), Semen Canavaliae (*Dao Dou*), Radix Albus Paeoniae Lactiflorae (*Bai Shao*), Flos Inulae Racemosae (*Xuan Fu Hua*)

This formula is for the treatment of liver-kidney yin vacuity with liver qi manifesting as belching and distention.

12. *Qi Wu Jiang Xia Tang* (Seven Materials Downbearing & Descending Decoction)

Ingredients: Radix Angelicae Sinensis (*Dang Gui*), cooked Radix Rehmanniae (*Shu Di*), Radix Albus Paeoniae Lactiflorae (*Bai Shao*), Radix Ligustici Wallichii (*Chuan Xiong*), Radix Astragali Membranacei (*Huang Qi*), Ramulus Uncariae Cum Uncis (*Gou Teng*), Cortex Phellodendri (*Huang Bai*)

This is a modern Japanese formula created by Otsuka Keisetsu for the treatment of hypertension, flushing, aching shoulders, tinnitus, and heaviness in the head. It nourishes liver blood and yin at the same time as it clears heat and harmonizes the liver.

13. Unnamed formula given by Guo Yuan

Ingredients: Radix Morindae Officinalis (*Ba Ji Tian*), Herba Ecliptae Prostratae (*Han Lian Cao*), Fructus Ligustri Lucidi (*Nu Zhen Zi*), Ramulus Loranthi Seu Visci (*Sang Ji Sheng*), Radix Dipsaci (*Xu Duan*), Radix Bupleuri (*Chai Hu*), Radix Scutellariae Baicalensis (*Huang Qin*), Radix Angelicae Sinensis (*Dang Gui*), Radix Albus Paeoniae Lactiflorae (*Bai Shao*),

Rhizoma Pinelliae Ternatae (*Ban Xia*), Radix Glycyrrhizae (*Gan Cao*), uncooked Rhizoma Zingiberis (*Sheng Jiang*), Fructus Zizyphi Jujubae (*Da Zao*)

Guo Yuan gives this formula for the treatment of liver yin vacuity-liver yang hyperactivity. I find it an interesting and useful formula.

14. *Qing Xuan Ping Gan Tang* (Clear Dizziness & Level the Liver Decoction)

Ingredients: Uncooked Radix Rehmanniae (*Sheng Di*), Folium Mori Albi (*Sang Ye*), Flos Chrysanthemi Morifolii (*Ju Hua*), Radix Scutellariae Baicalensis (*Huang Qin*), Radix Acyranthis Bidentatae (*Niu Xi*), Fructus Ligustri Lucidi (*Nu Zhen Zi*), Radix Angelicae Sinensis (*Dang Gui*), Herba Ecliptae Prostratae (*Han Lian Cao*)

This formula is given by Yao Shi-an for the treatment of yin vacuity-yang hyperactivity pattern perimenopausal syndrome. From its name and ingredients, one can see it is specifically designed to treat dizziness, red eyes, and headache due to liver yang hyperactivity above.

Yin vacuity, internal heat

Main symptoms: Night sweats, tidal fever, a red facial complexion, heart vexation, easy anger, reddish urination, a red tongue with thin, yellow; slimy, yellow; powdery white; or peeled, flowery (*i.e.*, geographic) fur, and a surging, rapid or bowstring, rapid, forceful pulse

In this case, internal heat refers to a stronger heat than vacuity heat. Typically, this heat is damp heat or depressive heat.

Treatment principles: Supplement yin, nourish the blood, and clear heat

Guiding formulas:

1. *Dang Gui Liu Huang Tang* (Dang Gui Six Yellows Decoction)

Ingredients: Radix Angelicae Sinensis (*Dang Gui*), uncooked Radix Rehmanniae (*Sheng Di*), cooked Radix Rehmanniae (*Shu Di*), Rhizoma Coptidis Chinensis (*Huang Lian*), Radix Scutellariae Baicalensis (*Huang Qin*), Cortex Phellodendri (*Huang Bai*), Radix Astragali Membranacei (*Huang Qi*)

Additions: For especially severe sweating, add Radix Ephedrae Sinensis (*Ma Huang Gen*), Radix Et Rhizoma Oryzae Glutinosae (*Nuo Mi Geng*), and Semen Levis Tritici Aestivi (*Fu Xiao Mai*). For tidal fever, dry mouth, and a strong pulse at the cubit position signifying stirring of ministerial fire, add Plastrum Testudinis (*Gui Ban*) and Rhizoma Anemarrhenae Aspheloidis (*Zhi Mu*).

2. *Wen Qing Yin* (Warming & Clearing Drink)

Ingredients: Uncooked Radix Rehmanniae (*Sheng Di*), Radix Angelicae Sinensis (*Dang Gui*), Radix Albus Paeoniae Lactiflorae (*Bai Shao*), Radix Ligustici Wallichii (*Chuan Xiong*), Rhizoma Coptidis Chinensis (*Huang Lian*), Radix Scutellariae Baicalensis (*Huang Qin*), Cortex Phellodendri (*Huang Bai*), Fructus Gardeniae Jasminoidis (*Zhi Zi*)

Additions: For night sweats and in order to more effectively engender blood, add Radix Astragali Membranacei (*Huang Qi*) and Radix Glycyrrhizae (*Gan Cao*).

3. *Qing Xin Yin* (Clear the Heart Drink)

Ingredients: Rhizoma Coptidis Chinensis (*Huang Lian*), Fructus Gardeniae Jasminoidis (*Zhi Zi*), Radix Gentianae Scabrae (*Long Dan Cao*), Folium Bambusae (*Zhu Ye*), Tuber Ophiopogonis Japonici (*Mai Dong*), Succinum (*Hu Po*)

This formula is given by Yao Shi-an for the treatment of heart-liver fire effulgence pattern climacteric syndrome. This is depressive fire of the liver accumulating in and disturbing the heart. In this case, the fire is replete and yin vacuity is minor.

4. *Dan Zhi Xiao Yao San Jia Wei* (Moutan & Gardenia Rambling Powder with Added Flavors)

Ingredients: Radix Bupleuri (*Chai Hu*), Radix Angelicae Sinensis (*Dang Gui*), Radix Albus Paeoniae Lactiflorae (*Bai Shao*), Rhizoma Atractylodis Macrocephalae (*Bai Zhu*), Sclerotium Poriae Cocos (*Fu Ling*), Radix Glycyrrhizae (*Gan Cao*), Cortex Radicis Moutan (*Dan Pi*), Fructus Gardeniae Jasminoidis (*Zhi Zi*), Flouritum (*Zi Shi Ying*), uncooked Os Draconis (*Long Gu*), uncooked Concha Ostreae (*Mu Li*), and Cortex Albizziae Julibrissin (*He Huan Pi*).

This formula is for depressive heat with blood vacuity but not marked yin vacuity.

Additions: If heart vexation and insomnia are severe, add Magnetitum (*Ci Shi*), Tuber Ophiopogonis Japonici (*Mai Dong*), and Fructus Schisandrae Chinensis (*Wu Wei Zi*). If there is chest and rib-side distention and oppression with a dry mouth and bitter taste in the mouth, add Radix Scutellariae Baicalensis (*Huang Qin*), uncooked Radix Rehmanniae (*Sheng Di*), and Fructus Citri Reticulatae Viride (*Qing Pi*). If there is headache and vertigo, add Concha Haliotidis (*Shi Jue Ming*), Flos Chrysanthemi Morifolii (*Ju Hua*), and Folium Mori Albi (*Sang Ye*) to clear the liver and drain fire.

Kidney yang vacuity

Main symptoms: A dark, dusky facial complexion, a withered and listless essence spirit, soreness and weakness of the low back and knees, dizziness, poor appetite, abdominal distention, a bland, tastelessness in the mouth, thin, loose stools, frequent urination which is clear and long or scanty urination with edematous swelling possibly of the face, profuse, pale colored menses, chilled extremities, profuse, white, watery vaginal discharge, a pale, white tongue with thin, white fur, and a deep, small, relaxed (retarded); deep, weak; or deep, fine, forceless pulse

Han Bai-ling calls this category spleen-kidney yang vacuity. The therapeutic principles Dr. Han gives are to warm and supplement the spleen and kidneys, boost fire and engender earth. The authors of *Concise Traditional Chinese Gynecology* list this pattern as kidney yang vacuity but then give therapeutic principles to warm kidney yang, fortify the spleen, and quiet the heart. This is based on the fact that spleen yang is rooted in kidney yang and that if one becomes vacuous, the other, over time, will likewise become vacuous. Han Bai-ling gives essentially the same or similar signs and symptoms but describes the tongue as white, pale, and moist with white, glossy fur and the pulse as deep and weak.

Treatment principles: Warm the kidneys and supplement yang

Guiding formulas:

1. *You Gui Wan* (Restore the Right [Kidney] Pills)

Ingredients: Cooked Radix Rehmanniae (*Shu Di*), Radix Lateralis Praeparatus Aconiti Carmichaeli (*Fu Zi*), Cortex Cinnamomi Cassiae (*Rou Gui*), Fructus Corni Officinalis (*Shan Zhu Rou*), Fructus Lycii Chinensis (*Gou Qi Zi*), Radix Dioscoreae Oppositae (*Shan Yao*), Cortex Eucommiae Ulmoidis (*Du Zhong*), Radix Angelicae Sinensis (*Dang Gui*), Semen Cuscutae (*Tu Si Zi*), Gelatinum Cornu Cervi (*Lu Jiao Jiao*)

Additions & subtractions: Song and Yu suggest adding Radix Codonopsitis Pilosulae (*Dang Shen*), Fructus Psoraleae Corylifoliae (*Bu Gu Zhi*), Rhizoma Curculiginis Orchioidis (*Xian Mao*), and Herba Epimedii (*Xian Ling Pi*). Han Bai-ling also suggests adding Psoralea and Curculigo. Zhu Cheng-han deletes the Eucommia, Deer Antler Glue, and Cuscuta and adds mix-fried Radix Glycyrrhizae (*Gan Cao*) and Radix Codonopsitis Pilosulae (*Dang Shen*). If there is diarrhea, abdominal distention, and abdominal pain due to liver-spleen disharmony, Zhu Cheng-han says to delete Dang Gui and Lycium and to add Rhizoma Atractylodis Macrocephalae (*Bai Zhu*), Pericarpium Citri Reticulatae (*Chen Pi*), stir-fried Radix Ledebouriellae Divaricatae (*Fang Feng*), and Radix Albus Paeoniae Lactiflorae (*Bai Shao*) to regulate the liver and to harmonize the spleen. Sun Jiu-ling recommends deleting

Eucommia, Cornus, and Dang Gui and adding Radix Codonopsitis Pilosulae (*Dang Shen*), Radix Dipsaci (*Chuan Xu Duan*), and Herba Epimedii (*Xian Ling Cao*). Zhang En-qin *et al.* in their version of this formula delete Lycium, Dang Gui, and Dioscorea and add Herba Epimedii (*Xian Ling Pi*), Radix Codonopsitis Pilosulae (*Dang Shen*), Rhizoma Atractylodis Macrocephalae (*Bai Zhu*), dry Rhizoma Zingiberis (*Gan Jiang*), and mix-fried Radix Glycyrrhizae (*Gan Cao*). And Liu Yan-chi, in *The Essential Book of Traditional Chinese Medicine*, deletes Aconite, Eucommia, Cuscuta, Deer Antler Glue, and Dang Gui and adds Radix Dipsaci (*Xu Duan*), Radix Codonopsitis Pilosulae (*Dang Shen*), Rhizoma Atractylodis Macrocephalae (*Bai Zhu*), Rhizoma Curculiginis Orchioidis (*Xian Mao*), and Herba Epimedii (*Xian Ling Pi*). Further, if accompanied by profuse menstruation or flooding and leaking, Liu adds Cacumen Biotae Orientalis (*Ce Bai Ye*), carbonized Folium Et Petriolus Trachycarpi (*Zong Lu Tan*), and Radix Pseudoginseng (*San Qi*). While for edema of the face and feet, Liu deletes cooked Rehmannia and adds Cortex Sclerotii Poriae Cocos (*Fu Ling Pi*), Radix Astragali Membranacei (*Huang Qi*), and Radix Stephaniae Tetrandrae (*Han Feng Ji*).

2. *Shen Ling Bai Zhu San Jia Wei* (Ginseng, Poria & Atractylodes Powder with Added Flavors)

Ingredients: Radix Panacis Ginseng (*Ren Shen*), Semen Nelumbinis Nuciferae (*Lian Zi Rou*), Radix Dioscoreae Oppositae (*Shan Yao*), Rhizoma Atractylodis Macrocephalae (*Bai Zhu*), Sclerotium Poriae Cocos (*Fu Ling*), Semen Dolichoris Lablab (*Bai Bian Dou*), Fructus Amomi (*Sha Ren*), Radix Platycodi Grandiflori (*Jie Geng*), mix-fried Radix Glycyrrhizae (*Gan Cao*), Semen Cuscutae (*Tu Si*), Radix Morindae Officinalis (*Ba Ji Tian*)

Han Bai-ling suggests this formula as opposed to *You Gui Wan* (Restore the Right [Kidney] Pills) if spleen yang vacuity is more prominent. This formula under this pattern underscores that, in clinical practice, spleen qi and kidney yang vacuity mostly occur simultaneously in perimenopausal women.

3. Unnamed formula from *Concise Traditional Chinese Gynecology*

Ingredients: Herba Epimedii (*Xian Ling Pi*), Rhizoma Curculiginis Orchioidis (*Xian Mao*), Rhizoma Atractylodis Macrocephalae (*Bai Zhu*), Radix Auklandiae Lappae (*Mu Xiang*), Radix Codonopsitis Pilosulae (*Dang Shen*), Ramulus Uncariae Cum Uncis (*Gou Teng*), Sclerotium Poriae Cocos (*Fu Ling*), Sclerotium Pararadicis Poriae Cocos (*Fu Shen*)

4. Unnamed formula given by Shang Xian-min *et al.*

Ingredients: Rhizoma Curculiginis Orchioidis (*Xian Mao*), Herba Ephedrae (*Ma Huang*), Radix Morindae Officinalis (*Ba Ji Tian*), Radix Codonopsitis Pilosulae (*Dang Shen*),

Gelatinum Cornu Cervi (*Lu Jiao Jiao*), Fructus Chaenomelis Lagenariae (*Ku Hu Lu*), Semen Cuscutae (*Tu Si Zi*)

Shang Xian-min *et al.* give this formula for kidney yang vacuity menopausal complaints characterized by a bearing down sensation in the pudenda, a tight sensation in the chest, a pale tongue, and a deep, weak pulse.

Additions & subtractions: For yin vacuity, delete Curculigo and Ephedra and add Herba Cistanchis Deserticolae (*Rou Cong Rong*), Radix Polygoni Multiflori (*He Shou Wu*), Os Draconis (*Long Gu*), and Concha Ostreae (*Mu Li*). For spleen yang vacuity and edema and diarrhea, delete Cistanches and add Rhizoma Atractylodis Macrocephalae (*Bai Zhu*) and Fructus Psoraleae Corylifoliae (*Bu Gu Zhi*).

5. *Rong Fu Yan Zhen Tang* (Pilose Deer Antler & Aconite Nourish the True Decoction)

Ingredients: Wine-washed dry Rhizoma Zingiberis (*Gan Jiang*), Cortex Cinnamomi Cassiae (*Rou Gui*), Radix Lateralis Praeparatus Aconiti Carmichaeli (*Fu Zi*), Radix Angelicae Sinensis (*Dang Gui*), wine-washed Cornu Cervi Parvum (*Lu Rong*), calcined Concha Ostreae (*Mu Li*), Radix Ledebouriellae Divaricatae (*Fang Feng*), Os Draconis (*Long Gu*)

Du Jie-hui says that this formula supplements the *chong* and *ren*, the defensive qi, and the blood. Du lists this formula for the treatment of kidney yang vacuity perimenopausal syndrome.

6. *Jin Gui Shen Qi Wan* (Golden Cabinet Kidney Qi Pills)

Ingredients: Cooked Radix Rehmanniae (*Shu Di*), Fructus Corni Officinalis (*Shan Zhu Yu*), Radix Dioscoreae Oppositae (*Shan Yao*), Sclerotium Poriae Cocos (*Fu Ling*), Rhizoma Alismatis (*Ze Xie*), Cortex Radicis Moutan (*Dan Pi*), Cortex Cinnamomi Cassiae (*Rou Gui*), Radix Lateralis Praeparatus Aconiti Carmichaeli (*Fu Zi Pian*)

7. *Wen Yang Chong Ren Fang* (Warm & Nourish the *Chong* & *Ren* Formula)

Ingredients: Cooked Radix Rehmanniae (*Shu Di*), Gelatinum Cornu Cervi (*Lu Jiao Jiao*), Fructus Psoraleae Corylifoliae (*Bu Gu Zhi*), Radix Morindae Officinalis (*Ba Ji Tian*), Cortex Eucommiae Ulmoidis (*Du Zhong*)

This formula is given by Yao Shi-an for spleen-kidney yang vacuity. However, personally, I feel it is mostly for kidney yang vacuity and needs to have additional spleen-fortifying medicinals added to it to treat spleen vacuity effectively.

Kidney yin & yang dual vacuity

Main symptoms: Dizziness, vertigo, tinnitus, lumbar soreness lacking strength, lack of warmth in the four extremities, alternating hot and cold sensations or hot above and cold below, a pale tongue and a deep, fine, bowstring pulse

Treatment principles: Supplement both kidney yin and yang aided by descending fire

Guiding formulas:

1. *Er Xian Tang* (Two Immortals Decoction)

Ingredients: Rhizoma Curculiginis Orchioidis (*Xian Mao*), Herba Epimedii (*Xian Ling Pi*), Radix Morindae Officinalis (*Ba Ji Tian*), Radix Angelicae Sinensis (*Dang Gui*), Rhizoma Anemarrhenae Aspheloidis (*Zhi Mu*), Cortex Phellodendri (*Huang Bai*)

This formula was created at the Shu Guang Hospital in Shanghai. It treats a wide range of menstrual problems and is perhaps the most useful formula for the treatment of perimeno-pausal complaints. Certainly, it is the guiding formula I tend to use the most. It can be modified in many ways. Some of this formula's indications are menopausal hypertension, hot flashes, night sweats, nervousness, fatigue, lassitude, depression, irritability, insomnia, heart palpitations, polyuria, and nocturia. It also is useful in the treatment of amenorrhea, polycystic ovarian disease, chronic breast lumps, nephritis, pyelonephritis, polycystic kidneys, hyperthyroidism, renal vascular disorder, urinary tract infections, and hypofunction of the anterior pituitary.

Additions & subtractions: During the summer or in women who are not particularly cold, one may delete either Curculigo or Morinda if the standard formula is too warm. Signs of the formula being too warm include mouth sores, sore throat, etc. Song and Yu suggest combining this formula with *Zuo Gui Wan* (Restore the Right [Kidney] Pills) whose ingredients are cooked Radix Rehmanniae (*Shu Di*), Radix Dioscoreae Oppositae (*Shan Yao*), Fructus Lycii Chinensis (*Gou Qi Zi*), Fructus Corni Officinalis (*Shan Zhu Yu*), Semen Cuscutae (*Tu Si Zi*), Radix Cyathulae Officinalis (*Chuan Niu Xi*), Colla Cornu Cervi (*Lu Jiao Jiao*), and Gelatinum Plastri Testudinis (*Gui Ban Jiao*). Zhang En-qin *et al.* suggest combining this formula with *Er Zhi Wan* (Two Ultimates [*i.e.*, Solstices] Pills) plus one added flavor. Their combined formula is composed of Rhizoma Curculiginis Orchioidis (*Xian Mao*), Herba Epimedii (*Xian Ling Pi*), Radix Morindae Officinalis (*Ba Ji Tian*), Fructus Ligustri Lucidi (*Nu Zhen Zi*), Herba Ecliptae Prostratae (*Han Lian Cao*), cooked Radix Rehmanniae (*Shu Di*), Radix Angelicae Sinensis (*Dang Gui*), Rhizoma Anemar-rhenae Aspheloidis (*Zhi Mu*), and Cortex Phellodendri (*Huang Bai*).

My own teacher, Dr. Yu Min at the Yue Yang Hospital in Shanghai, often combined this formula with *Gan Mai Da Zao Tang* (Licorice, Wheat & Red Dates Decoction). The ingredients of that formula are mix-fried Radix Glycyrrhizae (*Zhi Gan Cao*), Fructus Levis Tritici Aestivi (*Fu Xiao Mai*), and Fructus Zizyphi Jujubae (*Hong Zao*). This is a famous formula for the treatment of visceral agitation with hysteria, forgetfulness, emotional lability, loss of sleep and other symptoms of heart vacuity. The heart-nourishing and spirit-quieting effect of this formula can be increased by adding Semen Biotae Orientalis (*Bai Ren*), Semen Zizyphi Spinosae (*Zao Ren*), and Sclerotium Pararadicis Poriae Cocos (*Fu Shen*).

Dr. Yu also combined this formula with *Liu Wei Di Huang Wan* (Six Flavors Rehmannia Pills). Such a typical modification for a woman with night sweats, irritability, lumbar soreness, itchy skin, loss of sleep, and profuse dreaming might read: Rhizoma Curculiginis Orchioidis (*Xian Mao*), Herba Epimedii (*Xian Ling Pi*), Radix Morindae Officinalis (*Ba Ji Tian*), Radix Angelicae Sinensis (*Dang Gui*), Rhizoma Anemarrhenae Aspheloidis (*Zhi Mu*), Cortex Phellodendri (*Huang Bai*), uncooked Radix Rehmanniae (*Sheng Di*), Radix Dioscoreae Oppositae (*Shan Yao*), mix-fried Radix Glycyrrhizae (*Gan Cao*), Cortex Eucommiae Ulmoidis (*Du Zhong*), Fructus Levis Tritici Aestivi (*Fu Xiao Mai*), Fructus Zizyphi Jujubae (*Hong Zao*). In this case, Dr. Yu substituted mix-fried Licorice for Fructus Corni Officinalis (*Shan Zhu Yu*) since Morinda achieves the same astringing effects even more effectively and in order to take advantage of mix-fried Licorice's heart-nourishing, spirit-quieting ability.

Dr. Yu was also of the opinion that Fructus Akebiae Trifoliatae (*Ba Yue Zha*) is a good choice for addition to this formula for liver qi. This medicinal rectifies the qi, quickens the blood, and kills intestinal parasites. Since many women suffer from candidiasis and since one of the effects of this formula is to kill yeast and fungi due to the activity of Phellodendron and the immune-modulating effect of Epimedium, I find the use of this ingredient quite effective as well as thought-provoking. Often I combine this ingredient with Fructus Meliae Toosendanis (*Chuan Lian Zi*) which is also a good qi-rectifying ingredient when there is either damp heat or yin vacuity and which likewise has some parasite-killing ability.

Chen Ze-lin and Chen Mei-fang, in *A Comprehensive Guide to Chinese Herbal Medicine*, say to double the amount of Curculigo, Morinda, and Epimedium if yang vacuity is more prominent and to double the amount of Phellodendron and Anemarrhena if yin vacuity is more prominent.

2. *Shen Yu Si Wu Tang* (Ginseng & Evodia Four Materials Decoction)

Ingredients: Radix Angelicae Sinensis (*Dang Gui*), cooked Radix Rehmanniae (*Shu Di*), Radix Ligustici Wallichii (*Chuan Xiong*), Radix Albus Paeoniae Lactiflorae (*Bai Shao*), Radix Panacis Ginseng (*Ren Shen*), Fructus Evodiae Rutecarpae (*Wu Zhu Yu*), uncooked Rhizoma Zingiberis (*Sheng Jiang*), Fructus Zizyphi Jujubae (*Da Zao*)

This formula is given under perimenopausal syndrome by Du Jie-hui. Du says this formula treats older women whose menses have ceased but then start up again. Its ingredients nourish liver blood and, therefore, kidney essence, but the inclusion of Evodia both warms the uterus and supports yang.

3. Unnamed formula given by Guo Yuan

Ingredients: Radix Morindae Officinalis (*Ba Ji Tian*), Herba Ecliptae Prostratae (*Han Lian Cao*), Fructus Ligustri Lucidi (*Nu Zhen Zi*), Ramulus Loranthi Seu Visci (*Sang Ji Sheng*), Radix Dipsaci (*Xu Duan*), Radix Bupleuri (*Chai Hu*), Radix Scutellariae Baicalensis (*Huang Qin*), Radix Angelicae Sinensis (*Dang Gui*), Radix Albus Paeoniae Lactiflorae (*Bai Shao*), Rhizoma Pinelliae Ternatae (*Ban Xia*), Radix Glycyrrhizae (*Gan Cao*), uncooked Rhizoma Zingiberis (*Sheng Jiang*), Fructus Zizyphi Jujubae (*Da Zao*)

Guo Yuan gives this formula for the treatment of liver yin vacuity-liver yang hyperactivity. However, because it includes Morinda and Dipsacus, I would say that it treats both liver blood-kidney yin and yang vacuity.

Heart-spleen dual vacuity

Main symptoms: Heart palpitations, shortness of breath, impaired memory, loss of sleep, a sallow yellow facial complexion, listless spirit, fatigue, lack of strength, reduced appetite, stomach and abdominal distention, a pale tongue with thin fur, and a fine, soggy pulse

Han Bai-ling calls this pattern heart-spleen yang vacuity. In general, the signs and symptoms Dr. Han gives are very similar to the above. He adds emaciation, lack of warmth in the four extremities, and loose stools. He says the tongue is pale white with pale, moist fur and that the pulse is vacuous and relaxed (retarded).

Treatment principles: Nourish the heart, support the spleen, and boost the qi

Guiding formulas:

1. *Gui Pi Tang* (Restore the Spleen Decoction)

Ingredients: Radix Panacis Ginseng (*Ren Shen*), Radix Astragali Membranacei (*Huang Qi*), Radix Angelicae Sinensis (*Dang Gui*), Arillus Euphoriae Longanae (*Long Yan Rou*), Rhizoma Atractylodis Macrocephalae (*Bai Zhu*), Radix Auklandiae Lappae (*Mu Xiang*), Sclerotium Poriae Cocos (*Fu Ling*), Radix Polygalae Tenuifoliae (*Yuan Zhi*), Semen Zizyphi Spinosae (*Suan Zao Ren*), mix-fried Radix Glycyrrhizae (*Gan Cao*), uncooked Rhizoma Zingiberis (*Sheng Jiang*), Fructus Zizyphi Jujubae (*Da Zao*)

Additions: Song and Yu say that if the kidneys are vacuous as well to use *Hei Gui Pi Tang* (Black Restore the Spleen Decoction). This is merely the addition of cooked Radix Rehmanniae (*Shu Di*) to the standard formula. Han Bai-ling says that, if menstrual bleeding is profuse, add stir-fried Radix Sanguisorbae (*Di Yu*). If there is loss of sleep, add Os Draconis (*Long Gu*) and Concha Ostreae (*Mu Li*).

2. *Sheng Mai San He Gan Mai Da Zao Tang Jia Jian* (Engender the Pulse Powder plus Licorice, Wheat & Red Date Decoction with Additions & Subtractions)

Ingredients: Uncooked Radix Rehmanniae (*Sheng Di*), cooked Radix Rehmanniae (*Shu Di*), Bulbus Lilii (*Bai He*), Cortex Albizziae Julibrissin (*He Huan Pi*), Tuber Ophiopogonis Japonici (*Mai Dong*), mix-fried Radix Glycyrrhizae (*Gan Cao*), Fructus Levis Tritici Aestivi (*Fu Xiao Mai*), Fructus Zizyphi Jujubae (*Da Zao*), Plumula Nelumbinis Nuciferae (*Lian Xin*)

Shang Xian-min *et al.*, give this formula for the treatment of heart blood-spleen qi vacuity perimenopausal syndrome manifested by yawning, scanty tongue fur, and a fine, rapid pulse. In this case, heart blood vacuity is more prominent than spleen qi vacuity.

Liver depression

Main symptoms: Irritability, chest and epigastric fullness and oppression, rib-side distention and pain, a tendency to sigh frequently, a normal colored tongue with thin, white fur, and a bowstring pulse

Although these are the textbook signs and symptoms for this pattern, it is rarely seen in its discreet or simple form in perimenopausal syndrome. It is only given by Yao Shi-an amongst my Chinese sources. Nevertheless, in my experience, liver qi is a universally complicating factor in women with menopausal complaints as opposed to simple cessation of menstruation at seven times seven years. In clinical practice, it is more common to see liver depression transforming heat in perimenopausal women.

Treatment principles: Course the liver and rectify the qi

Guiding formula: *Xiao Yao San* **(Rambling Powder)**

Ingredients: Radix Bupleuri (*Chai Hu*), Radix Angelicae Sinensis (*Dang Gui*), Radix Albus Paeoniae Lactiflorae (*Bai Shao*), Rhizoma Atyractylodis Macrocephalae (*Bai Zhu*), Sclerotium Poriae Cocos (*Fu Ling*), mix-fried Radix Glycyrrhizae (*Gan Cao*), uncooked Rhizoma Zingiberis (*Sheng Jiang*), Herba Menthae Haplocalycis (*Bo He*)

If liver depression qi stagnation is the most prominent pattern in a woman's perimenopausal complaints, then this formula may be selected as one's guiding formula. However, it is more likely that one may simply need to add qi-rectifying medicinals to other guiding formulas for other, more marked patterns. It is possible for the dosage of Bupleurum to be only a single gram or less in order to protect against its tendency to damage yin but still make use of its upbearing of clear yang. One should remember that hyperactive yang is not the same as clear yang and that, according to Li Dong-yuan, upwardly counterflowing yang is due, at least in part, to failure to upbear clear yang.

Additions & subtractions: If liver depression transforms heat, then delete Ginger and Mentha and add Cortex Radicis Moutan (*Dan Pi*) and Fructus Gardeniae Jasminoidis (*Zhi Zi*), thus rendering *Dan Zhi Xiao Yao San* (Moutan & Gardenia Rambling Powder). If there is more serious blood and yin vacuity, one can add cooked Radix Rehmanniae (*Shu Di*), thus creating *Hei Xiao Yao San* (Black Rambling Powder).

Phlegm obstruction, qi stagnation

Main symptoms: Obesity, chest oppression, profuse phlegm, abdominal distention, belching, acid regurgitation, nausea, lack of appetite, edema, loose stools, white, slimy tongue fur, and a slippery or slippery, bowstring pulse

Treatment principles: Rectify the qi, transform phlegm, and fortify the spleen

Guiding formulas:

1. *Wen Dan Tang* **(Warm the Gallbladder Decoction)**

Ingredients: Rhizoma Pinelliae Ternatae (*Ban Xia*), Pericarpium Citri Reticulatae (*Chen Pi*), Sclerotium Poriae Cocos (*Fu Ling*), Fructus Immaturus Citri Aurantii (*Zhi Shi*), Caulis Bambusuae In Taeniis (*Zhu Ru*), Radix Glycyrrhizae (*Gan Cao*), Fructus Zizyphi Jujubae (*Da Zao*)

This formula is very effective for obese women with liver depression-depressive heat. In that case, use the modification given below. Some such women may have signs and symptoms of yin and yang dual vacuity. However, if there is phlegm and depressive heat, this formula is, in my experience, more effective than using a kidney-supplementing formula as one's base and modifying that for phlegm.

Additions: For a bitter taste in the mouth, add Rhizoma Coptidis Chinensis (*Huang Lian*). This then becomes *Huang Lian Wen Dan Tang* (Coptis Warm the Gallbladder Decoction). For headache, dizziness, vertigo, nausea, and vomiting, add Herba Agastachis Seu Pogostemi (*Huo Xiang*) and Rhizoma Acori Graminei (*Shi Chang Pu*). For dampness and heat, add Herba Artemisiae Apiaceae (*Qing Hao*) and Radix Scutellariae Baicalensis (*Huang Qin*). This is an interesting modification since Artemisia Apiacea also treats vacuity heat. If there is abdominal distention, add Percarpium Arecae Catechu (*Da Fu Pi*) and Semen Raphani Sativi (*Lai Fu Zi*). If there is indigestion due to food stagnation, add Massa Medica Fermentatae (*Liu Qu*) and Corneum Endothelium Gigeriae Galli (*Nei Jin*). If there is phlegm confounding the portals of the heart, add Rhizoma Arisaematis (*Nan Xing*) and Rhizoma Acori Graminei (*Chang Pu*).

2. *Wen Dan Tang Jia Wei* (Warm the Gallbladder Decoction with Added Flavors)

Ingredients: Rhizoma Pinelliae Ternatae (*Ban Xia*), Pericarpium Citri Reticulatae (*Chen Pi*), Sclerotium Poriae Cocos (*Fu Ling*), Fructus Immaturus Citri Aurantii (*Zhi Shi*), Caulis Bambusae In Taeniis (*Zhu Ru*), Radix Glycyrrhizae (*Gan Cao*), Fructus Zizyphi Jujubae (*Da Zao*), processed Rhizoma Arisaematis (*Nan Xing*), Semen Lepidii (*Ting Li Zi*), Rhizoma Anemarrhenae Aspheloidis (*Zhi Mu*), Tuber Ophiopogonis Japonici (*Mai Dong*), Caulis Polygoni Multiflori (*Ye Jiao Teng*)

Additions & subtractions: If phlegm is profuse and heat is heavy, remove the Caulis Bambusae and add fresh Succus Bambusae (*Zhu Li*).

3. *Ban Xia Hou Pu Tang* (Pinellia & Magnolia Decoction)

Ingredients: Rhizoma Pinelliae Ternatae (*Ban Xia*), Cortex Magnoliae Officinalis (*Hou Pu*), Sclerotium Poriae Cocos (*Fu Ling*), uncooked Rhizoma Zingiberis (*Sheng Jiang*), Folium Perillae Frutescentis (*Su Ye*)

This is a qi-rectifying formula which also transforms phlegm. It is indicated for the treatment of plum seed qi or the feeling as if there were something stuck in the throat. This feeling is known in Western medicine as neurotic esophageal stenosis or *globus hystericus*.

Additions: For more severe qi stagnation, add Radix Bupleuri (*Chai Hu*), Tuber Curcumae (*Yu Jin*), Rhizoma Cyperi Rotundi (*Xiang Fu*), and Pericarpium Citri Reticulatae Viride (*Qing Pi*). For vomiting, add Fructus Amomi (*Sha Ren*) and Fructus Cardamomi (*Bai Dou Kou*). For more severe oppression and fullness in the chest, add Tuber Curcumae (*Yu Jin*) and Fructus Citri Aurantii (*Zhi Qiao*). For chest pain, add Fructus Trichosanthis Kirlowii (*Gua Lou*) and Bulbus Allii (*Xie Bai*). For abdominal distention, add Fructus Amomi (*Sha Ren*). For rib-side pain, add Fructus Meliae Toosendan (*Chuan Lian Zi*) and Rhizoma Corydalis Yanhusuo (*Yan Hu Suo*). For pain and swelling in the throat, add Radix Scrophulariae Ningpoensis (*Yuan Shen*) and Radix Platycodi Grandiflori (*Jie Geng*).

Blood stasis

Main symptoms: Heart vexation, irritability, possible painful lumps in the breasts, possible flooding and leaking with dark colored blood containing clots, possible uterine myomas, rib-side and abdominal distention and pain, heart palpitations, insomnia, hot flashes, symptoms worse at night, a dark, dusky facial complexion, visible broken capillaries or varicosities, chloasma or "liver spots" on the face and skin, black spots or floating threads in the visual field, a purple or dark colored tongue with possible static spots or macules and thin, dry fur, and a bowstring, fine, choppy, and/or deep pulse

This pattern usually only complicates other patterns and mechanisms of perimenopausal syndrome. In that case, other guiding formulas appropriate for those other patterns should be modified with the addition of blood-quickening and stasis-transforming medicinals.

Treatment principles: Quicken the blood and dispel stasis

Guiding formula: *Gui Zhi Fu Ling Wan He Xue Fu Zhu Yu Tang* (Cinnamon Twig & Poria Pills plus Blood Mansion Dispel Stasis Decoction)

Ingredients: Ramulus Cinnamomi Cassiae (*Gui Zhi*), Sclerotium Poriae Cocos (*Fu Ling*), Radix Rubrus Paeoniae Lactiflorae (*Chi Shao*), Cortex Radicis Moutan (*Dan Pi*), Semen Pruni Persicae (*Tao Ren*), Flos Carthami Tinctorii (*Hong Hua*), Radix Angelicae Sinensis (*Dang Gui*), Radix Ligustici Wallichii (*Chuan Xiong*), Radix Cyathulae Officinalis (*Chuan Niu Xi*), Radix Bupleuri (*Chai Hu*), Radix Platycodi Grandiflori (*Jie Geng*), Fructus Citri Aurantii (*Zhi Ke*), uncooked Radix Rehmanniae (*Sheng Di*), Radix Glycyrrhizae (*Gan Cao*)

This formula is given by Yao Shi-an for blood stasis climacteric syndrome. If blood stasis is the main pattern and there are abdominal masses or mammary aggregations, this formula may be appropriate in its entirety. Otherwise, it should probably be paired down so as not to damage yin blood. *Gui Zhi Fu Ling Wan* is an interesting choice as a guiding formula for blood stasis as a perimenopausal pattern. Poria fortifies the spleen, Cinnamon Twigs warm yang, and Red Peony and Moutan clear liver heat as well as quicken the blood and transform stasis.

Additions & subtractions: If blood stasis is not substantial, delete Persica and Carthamus. If there is insomnia, add Succinum (*Hu Po*) and Caulis Polygoni Multiflori (*Ye Jiao Teng*). If there is heart vexation, add Fructus Gardeniae Jasminoidis (*Zhi Zi*) and Semen Praeparatus Sojae (*Dan Dou Chi*). If there are heart palpitations, add Radix Salviae Miltiorrhizae (*Dan Shen*) and Radix Polygalae Tenuifoliae (*Yuan Zhi*).

Discussion

Although all contemporary Chinese gynecology texts discriminate, more or less, the various patterns described above, in clinical practice, I find that most of my perimenopausal syndrome patients present a very consistent complicated pattern. This pattern is made up of liver depression, blood vacuity, and spleen qi-kidney yang vacuity. This may then be complicated by depressive heat, liver blood vacuity or heart blood vacuity, kidney yin vacuity with vacuity heat, yin vacuity with yang hyperactivity, internal stirring of liver wind, and/or damp heat. In addition, in some cases, spleen qi vacuity is more marked, while in other cases, kidney yang vacuity is more pronounced. This is nothing other than the same set of patterns seen in PMS and especially PMS in older women. This should not be surprising since the increase in incidence and severity of PMS as women age and the signs and symptoms of perimenopausal syndrome form, in fact, a continuum.

It is my experience that the following patterns form a more categorically complete picture of all the various permutations of perimenopausal disease mechanisms:

Liver blood-kidney yin vacuity
Heart blood-spleen qi vacuity
Yin vacuity, yang hyperactivity
Yin & yang vacuity
Liver depression
Heart-liver fire effulgence
Heart & kidneys not interacting
Internal stirring of liver wind
Phlegm confounding the orifices
Phlegm fire
Blood stasis
Damp heat

If one understands the interrelationships between these various disease mechanisms, one can diagnose and treat any woman's complaint occurring perimenopausally. Because liver blood with kidney yin and yang vacuity are often the most conspicuous elements of many women's perimenopausal pattern, I find *Er Xian Tang Jia Jian* (Two Immortals Decoction with Additions & Subtractions) the most common guiding formula I prescribe. However, I almost always modify it by adding medicinals to fortify the spleen and boost the qi, *i.e.*, Radix Panacis Ginseng (*Ren Shen*) and Radix Astragali Membranacei (*Huang Qi*), and medicinals to rectify the qi. These latter ingredients depend on the signs and symptoms of liver depression qi stagnation and whether or not there is depressive heat. This may include small doses of Radix Bupleuri (*Chai Hu*) notwithstanding its reputation for easily damaging yin. Interestingly, often the same or very similar formulas are commonly prescribed for women in their late 30s and 40s suffering from early menstruation due to a luteal phase defect and PMS.

One of the things I find so interesting about this is that these spleen-fortifying and qi-boosting as well as kidney-supplementing, yang-invigorating medicinals for treating perimenopasual complaints are the same medicinals that are also prescribed for treating other progesterone deficiency conditions, such as habitual miscarriage and luteal phase defect, or are prescribed for strengthening the sinews and bones and thus treating osteoporosis. Several years ago, most of the emphasis in Western medicine in treating perimenopausal syndrome centered on estrogen replacement therapy (ERT). However, more recent studies have begun to show the importance of progesterone supplementation for everything from PMS to hot flashes to osteoporosis. Chinese medicine has anticipated this shift in emphasis or added emphasis in the treatment of perimenopausal women by hundreds of years.

If a woman is 49, 50, or more years old, the goal of perimenopausal therapy is to merely eliminate any complicating symptoms, such as irritability, depression, hot flashes, hypertension, night sweats, etc. However, if the woman is in her mid to late 30s or early to mid-40s, the goal of therapy should also be to regulate and reestablish the menses if they have become scanty, delayed, or absent. Because the fundamental mechanism behind the cessation of the *tian gui* is the exhaustion of blood and essence and since essence controls the aging process, premature menopause means premature aging.

A person has two ages. There is biological age and chronological age. Everyone born on the same day of the same year is the same chronological age. However, amongst those people, various persons will be biologically older or younger. Premature menopause means that a woman who may be 39 has the energetic kidneys of a 49-year old. If the menses have stopped prematurely, this should be treated as blocked menstruation and an attempt should be made, I feel, to get them going again. Some women may object to this, saying that they are happy that the "fuss and muss" of menstruation is over and that they are just as happy not having it. But, if the difference between chronological and biological age is explained to the patient and also the relationship between the kidneys and the aging process, most women can understand why re-establishing the menses is a good thing. Whether one can, in fact, re-establish regular menstruation is another matter altogether. Nevertheless, treating for the mechanism causing premature menopause will benefit the overall health of the patient.

Just as it is necessay to determine each woman's normal menstrual cycle as opposed to the textbook norm, one must also determine a woman's normal age for menopause. One way of deciding when a woman is likely to go through menopause is to ask her when her mother, grandmothers, aunts, or older sisters went through their change in life. Typically, women will experience normal menopause at around the same age as their mother and other close female relatives. This is based on what the Chinese call one's natural or former heaven endowment. (As an aside, recent studies have shown that persons with prematurely grey hair are more likely to suffer from osteoporosis. The hair on the head is one of the efflorescences of the kidneys. Therefore, there does seem to be some connection between premature greying of the hair and constitutionally somewhat less exuberant kidneys.) In any case, if a woman's menses cease at the same age as her mother, this should be considered that woman's normal or constitutional age for menopause. If, on the other hand, a woman shows signs and symptoms of entering menopause considerably younger than her mother or other close female relatives, treatment should be given to try to forestall menopause.

When it comes to surgical menopause due to a complete hysterectomy taking the ovaries as well, I know of no natural therapy which can treat such women's hot flashes, night sweats, etc. with complete success. Either such natural therapies are not able to completely eliminate the symptoms or they are able to control the symptoms only as long as the person continues to regularly receive the therapy. Whereas, when perimenopausal complaints are due to the natural aging process, Chinese medicine can often completely eliminate those complaints in a matter of weeks without their return even after therapy is discontinued. It is important to remember that menopause itself is not a menstrual disease.

Over the years, I have had the opportunity to treat a number of women who have gone through surgical menopause and I have noticed that several of them have suffered from chronic sore throats and dry coughs which their estrogen replacement therapy does not benefit. Such dryness in the upper burner is consistent with TCM theory concerning the transportation of kidney yin upwards via the *bao luo-bao gong-bao mai* axis. It is similar to the dry cough and hoarse voice that some women develop in late pregnancy when the child's growing body literally blocks this same axis. If the uterus is removed, the pivot of this axis is missing and yin fluids from the kidneys do not seem to be able to ascend as efficiently as before. Such dry coughs and dry throats can be treated with formulas that enrich yin and clear heat such as *Qing Fei Tang* (Clear the Lungs Decoction).[31]

Chinese doctors began using hormones precipitated from urine as medicine as early as the Tang dynasty (618-907 CE). Therefore, hormone replacement therapy is not necessarily wrong or bad according to either Chinese medical theory or practice. However, many Western women are concerned about the long-term side effects of hormone replacement therapy. Although modern Western medicine continues to refine its use of estrogen replacement therapy or ERT, it has not eliminated all potential risks of such therapy. Chinese medicinal therapy, on the other hand, is extremely safe and effective and can, I believe, meet all the needs of the majority of menopausal and postmenopausal women.

Below I have added addenda on the Chinese medical diagnosis and treatment of osteoporosis and senile vaginitis. However, many Western women are also concerned about postmenopausal increases of risk for potentially fatal heart disease. Heart disease typically does not come out of nowhere. Everyone has heard stories, mostly concerning men, who suddenly drop dead from a heart attack without any prior warning or symptoms. However, my experience as a clinician is that most patients with incipient heart disease do have symptoms of rib-side pain and chest oppression; they just usually do not tell anyone about these because of the fear most people have around heart pain/heart attacks. This is why their symptoms are referred to as "secret anguish" in the menstrual movement disease chapter above. In addition, in women, heart disease is often heralded by shortness of breath. In Chinese medicine, such shortness of breath is usually a qi vacuity symptom. Most heart disease has its root cause in liver depression qi stagnation affecting the free flow of chest qi and, therefore, heart and lung blood. In women in particular, such liver depression is often complicated by qi vacuity. Chinese medicine has ways of both identifying and treating liver depression qi stagnation and qi vacuity. These include preventive treatments the patient can institute themselves as well as preventive and remedial treatments supplied by professional practitioners. Therefore, I believe that Chinese medicine is a good alternative to ERT for preventing heart disease in postmenopausal women.

One interesting fact concerning menopause is that, in cultures where women gain power and status, there are few if any menopausal complaints. Women go through this change in life

---

[31]   The ingredients in *Qing Fei Tang* are: Radix Scutellariae Baicalensis (*Huang Qin*), Semen Pruni Armeniacae (*Xing Ren*), Bulbus Fritillariae Thunbergii (*Bei Mu*), Caulis Bambusae In Taeniis (*Zhu Ru*), Tuber Ophiopogonis Japonicae (*Mai Dong*), Tuber Asparagi Cochinensis (*Tian Dong*), Fructus Gardeniae Jasminoidis (*Zhi Zi*), Radix Platycodi Grandiflori (*Jie Geng*), Folium Mori Albi (*Sang Ye*), Pericarpium Citri Reticulatae (*Chen Pi*), Sclerotium Poriae Cocos (*Fu Ling*), Fructus Schizandrae Chinensis (*Wu Wei Zi*), Radix Praeparatus Glycyrrhizae (*Zhi Gan Cao*), Radix Angelicae Sinensis (*Dang Gui*), Fructus Zizyphi Jujubae (*Hong Zao*), Rhizoma Recens Zingiberis (*Sheng Jiang*)

with a positive mental attitude, gaining stature within their community. Instead of being a climax from which everything is downhill from there, it is a climax similar to the transformation of a caterpillar into a butterfly. The woman awakens into a wider realm and larger role within her society and this is seen as the fruition or culmination of a woman's life. This underscores the fact that it is liver depression qi stagnation which is the root disease mechanism of perimenopausal complaints as opposed to simply the cessation of menstruation. Would that we could reintroduce this concept into modern Western culture.

Acupuncture & moxibustion

Because the root of menopausal complaints (as opposed to menopause itself) is liver depression and liver depression often is ameliorated by acupuncture, I believe acupuncture can be very useful in helping women through their change in life. This may be done preventively or remedially and may be as simple as frequently needling the Four Gates (*i.e.*, *He Gu* [LI 4] and *Tai Chong* [Liv 3]), remembering that *Tai Chong* refers to this point's relationship with the *chong mai*. In addition, direct, non-scarring thread moxa can be done at *Guan Yuan* (CV 4) and *Qi Hai* (CV 6) every year in the month of August in order to supplement the kidneys and strengthen the sinews and bones after menopause. To do this, one burns seven to fifteen tiny cones of moxa per day, every day for 30 days on the above two points. This was one of Golden Needle Wang Le-ting's acupuncture-moxibustion longevity techniques.

Prognosis

The vast majority of menopausal complaints are relatively easy to remedy using traditional Chinese internal medicine. Many cases only require two to six weeks of therapy. This is because we are only talking about facilitating a change which has gotten hung up in its process. If we can but nudge this process enough for it to complete itself, all negative signs and symptoms tend to resolve themselves automatically. It is my experience that the better able the woman is at dealing with stress and its subsequent liver depression qi stagnation, the less perimenopausal complaints she will have and the quicker and longer lasting therapy will be. When cases of perimenopausal syndrome are either recalcitrant to treatment or there is chronic recidivism, this is because of the woman's deep-seated liver depression. Therefore, practitioners should help their patients learn how to relax, encourage them to exercise regularly and eat well, and to develop a more positive outlook on life.

Addenda: Osteoporosis

Osteoporosis is typically not included in even modern Chinese gynecology texts. However, concerns over osteoporosis are one of the reasons many women are talked into ERT or

527

hormone replacement therapy (HRT). Although the Chinese gynecological textbook literature does not typically include discussions of osteoporosis, Chinese medicine does treat and prevent osteoporosis quite effectively. Therefore, I am including the following material on the Chinese treatment of osteoporosis in this book on so-called menstrual diseases.

(From "Experiences in the Treatment of 52 Cases of Senile Osteoporosis with *Qing E Wan Jia Wei* [Young Pretty Girl Pills with Added Flavors]" by Shen Lin *et al.*, *Hu Bei Zhong Yi Za Zhi [Hubei Journal of Traditional Chinese Medicine]*, #3, 1994, p. 16-18)

The authors of this clinical audit treated 52 patients with osteoporosis which had been previously confirmed by Western medical examination. Of these, 14 were men and 38 were women. They ranged in age from a young of 52 to an old of 78 years with an average age of 64.2 years old. All were seen as out-patients and all had some degree of upper and lower back pain. All the patients also were categorized as pertaining to various kidney vacuity patterns. There were 29 cases of kidney vacuity pattern, twelve cases of kidney yin vacuity pattern, four cases of kidney yang vacuity pattern, and seven cases of kidney yin and yang dual vacuity pattern.

Qing E Wan Jia Wei consisted of: Cortex Eucommiae Ulmoidis (*Du Zhong*), Semen Juglandis Regiae (*Hu Tao Rou*), Fructus Psoraleae Corylifoliae (*Bu Gu Zhi*), Herba Epimedii (*Yin Yang Huo*), dry Radix Rehmanniae (*Gan Di Huang*), Radix Achyranthis Bidentatae (*Huai Niu Xi*), 12g @. These were decocted down into a pure, thick liquid. This was then sterilized under high pressure and bottled. Each day, these patients took this liquid orally, 20ml per time, two times per day for three months. During this time, they were prohibited to take other Chinese or Western medicinals.

After 15 days of taking these medicinals, 15 patients or 28.85% felt that their lower and upper back aching and pain was decreased. After one month, 37 cases or 71.15% felt their back pain decreased. After two months, 45 cases or 86.53% felt their back pain decreased. And after taking these medicinals for three months, 46 cases or 88.46% felt their back pain eliminated or decreased. Measurements of bone density and x-ray analysis also showed statistically significant improvements from before to after this treatment.

The author cites the TCM statement of belief that the kidneys govern the bones as the rationale for this treatment's design and efficacy. *Qing E Wan* is an ancient formula for supplementing the kidneys and that is why it is capable of treating this disease with good results. It is comprised of Eucommia, Psoralea, and Walnuts. It is capable of treating kidney qi vacuity weakness and strengthening the sinews and bones. In addition, Epimedium boosts the essence qi and supplements the low back and knees, while Rehmannia nourishes yin blood and fulfills the bone marrow. Achyranthes leads the qi and blood to move downward, thus eliminating low back and knee bone pain. This formula is appropriate for the treatment of senile osteoporosis whether due to kidney vacuity, kidney yin vacuity, kidney yang vacuity, or kidney yin and yang dual vacuity.

Other research in Japan has shown that postmenopausal women using similar Chinese medicinals as above had greater bone density than a comparison group not using Chinese medicinals.[32] Since the prevention and treatment of osteoporosis is something which must be ongoing, I recommend *Ge Jie Da Bu Wan* (Gecko Greatly Supplementing Pills) to my postmenopausal patients who are concerned about osteoporosis. These pills are easy and convenient to take long-term. They are comprised of Gecko (*Ge Jie*), Radix Codonopsitis Pilosulae (*Dang Shen*), Radix Astragali Membranacei (*Huang Qi*), Fructus Lycii Chinensis (*Gou Qi Zi*), Radix Angelicae Sinensis (*Dang Gui*), Sclerotium Poriae Cocos (*Fu Ling*), cooked Radix Rehmanniae (*Shu Di*), Fructus Ligustri Lucidi (*Nu Zhen Zi*), Radix Glycyrrhizae (*Gan Cao*), Radix Dioscoreae Oppositae (*Shan Yao*), Fructus Chaenomelis Lagenariae (*Mu Gua*), Rhizoma Cibotii Barometsis (*Gou Ji*), Radix Morindae Officinalis (*Ba Ji Tian*), Rhizoma Atractylodis Macrocephalae (*Bai Zhu*), Radix Dipsaci (*Xu Duan*), Cortex Eucommiae Ulmoidis (*Du Zhong*), Rhizoma Polygonati (*Huang Jing*), Rhizoma Drynariae (*Gu Sui Bu*). This formula supplements both the qi and blood and both yin and yang. It also does not contain any medicinals from endangered species, such as Os Tigridis (*Hu Gu*) or Os Leopardis (*Bao Gu*), the way a number of Chinese patent medicines do which are designed specifically for chronic bone problems.

Senile Vaginitis

Senile vaginitis is commonly discussed in modern Chinese gynecology texts. However, when it is discussed, it is done so under diseases of the external genitalia *a la* Western medicine. It is categorically not considered a menstrual disease. However, because it too is an important concern for Western menopausal women, I have chosen to include information on the Chinese disease mechanisms and treatment of it as well.

After menopause, women's estrogen levels decrease and the vaginal tract's power of resistance diminishes and becomes weak. This may lead to the arising of vaginal tract inflammation. This is categorized under *dai xia* or abnormal vaginal discharge disease.

Disease causes, disease mechanisms

At seven times seven a woman's *tian gui* is exhausted and her *chong* and *ren* are debilitated and weak. The *dai mai* thus no longer restrains and hence this disease results. It is due to the

---

[32]   *Traditional Sino-Japanese Medicine*, #13, 1992, p. 38-43

righteous being vacuous and evils entering. Therefore, damp heat evils take advantage of vacuity to assail. Thus there is commonly simultaneous damp heat pouring downward with yin and possibly also yang vacuity.

Treatment based on pattern discrimination

Liver-kidney insufficiency

Main symptoms: Yellow or red-colored abnormal vaginal discharge, dryness and burning of the vaginal meatus, dizziness, blurred vision, heart vexation, easy anger, a dry mouth and red lips, a red tongue, and a fine pulse

Treatment principles: Enrich and supplement the liver and kidneys, clear heat and stop vaginal discharge

Guiding formulas:

1. *Zhi Bai Di Huang Tang Jia Jian* (Anemarrhena & Phellodendron Rehmannia Decoction with Additions & Subtractions)

Ingredients: Rhizoma Anemarrhenae Aspheloidis (*Zhi Mu*), Cortex Phellodendri (*Huang Bai*), uncooked Radix Rehmanniae (*Sheng Di*), Radix Dioscoreae Oppositae (*Shan Yao*), Cortex Radicis Moutan (*Dan Pi*), Sclerotium Poriae Cocos (*Fu Ling*), Herba Ecliptae Prostratae (*Han Lian Cao*), Fructus Cnidii Monnieri (*She Chuang Zi*), Herba Artemisiae Capillaris (*Yin Chen*), mix-fried Radix Glycyrrhizae (*Gan Cao*), Cortex Toonae Sinensis (*Chun Gen Pi*)

Additions: If there are hot flashes and a cold body with exiting of sweat (*i.e.*, yin and yang vacuity), use *Er Xian Tang* (Two Immortals Decoction) with Herba Artemisiae Capillaris (*Yin Chen*), Cortex Toonae Sinensis (*Chun Gen Pi*), Semen Coicis Lachryma-jobi (*Yi Ren*), Semen Euryalis Ferocis (*Qian Shi*), and Nodus Rhizomatis Nelumbinis Nuciferae (*Ou Jie*). If there is vexation and agitation and easy anger, add Fructus Gardeniae Jasminodis (*Shan Zhi*), Tuber Ophiopogonis Japonicae (*Mai Dong*), and Radix Albus Paeoniae Lactiflorae (*Bai Shao*). If there is lumbar pain, add Cortex Eucommiae Ulmoidis (*Du Zhong*), Ramulus Loranthi Seu Visci (*Sang Ji Sheng*), and Radix Achyranthis Bidentatae (*Niu Xi*). If there is urinary pain, add Herba Dianthi (*Qu Mai*) and *Liu Yi San* (Six to One Powder), wrapped.

2. *Zhi Bai Di Huang Wan Jia Wei* (Anemarrhena & Phellodendron Rehmannia Pills with Added Flavors)

Ingredients: Uncooked & prepared Radix Rehmanniae (*Sheng Shu Di*), Radix Dioscoreae Oppositae (*Shan Yao*), Sclerotium Poriae Cocos (*Fu Ling*), Fructus Corni Officinalis (*Shan*

Zhu Yu), Rhizoma Alismatis (*Ze Xie*), Cortex Radicis Moutan (*Dan Pi*), Fructus Ligustri Lucidi (*Nu Zhen Zi*), Fructus Lycii Chinensis (*Qi Zi*), Radix Polygoni Multiflori (*Shou Wu*), Fructus Rosae Laevigatae (*Jin Ying Zi*), Rhizoma Anemarrhenae Aspheloidis (*Zhi Mu*), Cortex Phellodendri (*Huang Bai*), Cortex Eucommiae Ulmoidis (*Du Zhong*), Radix Achyranthis Bidentatae (*Niu Xi*)

3. *Zhi Bai Di Huang Tang Jia Wei* (Anemarrhena & Phellodendron Rehmannia Decoction with Added Flavors)

Ingredients: Uncooked Radix Rehmanniae (*Sheng Di*), Cortex Radicis Moutan (*Dan Pi*), Fructus Corni Officinalis (*Shan Zhu Rou*), Rhizoma Alismatis (*Ze Xie*), Sclerotium Poriae Cocos (*Fu Ling*), Radix Dioscoreae Oppositae (*Shan Yao*), Rhizoma Anemarrhenae Aspheloidis (*Zhi Mu*), Cortex Phellodendri (*Huang Bai*), Rhizoma Smilacis Glabrae (*Tu Fu Ling*), Flos Lonicerae Japonicae (*Yin Hua*), Radix Rubrus Paeoniae Lactiflorae (*Chi Shao*)

4. *Zhi Bai Di Huang Tang Jia Jian* (Anemarrhena & Phellodendron Rehmannia Decoction with Additions & Subtractions)

Ingredients: Uncooked Radix Rehmanniae (*Sheng Di*), Cortex Phellodendri (*Huang Bai*), Rhizoma Anemarrhenae Aspheloidis (*Zhi Mu*), Fructus Lycii Chinensis (*Qi Zi*), Fructus Ligustri Lucidi (*Nu Zhen Zi*), Herba Ecliptae Prostratae (*Han Lian Cao*), Semen Coicis Lachryma-jobi (*Yi Ren*), Semen Euryalis Ferocis (*Qian Shi*), carbonized Flos Immaturus Sophorae Japonicae (*Huai Hua*), Nodus Rhizomatis Nelumbinis Nuciferae (*Ou Jie*)

This formula is suitable if there is a dilute, watery, but possibly reddish vaginal discharge.

5. *Si Wu Jia Wei Tang* (Four Materials Added Flavors Decoction)

Ingredients: Radix Angelicae Sinensis (*Dang Gui*), Radix Ligustici Wallichii (*Chuan Xiong*), Radix Rubrus Paeoniae Lactiflorae (*Chi Shao*), Cortex Radicis Moutan (*Dan Pi*), Radix Dioscoreae Oppositae (*Shan Yao*), Radix Dipsaci (*Chuan Duan*), uncooked Radix Rehmanniae (*Sheng Di*), Ramulus Loranthi Seu Visci (*Sang Ji Sheng*), Radix Salviae Miltiorrhizae (*Dan Shen*), processed Radix Polygoni Multiflori (*Shou Wu*), Radix Trichosanthis Kirlowii (*Hua Fen*), Rhizoma Smilacis Glabrae (*Tu Fu Ling*)

This formula is for chronic vaginal itching due to yin and blood vacuity.

Additions: If the spirit is listless and the facial complexion is yellow and if sleep at night is disquieted, add *Gui Pi Wan* (Restore the Spleen Pills). If there is lumbar pain, add Cortex Eucommiae Ulmoidis (*Du Zhong*) and Semen Cuscutae (*Tu Si Zi*). If there is yellow vaginal discharge, add Rhizoma Anemarrhenae Aspheloidis (*Zhi Mu*) and Cortex Phellodendri (*Huang Bai*). If the skin of the external vagina is dry and parched, add Radix Angelicae

Sinensis (*Dang Gui*), Rhizoma Polygonati (*Huang Jing*), Fructus Ligustri Lucidi (*Nu Zhen Zi*), and Tuber Ophiopogonis Japonici (*Mai Dong*).

6. *Zuo Gui Wan Jia Jian* (Restore the Left [Kidney] Pills with Additions & Subtractions)

Ingredients: Uncooked Radix Rehmanniae (*Sheng Di*), Radix Dioscoreae Oppositae (*Shan Yao*), Fructus Corni Officinalis (*Shan Zhu Yu*), Semen Cuscutae (*Tu Si Zi*), Fructus Lycii Chinensis (*Qi Zi*), Radix Achyranthis Bidentatae (*Niu Xi*), Fructus Meliae Toosendan (*Chuan Lian Zi*), Semen Litchi Sinensis (*Li Zhi He*), stir-fried Radix Albus Paeoniae Lactiflorae (*Bai Shao*), mix-fried Radix Glycyrrhizae (*Gan Cao*), Herba Cistanchis Deserticolae (*Rou Cong Rong*), Cortex Cinnamomi Cassiae (*Rou Gui*)

This formula is for dryness, astringency, aching and pain of the vaginal door, scanty vaginal discharge, and burning pain.

7. *Zuo Gui Yin Jia Wei* (Restore the Left [Kidney] Drink with Added Flavors)

Ingredients: Cooked Radix Rehmanniae (*Shu Di*), Radix Dioscoreae Oppositae (*Shan Yao*), Fructus Lycii Chinensis (*Gou Qi Zi*), mix-fried Radix Glycyrrhizae (*Gan Cao*), Sclerotium Poriae Cocos (*Fu Ling*), Fructus Corni Officinalis (*Shan Zhu Rou*), Fructus Foeniculi Vulgaris (*Xiao Hui*), Herba Cistanchis Deserticolae (*Rou Cong Rong*)

Additions: If there are hot flashes and sweating and vexatious heat in the five hearts, add Rhizoma Anemarrhenae Aspheloidis (*Zhi Mu*), Cortex Phellodendri (*Huang Bai*), uncooked Radix Rehmanniae (*Sheng Di*), and Cortex Radicis Moutan (*Dan Pi*).

8. *Dang Gui Yin Zi* (Dang Gui Drink)

Ingredients: Radix Angelicae Sinensis (*Dang Gui*), Radix Ligustici Wallichii (*Chuan Xiong*), Radix Albus Paeoniae Lactiflorae (*Bai Shao*), uncooked Radix Rehmanniae (*Sheng Di*), Radix Ledebouriellae Sesloidis (*Fang Feng*), Herba Schizonepetae Tenuifoliae (*Jing Jie*), Radix Astragali Membranacei (*Huang Qi*), Radix Glycyrrhizae (*Gan Cao*), Fructus Tribuli Terrestris (*Bai Ji Li*), Radix Polygoni Multiflori (*He Shou Wu*)

This formula is for the treatment of vaginal itching due to blood dryness engendering wind.

Additions: If there is simultaneous dizziness and blurred vision with vexatious heat in the five hearts due to yin vacuity, internal heat, add Cortex Phellodendri (*Huang Bai*), Plastrum Testudinis (*Gui Ban*), Carapax Amydae Sinensis (*Bie Jia*), and Cortex Radicis Lycii Chinensis (*Di Gu Pi*) to enrich yin and clear heat. If the menstruation is scanty in amount and pale in color, add cooked Radix Rehmanniae (*Shu Di*), Radix Codonopsitis Pilosulae

(*Dang Shen*), Fructus Lycii Chinensis (*Gou Qi*), Fructus Corni Officinalis (*Shan Zhu*), and Caulis Milletiae Seu Spatholobi (*Ji Xue Teng*) to supplement both the qi and the blood.

9. *Liu Wei Di Huang Wan Jia Jian* (Six Flavors Rehmannia Pills with Additions & Subtractions)

Ingredients: Cooked Radix Rehmanniae (*Shu Di*), Radix Dioscoreae Oppositae (*Shan Yao*), Fructus Corni Officinalis (*Shan Zhu*), Cortex Radicis Moutan (*Dan Pi*), Radix Angelicae Sinensis (*Dang Gui*), Radix Albus Paeoniae Lactiflorae (*Bai Shao*), Cortex Radicis Dictamni Dasycarpi (*Bai Xian Pi*), Radix Angelicae Dahuricae (*Bai Zhi*), Semen Cuscutae (*Tu Si Zi*), uncooked Radix Glycyrrhizae (*Sheng Cao*)

This formula is also for the treatment of blood dryness vaginal itching.

10. *Dang Gui Liu Huang Tang* (Dang Gui Six Yellows Decoction)

Ingredients: Radix Angelicae Sinensis (*Dang Gui*), Rhizoma Coptidis Chinensis (*Huang Lian*), Cortex Phellodendri (*Huang Bai*), Radix Astragali Membranacei (*Huang Qi*), Radix Scutellariae Baicalensis (*Huang Qin*), uncooked Radix Rehmanniae (*Sheng Di*)

This formula is for vaginal sweating due to a combination of yin vacuity and damp heat pouring downward. There may also be vaginal chilling, but this chilling is only a species of local cold. Damp heat prevents yang qi from warming the region. Generalized symptoms are of yin vacuity and damp heat, not yang vacuity.

11. Experiential formula

lgredients: Uncooked Radix Rehmanniae (*Sheng Di*), Fructus Ligustri Lucidi (*Nu Zhen Zi*), Gelatinum Corii Asini (*E Jiao*), Rhizoma Coptidis Chinensis (*Huang Lian*), Cortex Phellodendri (*Huang Bai*), Fructus Meliae Toosendan (*Chuan Lian Zi*), 8g each

12. *Shen Qi Wan Jia Jian* (Kidney Qi Pills with Additions & Subtractions)

Ingredients: Cortex Cinnamomi Cassiae (*Rou Gui*), Radix Lateralis Praeparatus Aconiti Carmichaeli (*Fu Zi*), cooked Radix Rehmanniae (*Shu Di*), Sclerotium Poriae Cocos (*Fu Ling*), Fructus Corni Officinalis (*Shan Zhu Rou*), Radix Dioscoreae Oppositae (*Shan Yao*), Os Draconis (*Long Gu*), Concha Ostreae (*Mu Li*), Radix Morindae Officinalis (*Ba Ji Tian*), Semen Cuscutae (*Tu Si Zi*), Herba Epimedii (*Xian Ling Pi*), Radix Polygalae Tenuifoliae (*Yuan Zhi*), Fructus Schisandrae Chinensis (*Wu Wei Zi*), Gelatinum Cornu Cervi (*Lu Jiao*), Fructus Rubi Chingii (*Fu Pen Zi*)

Liu Lan-fang and Liu Dian-gong, the authors of *Fu Ke San Bai Zheng (Three Hundred Gynecological Conditions),* give this formula for the treatment of vaginal atrophy due to decline of life gate fire. However, the formula contains ingredients for both yin and yang vacuity. The signs and symptoms Liu and Liu give are dryness and astringency of the vaginal tract during sexual intercourse, not a single pleasant sensation. At the beginning of intercourse, it is also possible for there to be an immediate, rapid, profuse discharge of yin fluids from the vaginal tract. This may be accompanied by dizziness, blurred vision, low back and knee soreness and weakness, lack of strength, profuse dreaming, a pale tongue with scanty coating, and a weak, fine, forceless pulse image.

External treatment methods:

1. Cortex Phellodendri (*Huang Bai*), 30g, Flos Lonicerae Japonicae (*Yin Hua*), 10g, Herba Epimedii (*Xian Ling Pi*), 30g. Douche and wash the vaginal tract or use as a sitz bath.

2. Radix Sophorae Flavescentis (*Ku Shen*), 30g, Fructus Cnidii Monnieri (*She Chuang Zi*), 30g, Herba Tougucao (*Tou Gu Cao*), 30g, Radix Glycyrrhizae (*Gan Cao*), 12g, Herba Taraxaci Mongolici Cum Radice (*Pu Gong Ying*), 15g, Radix Rubrus Paeoniae Lactiflorae (*Chi Shao*), 9g. Decoct in water and fumigate and wash, one *ji* each day. Use continuously for 10 times.

3. For vaginal sweating due to a combination of yin vacuity and damp heat, use equal amounts of powdered Lithargyum (*Mi Tuo Seng*) and Fructus Cnidii Monnieri (*She Chuang Zi*) applied externally.

4. For burning pain in the vagina, wash the external vagina with a decoction of Fructus Meliae Toosendan (*Chuan Lian Zi*). Then apply uncooked sesame seed oil (*Zhi Ma You*) to the inside of the vagina.

5. Radix Sophorae Flavescentis (*Ku Shen*), 30g, Fructus Cnidii Monnieri (*She Chuang Zi*), 39g, Pericarpium Zanthoxyli Bungeani (*Chuan Jiao*), 15g, Alum (*Ku Fan*), 30g, Flos Lonicerae Japonicae (*Jin Yin Hua*), 39g. If there is senile vaginitis, add Folium Artemisiae Argyii (*Ai Ye*), 29g, Radix Angelicae Sinensis (*Dang Gui*), 15g, Flos Carthami Tinctorii (*Hong Hua*), 15g. Boil the above medicinals into half a bowl and while still hot, first fumigate and then use as a sitz bath two times each day. This formula disperses heat and resolves toxins, dries dampness, kills worms, and stops itching. It is suitable for use in external vaginal itching conditions.

6. Fructus Cnidii Monnieri (*She Chuang Zi*), Radix Sophorae Flavescentis (*Ku Shen*), Radix Angelicae Sinensis (*Dang Gui*), 15g @, Cortex Radicis Dictamni Dasycarpi (*Bai*

Xian Pi), 12g, Flos Carthami Tinctorii (*Hong Hua*), 6g. Decoct in water two times and remove the dregs. First fumigate and then use as a sitz bath one time each day. This formula nourishes the blood, dries dampness, and stops itching. It is suitable for senile vaginitis.

7. Cortex Radicis Dictamni Dasycarpi (*Bai Xian Pi*), 30g, Caulis Milletiae Seu Spatholobi (*Ji Xue Teng*), 30g, Radix Polygoni Multiflori (*Shou Wu*), 30g, uncooked Radix Rehmanniae (*Sheng Di*), 30g, Herba Ephedrae (*Ma Huang*), 9g, Flos Carthami Tinctorii (*Hong Hua*), 6g, Herba Epimedii (*Xian Ling Pi*), 15g. Decoct in water and use as a sitz bath two times each day for 1/2 hour each time. This formula nourishes the blood, engenders fluids, and stops itching. It is used for senile vaginitis or vulvar leukoplakia.

Appendix 1:
Acupuncture & Moxibustion Formulas for Menstrual Diseases

The formulas given below correspond to the main patterns under the menstrual diseases discussed in the body of the text. Their composition is based on the contemporary TCM approach to Chinese acupuncture. Because most patients in clinical practice present with multifaceted patterns, practitioners should regard these formulas as only the basic building blocks for designing a TCM acupuncture protocol for any given Western gynecological patient. The theory behind the formulation of TCM acupuncture protocols is relatively straight-forward. After doing a pattern discrimination, one states the appropriate treatment principles for remedying that pattern. Then one chooses points whose functions and properties correspond to those principles. In general, one should choose several major transport points on the arms and legs corresponding to the major treatment principles. These are then combined with local points on the channels traversing the lower abdomen and lumbosacral region as well as extra-channel *a shi* points.

In my experience, the key issues in formulating and administering effective TCM acupuncture treatments for menstrual diseases primarily reside in 1) doing a correct pattern discrimination, 2) then stating the correct treatment principles, and 3) choosing the best and most effective time for administering treatment. Personally, I believe TCM acupuncture is most effective when several treatments are grouped together fairly closely. In China, the standard of care is usually every other day, three days per week for a course of treatment of 10-15 treatments. In the West, such repeated, intensive treatments are not always possible due to time and monetary constraints. However, when doing acupuncture for menstrual diseases, one does not necessarily need to treat throughout the entire cycle.

In other words, if the patient were willing to receive one treatment per week four times per month, it is my experience when treating menstrual diseases, she would be better served and her money would be spent in a more cost effective manner if she received three or four treatments spaced every other day in the correct phase of her cycle. This means that, for premenstrual complaints, it is more cost and therapeutically effective to give a treatment every other or every third day from the onset of the premenstrual signs and symptoms than it is to give one treatment per week throughout the entire cycle. Likewise, for painful menstruation, as long as this is not accompanied by midcycle, ovulatory pain, I believe that acupuncture and moxibustion really only needs to be begun several days before the onset of menstruation and then continued through the time when the pain is normally experienced.

During that time, it may mean that the patient receives one treatment every day or even more than one treatment per day.

Such intensive acupuncture is all the more appropriate when the practitioner is also treating the patient with some Chinese medicinals internally. These may be either bulk-dispensed, individually designed, water-based decoctions or they may be ready-made or so-called patent pills or powders. In that case, most of the cycle, the patient can be treated in the comfort of her own home by taking cyclically appropriate Chinese medicinals internally. Then, in addition to these, during certain phases of her monthly cycle, she may receive acupuncture daily, every other day, or every third day. If, for whatever reason, such cyclically phased intensive acupuncture is not possible, I nevertheless recommend designing acupuncture protocols keeping in mind what day of the patient's menstrual cycle it is and altering the protocol in order to work within and with this cycle.

Guiding acupuncture points for the treatment of menstrual disease

The formulas below are only meant as guides to treatment. They are not intended to be used without modification. Readers should consider the TCM rationale for each point in each formula. Since most cases area combination of two or more patterns occurring simultaneously, in clinical practice, one should choose one, two, or several points from each formula for each pattern present, thus crafting an individual treatment corresponding to the individual patient.

Menstruation Ahead of Schedule

Blood heat

Replete heat/damp heat: *Xue Hai* (Sp 10), *San Yin Jiao* (Sp 6), *He Gu* (LI 4), *Qu Chi* (LI 11), *Zhong Ji* (CV 3), *Yang Ling Quan* (GB 34) for replete heat, *Yin Ling Quan* (Sp 9) for damp heat

Depressive heat: *Xing Jian* (Liv 2) through to *Tai Chong* (Liv 3), *San Yin Jiao* (Sp 6), *Xue Hai* (Sp 10), *He Gu* (LI 4), *Qu Chi* (LI 11), *Qi Hai* (CV 6)

Vacuity heat: *Tai Xi* (Ki 3), *Yin Gu* (Ki 10), *San Yin Jiao* (Sp 6), *Xue Hai* (Sp 10), *Guan Yuan* (CV 4), *Shen Shu* (Bl 23)

Phlegm heat: *Tai Chong* (Liv 3), *He Gu* (LI 4), *Qu Chi* (LI 11), *Feng Long* (St 40), *San Yin Jiao* (Sp 6), *Xue Hai* (Sp 10), *Pi Shu* (Bl 20)

Qi vacuity

Spleen qi vacuity: *Zu San Li* (St 36), *San Yin Jiao* (Sp 6), *Pi Shu* (Bl 20), *Wei Shu* (Bl 21), *Qi Hai* (CV 6), *Bai Hui* (GV 20)

Kidney qi vacuity: *Tai Xi* (Ki 3), *Fu Liu* (Ki 7), *San Yin Jiao* (Sp 6), *Guan Yuan* (CV 4), *Shen Shu* (Bl 23)

Blood stasis: This only complicates other patterns above. When present, add *Gui Lai* (St 29), *Da Chang Shu* (Bl 25), and *Xue Hai* (Sp 10).

Menstruation Behind Schedule

Blood vacuity

Blood vacuity: *Zu San Li* (St 36), *San Yin Jiao* (Sp 6), *Guan Yuan* (CV 4), *Ge Shu* (Bl 17), *Gan Shu* (Bl 18), *Pi Shu* (Bl 20)

Vacuity cold: *Guan Yuan* (CV 4), *Shen Que* (CV 8), *Shui Dao* (St 28), *San Yin Jiao* (Sp 6), *Zu San Li* (St 36), *Xue Hai* (Sp 10)

Stasis & obstruction

Cold congelation: *Guan Yuan* (CV 4), *Shui Dao* (St 28), *San Yin Jiao* (Sp 6), *Zu San Li* (St 36), *Xue Hai* (Sp 10)

Qi stagnation: *Tai Chong* (Liv 3), *San Yin Jiao* (Sp 6), *Xue Hai* (Sp 10), *He Gu* (LI 4), *Tian Shu* (St 25), *Qi Hai* (CV 6)

Blood stasis: *Tai Chong* (Liv 3), *San Yin Jiao* (Sp 6), *Xue Hai* (Sp 10), *Zhong Ji* (CV 3), *Gui Lai* (St 29), *Da Chang Shu* (St 25)

Phlegm obstruction: *San Yin Jiao* (Sp 6), *Feng Long* (St 40), *Zhong Wan* (CV 12), *Pi Shu* (Bl 20), *Shui Dao* (St 28), *Tai Chong* (Liv 3), *Qi Hai* (CV 6)

(Sometimes) Early, (Sometimes) Late, No Fixed Schedule Menstruation

Liver depression qi stagnation: *Tai Chong* (Liv 3), *San Yin Jiao* (Sp 6), *He Gu* (LI 4), *Tian Shu* (St 25), *Qi Hai* (CV 6)

Spleen vacuity: *Zu San Li* (St 36), *San Yin Jiao* (Sp 6), *Guan Yuan* (CV 4), *Ge Shu* (Bl 17), *Gan Shu* (Bl 18), *Pi Shu* (Bl 20)

Kidney vacuity

Yin vacuity: *Tai Xi* (Ki 3), *San Yin Jiao* (Sp 6), *Guan Yuan* (CV 4), *Ge Shu* (Bl 17), *Gan Shu* (Bl 18), *Shen Shu* (Bl 23)

Yang vacuity: *Fu Liu* (Ki 7), *San Yin Jiao* (Sp 6), *Guan Yuan* (CV 4), *Ming Men* (GV 4), *Shen Shu* (Bl 23)

Profuse Menstruation

Blood heat

Replete heat/damp heat: *Xing Jian* (Liv 2), *Da Zhui* (GV 14), *Qu Chi* (LI 11), *San Yin Jiao* (Sp 6), *Xue Hai* (Sp 10), *Zhong Ji* (CV 3). Add *Yang Ling Quan* (Sp 9) if due to damp heat.

Depressive heat: *Xing Jian* (Liv 2) through to *Tai Chong* (Liv 3), *San Yin Jiao* (Sp 6), *Xue Hai* (Sp 10), *He Gu* (LI 4), *Qi Hai* (CV 6)

Vacuity heat: *Tai Xi* (Ki 3), *Yin Gu* (Ki 10), *San Yin Jiao* (Sp 6), *Xue Hai* (Sp 10), *Guan Yuan* (CV 4), *Shen Shu* (Bl 23)

Qi vacuity

Spleen qi vacuity: *Zu San Li* (St 36), *San Yin Jiao* (Sp 6), *Pi Shu* (Bl 20), *Wei Shu* (Bl 21), *Qi Hai* (CV 6), *Bai Hui* (GV 20)

Phlegm dampness: *Zu San Li* (St 36), *San Yin Jiao* (Sp 6), *Feng Long* (St 40), *Pi Shu* (Bl 20), *Wei Shu* (Bl 21), *Qi Hai* (CV 6)

Kidney qi vacuity: *Tai Xi* (Ki 3), *San Yin Jiao* (Sp 6), *Guan Yuan* (CV 4), *Ming Men* (GV 4), *Shen Shu* (Bl 23)

Blood stasis

Only complicates other patterns. If present, add *Xue Hai* (Sp 10), *Gui Lai* (St 29), *Zhong Ji* (CV 3).

Scanty Menstruation

Blood vacuity

Spleen vacuity: *Zu San Li* (St 36), *San Yin Jiao* (Sp 6), *Qu Quan* (Liv 8), *Guang Yuan* (CV 4), *Ge Shu* (Bl 17), *Gan Shu* (Bl 18), *Pi Shu* (Bl 20)

Kidney yin vacuity: *Tai Xi* (Ki 3), *Yin Gu* (Ki 10), *Qu Quan* (Liv 8), *San Yin Jiao* (Sp 6), *Guan Yuan* (CV 4), *Ge Shu* (Bl 17), *Gan Shu* (Bl 18), *Shen Shu* (Bl 23)

Kidney yang vacuity: *Fu Liu* (Ki 7), *San Yin Jiao* (Sp 6), *Guan Yuan* (CV 4), *Ming Men* (GV 4), *Shen Shu* (Bl 23)

Stasis & obstruction

Blood stasis: *Tai Chong* (Liv 3), *San Yin Jiao* (Sp 6), *He Gu* (LI 4), *Xue Hai* (Sp 10), *Zhong Ji* (CV 3), *Qi Hai* (CV 6)

Phlegm dampness: *Zu San Li* (St 36), *Feng Long* (St 40), *San Yin Jiao* (Sp 6), *Qi Hai* (CV 6), *Shui Dao* (St 28), *Pi Shu* (Bl 20), *Wei Shu* (Bl 21)

Mixed vacuity & repletion

Spleen-kidney vacuity with vacuity cold & stasis: *Guan Yuan* (CV 4), *Shen Que* (CV 8), *San Yin Jiao* (Sp 6), *Zu San Li* (St 36), *Xue Hai* (Sp 10), *Ming Men* (GV 4), *Shen Shu* (Bl 23)

Qi stagnation with spleen vacuity & blood vacuity: *Tai Chong* (Liv 3), *San Yin Jiao* (Sp 6), *Zu San Li* (St 36), *Guan Yuan* (CV 4), *Ge Shu* (Bl 17), *Gan Shu* (Bl 18), *Pi Shu* (Bl 20)

Flooding & Leaking

Blood heat

Replete heat: *San Yin Jiao* (Sp 6), *Xue Hai* (Sp 10), *Qu Chi* (LI 11), *Da Zhui* (GV 14), *Da Dun* (Liv 1), *Zhong Ji* (CV 3)

Depressive heat: *Da Dun* (Liv 1), *Tai Chong* (Liv 3), *San Yin Jiao* (Sp 6), *Xue Hai* (Sp 10), *Qi Hai* (CV 6), *Qu Chi* (LI 11)

Vacuity heat: *San Yin Jiao* (Sp 6), *Xue Hai* (Sp 10), *Tai Xi* (Ki 3), *Yin Gu* (Ki 10), *Guan Yuan* (CV 4), *Shao Fu* (Ht 8)

Damp heat: *Yin Bai* (Sp 1), *Yin Ling Quan* (Sp 9), *Xue Hai* (Sp 10), *Zhong Ji* (CV 3), *Qu Chi* (LI 11)

Qi vacuity

Spleen qi vacuity: *Yin Bai* (Sp 1), *San Yin Jiao* (Sp 6), *Zu San Li* (St 36), *Yang Chi* (TB 4), *Qi Hai* (CV 6), *Bai Hui* (GV 20), *Pi Shu* (Bl 20), *Wei Shu* (Bl 21)

Kidney qi vacuity: *Fu Liu* (Ki 7), *San Yin Jiao* (Sp 6), *Guan Yuan* (CV 4), *Yao Yang Guan* (GV 3), *Shen Shu* (Bl 23)

Spleen-kidney vacuity: *San Yin Jiao* (Sp 6), *Tai Xi* (Ki 3), *Zu San Li* (St 36), *Guan Yuan* (CV 4), *Shen Que* (CV 8), *Shen Shu* (Bl 23), *Ming Men* (GV 4)

Stasis & obstruction

Blood stasis: Usually only complicates other patterns. Therefore, add *Xue Hai* (Sp 10), *Zhong Ji* (CV 3), *Gui Lai* (St 29), *Da Chang Shu* (Bl 25)

Phelgm rheum: *Zu San Li* (St 36), *Feng Long* (St 40), *Yin Bai* (Sp 1), *San Yin Jiao* (Sp 6), *Shang Qiu* (Sp 5), *Qi Hai* (CV 6), *Pi Shu* (Bl 20), *Wei Shu* (Bl 21)

Blocked Menstruation

Blood vacuity

Qi & blood vacuity: *Zu San Li* (St 36), *San Yin Jiao* (Sp 6), *Guan Yuan* (CV 4), *Ge Shu* (Bl 17), *Gan Shu* (Bl 18), *Pi Shu* (Bl 20)

Liver-kidney vacuity: *Tai Xi* (Ki 3), *Qu Quan* (Liv 8), *San Yin Jiao* (Sp 6), *Guan Yuan* (CV 4), *Ge Shu* (Bl 17), *Gan Shu* (Bl 18), *Shen Shu* (Bl 23)

Lung yin & blood vacuity: *Lie Que* (Lu 7), *Zhao Hai* (Ki 6), *Guan Yuan* (CV 4), *San Yin Jiao* (Sp 6), *Fei Shu* (Bl 13), *Ge Shu* (Bl 17), *Shen Shu* (Bl 23)

Heart yin & blood vacuity: *Shen Men* (Ht 7), *San Yin Jiao* (Sp 6), *Zu San Li* (St 36), *Guan Yuan* (CV 4), *Xin Shu* (Bl 15), *Ge Shu* (Bl 17), *Shen Shu* (Bl 23)

Kidney vacuity: *Tai Xi* (Ki 3), *Yin Gu* (Ki 10), *San Yin Jiao* (Sp 6), *Qu Quan* (Liv 8), *Guan Yuan* (CV 4), *Shen Shu* (Bl 23)

Stasis & obstruction

Qi stagnation, blood stasis: *Tai Chong* (Liv 3), *San Yin Jiao* (Sp 6), *Xue Hai* (Sp 10), *He Gu* (LI 4), *Zhong Ji* (CV 3), *Qi Hai* (CV 6), *Tian Shu* (St 25), *Da Chang Shu* (Bl 25)

Cold damp congelation & stagnation: *San Yin Jiao* (Sp 6), *Xue Hai* (Sp 10), *Shui Dao* (St 28), *Guan Yuan* (CV 4), *Shen Que* (CV 8), *Zu San Li* (St 36), *Shen Shu* (Bl 23)

Phlegm dampness: *Feng Long* (St 40), *Zu San Li* (St 36), *San Yin Jiao* (Sp 6), *Shang Qiu* (Sp 5), *Qi Hai* (CV 6), *Shui Dao* (St 28), *Pi Shu* (Bl 20), *Wei Shu* (Bl 21)

Painful Menstruation

Stasis & obstruction

Qi stagnation: *Tai Chong* (Liv 3), *San Yin Jiao* (Sp 6), *He Gu* (LI 4), *Qi Hai* (CV 6), *Tian Shu* (St 25)

Liver depression-effuglent fire: *Xing Jian* (Liv 2) through to *Tai Chong* (Liv 3), *San Yin Jiao* (Sp 6), *He Gu* (LI 4), *Yang Ling Quan* (GB 34), *Qi Hai* (CV 6)

Blood stasis: *Tai Chong* (Liv 3), *San Yin Jiao* (Sp 6), *Xue Hai* (Sp 10), *He Gu* (LI 4), *Gui Lai* (St 29), *Zhong Ji* (CV 3), *Da Chang Shu* (Bl 25)

Cold damp congelation & stagnation: *San Yin Jiao* (Sp 6), *Zhong Ji* (CV 3), *Guan Yuan* (CV 4), *Shui Dao* (St 28), *Xue Hai* (Sp 10), *Zu San Li* (St 36), *Shen Shu* (Bl 23)

Stasis & heat: *San Yin Jiao* (Sp 6), *Xue Hai* (Sp 10), *Xing Jian* (Liv 2), *Yin Ling Quan* (Sp 9), *Gui Lai* (St 29), *Zu Lin Qi* (GB 41), *Dai Mai* (GB 26)

Vacuity

Qi & blood vacuity: *Zu San Li* (St 36), *San Yin Jiao* (Sp 6), *Guan Yuan* (CV 4), *Qu Quan* (Liv 8), *Ge Shu* (Bl 17), *Gan Shu* (Bl 18), *Pi Shu* (Bl 20)

Liver-kidney deficiency damage: *San Yin Jiao* (Sp 6), *Qu Quan* (Liv 8), *Yin Gu* (Ki 10), *Guan Yuan* (CV 4), *Ge Shu* (Bl 17), *Gan Shu* (Bl 18), *Shen Shu* (Bl 23)

543

Vacuity cold within the uterus: *San Yin Jiao* (Sp 6), *Zu San Li* (St 36), *Fu Liu* (Ki 7), *Guan Yuan* (CV 4), *Ming Men* (GV 4), *Shen Shu* (Bl 23)

Vacuity heat: *San Yin Jiao* (Sp 6), *Tai Xi* (Ki 3), *Yin Gu* (Ki 10), *Guan Yuan* (CV 4), *Shen Shu* (Bl 23), *Hou Xi* (SI 3)

Premenstrual Syndrome

Liver depression qi stagnation: *Tai Chong* (Liv 3), *San Yin Jiao* (Sp 6), *He Gu* (LI 4)

Liver depression transforming heat: *Xing Jian* (Liv 2) through to *Tai Chong* (Liv 3), *San Yin Jiao* (Sp 6), *He Gu* (LI 4), *Qu Chi* (LI 11)

Liver depression with spleen vacuity and depressive heat in the stomach & lungs: *Xing Jian* (Liv 2) through to *Tai Chong* (Liv 3), *San Yin Jiao* (Sp 6), *He Gu* (LI 4), *Qu Chi* (LI 11), *Nei Ting* (St 44), *Fei Shu* (Bl 13), *Pi Shu* (Bl 20)

Liver yang ascendant hyperactivity: *Xing Jian* (Liv 2), *Yang Ling Quan* (GB 34), *He Gu* (LI 4), *Qu Chi* (LI 11), *Zu San Li* (St 36), *Feng Chi* (GB 20)

Liver depression, spleen vacuity with counterflow chilling: *Tai Chong* (Liv 3), *He Gu* (LI 4), *Nei Guan* (Per 6), *San Yin Jiao* (Sp 6), *Zu San Li* (St 36)

Liver depression, spleen vacuity & kidney yang vacuity: *Tai Chong* (Liv 3), *San Yin Jiao* (Sp 6), *Zu San Li* (St 36), *Tai Xi* (Ki 3), *Quan Yuan* (CV 4), *Pi Shu* (Bl 20), *Shen Shu* (Bl 23), *Ming Men* (GV 4)

Menstrual Movement Breast Distention & Pain

Liver depression qi stagnation: *Tai Chong* (Liv 3), *Liang Qiu* (St 34), *San Yin Jiao* (Sp 6), *Nei Guan* (Per 6), *Ru Gen* (St 18), *Shan Zhong* (CV 17)

Liver depression, phlegm stasis: *Tai Chong* (Liv 3), *Zu San Li* (St 36), *Feng Long* (St 40), *San Yon Jiao* (Sp 6), *Nei Guan* (Per 6), *Ru Gen* (St 18), *Shan Zhong* (CV 17), encircling needling of lumps

Liver-stomach depressive heat: *Xing Jian* (Liv 2), *Nei Ting* (St 44), *Liang Qiu* (St 34), *He Gu* (LI 4), *San Yin Jiao* (Sp 6), *Ru Gen* (St 18), *Shan Zhong* (CV 17)

Chong & ren **disharmony:** *Tai Chong* (Liv 3), *San Yin Jiao* (Sp 6), *Tai Xi* (Ki 3) and/or *Fu Liu* (Ki 7), *Hou Xi* (SI 3), *Zu Lin Qi* (GB 41), *Nei Guan* (Per 6), *Shan Zhong* (CV 17), *Ling Xu* (Ki 22), *Shen Shu* (Bl 23)

Menstrual Movement Diarrhea and/or Vomiting

Spleen vacuity, dampness retained: *Zu San Li* (St 36), *Shang Qiu* (Sp 5), *San Yin Jiao* (Sp 6), *Zhong Wan* (CV 12), *Tian Shu* (St 25), *Pi Shu* (Bl 20), *Wei Shu* (Bl 21)

Phlegm rheum hidden in The stomach: *Feng Long* (St 40, *Zu San Li* (St 36), *San Yin Jiao* (Sp 6), *Zhong Wan* (CV 12), *Pi Shu* (Bl 20), *Wei Shu* (Bl 21)

Spleen yang vacuity: *Zu San Li* (St 36), *Zhong Wan* (CV 12), *Tian Shu* (St 25), *Pi Shu* (Bl 20), *Wei Shu* (Bl 21), moxa

Liver attacking the stomach: *Tai Chong* (Liv 3), *Zu San Li* (St 36), *Zhong Wan* (CV 12), *Shan Zhong* (CV 17), add *Nei Ting* (St 44) if there is depressive heat in the stomach

Liver wood exploiting The spleen: *Tai Chong* (Liv 3), *San Yin Jiao* (Sp 6), *Zu San Li* (St 36), *Tian Shu* (St 25), *Zhong Wan* (CV 12), *Pi Shu* (Bl 20), *Wei Shu* (Bl 21)

Liver channel damp heat: *Xing Jian* (Liv 2), *Nei Ting* (St 44), *Yang Ling Quan* (GB 34), *Tian Shu* (St 25), *Da Chang Shu* (Bl 25), *Zhong Ji* (CV 3)

Damp heat with spleen vacuity: *San Yin Jiao* (Sp 6), *Yin Ling Quan* (Sp 9), *Zu San Li* (St 36), *Zhong Wan* (CV 12), *Tian Shu* (St 25), *Da Chang Shu* (Bl 25), *Pi Shu* (Bl 20), *Wei Shu* (Bl 21)

Kidney yang vacuity: *San Yin Jiao* (Sp 6), *Fu Liu* (Ki 7), *Tian Shu* (St 25), *Qi Hai* (CV 6), *Guan Yuan (CV 4)*, *Pi Shu* (Bl 20), *Shen Shu* (Bl 23), *Da Chang Shu* (Bl 25), moxa

Menstrual Movement Body Pain

External invasion: *Feng Men* (Bl 12), *Fei Shu* (Bl 13), *Feng Chi* (GB 20), *He Gu* (LI 4), *Wai Guan* (Th 5), local points

Yang qi counterflowing upward: *Tai Chong* (Liv 3), *Kun Lun* (Bl 60), *Hou Xi* (SI 3), *Tai Xi* (Ki 3), *Zu Lin Qi* (GB 41), *Feng Chi* (GB 20), *Jian Jing* (GB 21), local points

Damp heat impediment: *Yin Ling Quan* (Sp 9), *Yang Ling Quan* (GB 34), *Da Chang Shu* (Bl 25), *Pang Guang Shu* (Bl 28), *Ba Liao* (Bl 31-34), local points

Yin & blood vacuity: *Ge Shu* (Bl 17), *Gan Shu* (Bl 18), *Pi Shu* (Bl 20) if blood vacuity, *Shen Shu* (Bl 23) if yin vacuity, *San Yin Jiao* (Sp 6), *Yang Ling Quan* (GB 34), local points

Blood stasis: *Xue Hai* (Sp 10), *San Yin Jiao* (Sp 6), *He Gu* (LI 4), *Da Chang Shu* (Bl 25), local points and/or network vessel needling

Menstrual Movement Headache

External invasion: *He Gu* (LI 4), *Lie Que* (Lu 7), *Feng Chi* (GB 20), *Feng Men* (Bl 12), *Fei Shu* (Bl 13), *Tai Yang* (M-HN-9), local points

Liver depression qi stagnation: *Tai Chong* (Liv 3), *San Yin Jiao* (Sp 6), *Tai Tang* (M-HN-9), *Feng Chi* (GB 20), *He Gu* (LI 4), local points

Liver yang ascendant hyperactivity: *Tai Chong* (Liv 3) through to *Xing Jian* (Liv 2), *Tai Xi* (Ki 3), *San Yin Jiao* (Sp 6), *Feng Chi* (GB 20), *Tai Yang* (M-HN-9), *Bai Hui* (GV 20), local points

Phlegm turbidity harassing above: *Feng Long* (St 40), *Zhong Wan* (CV 12), *Zu San Li* (St 36), *Pi Shu* (Bl 20), *Wei Shu* (Bl 21), local points

Depressive heat ascends phlegm: *Xing Jian* (Liv 20) *Lao Gong* (Per 8), *Feng Long* (St 40), *Zhong Wan* (CV 12), local points

Qi & blood vacuity: *Zu San Li* (St 36), *San Yin Jiao* (Sp 6), *Ge shu* (Bl 17), *Pi Shu* (Bl 20), *Shen Shu* (Bl 23), *Guan Yuan* (CV 4), *Qi Hai* (CV 6)

Central qi vacuity: *Zu San Li* (St 36), *Qi Hai* (CV 6), *Bai Hui* (GV 20), moxa

Liver-kidney yin vacuity: *Qu Quan* (Liv 8), *Tai Xi* (Ki 3), *San Yin Jiao* (Sp 6), *Ge Shu* (Bl 17), *Gan Shu* (Bl 18), *Shen Shu* (Bl 23), *Guan Yuan* (CV 4), massage local points

Blood stasis: *Xue Hai* (Sp 10), *San Yin Jiao* (Sp 6), *Xing Jian* (Liv 2), *He Gu* (LI 4), local points and/or network vessel needling

Menstrual Movement Fever

Cold damage: *Feng Men* (Bl 13), *Fei Shu* (Bl 13), *He Gu* (LI 4), *Qu Chi* (LI 11), *Feng Chi* (GB 20), *Da Zhui* (GV 14)

Wind heat: *Feng Men* (Bl 12), *Fei Shu* (Bl 13), *Feng Chi* (GB 20), *Da Zhui* (GV 14), *He Gu* (LI 4), *Wai Guan* (TB 5)

Retained evils: *Tai Xi* (Ki 3), *San Yin Jiao* (Sp 6), *He Gu* (LI 4), *Qu Chi* (LI 11), *Da Zhui* (GV 14)

Liver depression transforming heat: *Xing Jian* (Liv 2), *San Yin Jiao* (Sp 6), *He Gu* (LI 4), *Qu Chi* (LI 11), *Wai Guan* (TB 5), *Da Zhui* (GV 14)

Blood vacuity, internal heat: *Ge Shu* (Bl 17), *Pi Shu* (Bl 20), *San Yin Jiao* (Sp 6), *He Gu* (LI 4), *Qu Chi* (LI 11), *Da Zhui* (GV 14)

Yang qi insufficiency: *Zu San Li* (St 36), *San Yin Jiao* (Sp 6), *Fu Liu* (Ki 7), *Shen Shu* (Bl 23), *Da Zhui* (GV 14)

Food stagnation: *Nei Ting* (St 44), *Zhong Wan* (CV 12), *Liang Men* (St 21), *He Gu* (LI 4), *Qu Chi* (LI 11), *Da Zhui* (GV 14)

Blood stasis: *Xue Hai* (Sp 10), *San Yin Jiao* (Sp 6), *He Gu* (LI 4), *Qu Chi* (Li 11), *Da Zhui* (GV 14), bleed the last three points

Stools dry & replete: *Nei Ting* (St 44), *Zhi Gou* (Th 6), *He Gu* (LI 4), *Qu Chi* (LI 11), *Tian Shu* (St 25), *Da Chang Shu* (Bl 25), *Da Zhui* (GV 14)

Menstrual Movement Vertigo & Dizziness

Central qi fall: *Zu San Li* (St 36), *Qi Hai* (CV 6), *Bai Hui* (GV 20), moxa

Blood vacuity: *San Yin Jiao* (Sp 6), *Zu San Li* (St 36), *Feng Chi* (GB 20), *Ge Shu* (Bl 17), *Pi Shu* (Bl 20), *Shen Shu* (Bl 23), *Si Shen Cong* (M-HN-1)

Liver-kidney yin vacuity: *Tai Xi* (Ki 3), *Qu Quan* (Liv 8), *San Yin Jiao* (Sp 6), *Feng Chi* (GB 20), *Guan Yuan* (CV 4), *Ge Shu* (Bl 17), *Gan Shu* (Bl 18), *Shen Shu* (Bl 23)

Spleen vacuity mixed with phlegm: *Feng Long* (St 40), *Zu San Li* (St 36), *Zhong Wan* (CV 12), *Nei Guan* (Per 6), *San Yin Jiao* (Sp 6), *Pi Shu* (Bl 20), *Wei Shu* (Bl 21)

Menstrual Movement Edema

Devitalized spleen yang: *Zu San Li* (St 36), *Yin Ling Quan* (Sp 9), *San Yin Jiao* (Sp 6), *Pi Shu* (Bl 20), *Wei Shu* (Bl 21), *San Jiao Shu* (Bl 22), *Pang Guang Shu* (Bl 28)

Spleen vacuity-liver depression: *Tai Chong* (Liv 3), *San Yin Jiao* (Sp 6), *Zu San Li* (St 36), *Yin Ling Quan* (Sp 9), *Pi Shu* (Bl 20), *San Jiao Shu* (Bl 22)

Menstrual Movement Oral *Gan*

Heart-stomach fire flaring: *Shen Men* (Ht 7), *Lao Gong* (Per 8), *Nei Ting* (St 44), *He Gu* (LI 4), *Di Cang* (St 4)

Menstrual Movement Loss of Sleep

Yin vacuity-fire effulgence: *Shen Men* (Ht 7), *Nei Guan* (Per 6), *Tai Xi* (Ki 3), *San Yin Jiao* (Sp 6), *Xin Shu* (Bl 15), *Shen Shu* (Bl 23), *An Mian* (N-HN-54)

Heart-spleen dual vacuity: *Shen Men* (Ht 7), *Nei Guan* (Per 6), *San Yin Jiao* (Sp 6), *Zu San Li* (St 36), *Xin Shu* (Bl 15), *Ge Shu* (Bl 17), *Pi Shu* (Bl 20), *An Mian* (N-HN-54)

Heart-liver fire effulgence: *Shen Men* (Ht 7), *Nei Guan* (Per 6), *Xing Jian* (Liv 2), *San Yin Jiao* (Sp 6), *He Gu* (LI 4), *Feng Chi* (GB 20), *Bai Hui* (GV 20)

Menstrual Movement Acne

Liver-spleen damp heat: *Xing Jian* (Liv 2), *Yin Ling Quan* (Sp 9), *San Yin Jiao* (Sp 6), *Yang Ling Quan* (GB 34), *He Gu* (LI 4), *Qu Chi* (LI 11), *Xue Hai* (Sp 10)

Liver depression transforms heat: *Tai Chong* (Liv 3) through to *Xing Jian* (Liv 2), *Nei Ting* (St 44), *He Gu* (LI 4), *Qu Chi* (LI 11), *Xue Hai* (Sp 10), *San Yin Jiao* (Sp 6), *Fei Shu* (Bl 13)

Spleen vacuity, phlegm dampness: *Zu San Li* (St 36), *Feng Long* (St 40), *Shang Qiu* (Sp 5), *San Yin Jiao* (Sp 6), *Fei Shu* (Bl 13), *Pi Shu* (Bl 20)

Blood stasis: *Xue Hai* (Sp 10), *San Yin Jiao* (Sp 6), *He Gu* (LI 4), *Qu Chi* (LI 11), network vessel needling

Vacuity heat fuming the lungs: *Zhao Hai* (Ki 6), *Lie Que* (Lu 7), *Xue Hai* (Sp 10), *San Yin Jiao* (Sp 6), *Qu Chi* (LI 11), *Fei Shu* (Bl 13), *Shen Shu* (Bl 23)

Menstrual Movement Raving & Confused Vision

Heart blood insufficiency: *Shen Men* (Ht 7), *Nei Guan* (Per 6), *San Yin Jiao* (Sp 6), *Yin Tang* (M-HN-3), *Si Shen Cong* (M-HN-1), *Xin Shu* (Bl 15), *Ge Shu* (Bl 17), *Pi Shu* (Bl 20)

Liver depression-fire effulgence: *Shen Men* (Ht 7), *Nei Guan* (Per 6), *Xing Jian* (Liv 2), *San Yin Jiao* (Sp 6), *He Gu* (LI 4), *Feng Chi* (GB 20), *Bai Hui* (GV 20)

Phlegm qi depression & binding: *Feng Long* (St 40), *Zhong Wan* (CV 12), *Lao Gong* (Per 8), *Shen Men* (Ht 7), *San Yin Jiao* (Sp 6), *Xin Bao Shu* (Bl 14), *Xin Shu* (Bl 15)

Menstrual Movement Dull-wittedness & Stupidity

Kidney yang insufficiency & stasis: *Xue Hai* (Sp 10), *San Yin Jiao* (Sp 6), *Fu Liu* (Ki 7), *Shen Dao* (GV 11), *Tao Dao* (GV 13), *Shen Shu* (Bl 23), *Ming Men* (GV 4)

Menstrual Movement Addictive Papules

Liver effulgence, blood heat: *Xue Hai* (Sp 10), *San Yin Jiao* (Sp 6), *Xing Jian* (Liv 2), *He Gu* (LI 4), *Qu Chi* (LI 11), bleed the last two points

Blood vacuity engendering wind: *San Yin Jiao* (Sp 6), *Zu San Li* (St 36), *Feng Shi* (GB 31), *Xin Shu* (Bl 15), *Ge Shu* (Bl 17), *Pi Shu* (Bl 20)

Blood stasis obstructing & stagnating: *Xue Hai* (Sp 10), *San Yin Jiao* (Sp 6), *He Gu* (LI 4), *Qu Chi* (LI 11), bleed the last two points

Menstrual Movement Flowing Drool

Liver wood exploiting the spleen: *Tai Chong* (Liv 3), *San Yin Jiao* (Sp 6), *Zu San Li* (St 36), *He Gu* (LI 4), *Lian Quan* (CV 23), *Cheng Jiang* (CV 24)

Menstrual Movement Oral Thirst

Stomach heat: *Nei Ting* (St 44), *San Yin Jiao* (Sp 6), *He Gu* (LI 4), *Qu Chi* (LI 11), *Lian Quan* (CV 23)

Stasis & stagnation: *Xue Hai* (Sp 10), *San Yin Jiao* (Sp 6), *He Gu* (LI 4), *Qu Chi* (LI 11), *Lian Quan* (CV 23)

Menstrual Movement Hoarse Voice

Lung dryness: *Zhao Hai* (Ki 6), *Lie Que* (Lu 7), *San Yin Jiao* (Sp 6), *Fei Shu* (Bl 13), *Lian Quan* (CV 23)

Kidney vacuity: *Tai Yuan* (Lu 9), *Tai Xi* (Ki 3), *San Yin Jiao* (Sp 6), *Guan Yuan* (CV 4), *Lian Quan* (CV 23), *Shen Shu* (Bl 23)

Damp heat: *Yin Ling Quan* (Sp 9), *San Yin Jiao* (Sp 6), other points depending on the location of the damp heat: bladder, genitalia, large intestine, and/or muscles and skin

Menstrual Movement Eye Pain

Liver blood vacuity: *Guang Ming* (GB 37), *Qu Quan* (Liv 8), *San Yin Jiao* (Sp 6), *Ge Shu* (Bl 17), *Gan Shu* (Bl 18), *Shen Shu* (Bl 23), *Zan Zhu* (Bl 2), *Feng Chi* (GB 20)

Menstrual Movement Lumbar Pain

Liver-kidney yin vacuity: *San Yin Jiao* (Sp 6), *Qu Quan* (Liv 8), *Tai Xi* (Ki 3), *Yang Ling Quan* (GB 34), *Ge Shu* (Bl 17), *Gan Shu* (Bl 18), *Shen Shu* (Bl 23)

Kidney yang vacuity: *Fu Liu* (Ki 7), *San Yin Jiao* (Sp 6), *Shen Shu* (Bl 23), *Ming Men* (GV 4), *Qi Hai Shu* (Bl 24), moxa

Menstrual Movement Suspended Vagina Pain

Cold congelation: *Xue Hai* (Sp 10), *San Yin Jiao* (Sp 6), *Guan Yuan* (CV 4), *Qi Hai* (CV 6), local points, moxa

Damp heat in the liver channel: *Yin Ling Quan* (Sp 9), *Yang Ling Quan* (GB 34), *Zu Lin Qi* (GB 34), *Xing Jian* (Liv 2), *San Yin Jiao* (Sp 6), local points

Blood vacuity, qi binding: *Tai Chong* (Liv 3), *San Yin Jiao* (Sp 6), *Xin Shu* (Bl 15), *Ge Shu* (Bl 17), *Gan Shu* (Bl 18), local points

Menstrual Movement Nosebleed

Heat in both the exterior & interior: *He Gu* (LI 4), *Qu Chi* (LI 11), *Nei Ting* (St 44), *Yin Tang* (M-HN-3), *Xue Hai* (Sp 10), *San Yin Jiao* (Sp 6)

Liver channel depressive heat: *Xing Jian* (Liv 2), *Nei Ting* (St 44), *He Gu* (LI 4), *Qu Chi* (LI 11), *San Yin Jiao* (Sp 6), *Yin Yang* (M-HN-3), *Xue Hai* (Sp 10)

Stomach fire blazing & exuberant: *Nei Ting* (St 44), *Jie Xi* (St 41), *San Yin Jiao* (Sp 6), *He Gu* (LI 4), *Qu Chi* (LI 11), *Yin Tang* (M-HN-3), *Xue Hai* (Sp 10)

Lung-kidney yin vacuity: *Zhao Hai* (Ki 6), *Lie Que* (Lu 7), *San Yin Jiao* (Sp 6), *Xue Hai* (Sp 10), *He Gu* (LI 4), *Qu Chi* (LI 11), *Yin Tang* (M-HN-3)

Menstrual Movement Coughing Blood

Liver fire attacking the lungs: *Xing Jian* (Liv 2), *Yu Ji* (Lu 10), *San Yin Jiao* (Sp 6), *Xue Hai* (Sp 10), *He Gu* (LI 4), *Qu Chi* (LI 11), *Tian Tu* (CV 22)

Menstrual Movement Bloody Stool

Liver-stomach depressive heat: *Xing Jian* (Liv 2), *Nei Ting* (St 44), *He Gu* (LI 4), *Qu Chi* (LI 11), *San Yin Jiao* (Sp 6), *Xue Hai* (Sp 10), *Da Chang Shu* (Bl 25), *Cheng Qiang* (GV 1)

Vacuity heat: *Tai Xi* (Ki 3), *San Yin Jiao* (Sp 6), *Xue Hai* (Sp 10), *Qu Chi* (LI 11), *Shen Shu* (Bl 23), *Da Chang Shu* (Bl 25), *Cheng Qiang* (GV 1)

Menstrual Movement Bloody Urine

Heart fire blazing internally: *Xue Hai* (Sp 10), *Yin Ling Quan* (Sp 9), *San Yin Jiao* (Sp 6), *Shao Fu* (Ht 8), *Zhong Ji* (CV 3), *Xin Shu* (Bl 15), *Pang Guang Shu* (Bl 28), *Ci Liao* (Bl 32)

Liver-kidney yin vacuity: *Tai Xi* (Ki 3), *San Yin Jiao* (Sp 6), *Xue Hai* (Sp 10), *Zhong Ji* (CV 3), *Guan Yuan* (CV 4), *Ge Shu* (Bl 17), *Shen Shu* (Bl 23), *Pang Guang Shu* (Bl 28), *Ci Liao* (Bl 32)

Perimenopausal Syndrome

Liver depression: *Tai Chong* (Liv 3), *San Yin Jiao* (Sp 6), *He Gu* (LI 4), *Nei Guan* (Per 6)

Liver yang ascendant hyperactivity: *Xing Jian* (Liv 2), *Yang Ling Quan* (GB 34), *He Gu* (LI 4), *Qu Chi* (LI 11), *Zu San Li* (St 36), *San Yin Jiao* (Sp 6)

Liver fire harassing above: *Xing Jian* (Liv 2), *Nei Ting* (St 44), *He Gu* (LI 4), *Qu Chi* (LI 11), *Wai Guan* (Th 5)

Liver wind stirring internally: *Tai Chong* (Liv 3), *San Yin Jiao* (Sp 6), *Tai Xi* (Ki 3), *Guan Yuan* (CV 4), *Feng Chi* (GB 20), *Bai Hui* (GV 20)

Liver-kidney yin vacuity: *Tai Xi* (Ki 3), *San Yin Jiao* (Sp 6), *Tai Xi* (Liv 3), *Guan Yuan* (CV 4), *Ge Shu* (Bl 17), *Gan Shu* (Bl 18), *Shen Shu* (Bl 23)

Yin vacuity with vacuity heat: *Tai Xi* (Ki 3), *Yin Gu* (Ki 10), *San Yin Jiao* (Sp 6), *Guan Yuan* (CV 4), *Shen Shu* (Bl 23), *Hou Xi* (SI 3)

Yin vacuity with internal heat: *Tai Xi* (Ki 3), *San Yin Jiao* (Sp 6), *Shen Shu* (Bl 23), *Xing Jian* (Liv 2), *Qu Chi* (LI 11), *Wai Guan* (TB 5), *Da Zhui* (GV 14)

Kidney yang vacuity: *Fu Liu* (Ki 7), *San Yin Jiao* (Sp 6), *Guan Yuan* (CV 4), *Ming Men* (GV 4), *Shen Shu* (Bl 23)

Kidney yin & yang vacuity: *Tai Xi* (Ki 3), *Fu Liu* (Ki 7), *San Yin Jiao* (Sp 6), *Guan Yuan* (CV 4), *Shen Shu* (Bl 23), *Ming Men* (GV 4)

Heart-spleen vacuity: *Zu San Li* (St 36), *San Yin Jiao* (Sp 6), *Shen Men* (Ht 7), *Xin Shu* (Bl 15), *Pi Shu* (Bl 20)

Heart & kidneys not interacting: *Shen Men* (Ht 7), *Tai Xi* (Ki 3), *San Yin Jiao* (Sp 6), *Guan Yuan* (CV 4), *Xin Shu* (Bl 15), *Shen Shu* (Bl 23)

Phlegm obstruction, qi stagnation: *Feng Long* (St 40), *Tai Chong* (Liv 3), *San Yin Jiao* (Sp 6), *Zu San Li* (St 36), *He Gu* (LI 4), *Pi Shu* (Bl 20), *Wei Shu* (Bl 21)

Blood stasis: *Tai Chong* (Liv 3), *San Yin Jiao* (Sp 6), *Xue Hai* (Sp 10), *Zhong Ji* (CV 3), *Gui Lai* (St 29), *Da Chang Shu* (Bl 25)

Blood stasis with vacuity cold, spleen vacuity, and liver blood vacuity: *Tai Chong* (Liv 3), *San Yin Jiao* (Sp 6), *Xue Hai* (Sp 10), *Guan Yuan* (CV 4), *Shen Que* (CV 8), *Shui Dao* (St 28), *Zu San Li* (St 36), *Shen Shu* (Bl 23), *Ming Men* (GV 4)

In clinical practice, the above suggested main points should be combined with appropriate auxilliary points depending upon the signs and symptoms, the discrimination of root and branch, and the treatment of *a shi* points.

Appendix 2:
Ancient Formulas in Powdered Form for Menstrual Diseases

Within Chinese medicine, the medicinal formulas from the late Han and other dynasties in the first half of the first millenium are often referred to as *gu fang* or ancient formulas. The *locus classicus* of many of these is Zhang Zhong-jing's *Shan Han Lun/Jin Gui Yao Lue (Treatise on Cold Damage/Essentials of the Golden Cabinet)*. Others were created by Hua Tuo, Ge Hong, Sun Si-miao, etc. It is this group of formulas that later in Japan came to be known as and is the basic repertoire of *kanpo yaku*, Han or Chinese medicine. Therefore, it is this group of formulas that forms the major part of the Chinese herbal formulas manufactured in Japan and Taiwan[33] as desiccated, powdered extracts. These powdered extracts have become very popular among Western practitioners due to their ease of prescription and administration. Many Western practitioners assume that Western patients would not comply if asked to prepare and drink freshly brewed decoctions. In addition, many Western practitioners may not have easy access to bulk Chinese medicinals.

Therefore, although the use of such dessicated, powdered extracts is not considered the professional standard of care within Chinese TCM gynecology, I have included a list of such commercially available formulas corresponding to the patterns under the major menstrual diseases discussed in the text. When using these, practitioners should be aware that the recommended doses by their manufacturers tend to be quite low by modern Chinese standards. That being said, one can and, in emergency cases most definitely should, raise these doses. Further, when systematically combined with acupuncture and moxibustion and if the patient has been given good advice about diet and lifestyle, this lower potency may not be such an issue. It may simply mean that the patient must undergo treatment for a longer course.

Nevertheless, I strongly advise that, even if one uses such prepared Chinese medicinal, powdered, desiccated extracts, one should prescribe these based not only on the patient's individualized pattern discrimination but also on the phases of her menstrual cycle.

As the reader will see, in a few instances, there is no ready-made formula listed for a particular pattern in any of the catalogs of the companies that manufacture and market these

---

[33] Taiwan was a Japanese possession the entire first half of this century. Taiwanese youth were sent to Japan to study during this colonial period. Therefore, one can find both Chinese medicine as it is practiced in China and *kanpo yaku* practiced in Taiwan. The companies manufacturing powdered extracts in Taiwan have primarily been influenced by *kanpo yaku*.

desiccated extracts. In those cases, I have listed the appropriate individual ingredients. The companies that manufacture and market these desiccated extracts in the West are willing to either make up special formulas or sell desiccated extracts of the individual medicinals. In this latter case, the practitioner can then buy these individual extracts and mix up the formula by themselves. In several other cases, although there is a guiding formula available as a desiccated extract, I believe that it needs some further modification. In those cases, the reader will see that the name of the guiding formula is followed by one or more individual medicinals. Also, the reader should note that some of these formulas have more than one English name. When two names appear in parentheses after a single Pinyin name, the first name is the literal translation of the Chinese name and the second name is the English name commonly used by the manufacturers of these desiccated extracts.

Guiding ready-made formulas for the treatment of menstrual diseases

Menstruation Ahead of Schedule

Blood heat

Replete heat/damp heat: *Wen Qing Yin* (Warming & Clearing Drink, a.k.a. Tang-kuei & Gardenia Combination)

Depressive heat: *Dan Zhi Xiao Yao San* (Moutan & Gardenia Rambling Powder, a.k.a. Bupleurum & Peony Formula)

Vacuity heat: *Zhi Bai Di Huang Wan* (Anemarrhena & Phellodendron Rehmannia Pills, a.k.a. Anemarrhena, Phellodendron & Rehmannia Formula)

Phlegm heat: *Wen Dan Tang* (Warm the Gallbladder Decoction, a.k.a. Bamboo & Hoelen Combination) plus Rhizoma Coptidis Chinensis (*Huang Lian*). This formula is then called *Huang Lian Wen Dan Tang* (Coptis Warm the Gallbladder Decoction).

Qi vacuity

Spleen qi vacuity: *Gui Pi Tang* (Restore the Spleen Decoction, a.k.a. Ginseng & Longan Combination)

Kidney qi vacuity: *Ba Wei Di Huang Wan* (Eight Flavors Rehmannia Pills, a.k.a. Rehmannia Eight Formula). This formula is also simply known as *Shen Qi Wan* (Kidney Qi Pills).

Blood stasis: Only complicates other pattterns. Therefore, one can add Radix Pseudo-ginseng (*San Qi*, a.k.a. *Tian Qi*), Pollen Typhae (*Pu Huang*), and Feces Trogopterori Sei Pteromi (*Wu Ling Zhi*) to other appropriate formulas.

Menstruation Behind Schedule

Blood vacuity

Blood vacuity: *Ba Zhen Tang* (Eight Pearls Decoction, a.k.a. Tang-kuei & Ginseng Eight Combination)

Vacuity cold: *Wen Jing Tang* (Warm the Channels Decoction, a.k.a. Tang-kuei & Evodia Combination)

Stasis & obstruction

Cold congelation: *Dang Gui Si Ni Tang* (Dang Gui Four Counterflows Decoction, a.k.a. Tang-kuei & Jujube Combination)

Qi stagnation: *Xiao Yao San* (Rambling Powder, a.k.a. Bupleurum & Tang-kuei Formula)

Blood stasis: *Gui Zhi Fu Ling Wan* (Cinnamon Twig & Poria Pills, a.k.a. Cinnamon & Hoelen Formula)

Phlegm obstruction: *Er Chen Tang* (Two Aged [Ingredients] Decoction, a.k.a. Citrus & Pinellia Combination) plus Radix Angelicae Sinensis (*Dang Gui*) and Radix Ligustici Wallichii (*Chuan Xiong*). This then becomes *Xiong Gui Er Chen Tang* (Ligusticum & Dang Gui Two Aged [Ingredients] Decoction).

(Sometimes) Early, (Sometimes) Late, No Fixed Schedule Menstruation

Liver depression qi stagnation: *Xiao Yao San* (Rambling Powder, a.k.a. Bupleurum & Tang-kuei Formula)

Spleen vacuity: *Ba Zhen Tang* (Eight Pearls Decoction, a.k.a. Tang-kuei & Ginseng Combination)

Kidney vacuity

Kidney yin vacuity: *Zhi Bai Di Huang Wan* (Anemarrhena & Phellodendron Rehmannia Pills, a.k.a. Anemarrhena, Phellodendron & Rehmannia Formula)

Kidney yang vacuity: *Huan Shao Dan* (Return to Lesser [Years] Elixir, a.k.a. Lycium Formula)

Profuse Menstruation

Blood heat

Replete heat/damp heat: *Wen Qing Yin* (Warming & Clearing Drink, a.k.a. Tang-kuei & Gardenia Combination)

Depressive heat: *Dan Zhi Xiao Yao San* (Moutan & Gardenia Rambling Powder, a.k.a. Bupleurum & Peony Formula)

Vacuity heat: *Zhi Bai Di Huang Wan* (Anemarrhena & Phellodendron Rehmannia Pills, a.k.a. Anemarrhena, Phellodendron & Rehmannia Formula)

Qi vacuity

Spleen qi vacuity: *Gui Pi Tang* (Restore the Spleen Decoction, a.k.a. Ginseng & Longan Combination)

Phlegm dampness: *Liu Jun Zi Tang* (Six Gentlemen Decoction, a.k.a. Six Major Herb Combination) plus Radix Angelicae Sinensis (*Dang Gui*), Radix Albus Paeoniae Lactiflorae (*Bai Shao*), and Rhizoma Arisaematis (*Nan Xing*)

Kidney qi vacuity: *Ba Wei Di Huang Wan* (Eight Flavors Rehmannia Pills, a.k.a. Rehmannia Eight Formula)

Blood stasis: Typically only complicates other patterns. Therefore one can add *Shi Xiao San* (Sudden Smile Powder, a.k.a. Pteropus & Bulrush Formula) to other appropriate formulas. For even stronger effect, also add Radix Pseudoginseng (*San Qi* or *Tian Qi*).

Scanty Menstruation

Blood vacuity

Spleen vacuity: *Ba Zhen Tang* (Eight Pearls Decoction, a.k.a. Tang-kuei & Ginseng Eight Combination)

Kidney yin vacuity: *Liu Wei Di Huang Wan* (Six Flavors Rehmannia Pills, a.k.a. Rehmannia Six Formula) plus Radix Angelicae Sinensis (*Dang Gui*)

Kidney yang vacuity: *Huan Shao Dan* (Return to Lesser [Years] Elixir, a.k.a. Lycium Combination)

Stasis & obstruction

Blood stasis: *Si Wu Tang* (Four Materials Decoction, a.k.a. Four Major Herb Combination) plus Semen Pruni Persicae (*Tao Ren*) and Flos Carthami Tinctorii (*Hong Hua*). This then becomes *Tao Hong Si Wu Tang* (Persica & Carthamus Four Materials Decoction).

Phlegm dampness: *Er Chen Tang* (Two Aged [Ingredients] Decoction, a.k.a. Citrus & Pinellia Combination) plus Radix Angelicae Sinensis (*Dang Gui*) and Radix Ligustici Wallichii (*Chuan Xiong*). This then becomes *Xiong Gui Er Chen Tang* (Ligusticum & Dang Gui Two Aged [Ingredients] Decoction).

Mixed vacuity & repletion

Spleen-kidney vacuity with vacuity cold & stasis: *Wen Jing Tang* (Warm the Channels Decoction, a.k.a. Tang-kuei & Evodia Combination)

Qi stagnation with spleen vacuity & blood vacuity: *Xiao Yao San* (Rambling Powder, a.k.a. Bupleurum & Tang-kuei Formula)

Flooding & Leaking

Blood heat

Replete heat: *Wen Qing Yin* (Warming & Clearing Drink, a.k.a. Tang-kuei & Gardenia Formula)

Depressive heat: *Dan Zhi Xiao Yao San* (Moutan & Gardenia Rambling Powder, a.k.a. Bupleurum & Peony Formula)

Vacuity heat: *Zhi Bai Di Huang Wan* (Anemarrhena & Phellodendron Rehmannia Pills, a.k.a. Anemarrhena, Phellodendron & Rehmannia Formula)

Damp heat: *Dan Zhi Xiao Yao San* (Moutan & Gardenia Rambling Powder, a.k.a. Bupleurum & Peony Formula) plus Fructus Meliae Toosendan (*Chuan Lian Zi*), Radix Scutellariae Baicalensis (*Huang Qin*), Radix Sanguisorbae (*Di Yu*), Cacumen Biotae Orientalis (*Ce Bai Ye*), and Gelatinum Corii Asini (*E Jiao*)

Qi vacuity

Spleen qi vacuity: *Gui Pi Tang* (Restore the Spleen Decoction, a.k.a. Ginseng & Longan Combination)

Kidney qi vacuity: *Ba Wei Di Huang Wan* (Eight Flavors Rehmannia Pills, a.k.a. Rehmannia Eight Formula)

Spleen-kidney vacuity: *Gu Ben Zhi Xue Tang* (Secure the Root & Stop Bleeding Decoction): Cooked Radix Rehmanniae (*Shu Di*), Rhizoma Atractylodis Macrocephalae (*Bai Zhu*), Radix Codonopsitis Pilosulae (*Dang Shen*), Radix Astragali Membranacei (*Huang Qi*), Radix Angelicae Sinensis (*Dang Gui*), blast-fried Rhizoma Zingiberis (*Pao Jiang*)

Stasis & obstruction

Blood stasis: *Si Wu Tang* (Four Materials Decoction, a.k.a. Four Major Herb Combination) plus Semen Pruni Persicae (*Tao Ren*) and Flos Carthami Tinctorii (*Hong Hua*). This then becomes *Tao Hong Si Wu Tang* (Persica & Carthamus Four Materials Decoction). For better blood-stopping effect, add Radix Pseudoginseng (*San Qi* or *Tian Qi*).

Phelgm rheum: *Er Chen Tang* (Two Aged [Ingredients] Decoction, a.k.a. Citrus & Pinelliae Combination) plus Radix Angelicae Sinensis (*Dang Gui*), Radix Albus Paeoniae Lactiflorae (*Bai Shao*), and Fructus Citri Aurantii (*Zhi Ke*)

Blocked Menstruation

Blood vacuity

Qi & blood vacuity: *Ren Shen Yang Rong Tang* (Ginseng Nourish the Constructive Decoction, a.k.a. Ginseng Nutritive Combination)

Liver-kidney vacuity: *Liu Wei Di Huang Wan* (Six Flavors Rehmannia Pills, a.k.a. Rehmannia Six Formula) plus Radix Angelicae Sinensis (*Dang Gui*)

Lung yin & blood vacuity: *Bai He Gu Jin Tang* (Lily Secure Metal Decoction, a.k.a. Lily Combination)

Heart yin & blood vacuity: *Tian Wang Bu Xin Dan* (Heavenly Emperor Supplement the Heart Elixir, a.k.a. Ginseng & Zizyphus Formula)

Kidney vacuity: *Huan Shao Dan* (Return to Lesser [Years] Elixir, a.k.a. Lycium Formula)

Stasis & obstruction

Qi stagnation, blood stasis: *Si Wu Tang* (Four Materials Decoction, a.k.a. Four Major Herb Combination) plus Semen Pruni Persicae (*Tao Ren*) and Flos Carthami Tinctorii (*Hong Hua*). This then becomes *Tao Hong Si Wu Tang* (Persica & Carthamus Four Materials Decoction).

Cold damp congelation & stagnation: *Wen Jing Tang* (Warm the Channels Decoction, a.k.a. Tang-kuei & Evodia Combination)

Phlegm dampness: *Cang Fu Dao Tan Wan* (Atractylodis & Cyperus Abduct Phlegm Pills): Rhizoma Atractylodis (*Cang Zhu*), Rhizoma Cyperi Rotundi (*Xiang Fu*), Pericarpium Citri Reticulatae (*Chen Pi*), Sclerotium Poriae Cocos (*Fu Ling*), Fructus Citri Aurantii (*Zhi Ke*), Rhizoma Pinelliae Ternatae (*Ban Xia*), Rhizoma Arisaematis (*Nan Xing*), mix-fried Radix Glycyrrhizae (*Gan Cao*), uncooked Rhizoma Zingiberis (*Sheng Jiang*). This formula does have *Er Chen Tang* (Two Aged [Ingredients] Decoction, a.k.a. Citrus & Pinellia Combination) at its core.

Painful Menstruation

Stasis & obstruction

Qi stagnation: *Xiao Yao San* (Rambling Powder, a.k.a. Bupleurum & Tang-kuei Formula)

Liver depression-effulgent fire: *Dan Zhi Xiao Yao San* (Moutan & Gardenia Rambling Powder, a.k.a. Bupleurum & Peony Formula)

Blood stasis: *Gui Zhi Fu Ling Wan* (Cinnamon Twig & Poria Pills, a.k.a. Cinnamon & Hoelen Formula)

Cold damp congelation & stagnation: *Wen Jing Tang* (Warm the Channels Decoction, a.k.a. Tang-kuei & Evodia Combination)

Stasis & heat: *Xiao Yao San* (Rambling Powder, a.k.a. Bupleurum & Tang-kuei Formula) plus *Er Miao San* (Two Miracles Powder, *i.e.*, Rhizoma Atractylis [*Cang Zhu*] and Cortex Phellodendri [*Huang Bai*]) plus Rhizoma Cyperi Rotundi (*Xiang Fu*) and Rhizoma Corydalis Yanhusuo (*Yan Hu Suo*)

Vacuity

Qi & blood vacuity: *Ba Zhen Tang* (Eight Pearls Decoction, a.k.a. Tang-kuei & Ginseng Eight Combination) plus Herba Leonuri Heterophylli (*Yi Mu Cao*). This then becomes *Ba Zhen Yi Mu Tang* (Eight Pearls Leonurus Decoction).

Liver-kidney deficiency damage: *Huan Shao Dan* (Return to Lesser [Years] Elixir, a.k.a. Lycium Combination)

Vacuity cold within the uterus: *Wen Jing Tang* (Warm the Channels Decoction, a.k.a. Tang-kuei & Evodia Combination)

Vacuity heat: *Tong Jing Er Hao Fang* (Number 2 Painful Menstruation Formula): Uncooked Radix Rehmanniae (*Sheng Di*), cooked Radix Rehmanniae (*Shu Di*), Rhizoma Stellariae Dichotomae (*Yin Chai Hu*), Rhizoma Corydalis Yanhusuo (*Yan Hu Suo*), Cortex Radicis Moutan (*Dan Pi*), Fructus Meliae Toosendan (*Chuan Lian Zi*), Radix Angelicae Sinensis (*Dang Gui*), Radix Albus Paeoniae Lactiflorae (*Bai Shao*), Sclerotium Poriae Cocos (*Fu Ling*), Radix Glycyrrhizae (*Gan Cao*)

Premenstrual Syndrome

Liver depression qi stagnation: *Xiao Yao San* (Rambling Powder, a.k.a. Bupleurum & Tang-kuei Formula)

Liver depression transforming heat: *Dan Zhi Xiao Yao San* (Moutan & Gardenia Rambling Powder, a.k.a. Bupleurum & Peony Formula)

Liver depression with spleen vacuity and depressive heat in the stomach & lungs: *Xiao Chai Hu Tang* (Minor Bupleurum Decoction, a.k.a. Minor Bupleurum Combination)

Liver yang ascendant hyperactivity: *Chai Hu Jia Long Gu Mu Li Tang* (Bupleurum Plus Dragon Bone & Oyster Shell Decoction, a.k.a. Bupleurum & Dragon Bone Combination)

Liver depression, spleen vacuity with counterflow chilling: *Chai Hu Gui Zhi Tang* (Bupleurum & Cinnamon Twig Decoction, a.k.a. Bupleurum & Cinnamon Combination)

Liver depression, spleen vacuity & kidney yang vacuity: *Bu Zhong Yi Qi Tang* (Supplement the Center & Boost the Qi Decoction, a.k.a. Ginseng & Astragalus Combination) plus Rhizoma Curculiginis Orchiodis (*Xiang Mao*) and Herba Epimedii (*Xian Ling Pi*, a.k.a. *Yin Yang Huo*)

Perimenopausal Syndrome

Liver depression: *Xiao Yao San* (Rambling Powder, a.k.a. Bupleurum & Tang-kuei Formula)

Liver yang ascendant hyperactivity: *Chai Hu Jia Long Gu Mu Li Tang* (Bupleurum Plus Dragon Bone & Oyster Shell Decoction, a.k.a. Bupleurum & Dragon Bone Combination)

Liver fire harassing above: *Dang Gui Liu Huang Tang* (Dang Gui Six Yellows Decoction, a.k.a. Tang-kuei & Six Yellow Combination)

Liver wind stirring internally: *Tian Ma Gou Teng Yin* (Gastrodia & Uncaria Drink): Rhizoma Gastrodiae Elatae (*Tian Ma*), Ramulus Uncariae Cum Uncis (*Gou Teng*), Concha Haliotidis (*Shi Jue Ming*), Ramulus Loranthi Seu Visci (*Sang Ji Sheng*), Cortex Eucommiae Ulmoidis (*Du Zhong*), Radix Cyathulae (*Chuan Niu Xi*), Fructus Gardeniae Jasminoidis (*Shan Zhi Zi*), Radix Scutellariae Baicalensis (*Huang Qin*), Herba Leonuri Heterophylli (*Yi Mu Cao*), Sclerotium Pararadicis Poriae Cocos (*Fu Shen*)

Liver-kidney yin vacuity: *Liu Wei Di Huang Wan* (Six Flavors Rehmannia Pills, a.k.a. Rehmannia Six Formula)

Yin vacuity with vacuity heat: *Zhi Bai Di Huang Wan* (Anemarrhena & Phellodendron Rehmannia Pills, a.k.a. Anemarrhena, Phellodendron & Rehmannia Formula)

Yin vacuity with internal heat: *Wen Qing Yin* (Warming & Clearing Drink, a.k.a. Tang-kuei & Gardenia Formula)

Kidney yang vacuity: *Bai Wei Di Huang Wan* (Eight Flavors Rehmannia Pills, a.k.a. Rehmannia Eight Formula)

Kidney yin & yang vacuity: *Er Xian Tang* (Eight Immortals Decoction): Rhizoma Curculiginis Orchioidis (*Xian Mao*), Herba Epimedii (*Xiang Ling Pi* or *Yin Yang Huo*), Radix Morindae Officinalis (*Ba Ji Tian*), Radix Angelicae Sinensis (*Dang Gui*), Cortex Phellodendri (*Huang Bai*), Rhizoma Anemarrhenae Aspheloidis (*Zhi Mu*)

Heart-spleen vacuity: *Gui Pi Tang* (Restore the Spleen Decoction, a.k.a. Ginseng & Longan Combination)

Heart & kidneys not interacting: *Tian Wang Bu Xin Dan* (Heavenly Emperor Supplement the Heart Elixir, a.k.a. Ginseng & Zizyphus Formula)

Phlegm obstruction, qi stagnation: *Wen Dan Tang* (Warm the Gallbladder Decoction, a.k.a. Bamboo & Hoelen Combination). If there is also heat, add Rhizoma Coptidis Chinensis (*Huang Lian*). This then becomes *Huang Lian Wen Dan Tang* (Coptis Warm the Gallbladder Decoction).

Blood stasis: *Gui Zhi Fu Ling Wan* (Cinnamon Twig & Poria Pills, a.k.a. Cinnamon & Hoelen Formula)

Blood stasis with vacuity cold, spleen vacuity, and liver blood vacuity: *Wen Jing Tang* (Warm the Channels Decoction, a.k.a. Tang-kuei & Evodia Combination)

Appendix 3:
Abnormalities in the Color & Consistency of the Menstrual Water

The following discussion of the disease causes and mechanisms, treatment principles, and treatment protocols is from Zhang Jian-xiu's *Zhong Yi Zhi Liao Fu Nu Bing (The Chinese Medical Treatment of Gynecological Diseases)*. Other than discussions of various colored menstruates under the four examinations, it is the only discussion I have seen in the contemporary Chinese gynecological textbook literature specifically on the treatment of abnormalities of the color and consistency of the menstruate. Frankly, in my 16 years of practice specializing in gynecology, I have never come across most of these abnormalities.

Purple-colored menses

The menses come and are colored purple. If the menses come on time and are colored purple, this is due to wind. If the menses come and are colored black, this is mostly due to heat.

Disease causes: Menses which are colored purple are due to heat in the blood.

Main symptoms: The menses typically present with a purple color and are accompanied by abdominal pain and other such symptoms.

Treatment principles: One should clear heat unless there is wind chill, in which case use warm, hot formulas.

Guiding formula: Use *Si Wu Tang* (Four Materials Decoction) plus *Xiang Fu Huang Lian Tang* (Cyperus & Coptis Decoction): Extremitas Radicis Angelicae Sinensis (*Dang Gui Wei*), 12g, Radix Ligustici Wallichii (*Chuan Xiong*), 9g, Radix Rubrus Paeoniae Lactiflorae (*Chi Shao*), 9g, processed Rhizoma Cyperi Rotundi (*Xiang Fu*), 9g, uncooked Radix Rehmanniae (*Sheng Di*), 18g, Rhizoma Coptidis Chinensis (*Huang Lian*), 6g, Radix Glycyrrhizae (*Gan Cao*), Cortex Radicis Moutan (*Dan Pi*), 9g @. Decoct in water and take.

Pale-colored menses

When the menses come, they are pale red in color. This is called pale-colored menstruation. It is due to blood vacuity and excessive phlegm.

Disease causes: If the menses come and they are pale in color, this is due to blood vacuity.

Main symptoms: The menses are pale red in color and accompanied by dizziness, heart palpitations, lumbar and knee soreness and weakness, and lack of warmth in the hands and feet.

Treatment principles: Supplement both the qi and blood

Guiding formulas:

1. Radix Codonopsitis Pilosulae (*Dang Shen*), 15g, earth stir-fried Rhizoma Atractylodis Macrocephalae (*Bai Zhu*), 9g, Sclerotium Poriae Cocos (*Fu Ling*), 9g, mix-fried Radix Glycyrrhizae (*Gan Cao*), 9g, cooked Radix Rehmanniae (*Shu Di*), 15g, Radix Angelicae Sinensis (*Dang Gui*), 12g, Radix Ligustici Wallichii (*Chuan Xiong*), 9g, wine stir-fried Radix Albus Paeoniae Lactiflorae (*Bai Shao*), 9g, mix-fried Radix Astragali Membranacei (*Huang Qi*), 12g, processed Rhizoma Cyperi Rotundi (*Xiang Fu*), 9g, uncooked Rhizoma Zingiberis (*Sheng Jiang*), 3 slices, Fructus Zizyphi Jujubae (*Hong Zao*), 2 pieces. Decoct in water and administer.

2. Cooked Radix Rehmanniae (*Shu Di*), 240g, stir-fried Radix Dioscoreae Oppositae (*Shan Yao*), Fructus Corni Officinalis (*Shan Zhu Yu*), 120g @, Cortex Radicis Moutan (*Dan Pi*), Sclerotium Poriae Cocos (*Bai Fu Ling*), 90g @, earth stir-fried Rhizoma Alismatis (*Ze Xie*), processed Rhizoma Cyperi Rotundi (*Xiang Fu*), 60g @. Grind into a fine powder and make into pills with honey the size of Chinese parasol tree seeds. Take 9g each time on an empty stomach washed down with warm or hot water. Regular administration gets good results. If one cannot obtain these pills, one can use *Liu Wei Di Huang Wan* (Six Flavors Rehmannia Pills) plus processed Rhizoma Cyperi Rotundi (*Xiang Fu*), 15g, decocted in water and taken with the *Liu Wei Di Huang Wan*.

Menses like green water

The menses come like green water. There is entirely no red color.

Disease causes: If the menses come just like copper green water, this is due either to a great disease or enduring disease resulting in great vacuity or great cold.

Main symptoms: The menses come just like copper green water accompanied by muscular emaciation, vertigo and dizziness, a sallow yellow facial complexion, and lack of strength in the four limbs.

Treatment principles: Warm the menses and supplement the blood. Do not use cooling medicinals.

Guiding formula: Black-boned chicken meat (*Wu Ji Rou*; remove the skin and cook in wine), 90g, stir-fried Radix Dioscoreae Oppositae (*Shan Yao*), Cortex Cinnamomi Cassiae (*Rou Gui*), wine-washed Herba Cistanchis Deserticolae (*Rou Cong Rong*), stir-fried Pollen Typhae (*Pu Huang*), Radix Angelicae Sinensis (*Dang Gui*), Fructus Corni Officinalis (*Shan Zhu Yu*), Radix Albus Paeoniae Lactiflorae (*Bai Shao*), 30g @, cooked Radix Rehmanniae (*Shu Di*), 45g, large Radix Lateralis Praeparatus Aconiti Carmichaeli (*Da Fu Zi*), 9g, Cornu Parvum Cervi (*Lu Rong*), 3g, Radix Ligustici Wallichii (*Chuan Xiong*), 15g. Grind into fine powder and make into pills with polished rice paste the size of Chinese parasol tree seeds. Take 8g each time on an empty stomach washed down with wine.

Menses like yellow water

When the menses come, they are like yellow muddy water.

Disease causes: This is mostly due to great vacuity conditions.

Main symptoms: The menstruation is yellow colored like muddy water.

Treatment principles: Greatly warm the menses and blood. Do not use cool medicinals.

Guiding formula: Use *Jia Wei Si Wu Tang* (Added Flavors Four Materials Decoction): Radix Ligustici Wallichii (*Chuan Xiong*), 9g, Radix Angelicae Sinensis (*Dang Gui*), 12g, cooked Radix Rehmanniae (*Shu Di*), 12g, Radix Albus Paeoniae Lactiflorae (*Bai Shao*), 12g, Radix Linderae Strychnifoliae (*Wu Yao*), 6g, uncooked Rhizoma Zingiberis (*Sheng Jiang*), 3 slices, Fructus Zizyphi Jujubae (*Hong Zao*), 2 pieces. Decoct in water and take on an empty stomach.

Menses like house leaking water

When the menses come, their form is like house leaking water.

Disease causes: This is due to blood vacuity and heat.

Main symptoms: Dizziness, vertigo, lower abdominal pain, nausea, vomiting, bad breath smelling like fish

Treatment principles: Regulate the menses and supplement the blood

Guiding formulas:

1. Use *Li Jing Si Wu Tang* (Rectify the Menses Four Materials Decoction): Radix Angelicae Sinensis (*Dang Gui*), 12g, Radix Ligustici Wallichii (*Chuan Xiong*), wine stir-fried Radix Albus Paeoniae Lactiflorae (*Bai Shao*), uncooked Radix Rehmanniae (*Sheng Di*), 9g @,

honey mix-fried Rhizoma Atractylodis Macrocephalae (*Bai Zhu*), Radix Bupleuri (*Chai Hu*), processed Rhizoma Cyperi Rotundi (*Xiang Fu*), Rhizoma Corydalis Yanhusuo (*Yan Hu Suo*), 9g @, wine stir-fried Radix Scutellariae Baicalensis (*Huang Qin*), 9g, Rhizoma Sparganii (*San Leng*), 1.5g. Decoct in water.

2. Radix Dipsaci (*Xu Duan*), stir-fried Pollen Typhae (*Pu Huang*), stir-fried Gelatinum Corii Asini (*E Jiao*), Herba Cistanchis Deserticolae (*Rou Cong Rong*), ginger juice stir-fried Cortex Magnoliae Officinalis (*Hou Po*), Fructus Corni Officinalis (*Shan Zhu Yu*), Sclerotium Poriae Cocos (*Bai Fu Ling*), processed Rhizoma Cyperi Rotundi (*Xiang Fu*), Radix Angelicae Sinensis (*Dang Gui*), Radix Agnelicae Dahuricae (*Bai Zhi*), 60g @, Radix Ligustici Wallichii (*Chuan Xiong*), Radix Albus Paeoniae Lactiflorae (*Bai Shao*), 42g @, mix-fried Radix Glycyrrhizae (*Gan Cao*), dry Rhizoma Zingiberis (*Gan Jiang*), 30g @, cooked Radix Rehmanniae (*Shu Di*), 90g. Grind into fine powder and make into pills with honey the size of Chinese parasol tree seeds. Take 8g each time on an empty stomach washed down with hot water.

Menses like liver water

The menses are just like the water used for washing pig liver.

Disease causes: This is due to dual qi and blood vacuity.

Main symptoms: Vexatious heat in the heart, lumbar and abdominal aching and pain, a yellow face and emaciated muscles, no thought for food or drink

Treatment principles: Recede vexatious heat, regulate the qi and blood

Guiding formulas:

1. Radix Scutellariae Baicalensis (*Huang Qin*), 9g, Radix Angelicae Sinensis (*Dang Gui*), 15g, Radix Ligustici Wallichii (*Chuan Xiong*), 9g, wine stir-fried Radix Trichosanthis Kirlowii (*Tian Hua Fen*), Rhizoma Anemarrhenae Aspheloidis (*Zhi Mu*), Rhizoma Atractylodis (*Cang Zhu*), earth stir-fried Rhizoma Atractylodis Macrocephalae (*Bai Zhu*), wine stir-fried Radix Albus Paeoniae Lactiflorae (*Bai Shao*), 9g @. Decoct in water and administer.

2. Uncooked Radix Rehmanniae (*Sheng Di*), cooked Radix Rehmanniae (*Shu Di*), Radix Angelicae Sinensis (*Dang Gui*), Radix Albus Paeoniae Lactiflorae (*Bai Shao*), 90g @, Rhizoma Sparganii (*San Leng*), Rhizoma Curcumae Zedoariae (*E Zhu*), 15g, Rhizoma Corydalis Yanhusuo (*Xuan Hu Suo*), Sclerotium Poriae Cocos (*Bai Fu Ling*), 60g @, Radix Ligustici Wallichii (*Chuan Xiong*), Fructus Amomi (*Sha Ren*), Radix Linderae Strychni-

foliae (*Wu Yao*), 45g @, processed Rhizoma Cyperi Rotundi (*Xiang Fu*), 75g, Fructus Illicii Anisati (*Da Hui*), 60g. Grind into fine powder and make into pills with polished rice paste the size of Chinese parasol tree seeds. Take 9g each time washed down with aged wine.

3. If the menses contain clots the color of scallion bulbs (*Cong Bai*) and the blood is black in color like dead pig blood and if there is dizziness, dimming of vision, and numbness of the lips, this is a vacuity condition. In that case, use *Bu Nei Dang Gui Wan* (Supplement Internally Dang Gui Pills): Radix Angelicae Sinensis (*Dang Gui*), Radix Dipsaci (*Xu Duan*), Radix Angelicae Dahuricae (*Bai Zhi*), Cortex Magnoliae Officinalis (*Hou Po*), Sclerotium Poriae Cocos (*Fu Ling*), Herba Cistanchis Desrticolae (*Rou Cong Rong*), stir-fried till yellow-black Pollen Typhae (*Pu Huang*), Fructus Corni Officinalis (*Yu Rou*), 60g @, Radix Ligustici Wallichii (*Chuan Xiong*), 48g, cooked Radix Rehmanniae (*Shu Di*), 90g, Radix Glycyrrhizae (*Gan Cao*), dry Rhizoma Zingiberis (*Gan Jiang*), 30g, Radix Lateralis Praeparatus Aconiti Carmichaeli (*Fu Zi*), 12g. Grind into powder and make into pills with honey. Take 9g on an empty stomach washed down with warm wine. Simultaneously take *Bu Zhong Yi Qi Wan* (Supplement the Center & Boost the Qi Pills), 10g each time, 1 time per day.

Menses like rotten meat

When the menses come, they smell like putrefying meat in the summer.

Disease causes: There is blood vacuity with a debilitated body. Therefore, blood is scanty and new blood is not being engendered. Hence the menses are just like water in irrigation ditches when there has been a dry spell with no rain. After many days, it begins to smell foul.

Main symptoms: The menses smell like rotten meat which is difficult to smell.

Treatment principles: Open stasis and supplement the blood

Guiding formulas:

1. Calcined Os Draconis (*Long Gu*), Os Sepiae Seu Sepiellae (*Hai Piao Xiao*), uncooked Radix Rehmanniae (*Sheng Di*), 60g @, wine stir-fried Radix Albus Paeoniae Lactiflorae (*Bai Shao*), Radix Angelicae Sinensis (*Dang Gui*), 60g @, calcined Concha Ostreae (*Mu Li*), Radix Ligustici Wallichii (*Chuan Xiong*), wine stir-fried Radix Scutellariae Baicalensis (*Huang Qin*), Sclerotium Poriae Cocos (*Fu Ling*), 48g @. Grind into fine powder and make into pills with honey the size of Chinese parasol tree seeds. Take 9g on an empty stomach washed down with aged wine.

2. Radix Angelicae Sinensis (*Dang Gui*), 15g, Radix Rubrus Paeoniae Lactiflorae (*Chi Shao*), 9g, Rhizoma Sparganii (*San Leng*), Rhizoma Curcumae Zedoariae (*E Zhu*), 3g @, Cortex Radicis Moutan (*Dan Pi*), earth stir-fried Rhizoma Atractylodis Macrocephalae (*Bai Zhu*), processed Rhizoma Cyperi Rotundi (*Xiang Fu*), Sclerotium Polypori Umbellati (*Zhu Ling*), Pericarpium Citri Reticulatae (*Chen Pi*), Caulis Akebiae Mutong (*Mu Tong*), 9g @, uncooked Rhizoma Zingiberis (*Sheng Jiang*), 2 slices. Decoct in water and administer.

Menses like fish brains

When the menses come, they are like fish brain marrow.

Disease causes: This is due to lower origin vacuity chill with simultaneous wind evils.

Main symptoms: Both feet are aching and painful and are not able to move about.

Treatment principles: Mainly move the qi and blood

Guiding formula: Rhizoma Gastrodiae Elatae (*Tian Ma*), 12g, Bombyx Batryticatus (*Jiang Can*), 3g, Cortex Tripterygii Hypoglauci (*Zi Jin Pi*), 1g, Radix Linderae Strychnifoliae (*Wu Yao*), Radix Achyranthis Bidentatae (*Niu Xi*), Radix Angelicae Pubescentis (*Du Huo*), Radix Ligustici Wallichii (*Chuan Xiong*), 9g @, Radix Angelicae Sinensis (*Dang Gui*), 10g, Resina Olibani (*Ru Xiang*), Caulis Photiniae Serrulatae (*Shi Nan Teng*), Fructus Psoraleae Corylifoliae (*Bu Gu Zhi*), 3g @, uncooked Rhizoma Zingiberis (*Sheng Jiang*), 3 slices, Bulbus Allii Fistulosi (*Cong Bai*), 4 stalks. Decoct in water and alcohol and take on an empty stomach.

Menses like cow membrane

The menses come but do not stop. They precipitate a substance like pieces of cow membrane.

Disease causes: This is due to qi and blood binding and gathering.

Main symptoms: Loss of consciousness and falling down. Although this condition is frightening, it is not very harmful.

Treatment principles: Regulate the qi and scatter the blood

Guiding formula: Water-ground Cinnabar (*Zhu Sha*), Realgar (*Xiong Huang*), 6g @, Sclerotium Poriae Cocos (*Bai Fu Ling*), 120g. Grind into fine powder and make into pills with water the size of mung beans. Take 3g each time, 1 time per day, washed down with soup made from uncooked Rhizoma Zingiberis (*Sheng Jiang*).

Menses precipitate a meaty sack

The menses precipitate a bloody sack as large as a chicken egg. When it is cut open, inside it is like a pomegranate.

Disease causes: This is due to qi and blood deficiency and vacuity.

Main symptoms: The menses come and do not stop. Simultaneously a meaty sack is precipitated. There is also loss of consciousness, no arousal.

Treatment principles: Mostly administer supplementing formulas.

Guiding formula: Radix Codonopsitis Pilosulae (*Dang Shen*), 24g, earth stir-fried Rhizoma Atractylodis Macrocephalae (*Bai Zhu*), Sclerotium Poriae Cocos (*Fu Ling*), Radix Glycyrrhizae (*Gan Cao*), 9g @, cooked Radix Rehmanniae (*Shu Di*), Radix Angelicae Sinensis (*Dang Gui*), 15g @, Radix Ligustici Wallichii (*Chuan Xiong*), wine stir-fried Radix Albus Paeoniae Lactiflorae (*Bai Shao*), mix-fried Radix Astragali Membranacei (*Huang Qi*), 12g @, Cortex Cinnamomi Cassiae (*Rou Gui*), 3g, uncooked Rhizoma Zingiberis (*Sheng Jiang*), 3 slices, Fructus Zizyphi Jujubae (*Hong Zao*), 2 pieces. Decoct in water and administer warm.

Menses precipitate a white worm

When the menses come, within the blood there is a white worm, not several. In form it is like a chicken intestine.

Disease causes: This is due to lack of cleanliness within the vaginal meatus.

Main symptoms: Abdominal pain with the menstrual movement, a white worm within the precipitated blood, abdominal pain which is difficult to bear

Treatment principles: First treat by killing parasites. Once these have been discharged with the stools, then give warm supplementing medicinals.

Guiding formulas:

1. Radix Et Rhizoma Rhei (*Da Huang*), 10g, Semen Arecae Catechu (*Bing Lang*), 15g, Herba Cephalanoploris Segeti (*Da Ji*), 4g, Flos Daphnis Genkwae (*Yuan Hua*), 1.5g, Secretio Moschi Moschiferi (*She Xiang*), 0.1g. Grind into powder and make into pills with flour paste the size of Arillus Euphoriae Longanae kernels (*Long Yan Ke*). Take 1 pill each time washed down with warm wine. This formula kills parasites.

2. Radix Albus Paeoniae Lactiflorae (*Bai Shao*), 60g, honey mix-fried Radix Astragali Membranacei (*Huang Qi*), 60g, Cortex Cinnamomi Cassiae (*Rou Gui*), honey mix-fried Radix Glycyrrhizae (*Gan Cao*), 15g @. Grind into powder and take mixed in with rice drink soup, 9g each time, 1 time per day. This formula regulates and supplements the qi and blood.

Appendix 4: Li Dong-yuan's Gynecology

Because I find Li Dong-yuan's theories on yin fire so important in my clinical practice, I have included his section on regulating the menses from the *Lan Shi Mi Cang (The Secret Treasury of the Orchid Chamber)*. This translation is by Charles Chace.

Three types of blocked menstruation & failure of movement

"The Treatise on the Discrimination of Yin & Yang *(Yin Yang Bie Lun)*"[34] notes:

> Diseases of the second yang develop within the heart and spleen in such a manner that one cannot comprehend their hidden message, and a woman does not menstruate. It is said that [when this condition manifests in the context of] wind wasting thirst and inverted cup syndrome, it is fatal and cannot be treated.

When women experience a long-standing spleen-stomach vacuity or their bodies are emaciated such that the qi and blood are both debilitated, this results in expiry of the menstrual water which fails to move. [Another possibility is that] the disease may be one of wasting stomach heat where the patient likes food but, nonetheless, becomes emaciated and fluids and humors are not engendered. The menses are the product of the transformation of fluids and humors within the blood vessels and, if fluids and humors expire, heat then scorches the muscles and flesh, causing them to waste away and become emaciated. When we see [this condition with] thirsting and agitation, the sea of blood has become desiccated and this is [therefore] called blood desiccation menstrual expiry. [Thus] it is appropriate to clear dry heat from the stomach while supplementing and boosting the qi and blood. In this way, the menses move on their own. This pattern may be present in those cases where conception occurs during the course of menstruation or where fetal stirring disquietude causes illness during pregnancy.

[Another possible cause is that] the pericardium vessel may be surging and rapid and agitation may be apparent, accompanied by rough stool constipation[35], urination which is clear and inhibited, menstrual block expiry and failure to move. All this is a condition of desiccation of the sea of blood. It is appropriate to regulate the blood vessels and eliminate heat evils from within the *bao luo* and the menses will move on their own.

The *Nei Jing (Inner Classic)* notes:

---

[34] "The Treatise on the Differentiation of Yin and Yang" is a chapter seven of the *Simple Questions (Su Wen)*.

[35] This term suggests constipation and difficult evacuation resulting from fluid dryness.

When the small intestine transmits heat to the large intestine, this produces a deep-lying conglomeration causing [the menses] to disappear.[36] Since the vessels are astringed and inhibited, the menses are deeply stagnant and inhibited. Thus it is said that worrisome conglomerations produce a deeply [stagnant menstrual flow].

[Another possibility is that] the menses fail to arrive as a result of heart taxation and an ascending movement of heart fire. When one quiets the heart and drains fire, the menses flow of their own accord. The *Nei Jing (Inner Classic)* states:

> When the menses do not arrive, [this means that] the *bao mai* is blocked. The *bao mai* homes to the heart and diffusely connects [37] to the uterus. When the qi ascends to distress the lungs, the heart qi does not descend freely, and so the menses do not arrive.

Two types of incessant menstrual leaking[38]

"The Treatise on the Discrimination of Yin & Yang" says that when a vacuity of yin and yang strikes, this is called flooding. When women suffer from vacuity detriment of the spleen and stomach, the life gate pulse[39] becomes deep, fine, and rapid. On the other hand, it may be deep, bowstring, surging, large, and forceful. The inch and bar pulses may also have these [qualities]. All of these [pulse qualities] are due to a depletion of the spleen and stomach [which allows the qi to] sink down into the kidneys and combine with ministerial fire, thus producing a descending distress of damp heat which results in incessant menstrual leaking. Its color will be purple black which is like meat rotting during the summer months. If this is mixed with a white discharge, the pulse will be bowstring and fine. [This is indicative of] cold in the middle. If it is mixed with a red discharge, heat is evident provided there is a surging and rapid pulse. [This indicates] brilliant heat.[40] There will also be lumbar pain or subumbilical pain. When the menses are about to move, one will first see alternating

---

[36] *Chen,* literally means deep. In this context the implication is both that the menses go deep, *i.e.,* they disappear, and as the explanation the next sentence suggests, that the menses disappear because they are *chen zhi,* deeply stagnant.

[36] Wiseman renders *luo,* as connects or net. He describes the action of this word when used as a verb as diffusely connecting. I prefer his English description over his terminology.

[38] The original title was "Three Types of Incessant Menstrual Dribbling," although Li Dong-yuan actually mentions only two types in his discussion.

[39] The life gate pulse simply refers to the third or cubit position of the *cun kou* pulse on the radial aspect of either wrist.

[40] *I.e.,* intense heat

cold and heat and a sense of urgent contraction in the rib-side region. If there is a concurrent spleen-stomach pattern, the four limbs will feel hot, there will be heart vexation which prohibits lying down to sleep, and there will be a sense of subcardiac tension. [In this case,] it is appropriate to greatly supplement the spleen and stomach and to raise the blood and qi. With the administration of only one dose, the patient will be cured.

Another possible cause is that] a person of nobility may lose her status, being reduced to staying at home and not meeting friends, or she may have once been wealthy and then become impoverished. This disease is referred to as desertion of productivity. [It is the result of] an insufficiency of heart qi and fire blazing strongly to produce an effulgence within the blood vessels. Also, as a result of an irregularity of drink and food within the spleen and stomach, fire may overwhelm the middle. If the disposition of the form and flesh appears as if there is no disease, then the condition is a heart disease. Since one cannot diagnose through the form, if the drink and food within the spleen and stomach are unregulated, then the pattern will be evident.

In these cases the menstrual water descends [too] often. It suddenly arrives and suddenly terminates, or it may violently descend and [then] not cease. In treatment, one should first utter words of death and woe to urge her on, to make her fear death, and to urge her not to stir her heart [with things that are long past and cannot be changed]. One may then administer medicinals to greatly supplement the qi and blood and to raise and nourish the spleen and stomach. In addition, one should administer small amounts of medicinals to settle and downbear heart fire. Treat the heart by supplementing yin and draining yang and the menses will be arrested on their own.

Formulas

Sheng Yang Chu Shi Tang (Upbear Yang & Eliminate Dampness Decoction)

This formula is also called *Tiao Jing Sheng Yang Chu Shi Tang* (Regulate the Menses, Upbear Yang & Eliminate Dampness Decoction). It treats leaking of malign blood in women, menstrual irregularity, sudden incessant flooding [of menstrual blood], and copious discharge of viscous fluids. All of these conditions are due to unregulated intake of drink and food, taxation damaging the body, or simple heart qi insufficiency. This is because [unregulated intake of] drink and food or taxation and fatigue may cause heart fire to overwhelm the spleen. Thus the patient must suffer from lassitude and a desire to lie down, loss of the use of their limbs, and a lack of [physical] strength. When the qi does not stir, there is shortness of breath and ascension of qi, urgent counterflow and ascending surging. The pulse is relaxed and, when pressed, is surging and large. Yet is still present upon deeper palpation. [In this case,] spleen earth has contracted an evil. The spleen governs the nourishment of the entire body. The heart governs the blood, and the blood governs the vessels. Thus, when these two [the spleen and heart] contract a pathogen, the disease will always occur within the vessels as well. The vessels are the storehouse of the blood. The vessels are also a person's spirit. If the heart is unable to govern, then the *bao luo* substitute for it. Therefore, it is said that the government of the heart vessels pertains to the heart ligation. The heart ligation is the vessel of the *bao luo* and life gate and governs menstrual affairs. If there is a spleen-stomach vacuity and the pericardium overwhelms them, this results in an unregulated downward leaking of menstrual water. The condition of the spleen and stomach is the root and base[41] of the qi and blood and of yin and yang. One should, therefore, eliminate dampness, rid heat, and boost wind qi so that it extends upward and overcomes dampness. [The *Nei Jing*] also states that the [same condition] may develop when fire becomes depressed.

[This prescription contains] Radix Angelicae Sinensis (*Dang Gui*) which has been soaked in wine, and Radix Angelicae Pubescentis (*Du Huo*), 5 *fen* each, Fructus Viticis (*Man Jing Zi*), 7 *fen*, Radix Ledebouriellae Divaricatae (*Fang Feng*), Rhizoma Cimicifugae (*Sheng Ma*), and mix-fried Radix Glycyrrhizae (*Gan Cao*), Radix Et Rhizoma Ligustici Chinensis (*Gao Ben*), 1 *qian* each, Radix Bupleuri (*Chai Hu*), Radix Et Rhizoma Notopterygii (*Qiang Huo*), Rhizoma Atractylodis (*Cang Zhu*), and Radix Astragali Membranacei (*Huang Qi*), 1 *qian*, 5 *fen* each. Slice these into the size of sesame [seeds and mung] beans but do not powder the prescription. Administer this in a single dose using five large cups of pure, newly drawn water which are then cooked down to one large cup. Remove the dregs, administer hot on an empty stomach, and then wait a half hour before eating. One dose will produce a cure.

One may also moxa both *Xue Hai* (Sp 10) acupoints on the foot *tai yin* spleen channel seven times. [The above] medicinals use wind to overcome dampness, induce the stomach qi to sink, and induce the distressed qi to descend. This salvages the violent flooding of blood. Once one disposes of the malign blood condition[42], one may then use [medicinals such as] Radix Astragali Membranacei (*Huang Qi*), Radix Panacis Ginseng (*Ren Shen*), mix-fried Radix Glycyrrhizae (*Gan Cao*), and Radix Angelicae Sinensis (*Dang Gui*) to supplement [the qi and blood] with *Bu Qi Sheng Yang Tang* (Supplement the Qi & Upbear Yang Decoction).[43] To this, one may also add blood[-supplementing] medicinals. If the menstrual

---

[41] The allusion here is to the base of a piece of fruit.

[42] Malign blood is a synonym for static blood.

[43] There is no such formula. It is likely that Li Dong-yuan is referring to his *Yi Wei Sheng Yang Tang* (Boosting the Stomach & Upbearing Yang Decocton).

blood continues to contain malign substances and does not cease, it is still appropriate to investigate the root source. To treat the root of the menstrual [disorder], one need only boost the spleen and stomach and abate hyperactivity of heart fire as a means of treating the root. If, during the summer months, a white vaginal discharge and incessant leaking desertion[44] develops, then it is appropriate to use this decoction [*Bu Qi Sheng Yang Tang* or an analog. The vaginal discharge and the leaking] will be arrested with only one administration.

Liang Xue Di Huang Tang (Cool the Blood Rehmannia Decoction)

[This prescription] treats gynecological flooding of blood due to kidney water yin vacuity which is unable to settle and protect[45] ministerial fire in the *bao luo* which, in turn, results in blood traveling and flooding. [It contains] Radix Scutellariae Baicalensis (*Huang Qin*) and Herba Schizonepetae Tenufoliae (*Jing Jie*), 1 *fen* each, Cortex Phellodendri (*Huang Bai*), Rhizoma Anemarrhenae Asphodeloidis (*Zhi Mu*), Herba Cum Radice Asari (*Xi Xin*), and Radix Ligustici Wallichii (*Chuan Xiong*), 2 *fen* each, Rhizoma Coptidis Chinensis (*Huang Lian*), Radix Et Rhizoma Notopterygii (*Qiang Huo*), Radix Bupleuri (*Chai Hu*), Rhizoma Cimicifugae (*Sheng Ma*), and Radix Ledebouriellae Divaricatae (*Fang Feng*), 3 *fen* each, uncooked Radix Rehmanniae (*Sheng Di*), and Radix Angelicae Sinensis (*Dang Gui*), 5 *fen* each, Radix Glycyrrhizae (*Gan Cao*) 1 *qian*, and a small amount of Flos Carthami Tinctorii (*Hong Hua*). Grind up the formula and take it in a single dose in three cups [of water] cooked down to one cup. Remove the dregs and take it slightly warm on an empty stomach.

The two *Xue Hai* (Sp 10) points on the foot *tai yin* spleen channel lie above the inner angle of the kneecap, two *cun* within the border of the white flesh. [Sea of Blood] treats downward leaking of malign blood in women, irregularity of the menstrual affairs, counterflow of qi causing abdominal distention, all with a relaxed pulse. Moxa [this point] three times.

The two *Yin Gu* (Ki 10) points on the foot *shao yin* kidney channel are located on the inside of the knee behind the supporting bones, below the large sinew and above the small sinew. [To locate it,] press with the corresponding hand and stretch the knee. [Yin Valley] treats piercing [pain] in the knee[46], inability to stretch and flex [the knee], tongue loose and drooling, vexation counterflow and difficult urination, lower abdominal tension, drawing

---

[44] Low level uterine bleeding

[45] The image here is of a general controlling his troops.

[46] According to the commentary accompanying the text, this piercing pain is due to damp heat pouring down as opposed to blood stasis.

yin [genital] pain, and thigh and inner calf pain. [It also treats] incessant leaking of blood in women, abdominal distention and fullness, inability to breathe, yellow urination, and *ku*.[47] In women who are pregnant, it may be moxed three times.

Jiu Zhu Dang Gui Wan (Wine-cooked Dang Gui Pills)

[This prescription] treats *tui shan*, downward pouring of white vaginal discharge, leg qi, and a sensation in the lumbar region as if it were in an icy rain. In an effort to dry it out, [the patient] wears very thick clothing and covers their head. Yet the cold chill is still unbearable because [this is a condition of] utmost yin cold. The face is white like dried fish. The muscles and flesh feel as if they have been flayed with a knife and become quickly emaciated. There is uncontrolled urination, copious flow of white vaginal discharge that cannot be secured, unconsciousness, a white facial complexion, and greenish blue eyes like the color of vegetables. The vision is blurred and one cannot see. The body is heavy like a mountain, movement and walking is deviated, yet one cannot remain quiet. The legs and knees become withered and fine, and defecation is difficult. The mouth is unable to speak, and one is extremely listless. Food will not descend, there is glomus below the heart, heart vexation, and a burning sensation in the region of the heart which is unbearable. The facial complexion is dirty. The upper back is cold, and there is urinary incontinence which the patient is unaware of. These [symptoms lie in the] upper, middle, and lower three yang. The genuine qi is entirely vacuous and on the verge of exhaustion. There is vomiting and retching because the stomach is extremely vacuous. The pulse is deep and inverted, tense and choppy, yet it is empty and vacuous upon [deeper] palpation. If the pulse is surging, large, and choppy, it will lack strength upon [deeper] palpation. If this is a pattern of cold within, how is it that [the pulse] will be empty and vacuous upon palpation? If the pulse does respond upon palpation, this is yin cold and a condition due to an extreme vacuity of qi and blood.

[This formula contains] Fructus Foeniculi Vulgaris (*Hui Xiang*), 5 *qian*, blackened Radix Lateralis Praeparatus Aconiti Charmichaeli (*Hei Fu Zi*), Rhizoma Alpiniae Officinari (*Liang Jiang*), and Radix Angelicae Sinensis (*Dang Gui*), 1 *liang* each of the above. Take these four ingredients and slice them to the size of sesame [seeds and mung beans] and then cook them together in one and half cups of good wine. Next, draw off the wine and let them dry. Then take mix-fried Radix Glycyrrhizae (*Gan Cao*), Cortex Radicis Meliae Azerdachis (*Ku Lian Zi*), Flos Caryophyllae (*Ding Xiang*), and Rhizoma Cimicifugae (*Sheng Ma*), 1 *qian* each, Radix Bupleuri (*Chai Hu*), two *qian*, stir-fried yellow salt (*Huang Yan*), Buthus Martensis (*Chuan Xie*), 3 *qian* each, and Rhizoma Corydalis Yanhusuo (*Yan Hu Suo*), 4 *qian*. Mix these ingredients with the previous four ingredients and powder them finely.

---

[47] The meaning of *ku* in this context is unclear.

Cook this [powder] with wine down to a paste and form into pills the size of large parasol tree seeds. Take 50-70 pills each time on an empty stomach. Do not consume any oily, greasy, chilled foods, wine, or damp flour[48] during treatment.

Gu Zhen Wan (Secure the True Pills)

[This prescription] treats long-standing and incessant white vaginal discharge and chilly pain in the umbilicus and abdomen as well as in the yin [genitals]. There is a current of fire in the eyes due to an ascending obstruction. One sees things when there is nothing to be seen. If there is malign heat in the gums causing pain while eating, one must administer finely powdered Rhizoma Coptidis Chinensis (*Huang Lian*) topically to arrest the pain. One will desire to eat only dry foods and have a great aversion to soupy foods.

These illnesses are all due to cold damp overwhelming the interior of the uterus such that the patient prefers dry foods and has an aversion to damp. Yin fire within the liver channel ascends and spills over into the topmost branches where it stagnates above and produces a stream of fire in the eyes. Kidney water invades the liver and spills upward. Therefore the eyes are blurry and cannot see. The malign heat in the gums when eating is due to hidden heat in the *shao yin* and *yang ming*. Treatment methods should consist of greatly draining cold dampness using medicinals in pill form to treat this condition. Therefore, it is said that, in the case of cold in the lower warmer, it is appropriate to move slowly. Decoctions and powders are strongly cautioned against.

[This formula] uses wine-prepared Halloysitum Album (*Bai Shi Zhi*) and Os Draconis (*Bai Long Gu*) to dry dampness and dry Rhizoma Zingiberis (*Gan Jiang*) which is spicy and hot to drain cold water. The very cold Rhizoma Dioscoreae Bulbiferae (*Huang Yao*) is used for [its cold nature] to treat [a cold condition] and as a guiding [medicinal].[49] Therefore, as for treatment methods, it is said that even when the ancients convicted a man of a felony, his offspring were not executed. [In the same way,] they also recognized that that which governs [treatment] is hidden. [One must] first find the cause [of the disease and then one may] also drain malign heat rheum from the gums. Use Radix Bupleuri (*Chai Hu*) as an envoy to the root channel, and 5 *fen* of Radix Albus Paeoniae Lactiflorae (*Bai Shao*) as a guide, lest the acrid hot medicinals become detrimental to the liver channel. [In this manner,] one should use some slightly draining [medicinals]. Use the pungent warm body

---

[48] Damp flour refers to wheat products in general.

[49] While Li Dong-yuan is best known for his use of warm medicinals to treat warm diseases, he did not eschew the use of cold medicinals completely. In much the same way that he used warming medicinals to treat apparently hot conditions, on occasion he used cooling medicinals to treat cold symptoms.

of Radix Angelicae Sinensis (*Dang Gui Shen*) to greatly supplement the blood vessels. This is a complete method for the use of medicinals.

Use Radix Astragali Membranacei (*Huang Qi*), and wine-soaked Radix Albus Paeoniae Lactiflorae (*Bai Shao*), 5 *fen* each, Radix Bupleuri (*Chai Hu*), and Halloysitum Album (*Bai Shi Zhi*), 1 *qian* each. Fire [the Halloysitum Album] until it is red, spray it with water while it is finely ground, and dry it in the sun. Os Draconis (*Bai Long Gu*) is wine-cooked, sundried, sprayed with water, and powdered. Radix Angelicae Sinensis (*Dang Gui*) is wine-soaked. Two *qian* of each of the above are used. Dry Rhizoma Zingeberis (*Gan Jiang*), 4 *qian,* is blast-fried. Having water-sprayed the Hallyositum Album (*Bai Shi Zhi*) and Os Draconis (*Bai Long Gu*), grind [all of the ingredients] finely and mix them with water-boiled flour to form pills the size of Gorgon fruit seeds. Take 30 pills with each dose on an empty stomach with a substantial amount of boiled water. So that it will not stagnate in the stomach, wait a half hour before eating a meal, lest the hot medicinals attack the stomach. Uncooked and chilled [foods] are prohibited, as are tough substances[50], alcohol, and damp flour.

Wu Yao Tang (Lindera Decoction)

[This formula] treats pain and soreness in the sea of blood in women. It contains Radix Angelicae Sinensis (*Dang Gui*), Radix Glycyrrhizae (*Gan Cao*), Radix Auklandiae Lappae (*Mu Xiang*), 5 *qian* each, Radix Linderae Strychnifoliae (*Wu Yao*), 2 *qian*, Rhizoma Cyperi Rotundi (*Xiang Fu Zi*), 2 *liang,* stir-fried. Grind the above ingredients and take 5 *qian* per dose with two cups of water. Remove the dregs. Administer warm before meals.

Ju Yang Tang (Lift Yang Decoction)

This is also called *Sheng Yang Zao Shi Tang* (Upbear Yang & Dry Dampness Decoction). [It] treats white vaginal discharge, pain in the yin door [vagina], tense or cramping pain, a jaundiced body, and slack skin. The body is heavy like a mountain and the yin [genitals] are like ice. Slice the ingredients to the size of sesame [seeds] and mung [beans] and administer once daily in three cups of water cooked down to one cup. Take this before meals and slightly warm.

[This formula contains] uncooked Radix Scutellariae Baicalensis (*Huang Qin*), Pericarpium Citri Erythrocarpae (*Ju Pi*), 5 *fen* of each of the above, Radix Ledebouriellae Divaricatae (*Fang Feng*), Rhizoma Alpiniae Officinari (*Gao Liang Jiang*), dry Rhizoma Zingiberis (*Gan*

---

[50] Any food that is rather fibrous and does not easily break down is considered to be tough or chunky. This may even include carrots or potatoes.

Jiang), Semen Pruni (*Yu Li Ren*), and Radix Glycyrrhizae (*Gan Cao*), 1 *qian* of each of the above, Radix Bupleuri (*Chai Hu*), 1 *qian, 3 fen*, and Flos Helioanthi Annuae (*Bai Kua Hua*), 7 flowers. Slice [the above ingredients] to the size of sesame [seeds and mung] beans and divide them into two doses. Take each dose in two cups of water cooked down to one cup. Remove the dregs. Administer it warm and before eating.

Shui Fu Dan (Water Storage Elixir)

[This formula] treats long-standing vacuity with accumulated chill in women. The menses do not move. There are concretions and conglomerations in the abdomen accompanied by clots and sudden pain.The face looks dirty, dark, emaciated, and bony.

Cinnabar (*Nao Sha*),[51] separate with paper and cook in the froth of boiling water, Fructus Alpiniae Galangae (*Hong Tou*), 5 *qian* each, Cortex Cinnamomi Cassiae (*Gui Xin*), separated from the wood, Radix Auklandiae Lappae (*Mu Xiang*), dry Rhizoma Zingiberis (*Gan Jiang*), 1 *liang* each, Fructus Amomi (*Sha Ren*), calcined Ophicalcitum (*Hua Rui Shi*), 1 *liang, 5 fen*, Mylabris (*Ban Mao*) with the head and wings removed, the juice of uncooked Radix Rehmanniae (*Sheng Di Huang Zhi*), Urinae Hominis (*Tong Zi Xiao Bian*), 1 *sheng* each, Fellis Canis (*Gou Dan*) collected in deep winter, 7 gallbladders, and Cantharides (*Wan Qing*), three items with the head and feet removed, fried in 1 *sheng* of roasted glutinous rice until the rice is yellow. This is then removed and not used. Grind these nine ingredients to a fine powder and then together with the three juices cook them down into a paste. Form pills the size of Gorgon fruit seeds and coat them with Cinnabar. Take one pill daily, chewing it thoroughly with warm wine. Administer prior to meals or with rice gruel. This formula may not be taken in pregnancy.

Ding Xiang E Jiao Tang (Cloves & Donkey Skin Glue Decoction)

[This formula] treats incessant flooding and leaking, and heart qi insufficiency, due to taxation and unregulated intake of drink and food, as well as shortened duration between menstrual flows. The two cubit [pulses] are both bowstring, tense, and surging, yet upon pressure they lack strength. This pattern expresses itself as an ice-like sensation below the umbilicus and a preference for thick clothing to ward off the cold. There is white discharge and white slimy substances. However, intermixed with this is a downward leaking of [menstrual] water which is sometimes a fresh red color. The right cubit pulse may sometimes be slightly surging.

---

[51] *Nao Sha* is Sal Amoniacum. However a note in the text identifies this medicinal as Cinnabar (*Zhu Sha*).

Cooked Radix Rehmanniae (*Shu Di*), Radix Albus Paeoniae Lactiflorae (*Bai Shao*), 3 *fen* each, Radix Ligustici Wallichii (*Chuan Xiong*)[52], Flos Caryophyllii (*Ding Xiang*), 4 *fen* each, Gelatinum Corii Asini (*E Jiao*), 6 *fen*, uncooked Folium Artemisiae Argyii (*Ai Ye*), 1 *qian*, and Radix Angelicae Sinensis (*Dang Gui*), 1 *qian*, 2 *fen*. Grind the Ligusticum finely and soak the Dang Gui in wine and slice it. Powder finely the Rehmannia and Cloves, and slice the Mugwort as well. These are all taken in a single dose with five cups of water. First cook the five ingredients in one cup of water, two *fen*, and remove the dregs. Then add the Donkey Skin Glue and return the preparation to the fire. Cook this down to one large cup and administer it hot on an empty stomach.

Huang Qi Dang Gui Ren Shen Tang (Astragalus, Dang Gui & Ginseng Decoction)

During the winter, the Kuo Da Fang came to say she had developed a sudden and incessant flooding of her menstrual water. First she had experienced a bodily detriment [*i.e.,* miscarriage] with loss of blood, and thereafter, [her menstrual cycle] arrived ten days early. This time it would not stop. She had become overly worried and she was irritable and very frightened. My diagnosis was heart qi insufficiency and unregulated intake of drink and food. Da Fang stated her disagreement [with this diagnosis], however. Further examination revealed that there was cold in the palms. The pulse was deep, fine, and relaxed and intermittently deep and rapid. The nine portals were inhibited and the four extremities lacked strength. There was asthmatic ascension, shortness of breath and rough [respiration], and the qi of the nose and mouth was unregulated, all resulting in a pattern of insufficiency of heart qi and vacuity of the spleen and stomach. Her stomach and precordial region were painful, the left subcostal region was contracted, and there was an accumulation there. She was mindful of her umbilical region [and the sensation of] movement of qi there. There were sounds in her abdomen and she experienced a descension of qi[53] and difficult bowel movements.

This was a quintessential vacuity pattern and [the attendant symptoms] cannot be listed in their entirety. One must first decide to treat the root, the remains of the pattern will then be eliminated. One should quiet the heart and settle the mind, secure [the spirit] from collapse and bolster it, regulate and harmonize the spleen and stomach, greatly boost the original qi, supplement the blood vessels, and nourish the spirit with formulas for major warming to eliminate winter cold congelation from within the skin.

---

[52] Some sources say that these first three ingredients should each be one half *qian*.

[53] *I.e.,* flatulence

The addition of a small amount of uncooked Radix Rehmanniae (*Sheng Di*) eliminates ministerial fire from the life-gate and forestalls depletion atony in the four extremities. Rhizoma Coptidis Chinensis (*Huang Lian*), 1 *fen*, uncooked Radix Rehmanniae (*Sheng Di*), 3 *fen*, stir-fried Massa Medica Fermentata (*Shen Qu*), Pericartium Citri Erythrocarpae (*Ju Pi*), Ramulus Cinnamomi Cassiae (*Gui Zhi*), 5 *fen* each, Semen Alpiniae Katsumadae (*Cao Dou Kou Ren*), 6 *fen*, Radix Astragali Membranacei (*Huang Qi*), Radix Panacis Ginseng (*Ren Shen*), Herba Ephedrae (*Ma Huang*) with the nodes removed, 1 *qian* each, body of Radix Angelicae Sinensis (*Dang Gui Shen*), 1 *qian*, 5 *fen*, Semen Pruni Armeniacae (*Xing Ren*), 5 pieces, ground separately into a paste. Grind the above ingredients and administer in two doses [per day] in two and half large cups of water. Cook the Ephedra at a boil and remove the froth, cooking it down to two cups. Next, add the other ingredients and cook them together down to one large cup. Take it in the morning with a little food. One dose will arrest [the bleeding] on the spot.

If there is gastric duct pain and there is a visitation of cold in the stomach, then take 15 of the very hot medicinal, *Cao Dou Kou Ren Wan* (Alpinia Katsumada Pills), with boiling water and the pain will be arrested on the spot. This is also a medicinal for liver accumulation. It eliminates the root source of the accumulation and produces a cure.

Dang Gui Shao Yao Tang (Dang Gui & Peony Decoction)

Treats incessant downward leaking of the menses in women where the blood is a fresh red color. This tends to occur in the ninth month [*i.e.*, September] and is a concern during the summerheat. The initial cause is taxation [producing] spleen/stomach vacuity depletion. [The symptoms are] shortness of breath and qi counterflow, incessant spontaneous perspiration, generalized heat producing a sense of oppression and chaos, aversion to the sight of drink and food. Not only can one not eat, but one cannot even think of food. The four extremities lack strength and there is occasional diarrhea. Later, as a result of an insufficiency of heart qi, there is incessant menstrual movement. Although one may experience a downward desertion of qi, this condition is actually an ascending counterflow of original qi which has become completely absent. The patient may experience a sense of qi moving downward from the upper abdomen and may report a shortness of breath. The patient may be unable to speak, but this is due to a lack of strength to speak as opposed to some laziness in describing [her symptoms]. The following medicinals govern [this condition].

Radix Bupleuri (*Chai Hu*), 2 *fen*, mix-fried Radix Glycyrrhizae (*Zhi Gan Cao*), uncooked Radix Rehmanniae (*Sheng Di Huang*), 3 *fen*, Pericarpium Citri Reticulatae (*Ju Pi*) with the whites removed, cooked Radix Rehmanniae (*Shu Di Huang*), 5 *fen* each, Radix Astragali Membranacei (*Huang Qi*), 1 *qian*, 5 *fen*, Rhizoma Atractylodis (*Cang Zhu*) soaked in rice water and skinned, body of Radix Angelicae Sinensis (*Dang Gui Shen*), Radix Albus Paeoniae Lactiflorae (*Bai Shao Yao*), Rhizoma Atractylodis Macrocephelae (*Bai Zhu*), 2 *qian*. Take the above ten ingredients and slice them to the size of sesame [seeds and mung] beans. Administer this in two doses in two and a half cups of water cooked down to one cup. Discard the dregs and administer slightly warm on an empty stomach.

Chai Hu Tiao Jing Tang (Bupleurum Regulate the Menses Decoction)

[This formula] treats incessant flow of menstrual water which is bright red in color, distress of the neck sinews, brain pain and rigidity, and pain in the bones of the spine. [It contains] mix-fried Radix Glycyrrhizae (*Gan Cao*), body of Radix Angelicae Sinensis (*Dang Gui Shen*), Radix Peurariae (*Ge Gen*), 3 *fen* each, Radix Angelicae Pubescentis (*Du Huo*), Radix Et Rhizoma Ligustici Chinensis (*Gao Ben*), Rhizoma Cimicifugae (*Sheng Ma*), 5 *fen* each, Radix Bupleuri (*Chai Hu*), 7 *fen*, Rhizoma Atractylodis (*Cang Zhu*), 1 *qian* each, and a little bit of Flos Carthamii Tinctori (*Hong Hua*). Slice the above ingredients to the size of sesame [seeds and mung] beans and administer in a single dose in four large cups of water cooked down to one cup. Discard the dregs and administer slightly warm on an empty stomach. Once a slight perspiration is induced, [the bleeding] will be arrested on the spot.

A woman's menstrual indicators may reveal black blood which is congealed, bound, and containing clots, while, on the left side, there are blood conglomerations. [In addition,] there may be incessant watery diarrhea and grains may sometimes fail to be transformed. Subsequently, the blood clots then suddenly descend, accompanied by a pouring down of watery [diarrhea]. What is readily apparent in the region of both the anterior and posterior yin is the downward desertion of exhausted blood. If [this condition becomes] long-standing, not only are the menstrual indicators unregulated but one may observe a watery diarrhea two or three times per day. The consumption of food causes heart vexation, there is diminished intake of drink and food, and ultimately emaciation and weakness.

Old man Dong-yuan says: The sage who treats disease must root [himself] in the principles of the four seasons, ascension and descension, the floating and the sinking. He must weigh his priorities. He must first harvest the qi and not diminish the celestial harmony, producing no overcoming and no vacuity, leaving nowhere for death and disease [to afflict] a person. Thus, [the physician] does not produce an evil and does not lose the correct [qi]. Even a patient on the verge of expiring will live. Therefore, [Zhang] Zhong-jing said:

> When yang is exuberant and yin is vacuous, precipitation will produce a cure and diaphoresis will result in death. When yin is exuberant and yang is vacuous diaphoresis will produce a cure and precipitation will result in death.

The great sages established methods to nourish each [condition] naturally. Moreover, formulas for raising the yang or effusing and dispersing assist the yang qi of spring and summer. In promoting ascension and upbearing, one drains the perishing cold qi stored during the autumn and winter and the disease is arrested. Thus one should use this, the ultimate principle of raising and descending, floating and sinking as [the primary] treatment method. The qi of heaven and earth produces upbearing and downbearing, floating and sinking and acts in accordance with the four seasons. In treating disease, one cannot act in a manner contrary to this. The classic states, "When [one acts] in accordance with heaven, the result is prosperity, but, when [one acts] contrary to heaven, the result is loss." How can one fail to be in awe of this!

A person's body also has four seasons and the qi of heaven and earth and one cannot profess to be separate from these. A person's body is also the same as heaven and earth. When the menses leak incessantly, this is a downward desertion of the qi and blood of the anterior yin. When there is also watery diarrhea for a number of years, this reflects a downward sinking of the qi and blood of the posterior yin producing desertion. The posterior yin governs substance with form.[54] The anterior yin is the abode of the essence qi, and, when it becomes downwardly exhausted, it afflicts the qi and blood of the patient's entire body. This commonly occurs during the autumn and winter months, and, since the yin governs ominous [developments], the disease is stored. Yang engenderment and yin growth occur during the spring and summer. In the human body, this upbearing and floating of qi is the upward movement of grain qi. The grain qi cannot be victorious when there is no engenderment and growth of qi and blood within the entire body of a patient. The resulting wasting of the muscles and flesh reflects the complete expiry of these two polar qi. When the two yin of the lower source have completely deserted, the qi and blood become exhausted. Even though this is a heat pattern, chronic desertion in the lower burner transforms it to cold.

This disease is chronically deep and chronically downbearing, and there is a massive overwhelming of damp cold which must urgently be salvaged. To drain cold, use heat, and to eliminate dampness, use dryness with massive upbearing and elevation to assist in engenderment and growth in order to support and nourish the qi and blood so as to avoid a tendency toward their exhaustion.

The sages established a treatment method whereby, when there is a great overwhelming of damp qi, one should use [wind] to overwhelm and level dampness. One should first regulate and harmonize the stomach qi and then use medicinals such as Rhizoma Atractylodis Macrocephelae (*Bai Zhu*) to dry dampness and enrich the original qi. If this does not arrest [the bleeding and diarrhea], then use wind medicinals to overcome dampness. This is

---

[54] *I.e.*, defecation

achieved by greatly elevating and greatly upbearing and this assists in the ultimate treatment of the enduring descent of the twin dampnesses of spring and summer.

Yi Wei Sheng Yang Tang (Boost the Stomach & Upbear Yang Decoction)

In the case of blood desertion, boost the qi. This is the method of the ancient sages. First, boost the stomach qi to assist with the generation and production of qi. It is said that when yang engenders, this leads to the growth of yin. Sweet medicinals are a priority, and everyone understands that they supplement the qi. However, they really do not [also] know that sweet is able to engender blood. This is [based on] the principle of engendering yang resulting in growth of yin. Therefore, first rectify the stomach qi because, within a person's body, the stomach qi is most precious.

Radix Bupleuri (*Chai Hu*), Rhizoma Cimicifugae (*Sheng Ma*), 5 grams each, mix-fried Radix Glycyrrhizae (*Gan Cao*), body of Radix Angelicae Sinensis (*Dang Gui Shen*), wine-soaked, Pericarpium Citri Reticulatae (*Chen Pi*), 1 *qian* each, Radix Panacis Ginseng (*Ren Shen*), remove the calyx and delete this ingredient if there is cough, stir-fried Massa Medica Fermentata (*Shen Qu*), 1 *qian, 5 fen* each, Radix Astragali Membranacei (*Huang Qi*), 2 *qian*, Radix Atractylodis Macrocephelae (*Bai Zhu*), 3 *qian*, uncooked Radix Scutellariae Baicalensis (*Huang Qin*), a small amount. Grind the above ingredients and take two *qian* with each dose, cooking them in two large cups of water down to one cup. Then remove the dregs and administer slightly warm.

If there is abdominal pain, add 3 *fen* of Radix Albus Paeoniae Lactiflorae (*Bai Shao*) and a small amount of Cortex Cinnamoni Cassiae (*Gui*) to each dose. If there is thirst and oral dryness, add 2 *fen* of Radix Puerariae (*Ge Gen*) and take at any time.

Sheng Yang Sheng Jing Tang (Upbear the Yang & Elevate The Menses Decoction)

[This] treats incessant flow of menstrual water. If the left cubit pulse is empty and vacuous upon pressure, this [reflects] a pattern of a complete desertion of qi and blood and great cold. With a light [touch of the] hand the pulse is rapid and racing, and when one raises one's finger, it is bowstring and tense or choppy, all of which indicates a yang desertion pattern as well as a collapse [due to] yin fire. One may see a heat pattern in the mouth, nose, and eyes or thirst. This [is all due to an] agitation of yin which makes the yang want to be the first to leave. [In treatment,] one should warm it, elevate it, upbear it, float it, and dry it. These methods greatly upbear and float the blood and qi and precisely supplement the downward desertion of the life gate.

Cortex Cinnamomi Cassiae (*Rou Gui*) with the skin removed. Do not use in the exuberance of summer but it may be used in the autumn and winter. Radix Albus Paeoniae Lactiflorae (*Bai Shao*), Flos Carthami Tinctori (*Hong Hua*), 5 *fen* each, Herba Cum Radice Asari (*Xi Xin*), 6 *fen*, Radix Panacis Ginseng (*Ren Shen*) with the calyx removed, cooked Radix Rehmanniae (*Shu Di*), Radix Ligustici Wallichi (*Chuan Xiong*), 1 *qian*, Radix Angelicae Pubescentis (*Du Huo Gen*), blackened Radix Lateralis Praeparatus Aconiti Carmichaeli (*Fu Zi*), blast-fried with the skin removed, mix-fried Radix Glycyrrhizae (*Gan Cao*), 1 *qian*, 5 *fen*, Radix Et Rhizoma Notopterygii (*Qiang Huo*), Radix Et Rhizoma Ligustici Chinensis (*Gao Ben*), remove the earth, Radix Ledebouriellae Divaricatae (*Fang Feng*), 2 *qian* each of the above, Rhizoma Atractylodis Macrocephelae (*Bai Zhu*), Radix Angelicae Sinensis (*Dang Gui*), Radix Astragali Membranacei (*Huang Qi*), Radix Bupleuri (*Chai Hu*), 2 *qian* each of the above, and Semen Pruni Persicae (*Tao Ren*), 10 pieces, cooked and soaked to remove the skin and tips, then ground finely. Grind [the above ingredients] and administer three *qian* [per dose]. If the disease progresses, one may increase the dose up to five *qian*. Administer [each dose] in three cups of water cooked down to one *qian*. Take this warm on an empty stomach.

BIBLIOGRAPHY

Chinese Sources

"A Clinical Study of the Treatment of 68 Cases of Endometriosis by the Methods of Transforming Stasis & Softening the Hard", Chang Nuan & Ma Ping-chong, *Tian Jin Zhong Yi (Tianjin Chinese Medicine)*, #5, 1995, p. 11-12

"A Clinical Survey of 40 Cases of Endometriosis", Zhu Liang-yu, *Shang Hai Zhong Yi Yao Za Zhi (Shanghai Journal of Chinese Medicine & Medicinals)*, #1, 1994, p. 12-13

"An Analysis of the Treatment of 35 Cases of Endometriosis Using the Transforming Stasis, Supplementing the Kidneys Method", Yin Xiu-lan, *Shang Hai Zhong Yi Yao Za Zhi (Shanghai Journal of Chinese Medicine & Medicinals)*, #11, 1993, p. 21-22

"A Review of the Chinese Medical Literature on Climacteric Syndrome", Yao Shi-an, *Zhong Yi Za Zhi (Journal of Chinese Medicine)*, #2, 1994, p. 112-114

"A Study on the Treatment of Primary Dysmenorrhea with *Jia Wei Mo Jie Tang* (Added Flavors Myrrh & Dragon's Blood Decoction) and Its Effect on Prostaglandins & Related Factors)", Zhu Nan-sun *et al.*, *Zhong Yi Za Zhi (Journal of Chinese Medicine)*, #2, 1994, p. 99-101

Bai Ling Fu Ke (Bai-ling's Gynecology), Han Bai-ling, Heilongjiang Peoples Press, Harbin, 1983

"Chen Hui-lin's Experiences in Treating Uterine Myomas — Including an Analysis of the Clinical Data of 239 Cases", Zeng Zhen & Shen Xiao-heng, *Shang Hai Zhong Yi Yao Za Zhi (Shanghai Journal of Chinese Medicine & Medicinals)*, #12, 1995, p. 3-5

Cheng Dan An Zhen Jiu Xuan Ji (Cheng Dan-an's Selected Acupuncture & Moxibustion Works), ed. by Cheng Wei-fen *et al.*, Shanghai Science & Technology Press, Shanghai, 1986

Chu Zhen Zhi Liao Xue (A Study of Acupuncture Treatment), Li Zhong-yu, Sichuan Science & Technology Press, Chengdu, 1990

"Clinical Experiences in the Treatment of 56 Cases of Endometriosis with *Nei Yi Fang* (Endometriosis Formula)", Yu Chiao-qin & Zhai Mei-fu, *Zhe Jiang Zhong Yi Za Zhi (Zhejiang Journal of Chinese Medicine)*, #5, 1996, p. 209-210

"Clinical Experiences in the Treatment of 89 Cases of Endometriosis with the Methods of Quickening the Blood & Freeing the Flow of the Bowels", Li Ying, *Xin Zhong Yi (New Chinese Medicine)*, #3, 1996, p. 24-26

"Clinical Experiences in the Treatment of 120 Cases of Mammary Neoplasia with *Ru Tong Ling* (Breast Pain Efficacious [Remedy])", Ye Xiu-min & Zhang Geng-yang, *Tian Jin Zhong Yi (Tianjin Chinese Medicine)*, #3, 1994, p. 6

Dong Yuan Yi Ji (Dong-yuan's Collected Medical Works), ed. by Bao Zheng-fei *et al.*, People's Health & Hygiene Press, Beijing, 1993

"Experiences in the Chinese Medical Treatment of Endometriosis", Sha Ming-rong, *Zhong Yi Za Zhi (Journal of Chinese Medicine)*, #4, 1995, p. 213

"Experiences in the Treatment of Chronic Fibrocystic Breast Disease", Yang Hui-an, *Tian Jin Zhong Yi (Tianjin Chinese Medicine)*, #6, 1993, p. 9

Fu Ke Bing (Gynecological Diseases), California Certified Acupuncturists Association, Oakland, CA, 1988

Fu Ke Bing Liang Fang (Fine Formulas for Gynecological Diseases), He Yuan-lin & Jiang Chang-yun, Yunnan University Press, Chongqing, 1991

Fu Ke Lin Chuan Jing Hua (The Clinical Efflorescence of Gynecology), Wang Bu-ru & Wang Qi-ming, Sichuan Science & Technology Press, Chengdu, 1989

Fu Ke San Bai Zheng (Three Hundred Gynecological Conditions), Liu Lan-fang & Liu Dian-gong, Jiangxi Science & Technology Press, 1989

Fu Ke Yu Chi (The Jade Ruler of Gynecology), Shen Jin-ao, Shanghai Science & Technology Press, Shanghai, 1983

Fu Ke Zheng Zhi (Gynecological Patterns & Treatments), Sun Jiu-ling, Hebei People's Press, 1983

Fu Qing Zhu Nu Ke (Fu Qing-zhu's Gynecology), Fu Qing-zhu, Shanghai People's Press, Shanghai, 1979; available in English, trans. by Yang Shou-zhong & Liu Da-wei, Blue Poppy Press, Boulder, CO, 1992

Fu Ren Da Quan Liang Fang (A Great Compendium of Fine Formulas for Women), Chen Ze-ming, People's Government Press, Beijing, 1985

Gu Qin Fu Ke Zhen Jiu Miao Fa Da Cheng (A Great Compendium of Ancient & Modern Acupuncture & Moxibustion Miraculous Methods for Gynecology), Liu Ji, Chinese National Chinese Medicine & Medicinals Press, Beijing, 1993

Han Ying Chang Yong Yi Xue Ci Hui (Chinese-English Glossary of Commonly Used Medical Terms), Huang Xiao-kai, People's Health & Hygeine Press, Beijing, 1982

He Zi Huai Nu Ke Jing Yan Ji (A Collection of He Zi-huai's Experiences in Gynecology), ed. By Chen Shao-chun & Lu Zhi, Zhejiang Science & Technology Press, 1982

"Lai Chun-mao's Treatment of 38 Cases of Endometriosis", Cao Dong *et al.*, *Yun Nan Zhong Yi Za Zhi (Yunnan Journal of Chinese Medicine)*, #5, 194, p. 7

"Lu De-ming's Experiences Treating Mammary Hyperplasia Disease", Que Hua-fa, *Shang Hai Zhong Yi Yao Za Zhi (Shanghai Journal of Chinese Medicine & Medicinals)*, #2, 1994, p. 6-7

Nan Nu Bing Mi Yan Liang Fang (Secret, Proven, Fine Formulas for Men's & Women's Diseases), Du Jie-hui, Beijing Science & Technology Press, Beijing, 1991

Nu Bing Wai Zhi Liang Fang Miao Fa (Fine Formulas & Miraculous Methods for the External Treatment of Women's Diseases), Wang Jin-quan & Cai Yu-hua, Chinese National Chinese Medicine & Medicinals Press, Beijing, 1993

Nu Ke Bai Wen (100 Questions on Gynecology), Qi Chong-fu, Shanghai Ancient Chinese Medical Books Press, Shanghai, 1983

Nu Ke Ji Yao (The Collected Essentials of Gynecology), Yu Yao-feng, Peoples Government Press, Beijing, 1988

Nu Ke Jing Wei (Profundities from the Gynecological Classics), Lu Guo-zhi & Song Shu-de, Shanxi Science & Technology Press, Xian 1989

Nu Ke Mi Jue Da Quan (A Great Compendium of Secrets of Success in Gynecology), Chen Liang-fang, Beijing Daily Press, Beijing, 1989

Nu Ke Xian Fang (Immortal Formulas in Gynecology), Fu Shan, aka Fu Qing-zhu, Ancient Chinese Medical Book Press, Beijing, 1989

Nu Ke Yao Zhi (The Essentials of Gynecology), Yu Yo-yuan, Fujian Science & Technology Press, Fuzhou, 1982

Nu Ke Zong Yao (Gathered Essentials of Gynecology), Zhang Shou-qian, Hunan Science & Technology Press, Changsha, 1985

Ru Fang Ji Huan (Breast Diseases & Sufferings), Qiu Si-kang, People's Health & Hygiene Press, Beijing, 1985

Shang Hai Lao Zhong Yi Jing Yan Xuan Bian (A Collection of Shanghai Old Doctors' Experiences), Shanghai Science & Technology Press, Shanghai, 1984

Shi Yong Zhen Jiu Tui Na Zhi Liao Xue (A Study of Practical Acupuncture, Moxibustion & Tui Na Treatments), Xia Zhi-ping, Shanghai College of Chinese Medicine Press, Shanghai, 1990

Shi Yong Zhong Xi Yi Jie He Fu Chan Ke Zheng Zhi (Proven Treatments in Practical Integrated Chinese-Western Obstetrics & Gynecology), Guo Yuan, Shanxi People's Press, Xian, 1984

Tan Zheng Lun (Treatise on Phlegm Conditions), Hou Tian-yin & Wang Chun-hua, People's Army Press, Beijing, 1989

"The Pattern Discrimination Treatment of 90 Cases of Menstrual Movement Breast Distention", Wang Fa-chang & Wang Qu-an, *Shan Dong Zhong Yi Za Zhi (Shandong Journal of Chinese Medicine)*, #5, 1993, p. 24-25

"The Pattern Discrimination Treatment of 100 Cases of Mammary Hyperplasia", Fang Jian-ping, *Jiang Su Zhong Yi (Jiangsu Chinese Medicine)*, #2, 1993, p. 14

"The Treatment of 40 Cases of Endometriosis by Boosting the Qi & Transforming Stasis", He Shu-ying, *Si Chuan Zhong Yi (Sichuan Chinese Medicine)*, #9, 1993, p. 41

"The Treatment of 48 Cases of Endometriosis by the Methods of Quickening the Blood & Transforming Stasis", Hu Guo-zhen, *Shang Hai Zhong Yi Yao Za Zhi (Shanghai Journal of Chinese Medicine & Medicinals)*, #2, 1995, p. 38-40

"The Treatment of 63 Cases of Endometriosis with *Xiao Yi Tang* (Disperse the Abnormal Decoction)", Zhou Ying-hua, *Yun Nan Zhong Yi Za Zhi (Yunnan Journal of Chinese Medicine)*, #4, 1994, p. 17

"The Treatment of 50 Cases of Premenstrual Breast Distention & Pain with *Jie Yu Huo Xue Tang* [Resolve Depression & Quicken the Blood Decoction]", Gu Si-yun, *Shan Dong Zhong Yi Za Zhi (Shandong Journal of Chinese Medicine)*, #6, 1992, p. 27-28

"The Treatment of 24 Cases of Mammary Hyperplasia with *Ru Kuai Xiao Tang Jia Wei* [Breast Lump Dispersing Decoction with Added Flavors]", Hou Jian, *Shan Dong Zhong Yi Za Zhi (Shandong Journal of Chinese Medicine)*, #5, 1993, p. 33

"The Treatment of 128 Cases of Mammary Hyperplasia", Mi Yang, *Hu Nan Zhong Yi Za Zhi (Hunan Journal of Chinese Medicine)*, #1, 1993, p. 47

"The Treatment of 18 Cases of Uterine Myoma with *Gui Zhi Fu Ling Wan Jia Wei* (Cinnamon Twig & Poria Pills with Added Flavors)" by Zhang Shou-guo, *Hu Bei Zhong Yi Za Zhi (Hubei Journal of Chinese Medicine)*, #2, 1994, p. 52

"The Treatment of 42 Cases of Uterine Myoma with *Xiao Ji Tang* (Disperse Accumulation Decoction)", Zhang Yu-shen, *Shan Dong Zhong Yi Za Zhi (Shandong Journal of Chinese Medicine)*, #8, 1995, p. 356

"The Treatment of 45 Cases of Uterine Myoma with *Bu Zhong Yi Qi Tang Jia Jian* (Supplement the Center & Boost the Qi Decoction with Additions & Subtractions)", Wang Dao-qing *et al.*, *Zhe Jiang Zhong Yi Za Zhi (Zhejiang Journal of Chinese Medicine)*, #1, 1994, p. 15

"Use of Basal Body Temperature in Pattern Discrimination for Patients with Infertility and Blocked Menstruation", Xia Gui-cheng, *Shang Hai Zhong yi Yao Za Zhi (Shanghai Journal of Chinese Medicine & Medicinals)*, #10, 1992, p. 18-19

Wan Shi Fu Ren Ke (Master Wan's Gynecology), Wan Quan, a.k.a. Wan Mi-zhai, Hubei Science & Technology Press, 1984

Yi Zong Jin Jian (The Golden Mirror of Ancestral Medicine), Wu Qian *et al.*, Peoples Health & Hygeine Press, Beijing, 1985

Yu Xue Zheng Zhi (Static Blood Patterns & Treatments), Zhang Xue-wen, Shanxi Science & Technology Press, Xian, 1986

Zhen Jiu Da Cheng (A Great Compendium of Acupuncture & Moxibustion), Yang Ji-zhou, People's Health & Hygiene Press, Beijing, 1983

Zhen Jiu Xue (A Study of Acupuncture & Moxibustion), Qiu Mao-liang *et al.*, Shanghai Science & Technology Press, Shanghai, 1985

Zhen Jiu Yi Xue (An Easy Study of Acupuncture & Moxibustion), Li Shou-xian, People's Health & Hygiene Press, Beijing, 1990

Zhong Guo Min Jian Cao Yao Fang (Chinese Folk Herbal Medicinal Formulas), Liu Guang-rui & Liu Shao-lin, Sichuan Science & Technology Press, Chengdu, 1992

Zhong Guo Zhen Jiu Chu Fang Xue (A Study of Chinese Acupuncture & Moxibustion Prescriptions), Xiao Shao-qing, Ningxia People's Press, Yinchuan, 1986

Zhong Guo Zhong Yi Mi Fang Da Quan (A Great Compendium of Chinese National Chinese Medical Secret Formulas), ed. by Hu Zhao-ming, Literary Propagation Publishing Company, Shanghai, 1992

Zhong Yi Fu Chan Ke Xue (A Study of Chinese Medical Gynecology & Obstetrics), Heilonjiang College of TCM, People's Health and Hygiene Press, Beijing, 1991

Zhong Yi Fu Ke (Chinese Medical Gynecology), Zhu Cheng-han, People's Heath & Hygeine Press, Beijing, 1989

Zhong Yi Fu Ke Lin Chuang Shou Ce (A Clinical Handbook of Chinese Medical Gynecology), Shen Chong-li, Shanghai Science & Technology Press, Shanghai, 1990

Zhong Yi Fu Ke Shou Ce (A Handbook of Chinese Medical Gynecology), Song Guang-ji & Yu Xiao-zhen, Zhejiang Science & Technology Press, Hangzhou, 1984; available in English, fourth, revised edition, trans. by Zhang Ting-liang & Bob Flaws, Blue Poppy Press, Boulder, CO, 1995

Zhong Yi Fu Ke Xue (A Study of Chinese Medical Gynecology), Chengdu College of Chinese Medicine, Shanghai Science & Technology Press, Shanghai, 1983

Zhong Yi Fu Ke Xue (A Study of Chinese Medical Gynecology), Liu Min-ru, Sichuan Science & Technology Press, Chengdu, 1992

Zhong Yi Fu Ke Xue (A Study of Chinese Medical Gynecology), Luo Yuan-qi, *et al.*, Shanghai Science & Technology Press, Shanghai, 1987

Zhong Yi Fu Ke Zhi Liao Shou Ce (A Handbook of Chinese Medical Gynecological Treatments), Wu Shi-xing & Qi Cheng-lin, Shanxi Science & Technology Press, Xian, 1991

Zhong Yi Hu Li Xue (A Study of Chinese Medical Nursing), Lu Su-ying, People's Health & Hygiene Press, Beijing, 1983

Zhong Yi Lin Chuang Ge Ke (Various Clinical Specialties in Chinese Medicine), Zhang En-qin *et al.*, Shanghai College of Chinese Medicine Press, Shanghai, 1990

Zhong Yi Ling Yan Fang (Efficacious Chinese Medical Formulas), Lin Bin-zhi, Science & Technology Propagation Press, Beijing, 1991

Zhong Yi Zhi Liao Fu Nu Bing (The Chinese Medical Treatment of Gynecological Diseases), Zhang Jian-xiu, Hebei Science & Technology Press, 1988

Zhong Yi Zi Xue Cong Shu (The Chinese Medicine Self-study Series), Vol. 2, "*Gynecology*", Yang Yi-ya, Hebei Science & Technology Press, Shijiazhuang, 1987

English Sources

A Barefoot Doctor's Manual, revised & enlarged edition, Cloudburst Press, Mayne Isle, 1977

A Clinical Guide to Chinese Herbs and Formulae, Cheng Song-yu & Li Fei, Churchill & Livingstone, Edinburgh, 1993

A Compendium of TCM Patterns & Treatments, Bob Flaws & Daniel Finney, Blue Poppy Press, Boulder, CO, 1996

A Comprehensive Guide to Chinese Herbal Medicine, Chen Ze-lin & Chen Mei-fang, Oriental Healing Arts Institute, Long Beach, CA, 1992

A Glossary of Chinese Medical Terms & Acupuncture Points, Nigel Wiseman & Ken Boss, Paradigm Publications, Brookline, MA, 1990

Arisal of the Clear: A Simple Guide to Healthy Eating According to Traditional Chinese Medicine, Bob Flaws, Blue Poppy Press, Boulder, CO, 1991

A Handbook of Differential Diagnosis with Key Signs & Symptoms, Therapeutic Principles, and Guiding Prescriptions, Ou-yang Yi, trans. by C.S. Cheung, Harmonious Sunshine Cultural Center, SF, 1987

Chinese-English Terminology of Traditional Chinese Medicine, Shuai Xue-zhong *et al.*, Hunan Science & Technology Press, Changsha, 1983

Chinese-English Manual of Common-used Prescriptions in Traditional Chinese Medicine, ed. by Ou Ming, Joint Publishing Co., Ltd., Hong Kong, 1989

Chinese Herbal Medicine: Formulas & Strategies, Dan Bensky & Randall Barolet, Eastland Press, Seattle, 1990

Chinese Herbal Medicine: Materia Medica, Dan Bensky & Andrew Gamble, second, revised edition, Eastland Press, Seattle, 1993

Chinese Materia Medica, Vol. 1-6, Southern Materials Center Inc., Taipei, 1979

Chinese Self-massage, The Easy Way to Health, Fan Ya-li, Blue Poppy Press, Boulder, CO, 1996

Chong & Ren Imbalance, Cyclic Management of Menstrual Disorders, Cheng Jing, trans. by C.S. Cheung, Harmonious Sunshine Cultural Center, CA, undated

Concise Traditional Chinese Gynecology, Xia Gui-cheng *et al.*, Jiangsu Science & Technology Press, Nanjing, 1988

"Endometriosis: An Enigmatic Disease", Magdalen E. Hull & James Stelling, *Journal of Women's Health*, Vol. 5, #2, 1996, p. 111-120

English-Chinese Chinese-English Dictionary of Chinese Medicine, Nigel Wiseman, Hunan Science & Technology Press, Changsha, 1995

Extra Treatises Based on Investigation & Inquiry, Zhu Dan-xi, trans. by Yang Shou-zhong, Blue Poppy Press, Boulder, CO, 1993

Fundamentals of Chinese Acupuncture, Andrew Ellis, Nigel Wiseman & Ken Boss, Paradigm Publications, Brookline, MA, 1988

Fundamentals of Chinese Medicine, Nigel Wiseman & Andrew Ellis, Paradigm Publications, Brookline, MA, 1985

Glossary of Chinese Medical Terms and Acupuncture Points, Nigel Wiseman & Ken Boss, Paradigm Publications, Brookline, MA, 1990

Gynecology & Obstetrics: A Longitudinal Approach, ed. By Thomas R. Moore *et al.*, Churchill Livingstone, New York, 1993

Handbook of Chinese Herbs and Formulas, Yeung Him-che, Vol. 2, self-published, LA, 1985

Intractable Dysmenorrhea: Experiences of Master Physicians Shen Zhong Li and Ma Long Bai, trans. by C.S. Cheung, Harmonious Sunshine Cultural Center, Sunnyvale, CA, 1988

"Is Natural Progesterone the Missing Link in Osteoporosis Prevention & Treatment?", J.R. Lee, *Medical Hypotheses*, #35, 1991, p. 316-318

"Menopausal Hormone Replacement Therapy with Continuous Daily Oral Micronized Estradiol and Progesterone", Joel T. Hargrove *et al.*, *Gynecology & Obstetrics*, Vol. 73, #4, April 1989, p. 606-612

Oriental Materia Medica, A Concise Guide, Hong-yen Hsu, Oriental Healing Arts Institute, Long Beach, CA, 1986

"Osteoporosis Reversal: The Role of Progesterone", John R. Lee, *International Clinical Nutrition Review,* Vol. 10, #3, July 1990, p. 384-391

Pao Zhi: An Introduction to the Use of Processed Chinese Medicinals, Philippe Sionneau, trans. by Bob Flaws, Blue Poppy Press, Boulder, CO, 1995

Practical Traditional Chinese Medicine & Pharmacology: Clinical Experiences, Shang Xian-min et al., New World Press, Beijing, 1990

Practical Traditional Chinese Medicine & Pharmacology: Herbal Formulas, Geng Jun-ying, *et al.*, New World Press, Beijing, 1991

"Progesterone and Its Relevance for Osteoporosis", Jerilynn C. Prior, *Osteoporosis*, Vol. 2, #2, March 1993

"Progesterone and the Prevention of Osteoporosis", Jerilynn C. Prior *et al.*, *The Canadian Journal of Ob/Gyn & Women's Health Care*, Vol. 3, #4, 1991, p.178-184

"Progesterone as a Bone-trophic Hormone", J.C. Prior, *Endocrine Reviews*, Vol. 11, #2, 1990, p. 386-398

"Sexual Assault History and Premenstrual Distress in Two General Population Samples", Jaqueline M. Golding *et al.*, *Journal of Women's Health,* Vol. 5, #2, 1996, p. 143-152

"Spinal Bone Loss and Ovulatory Disturbances", Jerilynn C. Prior *et al.*, *The New England Journal of Medicine*, Volume 323, #18, November 1, 1990, 1221-1227

Symptoms and Treatment for Menses and Leukorrhea, Chen Yu-cang, trans. by Hor Ming Lee, Hor Ming Press, Victoria, BC, undated

The English-Chinese Encyclopedia of Practical Traditional Chinese Medicine, Vol. 12: Gynecology, Xuan Jia-sheng, ed., Higher Education Press, Beijing, 1990

The Essential Book of Traditional Chinese Medicine, Vol. 2: Clinical Practice, Liu Yan-chi, trans. by Fang Ting-yu & Chen Lai-di, Columbia University Press, NY, 1988

The Heart & Essence of Dan-xi's Methods of Treatment, Zhu Dan-xi, trans. by Yang Shou-zhong, Blue Poppy Press, Boulder, CO, 1993

The Merck Manual, 15th edition, ed. by Robert Berkow, Merck Sharp & Dohme Research Laboratories, Rahway, NJ, 1987

The Nanjing Seminars Transcript, Qiu Mao-lian & Su Xu-ming, The Journal of Chinese Medicine, UK, 1985

"The Role of the Liver in Menstrual Disorders", Wang Ru & Brian May, *The Pacific Journal of Oriental Medicine*, Australia, #77, p. 10-17

The Secret of the Chinese Pulse Diagnosis, Bob Flaws, Blue Poppy Press, Boulder, CO 1995

The Treatise on the Spleen & Stomach, Li Dong-yuan, trans. by Yang Shou-zhong, Blue Poppy Press, Boulder, CO 1993

"The Treatment of Fibrocystic Breast Disease with Chinese Herbs and Acupuncture", Deng Hui-ying & Liu Xin-ya, *The Journal of Chinese Medicine*, UK, #52, Sept. 1996, p. 28-30

The Yeast Connection, William G. Crook, Vintage Books, Random House, New York, 1986

The Yeast Syndrome, John Parks Towbridge & Morton Walker, Bantam Books, Toronto, 1988

Traditional Medicine in Contemporary China, Nathan Sivin, University of Michigan, Ann Arbor, 1987

Zang Fu: The Organ Systems of Traditional Chinese Medicine, second edition, Jeremy Ross, Churchill Livingstone, Edinburgh, 1985

Formula Index

A

Ai Fu Nuan Gong Wan 179
Ai Jian Wan 179
An Chong Tang 218

B

Ba Wei Di Huang Wan 426, 452, 556, 558, 560
Ba Wu Tang 341
Ba Zhen Jia Xiang Fu Tang 187
Ba Zhen Tang 163, 164, 181, 203, 204, 221, 326,
    408, 440, 441, 557, 559, 562
Ba Zhen Tang Jia Jian 408
Ba Zhen Tang Jia Wei 441
Ba Zhen Yi Mu Tang 352, 562
Ba Zheng San 496
Bai He Gu Jin Tang 303, 331, 490, 561
Bai He Gu Jin Tang Jia Jian 331
Bai He Gu Jin Tang Jia Wei 490
Bai Zi Ren Wan 301
Ban Xia Bai Zhu Tian Ma Tang Jia Wei 439, 459
Ban Xia Bai Zhu Tian Ma Wan 439
Ban Xia Hou Pu Tang 521
Ban Xia Xie Xin Tang 423, 424
Bao Yin Jian Jia Jian 254
Bao Yin Jian Jia Wei 215
Bu Shen Di Huang Tang Jia Jian 328
Bu Shen Di Huang Wan 302, 503
Bu Shen Gu Jing Tang 222
Bu Shen Tiao Jing Tang 237, 268
Bu Zhong Yi Qi Tang 162, 163, 169, 220, 227, 262,
    273, 274, 278, 290, 292, 297, 314, 352, 441, 563
Bu Zhong Yi Qi Tang Jia Jian 290, 292
Bu Zhong Yi Qi Tang Jia Wei 220, 227, 352
Bu Zhong Yi Qi Wan 291, 569

C

Cang Bai Er Chen Tang Jia Wei 271
Cang Fu Dao Tan Tang 191
Cang Fu Dao Tan Wan 192, 312, 313, 561
Cang Fu Dao Tan Wan Jia Jian 313
Cang Fu Dao Tan Wan Jia Wei 313
Cang Po Er Chen Tang Jia Wei 241
Chai Hu Gui Zhi Tang 392, 430, 562
Chai Hu Gui Zhi Tang Jia Ge Gen 430
Chai Hu Gui Zhi Tang Jia Wei 392
Chai Hu Jia Long Gu Mu Li Tang 465, 471, 562,
    563
Chai Hu Jia Long Gu Mu Li Tang Jia Wei 465, 471
Chai Hu Shu Gan San Jia Jian 325

Chai Hu Shu Gan Tang Jia Jian 403
Chai Hu Shu Gan Tang Jia Wei 437
Chai Hu Si Wu Tang Jia Wei 186
Chai Hu Tiao Jing Tang 584
Chen Xiang Jiang Qi Tang 187
Chu Tong San 346

D

Da Bu Yin Wan Jia Jian 406
Da Bu Yuan Jian 443
Da Huang Zhe Chong Wan 310, 332
Da Ying Jian 177
Dan Shen Gui Pi Tang 412
Dan Zhi Xiao Yao San 152, 203, 216, 229, 245,
    252, 256, 275, 351, 361, 404, 411, 412, 421,
    450, 465, 467, 471, 493, 512, 520, 556, 558-562
Dan Zhi Xiao Yao San Jia Jian 216, 256, 404, 467
Dan Zhi Xiao Yao San Jia Wei 465, 471, 493, 512
Dang Gui Bu Xue Tang Jia Qi Ju Di Huang Wan
    482
Dang Gui Chuan Xiong Tang 183
Dang Gui Di Huang Yin 237
Dang Gui Liu Huang Tang 158, 511, 533, 563
Dang Gui Shao Yao Tang 583
Dang Gui Si Ni Tang 185, 346, 484, 557
Dang Gui Si Ni Tang Jia Wei 346, 484
Dang Gui Yin 216, 532
Dang Gui Yin Zi 532
Dang Gui Yu Zhu San 303
Dao Chi San 496
Dao Zhi Tong Jing Tang Jia Wei 461
Di Gu Pi Yin 159, 253, 449, 450
Di Shao Liang Xue Tang Jia Wei 229
Di Tan Tang Jia Jian 326
Ding Jing Tang 202, 207
Ding Xiang E Jiao Tang 581

E, F

Er Chen Jia Xiong Gui Tang 241
Er Chen Tang Jia Wei 156, 241, 271, 272, 468
Er Huang Xiao Yao San 229
Er Xian Tang 164, 169, 204, 406, 516, 523, 530,
    563
Er Xian Tang Jia Jian 164, 523
Fen Li Wu Ling Tang Jia Wei 480
Fu Fang Shi Hui San 222
Fu Ke Tiao Li Fang 286, 287
Fu Pi Shu Gan Tang 257
Fu Tong Ning 381
Fu Zi Li Zhong Wan Jia Jian 298

G

Gan Cao Xie Xin Tang 424
Gan Mai Da Zao Tang Jia Bai He Di Huang Tang 470
Gan Mai Da Zao Tang Jia Xiao Yao San Jia Wei 485
Ge Jie Da Bu Wan 529
Ge Qi Si Wu Tang 429
Ge Xia Zhu Yu Tang 232, 330, 339
Ge Xia Zhu Yu Tang Jia Wei 232
Geng Nian An Tang 504
Gu Ben Zhi Beng Tang Jia Jian 264
Gu Ben Zhi Xue Tang 263, 560
Gu Chong Tang 265
Gu Jing Wan Jia Jian 230, 250
Gu Yin Jian 205, 207, 254, 305
Gu Yin Jian Jia Wei 205
Gu Zhen Wan 579
Gui Fu Wan Jia Wei 178
Gui Pi Tang 162, 184, 221, 227, 262, 263, 297, 298, 394, 412, 441, 457, 464, 518, 519, 556, 558, 560, 563
Gui Pi Tang Jia Jian 457, 464
Gui Pi Tang Jia Wei 184
Gui Pi Wan 184, 394, 475, 531
Gui Shao Di Huang Wan 503
Gui Shao Si Jun Zi Tang 190
Gui Shen Wan 165, 300, 326, 327, 483
Gui Shen Wan Jia Jian 300
Gui Shen Wan Jia Wei 483
Gui Xiong Di Huang Wan 191
Gui Zhi Fu Ling Chong Ji 288, 290
Gui Zhi Fu Ling Wan 280, 308, 345, 522, 557, 561, 564
Gui Zhi Fu Ling Wan He Xue Fu Zhu Yu Tang 522
Gui Zhi Si Wu Tang 429, 448, 454

H

Hai Zao Jing 285
He Xue Tong Jing Tang 311
Hei Pu Huang San Jia Jian 252
Hei Xiao Yao San 152, 239, 520
Hei Xiao Yao San Jia Wei 152
Hou Pu Er Chen Tang 313
Hu Po San 312
Huan Shao Dan 558, 559, 561, 562
Huang Lian E Jiao Tang 463, 506
Huang Lian E Jiao Tang Jia Wei 463
Huang Lian Wen Dan Tang 156, 420, 440, 472, 521, 556, 564
Huang Lian Wen Dan Tang Jia Wei 420
Huang Qi Dang Gui Ren Shen Tang 582

Huang Qi Jian Zhong Tang 432
Huo Xue Run Zao Sheng Jin Tang Jia Jian 490

J

Jia Jian Ba Zhen Tang 203
Jia Jian Chai Hu Shu Gan Tang 343
Jia Jian Cong Rong Tu Si Zi Wan 329
Jia Jian Dang Gui Bu Xue Tang 263
Jia Jian Jian Dan Dan 281
Jia Jian Niu Xi Tang 188
Jia Jian Si Wu Tang 219
Jia Jian Wen Jing Tang 354
Jia Jian Xiang Sha Liu Jun Zi Tang 314
Jia Jian Xiao Yao San 343
Jia Wei Bai Di Tang 217
Jia Wei Bu Zhong Yi Qi Tang 273
Jia Wei Chai Hu Shu Gan Tang 282
Jia Wei Dan Zhi Xiao Yao San 252
Jia Wei Di Gu Pi Yin 449
Jia Wei Er Chen Tang 157, 189
Jia Wei Gu Yin Jian 254
Jia Wei Gui Zhi Fu Ling Wan 280
Jia Wei Mai Men Dong Tang 491
Jia Wei Si Wu Er Chen Tang 313
Jia Wei Wu Yao Tang 185, 341
Jia Wei Xiang Fu Wan 186
Jia Wei Xiang Leng Wan 281
Jia Wei Yi Guan Jian 282
Jian Gu Tang 393, 426
Jian Gu Tang Jia Jian 393
Jian Gu Tang Jia Wei 393
Jian Ling Tang 508
Jiao Ai Ba Zhen Tang 221
Jiao Ai Tang 219, 270
Jiao Hong Yin 261
Jie Du Si Wu Tang 230, 251
Jie Du Si Wu Tang Jia Wei 251
Jin Gui Shen Qi Wan 270, 515
Jin Lian Hong Jiang Jie Du Tang 283
Jing Hou Fu Tong Fang 353
Jing Shui Guo Duo Fang 221
Jiu Zhu Dang Gui Wan 578
Ju Yang Tang 580
Ju Yuan Jian 162, 169, 220
Ju Yuan Jian Jia Wei 220

K, L

Kai Yu Er Chen Tang 240
Kan Li Ji Ji Wan 506
Li Jing Si Wu Tang 567
Li Yin Fu Yang Si Wu Tang 236
Li Zhong Tang 420

Liang Di Tang 159, 217, 228, 357
Liang Xu Gu Zhen Tang 219
Liang Xue Di Huang Tang 577
Ling Yang Gou Teng Tang 507
Liu Jun Zi Jia Gui Xiong Tang 190
Liu Jun Zi Tang Jia Wei 223
Liu Shen Tang 451
Liu Wei Di Huang Tang 267, 300, 506
Liu Wei Di Huang Tang He Huang Lian E Jiao Tang 506
Liu Wei Di Huang Tang Jia Jian 267
Liu Wei Di Huang Wan 64, 160, 182, 196, 206, 230, 276, 300, 302, 327, 442, 451, 502, 506, 517, 533, 559, 560, 563, 566
Liu Wei Di Huang Wan Jia Jian 230, 300, 533
Liu Wei Di Huang Wan Jia Wei 196, 206, 442, 451, 502, 506
Liu Wei Di Huang Wan Jia Wei Er Hao 442
Liu Wei Di Huang Wan Jia Wei Yi Hao 442
Liu Yuan San 266
Liu Zi Tang 324
Long Dan Xie Gan Tang 122, 423, 464, 466, 470, 474, 485
Long Dan Xie Gan Tang Jia Jian 464, 466, 470, 474
Long Dan Xie Gan Tang Jia Wei 485
Lu Jiao Shuang Yin 192
Lu Rong Wan 269

M, N

Ma Huang Si Wu Tang 429, 454
Miao Ying Wan 315
Nu Ke Ba Zhen Wan Jia Jian 296

P, Q

Ping Gan Kai Yu Zhi Beng Tang 260
Qi Ju Di Huang Tang Jia Wei 458, 509
Qi Ju Di Huang Wan 395, 482, 483
Qi Ju Di Huang Wan Jia Jian 483
Qi Li San 286
Qi Wei Bai Zhu San 418
Qi Wei Dou Qi Wan Jia Wei 480
Qi Wu Jiang Xia Tang 510
Qi Wu Tang 236
Qi Zhi Xiang Fu Wan 186, 391
Qiang Gui Si Wu Tang 433
Qin Jiao Si Wu Tang Jia Wei 432
Qin Jing Si Wu Tang 160
Qin Lian Si Wu Tang 150, 251
Qing E Wan 287, 528
Qing Gan Bu Shen Tang 330
Qing Gan Yin Jing Tang Jia Jian 487

Qing Gan Zhi Xue Tang 216
Qing Hai Tang 217
Qing Jing San Jia Jian 153
Qing Jing Si Wu Tang Jia Jian 488
Qing Jing Tang 159
Qing Liang San 245
Qing Re Gu Jing Tang 250, 254
Qing Re Tiao Xue Tang 341
Qing Xin Yin 512
Qing Xuan Ping Gan Tang 511
Qing Ying Jian Jia Jian 494
Qing Zao Jiu Fei Tang Jia Jian 479

R

Ren Shen Gu Ben Wan 180
Ren Shen Yang Rong Tang 180, 296, 452, 560
Ren Shen Yang Rong Tang Jia Jian 296
Ren Shen Zi Xue Tang 180, 234
Ren Shen Zi Xue Tang Jia Wei 234
Rong Fu Yan Zhen Tang 515
Ruan Jian Hua Yu Xiao Liu Fang 281

S

San Cai Da Bu Wan 353
San Huang San Bai Tang 349
San Huang Si Wu Tang 315, 487, 488, 492
San Huang Si Wu Tang Jia Jian 315
San Jia Fu Mai Tang 508
San Jie Fang 345
San Miao San 411
Sha Shen Mai Dong Tang Jia Jian 479
Shao Fu Zhu Yu Tang 184, 311, 344
Shao Ying Jian 218
Shen Ling Bai Zhu San 191, 202, 299, 393, 418, 421, 514
Shen Ling Bai Zhu San Jia Gui Xiong 191, 299
Shen Ling Bai Zhu San Jia Wei 514
Shen Qi Si Wu Tang Jia Wei 351
Shen Qi Wan Jia Jian 270, 533
Shen Xian Tai Yi Gao 409
Shen Yu Si Wu Tang 518
Shen Yu Tang 352
Sheng Hua Tang Jia Wei 342
Sheng Jiang Xie Xin Tang 424
Sheng Mai San He Gan Mai Da Zao Tang Jia Jian 519
Sheng Tie Luo Yin Jia Jian 472
Sheng Yang Chu Shi Tang 253, 575
Sheng Yang Chu Shi Tang Jia Wei 253
Sheng Yang Sheng Jing Tang 586
Sheng Yang Zao Shi Tang 580
Sheng Yu Tang Jia Wei 456

Shi Hui Wan 285, 475
Shi Quan Da Bu Tang 180, 235, 297, 321
Shi Quan Da Bu Tang Jia Jian 180, 321
Shi Quan Da Bu Wan 353
Shi Xiao San 223, 231, 259, 286, 370, 374, 391, 558
Shi Xiao San Jia Wei 231, 259
Shui Fu Dan 581
Shun Jing Liang An Tang 494
Shun Jing Tang 488, 490
Shun Jing Tang Jia Jian 490
Si Jun Zi Tang He Er Chen Tang Jia Wei 468
Si Ni San 308, 430
Si Ni San Jia Wei 430
Si Ni Tang Jia Wei 346, 473, 484
Si Qi Tang Jia Zuo Jin Wan 420
Si Shen Wan 426
Si Wu Chai Qin Tang 153
Si Wu Er Chen Tang 241, 313
Si Wu Jia Wei Tang 531
Si Wu Kan Li Wan Jia Wei 231
Si Wu Liang Ge San 489
Si Wu Tang He Shi Xiao San Jia Wei 259
Si Wu Tang Jia Duan Gua Yang 432
Si Wu Tang Jia Wei 178, 182, 186, 188, 235, 238, 251, 342, 351, 432, 433, 438, 444, 468, 475, 476
Suan Zao Ren Tang Jia Wei 465

T

Tao He Cheng Qi Tang 383, 385, 444
Tao Hong Er Chen Tang Jia Wei 156
Tao Hong Si Wu Tang Jia Jian 238, 322
Tao Hong Si Wu Tang Jia Wei 188, 238, 342, 433, 444, 468, 476
Tao Hong Si Wu Tang Jia Xiang Fu Wu Yao 208
Tian Ma Gou Teng Yin 438, 507, 563
Tian Wang Bu Xin Dan 302, 304, 505, 561, 564
Tiao Gan Tang 324, 356, 357, 395
Tiao Gan Tang Jia Jian 324
Tiao Gan Tang Jia Wei 357
Tiao Jing Wu Ji Wan 204
Tiao Jing Yang Rong Tang 183
Tiao Jing Yin 343
Tiao Yin Jian 206
Tong Jing Er Hao Fang 358, 562
Tong Jing Fang 286, 323, 332, 342
Tong Jing Huo Xue Tang 309
Tong Jing San Hao Fang 355
Tong Jing Shen Fang 355
Tong Xie Yao Fang 421
Tong Yu Jian 238
Tong Zhi Jian Jia Wei 309
Tu Niu Xi San 309
Tuo Mo Tang 375

W

Wen Bu Pi Shen Tang Jia Jian 407
Wen Dan Tang 156, 420, 440, 472, 520, 521, 556, 564
Wen Dan Tang Jia Wei 420, 521
Wen Jing Tang 177, 185, 242, 310, 345, 346, 354, 557, 559, 561, 562, 564
Wen Jing Tang Jia Jian 310
Wen Qing Yin 158, 218, 251, 512, 556, 558, 559, 563
Wen Shen Fu Yang Tang 204, 355
Wen Shen Tong Jing Fang Jia Wei 323
Wen Wei Yin 203
Wen Yang Chong Ren Fang 515
Wu Hu Tang Jia Wei 492
Wu Ling San 454, 460
Wu Ling San Jia Wu Pi Yin Jia Jian 460
Wu Mei Wan 358, 425
Wu Yao San 178, 307
Wu Yao San Jia Wei 178
Wu Yao Tang 185, 202, 341, 580
Wu Yao Tang Jia Jian 202
Wu Zhu Yu Tang 311, 345, 445

X

Xi Jiao Di Huang Tang 489, 492
Xia Ku Cao Gao 285
Xian Qi Tang 150, 215
Xiang Fu Bing 410
Xiang Gui Huo Xue Gao 286
Xiang Sha Liu Jun Zi Tang 190, 314, 418, 452
Xiao Chai Hu Tang 153, 187, 245, 391, 424, 428, 436, 467, 478, 562
Xiao Chai Hu Tang He Si Wu Tang 187, 428, 436
Xiao Chai Hu Tang Jia Wei 391, 478
Xiao Feng San 474
Xiao Feng San Jia Long Dan Xie Gan Tang Jia Jian 474
Xiao He San 405
Xiao Jin Dan 285
Xiao Yao Gua Lou San 404
Xiao Yao San 62, 152, 153, 186, 201, 203, 216, 229, 239, 245, 252, 256, 257, 275, 307, 321, 343, 344, 348, 351, 361, 390, 391, 401, 402, 404, 411-413, 421, 422, 437, 450, 465, 467, 471, 476, 485, 493, 512, 520, 556-563
Xiao Yao San He Ju He Wan 348
Xiao Yao San Jia Chuan Xiong Yu Jin 239
Xiao Yao San Jia Er Miao San 348
Xiao Yao San Jia Gua Lou Qiang Huo 402
Xiao Yao San Jia Jian 216, 256, 307, 321, 390, 391, 402, 404, 422, 467
Xiao Yao San Jia Wei 152, 201, 307, 401, 422, 437,

465, 471, 476, 485, 493, 512
Xing Su Si Wu Tang 449
Xiong Gui Er Chen Tang 189, 240, 557, 559
Xuan Fu Hua Dai Zhe Shi Tang Jia Wei 419
Xuan Yu Tong Jing Tang 349, 351
Xuan Yu Tong Jing Tang Jia Jian 349
Xue Beng Fang 195, 268, 356
Xue Beng Ji Yu Fang 266
Xue Beng Xiao Fang 254
Xue Fu Zhu Yu Tang 308, 340, 349, 443, 453, 522
Xue Fu Zhu Yu Tang Jia Jian 308, 340
Xue Fu Zhu Yu Tang Jia Wei 349

Y

Yao Tong Fang 287
Yi Guan Jian 161, 182, 282, 301, 304
Yi Guan Jian Jia Jian 161
Yi Guan Jian Jia Wei 301
Yi Hao Jiao Nang 286
Yi Huang Tang 411
Yi Mu Sheng Jin Dan 183
Yi Pi Wen Shen Tang 178
Yi Qi Tang Jia Wei 191, 220, 227, 352
Yi Shen Tang 350
Yi Shen Tiao Gan Tang 395
Yi Shen Yang Xin Tang 237
Yi Wei Sheng Yang Tang 576, 586
Yi Wei Zhu Yu Fang 369
Yin Jing Zhi Xue Tang 265
You Gui Wan 269, 275, 513, 514
You Gui Yin Jia Jian 273
Yu Nu Jian Jia Xie Xin Tang Jia Jian 462
Yu Yin Tang 267
Yu Zhu San 303, 453
Yue Ying Jian 494
Yun Nan Bai Yao 290, 291

Z

Ze Lan Tang 183
Zhen Gan Xi Feng Tang 438, 458, 508
Zhen Gan Xi Feng Tang Jia Jian 438
Zhen Gan Xi Feng Tang Jia Wei 458
Zhen Ling Dan 287
Zhi Bai Di Huang Tang Jia Jian 530, 531
Zhi Bai Di Huang Tang Jia Wei 531
Zhi Bai Di Huang Wan 206, 268, 462, 503, 530,
    556, 558, 560, 563
Zhi Dai Fang 287
Zhu Yu Zhi Beng Tang 231, 261
Zhu Yu Zhi Beng Tang Jia Jian 231
Zhu Yu Zhi Xue Tang 260
Zi Gong Ji Liu Fang 285, 286
Zi Lu Xian Zong Tang Jia Wei 301

Zong Hui San 221
Zuo Gui Wan 267, 275, 302, 516, 532
Zuo Gui Wan Jia Jian 267, 532
Zuo Gui Yin Jia Wei 532

General Index

A

A Clinical Handbook of Chinese Medical Gynecology 315, 320, 322, 323, 329

A Comprehensive Guide to Chinese Herbal Medicine 160, 517

A Great Compendium of Secrets of Success in Gynecology 145, 163

A Handbook of Differential Diagnosis with Key Signs & Symptoms, Therapeutic Principles, and Guiding Prescriptions 438

A Study of Chinese Medical Gynecology 57, 203, 206, 298, 418, 491

A Study of Chinese Medical Gynecology & Obstetrics 57

A Study of Chinese Medical Nursing 355, 358, 363

abdominal distention and pain, lower 30, 86, 88, 99, 103, 107, 128, 151, 153, 161, 171, 185, 238, 255-257, 322, 330, 339, 348, 390, 394, 401, 411, 461

abdominal distention and pain worse with emotional stress 239

abdominal downward heaviness or chill, lower 97, 101

abdominal masses 45, 46, 96, 104, 105, 265, 522

abdominal pain 68, 80, 83, 85-88, 100, 105, 108, 111, 122, 158, 160, 168, 202, 226, 261, 274, 284, 287, 290, 308, 337, 353, 358, 359, 368-374, 417, 421, 513, 565, 571, 586

abdominal pain, chilly 281

abdominal pain, cold *shan* 122

abdominal pain, lower 20, 46, 47, 83, 85-87, 105, 128, 149, 150, 154, 157, 168, 177, 180, 231, 249, 277, 282, 302, 341, 347, 348, 350, 355, 356, 361, 373, 374, 406, 412, 422, 425, 453, 475, 476, 488, 567

abdominal pain, lurking lower 128

abdominal pain refusing or resisting pressure 166, 188, 453, 487

abdominal pain, slight lower, desiring pressure 180

abdominal piercing pain, lower 485

abdominal sagging pain, lower 133

abdominal palpation 96

abdominal region, sensation of burning heat in the 369

abortions 34, 79, 80, 149, 170, 176, 214, 295, 338, 376, 380, 382

acid regurgitation 121, 151, 520

acne, facial 151

addictive papules 100, 104, 473, 549

agalactia 112

amenorrhea 29, 69, 224, 274, 293, 306, 313, 317-319, 323, 326, 327, 331, 516

amenorrhea, contraceptive medicinals leading to 323

amenorrhea, obesity condition 326

amenorrhea, Stein-Leventhal syndrome 327

amenorrhea, tubercular 331

anal sagging and distention 369, 370

anemia 287-289

anger, easy 99, 122, 275, 282, 284, 306, 315, 327, 330, 369, 411, 458, 464, 470, 476, 487, 493, 502, 506, 508, 511, 530

anterior pituitary, hypofunction of the 516

antibiotics 34, 55, 79, 80

appetite, diminished 101, 109, 110, 121, 164, 190, 204, 241, 271, 272, 295, 298, 299, 319, 320, 325, 326, 332, 358, 390, 392, 412, 459, 476, 518

appetite, increased 151

Arisal of the Clear: A Simple Guide to Healthy Eating According to Chinese Medicine 427

B

Baby Boom generation 55, 193

back, arched, rigidity 110, 123

Bai Ling Fu Ke 55, 224, 259

Bai-ling's Gynecology 224, 259

bao gong 3-5, 12, 39, 331, 368, 373, 414, 500, 525

bao luo 3-6, 50, 326, 331, 525, 573, 576, 577

bao mai 3-6, 10, 38, 39, 41, 42, 46, 48, 50, 295, 297, 305, 375, 414, 501, 525, 574

basal body temperature 19, 21, 22, 140, 149, 171, 194, 286

bedroom taxation 38, 48

belching 78, 151, 321, 421, 430, 437, 452, 510, 520

Ben Cao Gang Mu 372

beng lou 69, 247, 274

Bensky and Barolet 359, 496, 507

bian bing lun zhi 59

bian zheng lun zhi 59, 60

Bie Lu 372

birth control pills, oral 34, 149, 234

bleeding, dribbling and dripping without cease 103, 282

bleeding, midcycle 30, 99, 106

bleeding, profuse uterine 39, 279

bleeding, subdermal 104

blindness, night 431, 451

bodily emaciation and weakness 180, 333, 358, 405, 417, 476

body aches and pain 168, 427, 428, 436, 448

body, scorching hot 105

bones, steaming 458

borborygmus 359, 417, 419, 422

breast abscess 102

breast distention 9, 11, 13, 33, 40, 46, 48, 51, 77, 81, 85, 90, 99, 103, 105, 109, 120, 125, 139, 160, 171, 185, 201, 242, 284, 306, 321, 322, 325, 370, 387, 399, 401, 402, 404, 408-413, 467, 476, 544

breast fluids, spontaneous discharge of 99, 101, 103, 106

breast pain 30, 35, 85, 171, 340, 401, 402, 412

breast pain, mild, insidious 412

breast-feeding 116, 297, 479

breath, bad 452, 567

breath, shortness of 101, 103, 106, 110, 111, 161, 189, 192, 204, 218, 220, 227, 241, 257, 261, 272, 279, 284, 295, 303, 320, 321, 329, 351, 365, 407, 440, 441, 457, 475, 494, 518, 526, 575, 582, 583

breathing, rapid 103, 492

burping 78, 109, 151, 452

C

cancer, cervical 89

Candida albicans 36, 148, 359

candidiasis 37, 158, 168, 358, 359, 365, 425, 517

Cao Dong 372

Cao Ling-xian 359
cervical cancer 89
CFIDS 365, 447, 454, 455
Chang Nuan 380
Charles Chace 573
cheeks, flushing of the 74, 98, 103, 109, 266 299, 304, 331, 431, 442, 451, 469, 482, 502
Chen and Chen 160
Chen Hui-lin 284
Chen Mei-fang 517
Chen Wei 265
Chen Yu-cang 19, 28
Chen Ze-lin 517
Cheng Jing 24
chest and epigastric glomus and oppression 101
chest and rib-side fullness and oppression 100, 312, 330, 461
chest oppression 90, 103, 109, 112, 155, 189, 192, 209, 223, 284, 310, 326, 327, 405, 406, 411-413, 421, 422, 430, 439, 440, 450, 459, 472, 520, 526
chest pain 303, 522
Cheung, C.S. 357, 359
Chinese Herbal Medicine: Formulas & Strategies 359
Chinese Materia Medica 155
Chinese Medical Gynecology 57, 69, 156, 161, 203, 206, 228-230, 232, 259, 264, 298, 305, 315, 320, 322, 323, 325, 328, 329, 354, 388, 418, 491
Chinese Medical Treatments for Women's Diseases 333, 334
Chinese Self-massage, The Easy Way to Health 410
chloasma 522
chong and *ren* 12, 13, 27, 33, 38-40, 42, 44-51, 55, 57, 77, 80, 81, 95, 116, 126, 134, 160, 191, 193, 199, 201, 203, 214, 219, 226, 227, 229, 231, 234, 241, 242, 248, 255, 265, 271, 284, 305, 310, 315, 323, 326, 331, 344, 348, 368, 369, 375, 376, 401, 403, 406, 408, 410, 413-416, 462, 493, 500, 515, 529
chong mai 5, 13, 18, 148, 305, 408, 411, 414, 415, 462, 500, 501, 527
chong medicinals 131
chronic fatigue immune deficiency syndrome 365, 447
cold, aversion to 184
cold, fear of 98, 109, 110, 129, 237, 263, 269, 273, 281, 284, 299, 306, 310, 328, 346, 368, 427-429, 436, 448, 449
Compendium of TCM Patterns & Treatments 398
compresses 132, 141, 196, 197, 362, 409
Concise Traditional Chinese Gynecology 181, 216, 236, 237, 240, 250, 259, 265, 268, 270, 297, 301, 309, 345, 349, 352, 488, 491, 509, 513, 514
consciousness, loss of 110, 124, 570, 571
confusion 79, 464
constipation 129, 149, 151, 249, 258, 299, 303, 304, 306, 308, 340, 358, 359, 362, 377, 392, 416, 423, 444, 448, 453, 455, 467, 489, 494-496, 502, 505, 509, 573
constipation and diarrhea, alternating 358
constipation, dry, knotted 149
constitutional insufficiency 122, 148
controlling vessel 8, 12, 13, 18
convulsive spasms 110, 123, 124
corneal opacity 481
corpus luteum 22
corticosteroids 37

cough 43, 45, 91, 103, 110, 302, 303, 331, 422, 436, 448, 469, 479, 525, 586
cough, dry 303, 331, 469, 479, 525
cough, dry, with blood in the spittle 303
cravings 30, 151, 358, 423
cravings for sweets 151, 423
cry for little reason, tendency to 467

D

D & Cs 275
dai mai 12, 49, 107, 362, 529, 543
dai xia 12, 29, 95, 109-112, 529
debility, premature 98
delivery, difficult 105
diarrhea, alternating constipation and 358
diarrhea, cock-crow 98
diarrhea like duck droppings 419
diarrhea, yellowish 422
dilation and curettage 80
Divergent Records 372
dizziness 30, 42, 97-101, 104, 106, 109-112, 122-124, 154, 155, 158, 161, 177, 180, 189, 203-205, 207, 222, 234, 242, 252, 253, 255, 258, 261, 263, 266, 268, 272, 274, 284, 295, 298, 306, 314, 319-321, 323, 324, 326, 328, 329, 331, 332, 337, 350, 351, 356, 369, 370, 392, 405, 407, 412, 419, 420, 437-440, 442, 449, 451, 453, 456-459, 464, 471, 480-482, 487, 490, 494, 495, 501, 502, 504-508, 511, 513, 516, 521, 530, 532, 534, 547, 566, 567, 569
dizziness and a heavy head 459
dizziness and tinnitus 203, 236, 299, 304, 404, 437, 504, 505
dizziness and vertigo 86, 100, 123, 124, 258, 269, 295, 419, 456-458, 499
dizziness when standing up 279
dreaming, profuse 249, 258, 282, 412, 420, 464, 504, 508, 509, 517, 534
Du Jie-hui 153, 165, 179, 183, 187, 218, 219, 236, 239-241, 254, 260, 261, 266, 270, 309, 314, 343, 346, 350, 353, 506, 515, 518
dysmenorrhea 69, 84, 337, 357, 359, 382, 385, 500

E

edema 68, 73, 98, 109, 110, 241, 252, 298, 299, 312, 350, 351, 391, 392, 403, 417, 431, 460, 461, 514, 515, 520, 548
emotional depression 40, 99, 282, 284, 319, 321, 326, 330, 368, 401, 471, 485
emotional lability 30, 100, 469, 499, 501, 502, 517
endometrium 22, 331, 360, 486
enemas 141, 168, 362, 363
epistaxis 33, 43, 45, 55, 57, 68, 87, 99, 100, 103, 104, 109, 110, 122, 487, 488, 490-492
ERT 37, 524, 526, 527
eructations, sour 452
essence spirit, abnormalities in the 42
essence spirit abstraction 470
essence spirit listlessness, debility and dullness 98, 329, 513

Essentials for Absorbing Gynecology 301
Essentials from the Golden Cabinet 295, 346, 371
estrogen replacement therapy 37, 524, 525
external injury to the reproductive organs 105
extremities, lack of strength in the 161
extremities, swollen and distended four 417,461
eyeballs, swelling and pain of the 99
eyelids, dry, astringent 299
eyelids, edema of, and four extremities 417
eyes and face red 100
eyes, heavy sensation in the 439
eyes, inability to open the 439
eyes, soreness and pain in the supraorbital region above
 the 442

F

face, pale, which is flushed red 303
face, puffy, red 451
facial acne 151
facial complexion, dark, dusky 255, 425, 513, 522
facial complexion. darkish, blackish 97
facial complexion, greenish blue, yellowish 244
facial complexion, greenish bluish white 105
facial complexion,. grey or ashen 281
facial complexion, lusterless 234, 476
facial complexion, pale red 449
facial complexion, pale white 161, 177, 355, 407, 454
facial complexion, red 100, 207, 215, 258, 266, 334, 357,
 422, 437, 449, 450, 453, 488, 495, 496, 502, 505, 511
facial complexion, sallow yellow or wan 73, 98, 100,
 104, 133, 180, 241, 279, 321, 369, 417, 461, 475, 518,
 566
facial complexion, yellowish white 227
fainting and dizziness 106
fainting and inversion, postpartum 105
falling fetus 105, 372
fallopian tube inflammation 129
fatigue 30, 41, 47, 48, 55, 89, 91, 101, 103, 110, 111,
 122, 133, 151, 161, 190, 214, 218, 220, 225, 227, 233,
 240, 257, 261, 272, 274, 278, 279, 294, 312, 314, 334,
 351, 358, 365, 366, 407, 408, 417, 424, 428, 435,
 439-441, 447, 454, 456, 460, 464, 471, 473, 475, 494,
 499, 516, 518, 575
feet and lower limbs sore and weak 240
feet, cold 35, 89, 98, 278, 330, 501
feet, numbness of the hands and 104
fetus, stirring, disquietude 270
fever 10, 68, 80, 84, 103, 104, 110-112, 129, 134, 158,
 168, 207, 244, 266, 282, 294, 295, 298, 299, 302, 324,
 331-333, 347, 348, 350, 357, 369, 391, 405, 427-429,
 431, 436, 442, 447-456, 458, 482, 484, 487, 496, 502,
 505, 507, 511, 547
fever and chills, alternating 244, 428
fever and sweating 451, 452
fever, constant low-grade 369
fever, high 487, 507
fever in the afternoon, low 324, 332
fever, tidal 103, 104, 110, 112, 158, 208, 266, 295, 299,
 302, 331, 333, 357, 431, 442, 449, 451, 458, 482, 496,
 502, 505, 511
fibrocystic breast disease 399

fibroids 96, 130, 226, 277, 280, 337
Fine Formulas for Women 185, 226, 345
flooding and leaking 10, 30, 33, 36, 38, 39, 41, 42, 44,
 45, 47, 50, 51, 55, 57, 68, 69, 74-77, 80-83, 88, 93,
 94, 98-101, 103-107, 134, 158, 213, 218, 224, 226,
 247-249, 253-257, 259, 261-266, 268-270, 272,
 274-278, 280, 293, 514, 522, 581
food, lack of flavor for 464
forgetfulness 499, 517
Fu Ke San Bai Zheng 230, 244, 477, 478, 534
Fu Qing Zhu Nu Ke 4, 351, 357, 426
Fu Qing-zhu 4, 27, 125, 260, 263-265
Fu Qing-zhu's Gynecology 351, 357, 426
Fu Ren Liang Fang 226

G

galactorrhea-amenorrhea 317, 319
galactorrhea 102, 103, 316, 317, 319
Gathered Essentials of Gynecology 8
Ge Hong 555
General Collection for Sage-like Relief 413
genital atrophy 97, 98
Great Outline of the Materia Medica 372
Guo Yuan 164, 226, 297, 299, 302, 314, 418, 429, 510,
 511, 518

H

hair, falling 98, 328
hair, lusterless 295
Han Bai-ling 55, 57, 159, 162, 175, 182, 185, 186, 202,
 207, 224, 250, 254, 256, 258, 262, 263, 269, 295, 296,
 298, 302, 307, 308, 339, 417, 418, 420, 423, 426, 447,
 448, 451-454, 495, 496, 505, 513, 514, 518, 519
Handbook of Chinese Herbs and Formulas 359
hands and feet, numbness of the 104
hands and feet, tightness in the 356
He Shu-ying 376
head, pain on the top of the 437
headache 30, 33, 41, 45, 48, 68, 85, 91, 99, 100, 103,
 104, 109, 110, 122, 123, 168, 184, 282, 310, 327, 337,
 345, 350, 388, 391, 392, 394, 403, 405, 425, 429, 430,
 434-447, 464, 474, 481, 502, 504, 507, 508, 511, 512,
 521, 546
headache, dull, persistent 441
headache, intolerable 440
headache, neurovascular 434
headache, one-sided 437
headache, premenstrual 33, 123, 430
headache, splitting 437
heart, heat in the centers of the hands, feet, and 158, 431
heart pain 279, 526
heart pain, killed blood 279
heart palpitations 101, 104, 110-112, 123, 154, 158, 161,
 163, 180, 189, 192, 204, 220, 227, 234, 242, 253, 258,
 261, 262, 266, 291, 295, 298, 299, 320, 321, 329, 351,
 393, 412, 422, 440, 441, 449, 451, 457, 470, 475, 499,
 501, 505, 508, 509, 516, 518, 522, 523, 566
heart palpitations on exertion 102
heart palpitations when scared 304

heart, racing 102, 242, 329, 470, 499
heart vexation 41, 90, 99, 100, 102, 104, 109, 111, 153, 215, 249, 258, 275, 302, 306, 315, 324, 328, 334, 369, 373, 404, 405, 411-413, 430, 431, 442, 453, 454, 462-464, 470, 487, 493-495, 502, 504, 506, 508, 511, 512, 522, 523, 530, 575, 578, 584
heels, pain in the 236, 266, 356
hematuria 33, 68, 480, 481, 495, 496
hemophilus vaginitis 89
hemoptysis 33, 43, 45, 55, 57, 68, 87, 99, 100, 103, 104, 122, 488, 491, 492
hemorrhoids 42, 78, 101
Herxheimer reaction 168, 425
hiatal hernia 78
hiccup 103, 121, 430, 437, 476
hives 158, 473, 475
hormone replacement therapy 526, 528
hot flashes 158, 206, 401, 447, 499-502, 516, 522, 524, 525, 530, 532
Hou Tian-yin 200
HRT 528
Hu Guo-zhen 368
Hua Tuo 555
hunger 11, 102, 426
hypertension 206, 218, 499, 501, 507, 508, 510, 516, 524
hyperthermal phase 22-24, 171
hyperthyroidism 516
hypotension 101, 365, 441
hypothermal phase 21-25, 171, 196
hypothyroidism 421

I

iatrogenesis 33, 34, 176, 234, 294, 500
infertility 35, 38, 84, 97, 98, 104-107, 109-111, 120-122, 126, 140, 166, 286, 330, 368, 371, 372, 374, 378-381, 384, 385, 399, 401, 404
Inner Classic 5, 6, 8, 18, 27, 32, 43, 46, 51, 54, 295, 297, 298, 306, 500, 573, 574
Inner Classic Simple Questions 5, 6, 8, 18, 32, 43, 46, 295, 500
insomnia 41, 42, 45, 80, 98, 100, 102, 104, 109, 110, 122, 184, 315, 329, 437, 440, 442, 457, 462-464, 496, 499, 501-504, 509, 512, 516, 522, 523
intercourse during menses 149
intercourse, poking pain with 71, 84
internal medicine 52, 53, 73, 91, 132, 140, 141, 224, 278, 527
intestinal noises 419
Intractable Dysmenorrhea: Experiences of Master Physicians Shen Zhong Li and Ma Long Bai 357
intrauterine devices 34
irritability 90, 104, 171, 201, 239, 330, 401, 499, 507, 516, 517, 519, 522, 524

J, K

Jin Gui Yao Lue 295, 346, 371, 555
Jing Dai Zheng Zhi 19
Jing Yue Quan Shu 206, 309, 371, 443
Jing-yue's Complete Book 309

joints, pain and stiffness in the 431
joints, red, hot, swollen 431
Journal of Integrated Chinese-Western Medicine 380
Journal of the American College of Traditional Chinese Medicine 358, 359
kanpo yaku 555
kidneys, polycystic 516
knee or lower leg aching or weakness 97
knees, lack of strength in the low back and 177, 261

L

Lan Shi Mi Cang 573
lassitude and fatigue 261, 312
leaking which dribbles and drips 103
leg, lower, or knee aching or weakness 97
Li Dong-yuan 53, 54, 162, 448, 520, 574, 576, 579
Li Xiang-yun 368
Li Ying 382
Lian Fang 21, 172, 217, 251, 270, 276
libido, decreased 89, 97, 98, 164, 278, 365
limbs, chilled 88, 104, 110-112, 129, 134, 184, 222, 274, 284, 328, 368
limbs, weakness of the 30, 220
lin zheng 145
lips, pale, whitish 104
lips, red 74, 228, 303, 350, 474, 495, 530
Liu Dian-gong 230, 534
Liu He-jian 33
Liu Lan-fang 230, 534
Liu Min-ru 57
Liu Wan-su 52, 53
Liu Yan-chi 514
liver spots 74
low back and abdominal distention and pain 215
low back and buttock soreness and pain 134
low back region, aching and pain in 483
low back and knee soreness and weakness 87, 89, 97, 177, 207, 234, 236, 261, 263, 266, 273, 274, 284, 299, 319, 323, 331, 344, 355, 379, 425, 480, 494, 506, 513, 534
lower/upper back aching and chill 98
Lu De-ming 413
Lu Guo-zhi 154, 257
lumbar pain 83, 97, 98, 107, 134, 160, 164, 165, 178, 184, 202, 207, 208, 222, 258, 266, 271, 274, 278, 283, 287-289, 302, 306, 312, 320, 329, 347, 350, 354, 356, 365, 369, 370, 380, 381, 392, 394, 402, 406, 408, 412, 449, 464, 482, 483, 499, 501, 503, 516, 517 530, 531, 550, 574
luteal phase 21, 22, 24, 25, 140, 171, 524

M

Ma Long-bai 357
Ma Ping-chong 380
malar flushing 207, 357
mania 373, 374, 470, 471
Master Wan 151, 154, 157, 160, 181, 262, 490
memory, impaired 205, 222, 253, 298, 329, 505, 508, 518
menarche 6, 18, 28, 77, 79, 88, 97, 195, 316, 414, 500

menstrual cycle abnormalities 282
menstrual disease, causes of 31
menstrual disease, mechanisms of 37, 81
menstrual disease, prevention of 55
menstrual history 78, 79
menstrual irregularity 38, 93, 102, 104, 106, 122, 280, 368, 378, 380, 381, 394, 575
menstrual movement abdominal distention 68
menstrual movement abdominal pain 68, 284, 337, 369, 371, 372
menstrual movement acne 465, 548
menstrual movement bloody stool 493, 495, 551
menstrual movement bloody urine 495, 552
menstrual movement body pain 68, 427, 429, 432, 433, 435, 447, 482, 545
menstrual movement breast distention & pain 399, 544
menstrual movement coughing blood 492, 551
menstrual movement diarrhea 68, 98, 101, 109, 110, 125, 387, 416-419, 421, 423, 426, 545
menstrual movement dull-wittedness & stupidity 472, 549
menstrual movement edema 460, 548
menstrual movement epistaxis & hemoptysis 68
menstrual movement essence spirit abnormality 102
menstrual movement eye pain 481, 550
menstrual movement fever 68, 447, 448, 453-456, 547
menstrual movement flowing drool 476, 550
menstrual movement headache 41, 45, 68, 85, 100, 104, 388, 434-436, 445, 446, 546
menstrual movement hemafecia 68
menstrual movement hoarse voice 478, 550
menstrual movement loss of sleep 463, 548
menstrual movement lumbar pain 482, 550
menstrual movement nosebleed 486, 551
menstrual movement oral gan 461, 548
menstrual movement oral thirst 477, 550
menstrual movement raving & confused vision 469, 549
menstrual movement suspended vagina pain 484, 551
menstrual movement vertigo & dizziness 456, 547
menstrual movement water swelling 101
menstruation ahead of schedule 20, 23, 25, 33, 39, 67, 74, 76, 77, 80, 81, 86, 93, 94, 98, 99, 101, 103, 104, 106, 109-112, 122, 125, 133, 140, 145-152, 153-172, 193, 200, 213, 215, 218, 219, 247, 357, 369, 449, 487, 524, 538, 556
menstruation behind schedule 29, 67, 86, 99, 175, 177, 179, 183-185, 187, 188, 191, 193, 195, 209, 299, 539, 557
menstruation, blocked 19, 29, 32, 33, 36, 38, 39, 41-51, 55, 57, 68, 74, 76, 77, 79, 82, 88, 93-100, 102-106, 109-112, 121, 126, 127, 130, 183, 193, 224, 233, 240, 241, 276, 293-300, 302-304, 307, 309, 310, 312, 314-322, 326-334, 350, 372, 405, 452, 505, 524, 542, 560, 573
menstruation, ceased in a young girl 333
menstruation comes, starts & stops 244
menstruation, delayed 10, 19, 33, 35, 38, 44, 46, 74, 76, 77, 82, 94, 95, 100, 103, 104, 106, 111, 133, 140, 175-177, 182, 183, 185, 187, 189, 190, 192-194, 196, 197, 200, 233, 239, 241, 293, 303, 330, 390, 419
menstruation, enduring blocked 302, 333
menstruation, lengthened 99-101, 103, 104, 106, 137, 228, 288, 289

menstruation, normal 23, 28, 29
menstruation, painful 9, 19, 33, 35, 36, 38, 40, 41, 46, 47, 50, 51, 55, 57, 68, 71, 74, 76-79, 81, 82, 84, 91, 93, 94, 96, 99, 100, 104-107, 109, 111, 112, 130, 132, 137, 166, 172, 195, 210, 280, 283, 286, 288, 289, 318, 337, 338, 342-346, 350, 354-365, 367, 368, 378, 380, 381, 384, 385, 401, 404, 417, 430, 432, 443, 450, 453, 468, 537, 543, 561, 562
menstruation, profuse 10, 20, 33, 36, 38, 41, 42, 50, 55, 74-77, 81, 82, 87, 94, 95, 99-101, 103, 104, 106, 122, 125, 137, 146, 153, 158, 213-219, 222-226, 230, 247, 256, 275, 277, 278, 288-290, 356, 360, 475, 480, 514, 540, 558
menstruation, pulses of 92
menstruation, scanty 19, 33, 44, 46, 49, 51, 74, 76, 82, 83, 87, 93, 94, 100, 103, 104, 106, 121, 133, 137, 167, 183, 187, 193, 224, 233-236, 239-241, 243, 245, 293, 315, 369, 411, 430, 454, 467, 470, 541, 559
menstruation sometimes early, sometimes late, no fixed schedule 39, 40, 67, 199-206, 209, 210, 539, 557
midcycle bleeding 30, 99, 106
migraines 434, 446
miscarriage 80, 97, 101, 103, 106, 107, 125, 524
miscarriage, habitual 97, 106, 107, 524
mittelschmerz 140
mouth, bitter taste in the 99, 100, 153, 284, 330, 350, 391, 422, 430, 437, 440, 450, 453, 464, 487, 495, 512, 521
mouth, bland taste in the 101, 208
mouth, dry, and parched throat 299, 302, 324, 451, 463, 467, 488
mouth, dry, and sore throat 268, 469
mouth, dry but no increased tendency to drink 158, 266
mouth, dry, with a bitter taste 151, 347
mouth sores 43, 102, 206, 516
muscles and flesh withered 417
muscles, twitching facial 100
muscular spasms 100

N

Nan Nu Bing Mi Yan Liang Fang 153, 165
nasal discharge, clear, thin 448
nausea 11, 40, 45, 84, 91, 100, 101, 110, 112, 121, 151, 168, 312, 325, 337, 345, 358-361, 403, 416, 420, 423, 425, 434, 439, 445, 446, 459, 476, 520, 521, 567
nausea and vomiting 11, 40, 151, 358, 359, 403, 425, 445
navel, palpitations above the 271
Nei Jing 5, 6, 8, 18, 27, 32, 46, 51, 54, 295, 297, 298, 306, 500, 573, 574
nephritis 516
nervousness 304, 516
nettle rash 473
night blindness 431, 451
night sweats 80, 98, 109, 110, 112, 158, 207, 266, 295, 299, 302, 304, 331, 332, 357, 401, 431, 442, 449, 451, 482, 496, 499, 500, 502, 505, 511, 512, 516, 517, 524, 525
nocturia 89, 98, 109, 202, 501, 516
nose, runny 429
nose, stuffy 428, 429, 436, 448
nosebleeds 149

Nu Ke Ji Yao 7
Nu Ke Jing Wei 154, 155, 161, 179, 187, 203, 208, 255, 257, 270, 347, 354
Nu Ke Mi Jue Da Quan 145, 153, 163
Nu Ke She Yao 301
Nu Ke Xian Fang 260
Nu Ke Zong Yao 8
numbness of the hands and feet 104

O

obesity condition amenorrhea 326
old age 51, 123, 499
oral cavity sores and ulcers 102
oral contraceptives 79, 214, 234
oral thirst 373, 453, 454, 469, 477, 480, 550
osteoporosis 524, 525, 527-529
Otsuka Keisetsu 510
ovarian cyst 71
ovulation 19, 20, 22-25, 29, 140, 171, 172, 194, 196, 197, 211, 274, 318, 396
ovulatory bleeding 30

P

palpitations above the navel 271
papules, addictive 100, 104, 473, 549
parasites 34, 36, 37, 49, 75, 148, 157, 358, 359, 425, 517, 571
pelvic inflammatory disease 71, 122, 168, 331, 347, 350
perianal burning 422, 423
perimenopausal syndrome 39, 45, 69, 98, 100, 102, 105, 123, 125, 447, 499, 501, 502, 506, 511, 515, 518, 519, 522-524, 527, 552, 563
perspiration, spontaneous 103, 111, 161, 225, 241, 252, 279, 334, 361, 583
PGE$_2$ 385
PGF$_2$ 385
phlegm, profuse 101, 189, 191, 192, 223, 271, 312, 326, 365, 439, 472, 520
physiologic *dai xia* 29
Pi Wei Lun 53
PID 71, 347, 350
pituitary, hypofunction of the anterior 516
placenta, non-descension of the 105
plasters 132, 141, 362, 363, 371, 409
PMS 35, 36, 69, 94, 138, 166, 170-172, 366, 367, 387-390, 392, 395, 396, 398, 399, 416, 426, 433, 434, 447, 482, 500, 523, 524
polyuria 64, 109, 134, 222, 501, 516
postpartum fainting and inversion 105
poultices 132, 141, 409
prednisone 37
premenstrual tension 51, 125, 280, 469
pregnancy, pulses of 95, 96
pressure pain 128, 129, 134
Profundities from the Gynecological Classics 154, 155, 161, 179, 187, 203, 208, 255, 257, 270, 347, 354
progesterone 22, 524
puberty 18, 50, 51, 434
pulse, normal female 92

pulses of menstruation 92
pulses of pregnancy 95, 96
pyelonephritis 516

Q, R

Qian Jia Miao Fang 403
Qian Jin Yao Fang 489
Qin Bo-wei 48, 64
Que Hua-fa 413
rebound pain 129
renal vascular disorder 516
reproductive organs, external injury to the 105
reproductive tract infections 129
rib-side pain 46, 85, 86, 90, 99, 103, 105, 192, 330, 356, 405, 437, 522, 526
runny nose 429

S

sacral pain 84
sadness, spontaneous 471
saliva, excessive 476
scars, purplish 468
sciatic pain with swelling and redness 157
sea of blood 4, 8, 11, 12, 18, 19, 27, 41, 42, 44-46, 95, 116, 201, 214, 226, 229, 234, 248, 249, 293, 298, 319, 323, 327, 331, 414, 415, 573, 580
sexual abuse 37, 149
sexual activity, unrestrained 479
sexual desire, diminished 35, 109, 329, 369, 379
sexual intercourse during menstruation 227
sexual taxation 36
sexually transmitted evils 148
shan abdominal pain, cold 122
Shang Han Lun 185, 373
Shang Xian-ming 510
Shen Lin 528
Shen Shi Zun Sheng Shu 450
Shen Xiao-heng 284
Shen Yao-fang 8
Shen Zhong-li 315
Sheng Ji Zong Lu 413
shoulders, aching 510
sighing 77, 99, 109, 255, 275, 284, 437, 519
Sionneau, Philippe 181, 277
six depressions 51, 52, 81, 397, 448, 456
skin, dry 51, 180, 299, 302, 366, 501
sleep, excessive 459
sleep, loss of 123, 262, 266, 283, 304, 393, 405, 412, 457, 463, 505, 508, 517-519, 548
sleep, none the entire night 464
sleep, scanty 111, 112, 242, 457, 479, 494
sneezing 429, 436, 448
somnolence 326, 471, 473
Song and Yu 156, 161, 175, 198, 202, 214, 216, 250, 253, 263, 270, 276, 297, 300, 301, 307, 311, 312, 345, 348, 352, 499, 513, 516, 519
Song Guang-ji 34
Song Shu-de 154, 257
spasms, convulsive 110, 123, 124

speak, disinclination to 77, 111, 279, 457, 470
speech, delirious 104
speech, raving 469
spirit, lassitude of the 101, 240, 257, 274, 279, 284, 295, 326, 328, 332, 333, 351, 369, 393, 405, 407, 412, 456, 460, 464, 475, 494
Static Blood Patterns & Treatments 94, 261
steaming bones 458
Stein-Leventhal syndrome amenorrhea 327
stomach and epigastric glomus and fullness 419
stomach, sound of water in the 419
stools, dry, bound 98, 102, 104, 111, 125, 127, 215, 303, 315, 328, 369, 467, 469, 474, 479, 487
stools, loose 89, 91, 97, 100, 101, 107, 110, 111, 155, 163, 164, 168, 190, 193, 203, 241, 269, 271-273, 284, 295, 298, 299, 306, 314, 319, 320, 324, 326, 329, 351, 365, 392, 416, 419, 422, 424, 426, 451, 468, 513, 518, 520
stools, watery, thin 425
strength, lack of 110, 122, 133, 161, 177, 192, 204, 218, 261, 272, 279, 284, 291, 312, 320, 326, 328, 329, 332, 333, 351, 365, 369, 393, 407, 412, 456, 457, 460, 475, 483, 518, 534, 566, 583
Sun Jiu-ling 162, 177, 186, 202, 215, 267, 269, 301, 310, 344, 388, 513
Sun Si-miao 141, 555
supraorbital region, soreness and pain in the 442
surgery 34, 49, 176, 226, 278, 338, 369, 375, 376
sweating, spontaneous, on movement 161
sweats, cold 337
sweats, night 80, 98, 109, 110, 112, 158, 207, 266, 295, 299, 302, 304, 331, 332, 357, 401, 431, 442, 449, 451, 482, 496, 499, 500, 502, 505, 511, 512, 516, 517, 524, 525

T

Tan Zheng Lun 200
Tang Ji-fu 358
Tang Rong-chuan 25, 27
teeth, clenched 123
teeth, withered 98
The Chinese Medicine Self-study Series 200
The Clinical Efflorescence of Chinese Medical Gynecology 354
The Collected Essentials of Gynecology 7
The Golden Mirror of Ancestral Medicine 387, 417, 427, 429, 432, 433, 447, 449, 451, 489, 491
The Journal of Chinese Medicine 21
The Merck Manual 67
The Secret Treasury of the Orchid Chamber 573
thirst, vexatious, leading to drinking 487
thirst with a preference for cold drinks 149
thirsty mouth 102
thoughts, chaotic 412, 413
Three Hundred Gynecological Conditions 230, 244, 477, 478, 534
throat, dry 99, 106, 109, 110, 112, 306, 422, 449, 450, 453, 464, 478, 480, 487, 490, 495, 505, 508
throat, dry, red 98
throat, dry, with a desire to drink 452
throat, scratchy 356

throat, sore 161, 205, 268, 350, 428, 450, 469, 516
throat, sore, dry 449
thyroid, enlarged 421
tian gui 4, 6-9, 12, 18, 21, 33, 38, 116, 264, 414, 500, 524, 529
timidity 304
tinnitus 97, 98, 109, 110, 122, 188, 203, 205, 222, 234, 236, 263, 266, 274, 299, 304, 323, 324, 328, 329, 331, 356, 369, 379, 394, 404, 412, 437, 440, 442, 449, 480, 482, 487, 490, 499, 501, 502, 504, 505, 507, 508, 510, 516
trauma 33, 34, 37, 146, 149, 176, 213, 214, 234, 294, 338, 432, 443
Treatise on Bleeding Disorders 25
Treatise on Cold Damage 185, 373, 555
Treatise on the Spleen & Stomach 53
trichomoniasis vaginitis 89

U

urinary strangury 85, 100
urinary tract infections 516
urination at night, excessive 98
urination, burning 431
urination, clear 193, 284, 329
urination, frequent, scanty, yellow 482
urination, frequent, short 394
urination, inhibited 103, 425, 454, 461
urination, nighttime 97, 165
urination, short, yellow 98, 102, 104
urination, terminal dribbling after 269
urination scanty, reddish 299, 453
urine, reddish 249, 306, 328, 422
urticaria 218, 473-475
uterine bleeding, profuse 39, 279
uterine concretions and lumps 280
uterine myomas 80, 96, 130, 226, 275, 280, 284, 285, 288, 337, 522
uterine prolapse 42, 55, 97, 103, 106, 107, 109, 110

V

vaginal discharge, continuous abnormal 128, 189
vaginal discharge, profuse, thick, foul-smelling, possibly yellow 431
vaginal discharge pulses, abnormal 95
vaginal discharge, yellowish white or like pus 485
vaginal flatulence 107
vaginal irritation preceding the period 157
vaginal itching 41, 100, 104, 107, 109, 110, 112, 411, 531-534
vaginal meatus dry, burning, and astringent 329, 530
vaginal pain 85, 484
vaginal sores 41, 85, 107, 109
vaginal sweating 533, 534
vaginal tract, pulling, draining painful sensation in the 485
vaginitis 89, 347, 359, 431, 481, 501, 526, 529, 534, 535
vaginitis, hemophilus 89
vaginitis, senile 501, 526, 529, 534, 535
vaginitis, trichomoniasis 89

Valium 78
varicosities 522
Various Clinical Specialties in Traditional Chinese 163
veins, engorged 443
vertigo 86, 99, 100, 109-111, 123, 124, 154, 258, 269,
    295, 319, 329, 419, 456-458, 481, 494, 499, 506-508,
    512, 516, 521, 547, 566, 567
vexation and agitation 104, 122-124, 151, 154, 188, 282,
    284, 330, 347, 391, 431, 458, 467, 530
vexatious heat in the five hearts 98, 106, 125, 134, 208,
    266, 274, 458, 492, 532
vexatious thirst leading to drinking 487
visceral agitation 41, 120, 123, 501, 517
vision, blurred 100, 104, 110, 111, 180, 207, 234, 242,
    253, 322, 394, 407, 431, 451, 502, 530, 532, 534
vision, confused 469, 549
visual acuity, loss of 481
visual field, black spots or floating threads in the 522
voice, feeble 101, 103
vomiting 10, 11, 40, 64, 84, 99-101, 103, 151, 152, 168,
    175, 312, 337, 345, 347, 358, 359, 361, 364, 403,
    416-423, 425, 434, 445, 446, 521, 545, 567, 578
vomiting and nausea with profuse phlegm 312

W

Wai Ke Yi An Hui Bian 413
Wan Mi-zhai 151, 160, 181, 183, 187, 191, 205, 273, 490
Wan Quan 187
Wang Bo-jiu 280
Wang Chun-hua 201
Wang Dao-qing 290
Wang Fa-Chang 411
Wang Ken-tang 190
Wang Qi-ming 280
Wang Zi-heng 19
weariness and fatigue 161
weeping, spontaneous 467, 471
Wu Ben-li 145, 181
Wu Qian 417-419, 432, 433, 447, 449, 451, 491
Wu Shu-qing 298

X, Y

Xia Gui-cheng 22, 181
Xu Da-Chun 415
Xu Ling-tai 415
Xu Sheng-yang 403
Xue Li-zhai 153, 163, 181, 182
Xue Zheng Lun 25
Yang Shi-xing 229
Yang Shou-zhong 5
Yang Yi-ya 200, 227, 489
Yao Shi-an 511, 512, 515, 519, 522
Ye Gui 414
Ye Tian Shi Nu Ke 489
Ye Tian-shi 275, 414
yeast die-off 425
Yeung Him-che 359
Yi Xue Zheng Zhuan 8
Yi Xue Zhong Zhong Can Xi Lu 491
Yi Zong Jin Jian 387, 417, 427, 429, 432, 433, 447, 449,
    451, 489, 491
yin fire 53-55, 65, 163, 573, 579, 586
Yin Xiu-lan 378
Yu Min 517
Yu Xiao-zhen 34
Yu Xue Zheng Zhi 94, 261, 350
Yu Yao-feng 7
Yu Yo-yuan 298
Yue Yang Hospital 517

Z

Zeng Zhen 284
Zhang En-qin 163, 250, 258, 263, 296, 306, 308, 313,
    342, 346, 352, 356, 509, 514, 516
Zhang Jie-bin 8
Zhang Jing-yue 8
Zhang Xue-wen 94, 261, 350
Zheng Zhi Zheng Sheng 371
Zhong Xi Yi Jie He Za Zhi 380
Zhong Yi Fu Chan Ke Xue 57
Zhong Yi Fu Ke 34, 57, 69, 156, 161, 203, 206, 228-230,
    232, 259, 264, 280, 298, 305, 315, 320, 322, 323, 325,
    328, 329, 354, 388, 418, 457-459, 491
Zhong Yi Fu Ke Lin Chuang Jing Hua 280, 354
Zhong Yi Fu Ke Lin Chuang Shou Ce 315, 320, 322, 323,.
    325, 328, 329
Zhong Yi Fu Ke Shou Ce 34, 69, 156, 161
Zhong Yi Fu Ke Xue 57, 203, 206, 298, 491
Zhong Yi Fu Ke Zhi Liao Shou Ce 228-230, 232, 457-459
Zhong Yi Lin Chuang Ge Ke 163, 250
Zhong Yi Xue Cong Shu 200
Zhong Yi Zhi Liao Fu Nu Bing 279, 332-334, 565
Zhu Cheng-han 259, 264, 302, 305, 311, 312, 388, 390,
    391, 393-395, 504, 509, 513
Zhu Dan-xi 52, 156, 175, 182, 295, 491

GOLDEN NEEDLE WANG LE-TING:
A 20th Century Master's Approach
to Acupuncture
by Yu Hui-chan and Han Fu-ru,
 trans. by Shuai Xue-zhong
ISBN 0-936185-78-3

A GUIDE TO GYNECOLOGY
by Ye Heng-yin,
trans. by Bob Flaws and Shuai Xue-zhong
ISBN 1-891845-19-5

A HANDBOOK OF TCM PATTERNS
& TREATMENTS
by Bob Flaws & Daniel Finney
ISBN 0-936185-70-8

A HANDBOOK OF TRADITIONAL
CHINESE DERMATOLOGY
by Liang Jian-hui,
trans. by Zhang Ting-liang & Bob Flaws
ISBN 0-936185-07-4

A HANDBOOK OF TRADITIONAL
CHINESE GYNECOLOGY
by Zhejiang College of TCM, trans. by
Zhang Ting-liang & Bob Flaws
ISBN 0-936185-06-6 (4th edit.)

A HANDBOOK OF CHINESE
HEMATOLOGY
by Simon Becker
ISBN 1-891845-16-0

A HANDBOOK OF MENSTRUAL
DISEASES IN CHINESE MEDICINE
by Bob Flaws
ISBN 0-936185-82-1

A HANDBOOK of TCM PEDIATRICS
by Bob Flaws
ISBN 0-936185-72-4

A HANDBOOK OF TCM UROLOGY &
MALE SEXUAL DYSFUNCTION
by Anna Lin, OMD
ISBN 0-936185-36-8

THE HEART & ESSENCE OF DAN-
XI'S METHODS OF TREATMENT
by Xu Dan-xi, trans. by Yang Shou-zhong
ISBN 0-926185-49-X

THE HEART TRANSMISSION
OF MEDICINE
by Liu Yi-ren, trans. by Yang Shou-zhong
ISBN 0-936185-83-X

HIGHLIGHTS OF ANCIENT
ACUPUNCTURE PRESCRIPTIONS
trans. by Honora Lee Wolfe & Rose
Crescenz
ISBN 0-936185-23-6

IMPERIAL SECRETS OF
HEALTH & LONGEVITY
by Bob Flaws
ISBN 0-936185-51-1

INSIGHTS OF A SENIOR
ACUPUNCTURIST
by Miriam Lee
ISBN 0-936185-33-3

KEEPING YOUR CHILD HEALTHY
WITH CHINESE MEDICINE
by Bob Flaws
ISBN 0-936185-71-6

THE LAKESIDE MASTER'S
STUDY OF THE PULSE
by Li Shi-zhen, trans. by Bob Flaws
ISBN 1-891845-01-2

Li Dong-yuan's TREATISE ON THE
SPLEEN & STOMACH, A Translation
of the Pi Wei Lun
trans. by Yang Shou-zhong
ISBN 0-936185-41-4

MASTER HUA'S CLASSIC OF
THE CENTRAL VISCERA
by Hua Tuo, trans. by Yang Shou-zhong
ISBN 0-936185-43-0

MASTER TONG'S ACUPUNCTURE
by Miriam Lee
ISBN 0-926185-37-6

THE MEDICAL I CHING:
Oracle of the Healer Within
by Miki Shima
ISBN 0-936185-38-4

MANAGING MENOPAUSE
NATURALLY with Chinese Medicine
by Honora Lee Wolfe
ISBN 0-936185-98-8

PAO ZHI: Introduction to Processing
Chinese Medicinals to Enhance Their
Therapeutic Effect
by Philippe Sionneau
ISBN 0-936185-62-1

PATH OF PREGNANCY, VOL. I,
Gestational Disorders
by Bob Flaws
ISBN 0-936185-39-2

PATH OF PREGNANCY, Vol. II,
Postpartum Diseases
by Bob Flaws
ISBN 0-936185-42-2

THE PULSE CLASSIC:
A Translation of the Mai Jing
by Wang Shu-he, trans. by Yang Shou-zhong
ISBN 0-936185-75-9

RECENT TCM RESEARCH
FROM CHINA
by Bob Flaws and Charles Chase
ISBN 0-936185-56-2

THE SECRET OF CHINESE
PULSE DIAGNOSIS
by Bob Flaws
ISBN 0-936185-67-8

SEVENTY ESSENTIAL CHINESE
HERBAL FORMULAS
by Bob Flaws
ISBN 0-936185-59-7

SHAOLIN SECRET FORMULAS for
Treatment of External Injuries
by De Chan, trans. by Zhang Ting-liang &
Bob Flaws
ISBN 0-936185-08-2

STATEMENTS OF FACT IN
TRADITIONAL CHINESE MEDICINE
by Bob Flaws
ISBN 0-936185-52-X

STICKING TO THE POINT 1: A
Rational Methodology for the Step by
Step Formulation & Administration of
an Acupuncture Treatment
by Bob Flaws
ISBN 0-936185-17-1

STICKING TO THE POINT 2: A
Study of Acupuncture & Moxibustion
Formulas and Strategies
by Bob Flaws
ISBN 0-936185-97-X

THE TAO OF HEALTHY EATING
ACCORDING TO CHINESE
MEDICINE
by Bob Flaws
ISBN 0-936185-92-9

TEACH YOURSELF TO READ
MODERN MEDICAL CHINESE
by Bob Flaws
ISBN 0-936185-99-6

THE SYSTEMATIC CLASSIC OF
ACUPUNCTURE & MOXIBUSTION
A translation of the Jia Yi Jing
by Huang-fu Mi, trans. by Yang Shou-zhong
& Charles Chace
ISBN 0-936185-29-5

THE TREATMENT OF DISEASE IN
TCM Vol I: Diseases of the Head &
Face Including Mental/Emotional
Disorders
by Philippe Sionneau & Lü Gang
ISBN 0-936185-69-4

THE TREATMENT OF DISEASE IN
TCM, Vol. II: Diseases of the Eyes,
Ears, Nose, & Throat
by Sionneau & Lü
ISBN 0-936185-73-2

THE TREATMENT OF DISEASE, Vol.
III: Diseases of the Mouth, Lips,
Tongue, Teeth & Gums
by Sionneau & Lü
ISBN 0-936185-79-1

THE TREATMENT OF DISEASE, Vol
IV: Diseases of the Neck, Shoulders,
Back, & Limbs
by Philippe Sionneau & Lü Gang
ISBN 0-936185-89-9

THE TREATMENT OF DISEASE, Vol
V: Diseases of the Chest & Abdomen
by Philippe Sionneau & Lü Gang
ISBN 1-891845-02-0

THE TREATMENT OF DISEASE, Vol
VI: Diseases of the Urogential System
& Proctology
by Philippe Sionneau & Lü Gang
ISBN 1-891845-05-5

THE TREATMENT OF DISEASE, Vol
VII: General Symptoms
by Philippe Sionneau & Lü Gang
ISBN 1-891845-14-4

THE TREATMENT OF EXTERNAL
DISEASES WITH ACUPUNCTURE
& MOXIBUSTION
by Yan Cui-lan and Zhu Yun-long, trans. by
Yang Shou-zhong
ISBN 0-936185-80-5

160 ESSENTIAL CHINESE HERBAL
PATENT MEDICINES
by Bob Flaws
ISBN 1-891945-12-8

630 QUESTIONS & ANSWERS
ABOUT CHINESE HERBAL MEDI-
CINE: A Workbook & Study Guide
by Bob Flaws
ISBN 1-891845-04-7

230 ESSENTIAL CHINESE
MEDICINALS
by Bob Flaws
ISBN 1-891845-03-9

A Handbook
of TCM Pediatrics

*A Practitioner's Guide to Care and Treatment
of Common Childhood Diseases*
by Bob Flaws

This book is a clinical manual of Chinese medical pediatrics. It covers the disease causes and mechanisms, pattern discrimination, treatment principles, and Chinese herbal and acupuncture treatments of 46 of the most commonly encountered childhood diseases. These diseases are arranged in a longitudinal manner corresponding to the typical ages at which these conditions tend to occur. Also included are discussions of immunizations, antibiotics, and the primary importance of diet in keeping children healthy and well. This book is a must for any practitioner who wishes to treat children with Chinese medicine.

$49.95 US plus **$7.25 shipping**

Available from Blue Poppy Press.
☐ Yes! I'd like to order __ copy(ies) of
A Handbook of TCM Pediatrics
☐ *Check/money order enclosed* ☐ *Please charge my credit card*

Name

Address

City/State/Zip

Daytime Phone

Credit Card #

Expiration Date

Send to Blue Poppy 5441 Western Ave. Boulder, CO 80301
*Or order toll free at 1-800-487-9296
or Fax your order to 303-245-8362*